Recent Advances in Deep Learning and Medical Imaging for Cancer Treatment

Recent Advances in Deep Learning and Medical Imaging for Cancer Treatment

Editors

Muhammad Fazal Ijaz
Marcin Woźniak

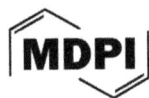

Basel • Beijing • Wuhan • Barcelona • Belgrade • Novi Sad • Cluj • Manchester

Editors
Muhammad Fazal Ijaz
School of Engineering and
Information Technology,
Melbourne Institute of
Technology
Melbourne
Australia

Marcin Woźniak
Silesian University of
Technology
Gliwice
Poland

Editorial Office
MDPI
St. Alban-Anlage 66
4052 Basel, Switzerland

This is a reprint of articles from the Special Issue published online in the open access journal *Cancers* (ISSN 2072-6694) (available at: https://www.mdpi.com/journal/cancers/special_issues/Recent_Advances_Deep_Learning_Medical_Imaging_Cancer_Treatment).

For citation purposes, cite each article independently as indicated on the article page online and as indicated below:

Lastname, A.A.; Lastname, B.B. Article Title. *Journal Name* **Year**, *Volume Number*, Page Range.

ISBN 978-3-7258-0711-6 (Hbk)
ISBN 978-3-7258-0712-3 (PDF)
doi.org/10.3390/books978-3-7258-0712-3

© 2024 by the authors. Articles in this book are Open Access and distributed under the Creative Commons Attribution (CC BY) license. The book as a whole is distributed by MDPI under the terms and conditions of the Creative Commons Attribution-NonCommercial-NoDerivs (CC BY-NC-ND) license.

Contents

About the Editors ix

Muhammad Fazal Ijaz and Marcin Woźniak
Editorial: Recent Advances in Deep Learning and Medical Imaging for Cancer Treatment
Reprinted from: *Cancers* 2024, 16, 700, doi:10.3390/cancers16040700 1

Miguel Mascarenhas Saraiva, Tiago Ribeiro, Mariano González-Haba, Belén Agudo Castillo, João P. S. Ferreira, Filipe Vilas Boas, et al.
Deep Learning for Automatic Diagnosis and Morphologic Characterization of Malignant Biliary Strictures Using Digital Cholangioscopy: A Multicentric Study
Reprinted from: *Cancers* 2023, 15, 4827, doi:10.3390/cancers15194827 6

Zaenab Alammar, Laith Alzubaidi, Jinglan Zhang, Yuefeng Li, Waail Lafta and Yuantong Gu
Deep Transfer Learning with Enhanced Feature Fusion for Detection of Abnormalities in X-ray Images
Reprinted from: *Cancers* 2023, 15, 4007, doi:10.3390/cancers15154007 19

Jose Luis Diaz Resendiz, Volodymyr Ponomaryov, Rogelio Reyes Reyes and Sergiy Sadovnychiy
Explainable CAD System for Classification of Acute Lymphoblastic Leukemia Based on a Robust White Blood Cell Segmentation
Reprinted from: *Cancers* 2023, 15, 3376, doi:10.3390/cancers15133376 55

Suryadipto Sarkar, Kong Min, Waleed Ikram, Ryan. W. Tatton, Irbaz B. Riaz, Alvin C. Silva, et al.
Performing Automatic Identification and Staging of Urothelial Carcinoma in Bladder Cancer Patients Using a Hybrid Deep-Machine Learning Approach
Reprinted from: *Cancers* 2023, 15, 1673, doi:10.3390/cancers15061673 77

Salem Alkhalaf, Fahad Alturise, Adel Aboud Bahaddad, Bushra M. Elamin Elnaim, Samah Shabana, Sayed Abdel-Khalek and Romany F. Mansour
Adaptive Aquila Optimizer with Explainable Artificial Intelligence-Enabled Cancer Diagnosis on Medical Imaging
Reprinted from: *Cancers* 2023, 15, 1492, doi:10.3390/cancers15051492 92

Bofan Song, Chicheng Zhang, Sumsum Sunny, Dharma Raj KC, Shaobai Li, Keerthi Gurushanth, et al.
Interpretable and Reliable Oral Cancer Classifier with Attention Mechanism and Expert Knowledge Embedding via Attention Map
Reprinted from: *Cancers* 2023, 15, 1421, doi:10.3390/cancers15051421 112

Marwa Obayya, Mashael S. Maashi, Nadhem Nemri, Heba Mohsen, Abdelwahed Motwakel, Azza Elneil Osman, et al.
Hyperparameter Optimizer with Deep Learning-Based Decision-Support Systems for Histopathological Breast Cancer Diagnosis
Reprinted from: *Cancers* 2023, 15, 885, doi:10.3390/cancers15030885 124

Mehmet Ali Balcı, Larissa M. Batrancea, Ömer Akgüller and Anca Nichita
A Series-Based Deep Learning Approach to Lung Nodule Image Classification
Reprinted from: *Cancers* 2023, 15, 843, doi:10.3390/cancers15030843 143

Prabhu Kavin Balasubramanian, Wen-Cheng Lai, Gan Hong Seng, Kavitha C and Jeeva Selvaraj
APESTNet with Mask R-CNN for Liver Tumor Segmentation and Classification
Reprinted from: *Cancers* 2023, 15, 330, doi:10.3390/cancers15020330 157

Zubaira Naz, Muhammad Usman Ghani Khan, Tanzila Saba, Amjad Rehman, Haitham Nobanee and Saeed Ali Bahaj
An Explainable AI-Enabled Framework for Interpreting Pulmonary Diseases from Chest Radiographs
Reprinted from: *Cancers* 2023, 15, 314, doi:10.3390/cancers15010314 176

Vinayakumar Ravi
Attention Cost-Sensitive Deep Learning-Based Approach for Skin Cancer Detection and Classification
Reprinted from: *Cancers* 2022, 14, 5872, doi:10.3390/cancers14235872 192

Niharika Mohanty, Manaswini Pradhan, Annapareddy V. N. Reddy, Sachin Kumar and Ahmed Alkhayyat
Integrated Design of Optimized Weighted Deep Feature Fusion Strategies for Skin Lesion Image Classification
Reprinted from: *Cancers* 2022, 14, 5716, doi:10.3390/cancers14225716 218

Russ A. Kuker, David Lehmkuhl, Deukwoo Kwon, Weizhao Zhao, Izidore S. Lossos, Craig H. Moskowitz, et al.
A Deep Learning-Aided Automated Method for Calculating Metabolic Tumor Volume in Diffuse Large B-Cell Lymphoma
Reprinted from: *Cancers* 2022, 14, 5221, doi:10.3390/cancers14215221 243

Fazal Subhan, Muhammad Adnan Aziz, Inam Ullah Khan, Muhammad Fayaz, Marcin Wozniak, Jana Shafi and Muhammad Fazal Ijaz
Cancerous Tumor Controlled Treatment Using Search Heuristic (GA)-Based Sliding Mode and Synergetic Controller
Reprinted from: *Cancers* 2022, 14, 4191, doi:10.3390/cancers14174191 255

K. Shankar, Ashit Kumar Dutta, Sachin Kumar, Gyanendra Prasad Joshi and Ill Chul Doo
Chaotic Sparrow Search Algorithm with Deep Transfer Learning Enabled Breast Cancer Classification on Histopathological Images
Reprinted from: *Cancers* 2022, 14, 2770, doi:10.3390/cancers14112770 277

Rytis Maskeliūnas, Audrius Kulikajevas, Robertas Damaševičius, Kipras Pribuišis, Nora Ulozaitė-Stanienė and Virgilijus Uloza
Lightweight Deep Learning Model for Assessment of Substitution Voicing and Speech after Laryngeal Carcinoma Surgery
Reprinted from: *Cancers* 2022, 14, 2366, doi:10.3390/cancers14102366 295

Anita Froń, Alina Semianiuk, Uladzimir Lazuk, Kuba Ptaszkowski, Agnieszka Siennicka, Artur Lemiński, et al.
Artificial Intelligence in Urooncology: What We Have and What We Expect
Reprinted from: *Cancers* 2023, 15, 4282, doi:10.3390/cancers15174282 313

Navneet Melarkode, Kathiravan Srinivasan, Saeed Mian Qaisar and Pawel Plawiak
AI-Powered Diagnosis of Skin Cancer: A Contemporary Review, Open Challenges and Future Research Directions
Reprinted from: *Cancers* 2023, 15, 1183, doi:10.3390/cancers15041183 336

Mohammad Madani, Mohammad Mahdi Behzadi and Sheida Nabavi
The Role of Deep Learning in Advancing Breast Cancer Detection Using Different Imaging Modalities: A Systematic Review
Reprinted from: *Cancers* **2022**, *14*, 5334, doi:10.3390/cancers14215334 . . . . **372**

About the Editors

Muhammad Fazal Ijaz

Muhammad Fazal Ijaz received a Dr. Eng. from Dongguk University, Seoul, South Korea. He was a research assistant, a visiting guest professor, and an assistant professor with tertiary institutes, including the Dongguk University, Technology De Monterrey, Campus Mexico City and Guadalajara, Mexico; Sejong University, Seoul; and the University of Melbourne, Australia. He has published numerous research articles in several international peer-reviewed journals, including IEEE Transactions on Industrial Informatics, *IEEE Internet of Things Journal*, Scientific Reports (*Nature*), Cancers, Biomedical Signal Processing and Control, Computational Intelligence, and Human-centric Computing and Information Science. His research interests include the Internet of Things, medical informatics, machine learning, AI, and data science. From 2021 to 2023, each year, Dr. Muhammad Fazal Ijaz was presented among the "TOP 2% Scientists in the World" by Stanford University for his career achievements. He is an Editorial Board member for *Sensors, Diagnostics, Archives of Artificial Intelligence*, and *Frontiers in Human Neuroscience*.

Marcin Woźniak

Marcin Woźniak is a Full Professor at the Faculty of Applied Mathematics, Silesian University of Technology. He is a Scientific Supervisor in editions of "The Diamond Grant" and "The Best of the Best" programs for highly talented students from the Polish Ministry of Science and Higher Education. He participated in various scientific projects at Polish, Italian, and Lithuanian universities and projects with applied results in the IT industry. He was a Visiting Researcher with universities in Italy, Sweden, and Germany. He has authored/co-authored over 200 research papers in international conferences and journals. His current research interests include neural networks and fuzzy logic control systems, their applications, and various aspects of applied computational intelligence accelerated by evolutionary computation and federated learning models. In 2021, he received an award from the Polish Ministry of Science and Higher Education for research achievements. From 2020 to 2023, each year, Prof. M. Woźniak was presented among the "TOP 2% Scientists in the World" by Stanford University for his career achievements. Prof. Woźniak was the Editorial Board member or an Editor for Sensors, Machine Learning with Applications, Pattern Analysis and Applications, IEEE ACCESS, Measurement, Sustainable Energy Technologies and Assessments, Frontiers in Human Neuroscience, Frontiers in Plan Science, PeerJ CS, International Journal of Distributed Sensor Networks, Computational Intelligence and Neuroscience, Journal of Universal Computer Science, etc., and a Session Chair at various international conferences and symposiums, including IEEE Symposium Series on Computational Intelligence, IEEE Congress on Evolutionary Computation, International Joint Conference on Neural Networks, etc.

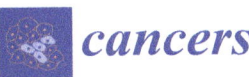

Editorial

Editorial: Recent Advances in Deep Learning and Medical Imaging for Cancer Treatment

Muhammad Fazal Ijaz [1,*] and Marcin Woźniak [2,*]

1. School of Engineering and Information Technology, Melbourne Institute of Technology, Melbourne 3000, Australia
2. Faculty of Applied Mathematics, Silesian University of Technology, Kaszubska 23, 44100 Gliwice, Poland
* Correspondence: mfazal@mit.edu.au (M.F.I.); marcin.wozniak@polsl.pl (M.W.)

Citation: Ijaz, M.F.; Woźniak, M. Editorial: Recent Advances in Deep Learning and Medical Imaging for Cancer Treatment. *Cancers* **2024**, *16*, 700. https://doi.org/10.3390/cancers16040700

Received: 4 February 2024
Accepted: 6 February 2024
Published: 7 February 2024

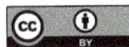

Copyright: © 2024 by the authors. Licensee MDPI, Basel, Switzerland. This article is an open access article distributed under the terms and conditions of the Creative Commons Attribution (CC BY) license (https:// creativecommons.org/licenses/by/ 4.0/).

In the evolving landscape of medical imaging, the escalating need for deep-learning methods takes center stage, offering the capability to autonomously acquire abstract data representations crucial for early detection and classification for cancer treatment. The complexities in handling diverse inputs, high-dimensional features, and subtle patterns within imaging data are acknowledged as significant challenges in this technological pursuit. This Special Issue, "Recent Advances in Deep Learning and Medical Imaging for Cancer Treatment", has attracted 19 high-quality articles that cover state-of-the-art applications and technical developments of deep learning, medical imaging, automatic detection, and classification, explainable artificial intelligence-enabled diagnosis for cancer treatment. In the ever-evolving landscape of cancer treatment, five pivotal themes have emerged as beacons of transformative change. This editorial delves into the realms of innovation that are shaping the future of cancer treatment, focusing on five interconnected themes: use of artificial intelligence in medical imaging, applications of AI in cancer diagnosis and treatment, addressing challenges in medical image analysis, advancements in cancer detection techniques, and innovations in skin cancer classification.

In the realm of medical sciences, particularly within the field of cancer treatment, groundbreaking advancements have been achieved through the integration of deep learning and medical imaging technologies. This dynamic landscape has witnessed substantial progress, thanks to pioneering research endeavors that leverage the capabilities of artificial intelligence to revolutionize the detection and treatment of cancer. Authors in [1] utilized digital single-operator cholangioscopy (D-SOC) and artificial intelligence (AI) to enhance the diagnosis of indeterminate biliary strictures (BSs). Their study employed a convolutional neural network (CNN) trained on 84,994 images from 129 D-SOC exams in Portugal and Spain, achieving an impressive overall accuracy of 82.9%, with a sensitivity of 83.5% and specificity of 82.4%. The findings highlight the potential of integrating AI into D-SOC for substantial improvement in identifying malignant strictures.

In a parallel effort, authors in [2] tackled challenges in medical image classification, particularly with musculoskeletal radiographs (MURA), using a novel transfer learning (TL) approach. Their method involved pre-training deep-learning (DL) models on similar medical images, addressing limitations associated with TL on ImageNet datasets, and fine-tuning with a small set of annotated images. Focusing on humerus and wrist classification, their TL approach outperformed traditional ImageNet TL methods and showcased robustness and potential reusability across diverse medical image applications, effectively addressing the scarcity of labeled training data. In addressing leukemia challenges, authors in [3] proposed an explainable AI (XAI) leukemia classification method to overcome the "black box problem" in deep-learning approaches. Their approach incorporated a strong white blood cell (WBC) nuclei segmentation as a robust attention mechanism, resulting in an intersection over union (IoU) of 0.91. With a testing accuracy of 99.9%, the deep-learning classifier showcased the potential of the visual explainable CAD system to enhance leukemia diagnosis reliability and patient outcomes. Authors in [4] developed the adaptive Aquila optimizer with explainable artificial intelligence-enabled cancer diagnosis (AAOXAI-CD) technique, leveraging the faster SqueezeNet model, AAO algorithm for hyperparameter tuning, and a majority-weighted voting ensemble model with RNN, GRU, and BiLSTM classifiers. The integration of the XAI approach LIME enhanced the interpretability of the black-box method in cancer detection, demonstrating promising results in simulation evaluations on medical cancer imaging databases compared to existing approaches. The study focused on improving colorectal and osteosarcoma cancer classification through this methodology.

In a related study, authors in [5] emphasize the significance of early breast cancer detection, focusing on the role of artificial intelligence, specifically deep learning. The paper highlights the limitations of manual screening by radiologists, advocating for automated methods and discussing recent studies using AI for improved early detection. Acknowledging the crucial role of datasets in training AI algorithms for breast cancer analysis, the review aims to be a comprehensive resource for researchers, recognizing AI's potential in enhancing outcomes for women with breast cancer.

In the realm of applications of artificial intelligence in cancer diagnosis and treatment, authors in [6] highlight the global concern of skin cancer, emphasizing the crucial role of early detection for successful treatment. The current limitation of specialized skin cancer professionals in developing countries leads to expensive and inaccessible diagnoses. The paper explores the potential of AI, particularly machine learning and deep learning, in automating skin cancer diagnosis to enhance early detection and reduce associated morbidity and mortality rates, drawing insights from previous works and proposing future directions for overcoming challenges in this field. Authors in [7] emphasized AI's transformative role in healthcare, focusing on its impact on urological cancer diagnosis, treatment planning, and monitoring. The study, based on a comprehensive review until 31 May 2022, identified various AI forms, such as machine learning and computer vision. The findings suggest that AI has significant potential to enhance uro-oncology, revolutionizing cancer care for improved patient outcomes and overall tumor management in the future.

On the other hand, authors in [8] highlighted that laryngeal carcinoma is the most common upper respiratory tract malignant tumor, leading to postoperative voice loss after total laryngectomy. They suggested employing modern deep learning, specifically convolutional neural networks (CNNs) applied to Mel-frequency spectrogram (MFCC) inputs, to objectively analyze substitution voicing in audio signals following laryngeal oncosurgery. Their approach achieved the highest true-positive rate and an overall accuracy of 89.47% compared to other state-of-the-art methods. Authors in [9] discussion on breast cancer as a leading cause of death among women globally, they highlighted the time-consuming nature and subjectivity of histopathological diagnosis. Their paper introduced the CSSADTL-BCC model, utilizing Gaussian filtering for noise reduction, a MixNet-based feature extraction model, and a stacked gated recurrent unit (SGRU) classification approach with hyperparameter tuning using the CSSA. The CSSADTL-BCC model exhibited superior performance in breast cancer classification on histopathological images compared to recent state-of-the-art approaches.

In the realm of addressing challenges in medical image analysis, authors in [10] explore the complexities in diagnosing and treating liver tumors, emphasizing the vital role of accurate segmentation and classification in conditions like hepatocellular carcinoma or metastases. Despite challenges posed by unclear borders and diverse tumor characteristics, the paper introduces a transformative solution by adapting the transformer paradigm from natural language processing (NLP) to computer vision (CV). Their three-stage approach, involving pre-processing, enhanced Mask R-CNN for liver segmentation, and classification using enhanced swin transformer network with adversarial propagation (APESTNet), demonstrates superior performance, efficiency, and noise resilience in experimental findings.

On the other hand, authors in [11] discuss the challenges faced by computer-aided diagnosis (CAD) methods in medical imaging due to diverse imaging modalities and clinical pathologies. Despite recognizing deep learning's efficacy, they propose an innovative hybrid approach that integrates medical image analysis and radial scanning series features, utilizing a U-shape convolutional neural network for classifying 4D data from lung nodule images. The results demonstrate a notable accuracy of 92.84%, outperforming recent classifiers and underscoring the efficiency of this novel method.

In a parallel effort, authors in [12] highlights the pivotal role of precise clinical staging in enhancing decision making for bladder cancer treatment. To overcome the constraints of current radiomics methods with grayscale CT scans, the suggested hybrid framework combines pre-trained deep neural networks for feature extraction with statistical machine learning for classification. This approach excels in distinguishing bladder cancer tissue from normal tissue, differentiating muscle-invasive bladder cancer (MIBC) and non-muscle-invasive bladder cancer (NMIBC), as well as discerning post-treatment changes (PTC) versus MIBC. Authors in [13] enhance breast cancer diagnosis through their AOADL-HBCC technique, which combines the arithmetic optimization algorithm with deep-learning-based histopathological breast cancer classification. The approach employs median filtering for noise removal and contrast enhancement and features a SqueezeNet model and a deep belief network classifier optimized with Adamax. Comparative studies demonstrate that the AOADL-HBCC technique surpasses recent methodologies, achieving a maximum accuracy of 96.77% in breast cancer classification.

In realm of advancements in cancer detection techniques, a study by authors in [14] enhance their automated method for calculating metabolic tumor volume (MTV) in diffuse large B-cell lymphoma (DLBCL), addressing the limitations of the current semiautomatic software. The updated method utilizes an improved deep convolutional neural network to segment structures from CT scans with avidity on PET scans, demonstrating high concordance in MTV calculations through rigorous validation against nuclear medicine readers. This advancement supports the potential integration of PET-based biomarkers in clinical trials, offering a more efficient and accurate approach to prognostic assessments in DLBCL.

Authors in [15], addresses limitations in deep-learning models for rare skin disease detection by emphasizing challenges related to imbalanced datasets and identifying tiny, affected skin portions in medical images. He proposes an evolved attention-cost-sensitive deep-learning-based feature fusion ensemble meta-classifier approach that incorporates refined cost weights to combat data imbalance and enhances attention mechanisms for optimal feature capture. The updated two-stage ensemble meta-classifier achieves an impressive 99% accuracy for both skin disease detection and classification, outperforming existing methods by 6% and 11%, respectively, positioning itself as a valuable computer-aided diagnosis tool for early and accurate skin cancer detection in medical environments. Authors in [16] expand the exploration of explainable artificial intelligence (XAI) for classifying pulmonary diseases from chest radiographs. They enhance their CNN-based transfer learning approach using the ResNet50 neural network, trained on a more extensive dataset that includes a comprehensive collection of COVID-19-related radiographs. The updated study demonstrates an improved classification accuracy of 95% and 98%, reinforcing the potential of XAI in enhancing disease detection and providing crucial interpretable explanations for early-stage diagnosis and treatment of pulmonary diseases. This underscores the ongoing commitment to refining models for accurate and transparent chest radiograph classification.

In the realm of innovations in skin cancer classification, authors in [17] delve into skin cancer classification, refining the analysis of HAM10000 and BCN20000 datasets to enhance classification accuracy. They employ three feature fusion methods with CNN models (VGG16, EfficientNet B0, and ResNet50), forming adaptive weighted feature sets (AWFS). Introducing two optimization strategies, MOWFS and FOWFS, leveraging an artificial jellyfish (AJS) algorithm, the authors showcase the superiority of FOWFS-AJS, achieving the highest accuracy, precision, sensitivity, and F1 score, particularly with SVM classifiers attaining 94.05% and 94.90% accuracy for HAM10000 and BCN20000 datasets, respectively. The non-parametric Friedman statistical test reinforces FOWFS-AJS as the top-performing strategy, emphasizing its efficiency due to the quick converging nature facilitated by AJS. Authors in [18] advance oral cancer detection by introducing the attention branch network (ABN), addressing interpretability concerns of their prior work on convolutional neural networks (CNNs). The ABN incorporates visual explanation, attention mechanisms, and expert knowledge through manually edited attention maps, outperforming the baseline network and achieving an accuracy of 0.903 with the integration of squeeze-and-excitation (SE) blocks for improved cross-validation accuracy. The study establishes a reliable and interpretable oral cancer computer-aided diagnosis system.

Finally, in the realm of mathematical modeling for cancer cell growth control, authors in [19] address the challenge of cancer cell growth control through mathematical modeling. The study advocates for optimal medications to counter chemotherapy's destructive effects, employing techniques like Bernstein polynomial with genetic algorithm and synergetic control for stability. The simulation results highlight synergetic control's effectiveness in eliminating cancerous cells within five days, presenting a promising early reduction approach.

Author Contributions: M.F.I.: Project administration, Supervision, Writing—original draft, Writing—review and editing. M.W.: Project administration, Supervision, Writing—original draft, Writing—review and editing. All authors have read and agreed to the published version of the manuscript.

Acknowledgments: We would like to acknowledge the help of the reviewers and thank the authors for their contributions.

Conflicts of Interest: The authors declare that the research was conducted in the absence of any commercial or financial relationships that could be construed as a potential conflict of interest.

References

1. Saraiva, M.M.; Ribeiro, T.; González-Haba, M.; Agudo Castillo, B.; Ferreira, J.P.; Vilas Boas, F.; Afonso, J.; Mendes, F.; Martins, M.; Cardoso, P.; et al. Deep Learning for Automatic Diagnosis and Morphologic Characterization of Malignant Biliary Strictures Using Digital Cholangioscopy: A Multicentric Study. *Cancers* **2023**, *15*, 4827. [CrossRef]
2. Alammar, Z.; Alzubaidi, L.; Zhang, J.; Li, Y.; Lafta, W.; Gu, Y. Deep transfer learning with enhanced feature fusion for detection of abnormalities in x-ray images. *Cancers* **2023**, *15*, 4007. [CrossRef] [PubMed]
3. Diaz Resendiz, J.L.; Ponomaryov, V.; Reyes Reyes, R.; Sadovnychiy, S. Explainable CAD System for Classification of Acute Lymphoblastic Leukemia Based on a Robust White Blood Cell Segmentation. *Cancers* **2023**, *15*, 3376. [CrossRef] [PubMed]
4. Alkhalaf, S.; Alturise, F.; Bahaddad, A.A.; Elnaim, B.M.E.; Shabana, S.; Abdel-Khalek, S.; Mansour, R.F. Adaptive Aquila Optimizer with explainable artificial intelligence-enabled cancer diagnosis on medical imaging. *Cancers* **2023**, *15*, 1492. [CrossRef] [PubMed]
5. Madani, M.; Behzadi, M.M.; Nabavi, S. The role of deep learning in advancing breast cancer detection using different imaging modalities: A systematic review. *Cancers* **2022**, *14*, 5334. [CrossRef]
6. Melarkode, N.; Srinivasan, K.; Qaisar, S.M.; Plawiak, P. AI-Powered Diagnosis of Skin Cancer: A Contemporary Review, Open Challenges and Future Research Directions. *Cancers* **2023**, *15*, 1183. [CrossRef] [PubMed]
7. Froń, A.; Semianiuk, A.; Lazuk, U.; Ptaszkowski, K.; Siennicka, A.; Lemiński, A.; Krajewski, W.; Szydełko, T.; Małkiewicz, B. Artificial Intelligence in Urooncology: What We Have and What We Expect. *Cancers* **2023**, *15*, 4282. [CrossRef]
8. Maskeliūnas, R.; Kulikajevas, A.; Damaševičius, R.; Pribuišis, K.; Ulozaitė-Stanienė, N.; Uloza, V. Lightweight deep learning model for assessment of substitution voicing and speech after laryngeal carcinoma surgery. *Cancers* **2022**, *14*, 2366. [CrossRef]
9. Shankar, K.; Dutta, A.K.; Kumar, S.; Joshi, G.P.; Doo, I.C. Chaotic Sparrow Search Algorithm with Deep Transfer Learning Enabled Breast Cancer Classification on Histopathological Images. *Cancers* **2022**, *14*, 2770. [CrossRef] [PubMed]
10. Balasubramanian, P.K.; Lai, W.C.; Seng, G.H.; Selvaraj, J. Apestnet with mask r-cnn for liver tumor segmentation and classification. *Cancers* **2023**, *15*, 330. [CrossRef] [PubMed]
11. Balcı, M.A.; Batrancea, L.M.; Akgüller, Ö.; Nichita, A. A Series-Based Deep Learning Approach to Lung Nodule Image Classification. *Cancers* **2023**, *15*, 843. [CrossRef] [PubMed]
12. Sarkar, S.; Min, K.; Ikram, W.; Tatton, R.W.; Riaz, I.B.; Silva, A.C.; Bryce, A.H.; Moore, C.; Ho, T.H.; Sonpavde, G.; et al. Performing Automatic Identification and Staging of Urothelial Carcinoma in Bladder Cancer Patients Using a Hybrid Deep-Machine Learning Approach. *Cancers* **2023**, *15*, 1673. [CrossRef] [PubMed]

13. Obayya, M.; Maashi, M.S.; Nemri, N.; Mohsen, H.; Motwakel, A.; Osman, A.E.; Alneil, A.A.; Alsaid, M.I. Hyperparameter optimizer with deep learning-based decision-support systems for histopathological breast cancer diagnosis. *Cancers* **2022**, *15*, 885. [CrossRef] [PubMed]
14. Kuker, R.A.; Lehmkuhl, D.; Kwon, D.; Zhao, W.; Lossos, I.S.; Moskowitz, C.H.; Alderuccio, J.P.; Yang, F. A Deep Learning-Aided Automated Method for Calculating Metabolic Tumor Volume in Diffuse Large B-Cell Lymphoma. *Cancers* **2022**, *14*, 5221. [CrossRef] [PubMed]
15. Ravi, V. Attention cost-sensitive deep learning-based approach for skin cancer detection and classification. *Cancers* **2022**, *14*, 5872. [CrossRef] [PubMed]
16. Naz, Z.; Khan, M.U.; Saba, T.; Rehman, A.; Nobanee, H.; Bahaj, S.A. An Explainable AI-Enabled Framework for Interpreting Pulmonary Diseases from Chest Radiographs. *Cancers* **2023**, *15*, 314. [CrossRef] [PubMed]
17. Mohanty, N.; Pradhan, M.; Reddy, A.V.N.; Kumar, S.; Alkhayyat, A. Integrated design of optimized weighted deep feature fusion strategies for skin lesion image classification. *Cancers* **2022**, *14*, 5716. [CrossRef] [PubMed]
18. Song, B.; Zhang, C.; Sunny, S.; Kc, D.R.; Li, S.; Gurushanth, K.; Mendonca, P.; Mukhia, N.; Patrick, S.; Gurudath, S.; et al. Interpretable and Reliable Oral Cancer Classifier with Attention Mechanism and Expert Knowledge Embedding via Attention Map. *Cancers* **2023**, *15*, 1421. [CrossRef] [PubMed]
19. Subhan, F.; Aziz, M.A.; Khan, I.U.; Fayaz, M.; Wozniak, M.; Shafi, J.; Ijaz, M.F. Cancerous tumor controlled treatment using search heuristic (GA)-based sliding mode and synergetic controller. *Cancers* **2022**, *14*, 4191. [CrossRef] [PubMed]

Disclaimer/Publisher's Note: The statements, opinions and data contained in all publications are solely those of the individual author(s) and contributor(s) and not of MDPI and/or the editor(s). MDPI and/or the editor(s) disclaim responsibility for any injury to people or property resulting from any ideas, methods, instructions or products referred to in the content.

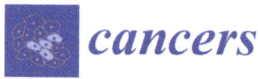

Article

Deep Learning for Automatic Diagnosis and Morphologic Characterization of Malignant Biliary Strictures Using Digital Cholangioscopy: A Multicentric Study

Miguel Mascarenhas Saraiva [1,2,3,*], Tiago Ribeiro [1,2], Mariano González-Haba [4], Belén Agudo Castillo [4], João P. S. Ferreira [5,6], Filipe Vilas Boas [1,2,3], João Afonso [1,2], Francisco Mendes [1,2], Miguel Martins [1,2], Pedro Cardoso [1,2], Pedro Pereira [1,2,3] and Guilherme Macedo [1,2,3]

1 Department of Gastroenterology, São João University Hospital, Alameda Professor Hernâni Monteiro, 4200-427 Porto, Portugal
2 WGO Gastroenterology and Hepatology Training Center, 4200-319 Porto, Portugal
3 Faculty of Medicine, University of Porto, Alameda Professor Hernâni Monteiro, 4200-427 Porto, Portugal
4 Department of Gastroenterology, Hospital Universitario Puerta de Hierro Majadahonda, C/Joaquín Rodrigo, 28220 Majadahonda, Madrid, Spain
5 Department of Mechanical Engineering, Faculty of Engineering, University of Porto, Rua Dr. Roberto Frias, 4200-465 Porto, Portugal
6 DigestAID—Digestive Artificial Intelligence Development, Rua Alfredo Allen n.º 455/461, 4200-135 Porto, Portugal
* Correspondence: miguelmascarenhassaraiva@gmail.com; Tel.: +351-912492511

Citation: Saraiva, M.M.; Ribeiro, T.; González-Haba, M.; Agudo Castillo, B.; Ferreira, J.P.S.; Vilas Boas, F.; Afonso, J.; Mendes, F.; Martins, M.; Cardoso, P.; et al. Deep Learning for Automatic Diagnosis and Morphologic Characterization of Malignant Biliary Strictures Using Digital Cholangioscopy: A Multicentric Study. *Cancers* 2023, 15, 4827. https://doi.org/10.3390/cancers15194827

Academic Editors: Muhammad Fazal Ijaz, Marcin Woźniak and Dania Cioni

Received: 3 August 2023
Revised: 22 September 2023
Accepted: 28 September 2023
Published: 1 October 2023

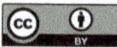

Copyright: © 2023 by the authors. Licensee MDPI, Basel, Switzerland. This article is an open access article distributed under the terms and conditions of the Creative Commons Attribution (CC BY) license (https://creativecommons.org/licenses/by/4.0/).

Simple Summary: Diagnosis and characterization of biliary strictures is challenging, even after the introduction of digital single-operator cholangioscopy (D-SOC). The endoscopist's visual impression has a suboptimal accuracy and there is a significant interobserver variability. Artificial intelligence tools for image analysis have presented important contributions in several fields of gastroenterology. Convolutional neural networks are highly efficient multi-layered deep neural networks for image analysis, with great results in several fields of medicine. Nevertheless, the role of these deep learning models in digital cholangioscopy is still in a premature phase. With this bicentric international study, the authors aimed to create a deep learning-based algorithm for digital cholangioscopy capable of distinguishing benign from malignant biliary lesions. The present model accurately detected malignant biliary lesions with an image processing rate that favors its clinical applicability. The authors believe that the use of an AI-based model may change the landscape in the digital cholangioscopy diagnostic yield.

Abstract: Digital single-operator cholangioscopy (D-SOC) has enhanced the ability to diagnose indeterminate biliary strictures (BSs). Pilot studies using artificial intelligence (AI) models in D-SOC demonstrated promising results. Our group aimed to develop a convolutional neural network (CNN) for the identification and morphological characterization of malignant BSs in D-SOC. A total of 84,994 images from 129 D-SOC exams in two centers (Portugal and Spain) were used for developing the CNN. Each image was categorized as either a normal/benign finding or as malignant lesion (the latter dependent on histopathological results). Additionally, the CNN was evaluated for the detection of morphologic features, including tumor vessels and papillary projections. The complete dataset was divided into training and validation datasets. The model was evaluated through its sensitivity, specificity, positive and negative predictive values, accuracy and area under the receiver-operating characteristic and precision-recall curves (AUROC and AUPRC, respectively). The model achieved a 82.9% overall accuracy, 83.5% sensitivity and 82.4% specificity, with an AUROC and AUPRC of 0.92 and 0.93, respectively. The developed CNN successfully distinguished benign findings from malignant BSs. The development and application of AI tools to D-SOC has the potential to significantly augment the diagnostic yield of this exam for identifying malignant strictures.

Keywords: cholangioscopy; artificial intelligence; biliary strictures

1. Introduction

Biliary strictures (BSs) are a concerning finding, often confronting patients with a poor prognosis. The primary focus in the presence of a BS is to exclude malignancy, which is responsible for the majority of BS cases. Malignant BSs typically result from primary (cholangiocarcinoma) or secondary neoplasia with biliary tract extension (gallbladder, pancreatic, hepatocellular carcinoma) [1,2]. On the other hand, around 30% of all BS cases are benign, with the need to consider iatrogenic causes, biliary lithiasis, primary and IgG4-related sclerosing cholangitis [2,3]. Therefore, it is crucial to differentiate between benign and malign BSs, as the treatment and prognosis greatly differ between the different etiologies [4,5].

Endoscopic retrograde cholangiopancreatography (ERCP) has historically been the primary diagnostic modality in patients with biliary strictures. This technique allows the observation of indirect signs that may suggest the malignant nature of BSs (surface irregularity, stricture length), together with tissue sampling, either by brush cytology or fluoroscopy-guided transpapillary biopsy. However, the diagnostic performance of ERCP combined with brush cytology or biopsy is poor [6]. Indeed, a meta-analysis reported a sensitivity of 45% for brush cytology and 48% for ERCP-guided biopsies. The combination of both methods modestly increased the sensitivity for detection of malignant biliary strictures [7].

Digital single-operator cholangioscopy (D-SOC) allows high-resolution inspection of the bile duct, enabling its application for diagnostic and therapeutic purposes. Direct visualization allows for more accurate morphologic characterization of BSs as well as the possibility for targeted biopsies [8]. A recent multicentric randomized trial demonstrated the higher sensitivity of D-SOC for the visual identification of malignant strictures, compared to standard ERCP cholangiographic impression (96% vs. 67%, $p = 0.02$) [9]. Nonetheless, the specificity of the visual impression remains suboptimal (89%) [10]. In fact, the accuracy is diminished when evaluating extrinsic BSs (most commonly pancreatic adenocarcinoma or metastatic disease) [11]. Additionally, the presence of traumatic lesions after stent removal or even the passage of the scope may be mistaken with malignant lesions. Lastly, the presence of diseases associated with chronic biliary duct inflammation (namely primary sclerosing cholangitis) is associated with a decreased diagnostic yield for diagnosing malignant BSs.

Several morphological features are associated with an increased malignancy risk [12,13]. The identification of papillary projections is associated with a seven-times increased risk of malignancy in a multivariate analysis [14]. Nevertheless, a significant lack of interobserver agreement in this morphologic feature identification was observed. On the other hand, abnormal dilated tumor vessels are commonly visualized in malignant BSs [12]. These vessels are developed during tumoral angiogenesis and are associated with an accurate detection of malignant BSs [15]. However, chronic inflammation can diminish the diagnostic accuracy of D-SOC for tumoral vessels. Therefore, classification systems for prediction of BS malignancy have been tested, namely systems based on morphological features [14,16]. Sethi et al. developed the Monaco Classification System for indeterminate BSs, reporting an overall accuracy of 70% for malignant BSs and relevant interobserver agreement for papillary projection ($k = 0.43$) and abnormal vessels identification ($k = 0.26$) [14]. However, there is no universally accepted classification system for D-SOC findings and interobserver agreement between different endoscopists remains poor [17].

The development of artificial intelligence (AI) models suited for the analysis of large image datasets is a matter of great scientific interest, specially using deep learning algorithms. Convolutional neural networks (CNN) are a human visual cortex inspired multilayered deep learning model suitable to increase the diagnostic yield in several medical fields [18–20]. Additionally, there are several published studies about the impact of these models in the diagnostic performance of several endoscopic techniques [21–23].The impact of AI for the evaluation of cholangioscopy images has recently started to be investigated. However, a tool providing categorization (i.e., discriminating malignant from non-malignant strictures) as well as morphologic classification has scarcely been assessed. Given the current limitations in the diagnostic approach to biliary strictures and the potential of AI to provide effective image analysis, our group aimed to develop and validate a CNN model for automatic detection and differentiation between benign and malignant BSs in D-SOC. Additionally, our group assessed the capacity of the CNN to provide accurate identification of significant morphological features of malignant BSs.

2. Materials and Methods

2.1. Patient Population and Study Design

For the development of the study, our group included D-SOC exams performed between August 2017 and November 2022 at two centers in Portugal (Centro Hospitalar Universitário de São João (CHUSJ), Porto, Portugal) and Spain (Hospital Universitario Puerta de Hierro Majadahonda (HUPHM), Madrid, Spain). A total of 124 patients (CHUSJ, n = 106; HUPHM, n = 18), corresponding to 129 D-SOC exams (CHUSJ, n = 111; HUPHM, n = 18), were enrolled. A total of 84,994 still-frame images were used for the development, training and validation phases of the CNN for automatic differentiation between malignant and benign BSs. The still-frame images were obtained during the exam, mainly through decomposition of the procedure videos into frames, using a VLC media player (VideoLAN, Paris, France).

The study was performed after approval by the ethics committee of Centro Hospitalar Universitário de São João/Faculdade de Medicina da Universidade do Porto (CE 41/2021) and Hospital Universitario Puerta de Hierro Majadahonda (PI 153/22). This was a retrospective non-interventional study, performed with respect for the Declaration of Helsinki. An adequate omission of potentially identifiable patient information was assured, with each individual patient being assigned with a random number, guaranteeing data anonymization. The non-traceability of the data and respect to the general data protection regulation (GDPR) was assured by a team with a Data Protection Officer (DPO).

2.2. Digital-Single Operator Cholangioscopy Procedure and Definitions

All of the D-SOC exams included in the study were performed with the SpyGlass™ DS II system (Boston Scientific Corp., Marlborough, MA, USA). The procedures were performed by expert gastroenterologists (P.P., F.V.B., M.G.-H., and B.A.G), each with experience of more than 2000 ERCPs and 100 cholangioscopies prior to this study. For the performance of the exams the Olympus TJF-160V or TFJ-Q180V duodenoscopes (Olympus Medical Systems, Tokyo, Japan) were used. Additionally, the SpyBite™ forceps (Boston Scientific Corp., Marlborough, MA, USA) were utilized for obtaining the biopsy specimens with direct visual guidance, assuring a minimum of 4 biopsies in all the study exams.

A total of 84,994 D-SOC biliary images were classified as benign or malignant. Benign biliary findings typically included normal bile ducts, stone disease and benign BSs. A benign BS-confirmed diagnosis implied a negative histopathology (biopsy or surgically obtained) with absence of malignancy after 6 months of follow up. Stone disease was diagnosed upon direct observation and in the absence of other findings. A malignant diagnosis implied a malign histopathology, obtained either through D-SOC biopsy or other tissue sampling exams (namely brush cytology, fluoroscopic or endoscopic ultrasound-guided biopsy or even surgical specimen).

2.3. Development of the Convolutional Neural Network

We developed a deep learning-based CNN to automatically detect and differentiate malignant biliary strictures from benign biliary conditions, the latter including benign strictures, stone disease and normal bile ducts. A total of 84,994 frames were included:

malignant strictures were seen in 44,743 images; whereas the remaining 40,521 showed benign biliary conditions.

The total data was separated into two sets: training and validation. The first comprised 80% of the frames (n = 67,678), while the second used 20% of the remaining images (n = 17,316) using a patient-split design, ensuring that no data from the same patient overlapped in both the datasets. The validation dataset was used to assess the model's performance. A graphical flowchart of the study design is shown in Figure 1. Additionally, in a subset of exams (n = 62) we evaluated the performance of the CNN for the detection of morphologic features associated with bile duct malignancy ("tumor vessels" and "papillary projections"). Tumor vessels were defined as abnormal, dilated, tortuous vessels associated with bile duct malignancy (n = 18,388). Papillary projections (n = 18,388) were represented as finger-like projections associated with bile duct malignancy.

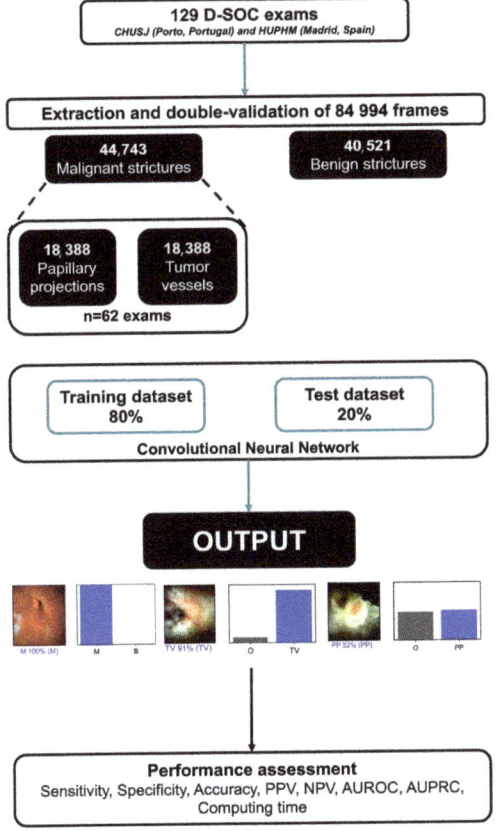

Figure 1. Study flowchart for the training and validation phases. AUC—area under the receiving operator characteristic curve; B—benign biliary findings; D-SOC—digital single-operator cholangioscopy; M—malignant stricture; NPV—negative predictive value; PP—papillary projections; O—other; PPV—positive predictive value; TV—tumor vessels.

The Resnet model was used to build this CNN. ImageNet, a large-scale collection of images used for object recognition software development, was used to train weights between units. We preserved its convolutional layers to impart its learning to our model. The final fully connected layers were deleted and replaced with new fully connected layers according to the number of classes we used to categorize our endoscopic frames. There was an initial fully connected layer in each of the two blows that we used, followed by dropout layers with a drop rate of 0.1. After that, we added a dense layer whose size defined the number of classification groups (two: malignant strictures and benign biliary conditions). The learning rate was 0.00015, the batch size was 128 and the number of epochs was 10. PyTorch was used to prepare and run the model. Performance analyses was carried out with a computer equipped with a 2.1 GHz Intel® Xeon® Gold 6130 processor (Intel, Santa Clara, CA, USA) and a double NVIDIA Quadro® RTX™ 4000 graphic processing unit (NVIDIA Corporate, Santa Clara, CA, USA).

2.4. Model Performance and Statistical Analysis

The assessment of CNN's performance was performed using an independent validation dataset (20% of all the data). For each frame, the algorithm calculated the probability of having a malignant stricture and the probability of being considered a benign biliary condition (Figure 2). Since a higher probability translated into greater confidence of the CNN prediction, the model selected the category with the highest probability as its final classification. Then, the final classification of the CNN was compared with the corresponding histopathological evaluation, which was regarded as the gold standard. Sensitivity, specificity, positive predictive value (PPV), negative predictive value (NPV) and accuracy in distinguishing malign strictures from benign biliary conditions were our primary outcomes. Additionally, we performed receiver operating characteristic (ROC) curves analysis and calculated the area under the ROC curves (AUROC) to evaluate the discriminatory capacity of our model. Moreover, the precision-recall (PR) curve and the area under the precision-recall curve (AUPRC) were used to measure the performance of the model, accounting for potential data imbalance. Finally, we evaluated the computational performance of the algorithm by measuring the time required for the CNN to process and generate output for all the frames included in the validation dataset. We performed statistical analysis using Sci-Kit learn v0.22.2 [24].

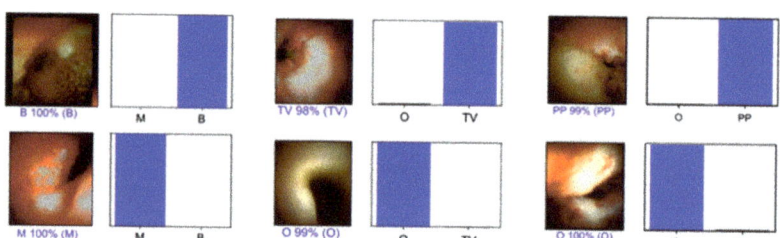

Figure 2. Output obtained during the training and development of the convolutional neural network. The bars represent the probability estimated by the network. The finding with the highest probability was output as the predicted classification. A blue bar represents a correct prediction. B—benign biliary findings; M—malignant stricture; O—other; PP—papillary projections; PPV—positive predictive value; TV—tumor vessels.

3. Results

3.1. Performance of the Convolutional Neural Network

In total, 129 D-SOC exams were performed in 124 patients, from August 2017 to November 2022. In 73 patients, a diagnosis of malignancy was established. Benign findings were established in 51 patients. We included 84,994 frames for development of this CNN, of which 44 743 were malignant strictures. The remaining 40,521 images were benign biliary conditions (benign strictures, stone disease and normal bile ducts).

The model was trained and developed using 80% of the total dataset (n = 67,678). The remaining 20% (n = 17,316) was used to test the algorithm's performance. Table 1 shows the confusion matrix between the CNN's predictions in validation set versus the histopathologic characterization. In terms of detecting and distinguishing malign strictures from benign conditions, the CNN was associated with a sensitivity of 83.5%, a specificity of

82.4% and an accuracy of 82.9%. PPV and NPV were, 79.6% and 85.8%, respectively. The model's AUROC and AUPRC for differentiating between the malignant lesions and benign biliary conditions were 0.92 and 0.93, respectively, as shown in Figure 3.

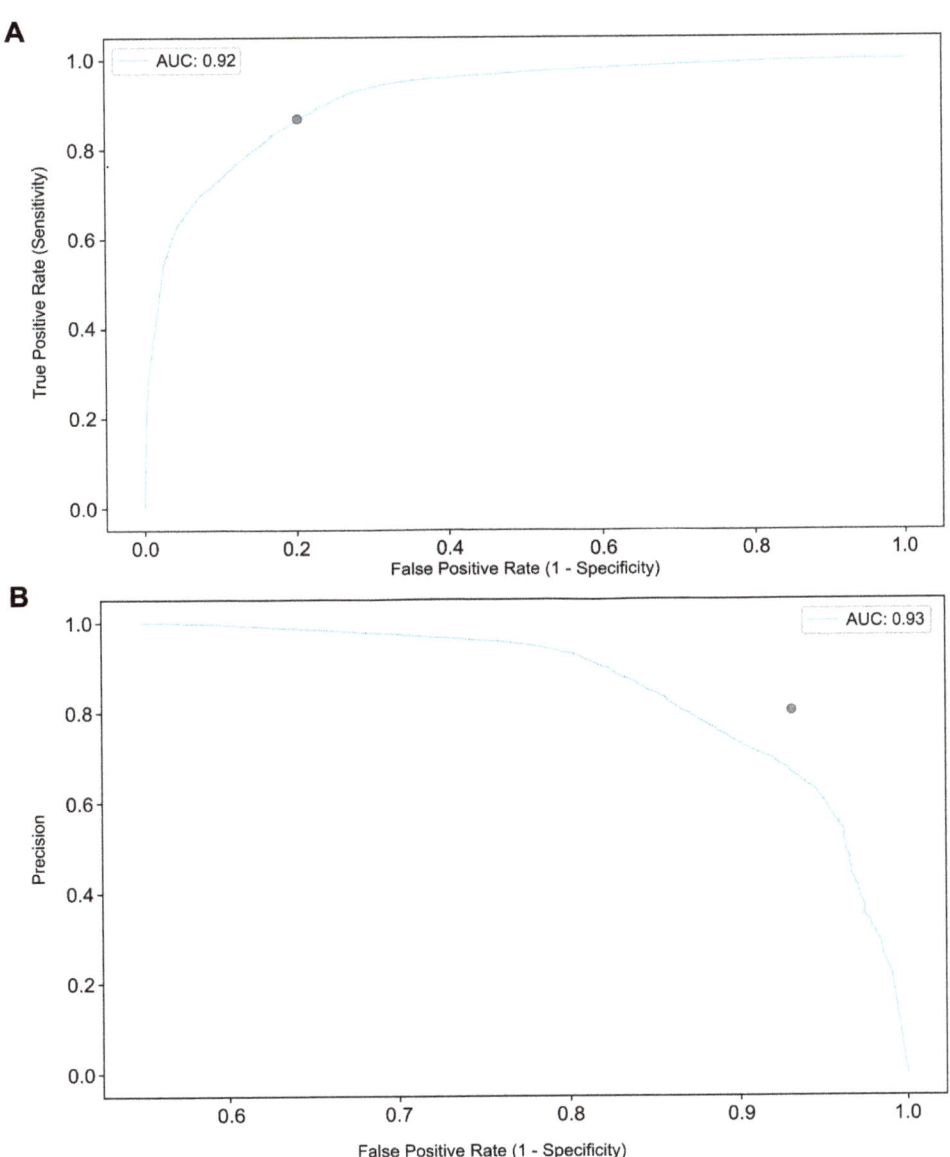

Figure 3. Receiver operating characteristic (**A**) and precision-recall (**B**) analyses of the network's performance in the detection of malignant biliary strictures or benign biliary conditions.

Table 1. Confusion matrix of the automatic detection versus final diagnosis, CNN—convolutional neural network; Malignant—malignant biliary strictures; Benign—normal bile ducts or benign biliary findings.

		Final Diagnosis	
		Malignant	Benign
CNN classification	Malignant	6527	1673
	Benign	1293	7823

3.2. Detection of Morphological Characteristics Associated with Biliary Malignancy

The CNN's performance for the detection of morphological features associated with malignancy of the biliary tract (tumor vessels and papillary projections) were also assessed on a subset of 62 D-SOC exams of patients with malignant biliary strictures. Two sets of 18,388 images were used for the constitution of the CNNs for the automatic detection of TV and PP, respectively. Heatmap analysis was performed for the identification of features contributing to the predictions of the CNN (Figure 4). Regarding tumor vessel detection, the CNN sensitivity and specificity were 95.7% and 88.6%, respectively, with an accuracy of 93.0%. In terms of papillary projection identification, the model's sensitivity, specificity and accuracy were 74.1%, 94.5% and 91.2%, respectively. The AUROC for the detection and differentiation of tumor vessels and papillary projections by the CNN was 0.98 and 0.96, respectively (Figure 5).

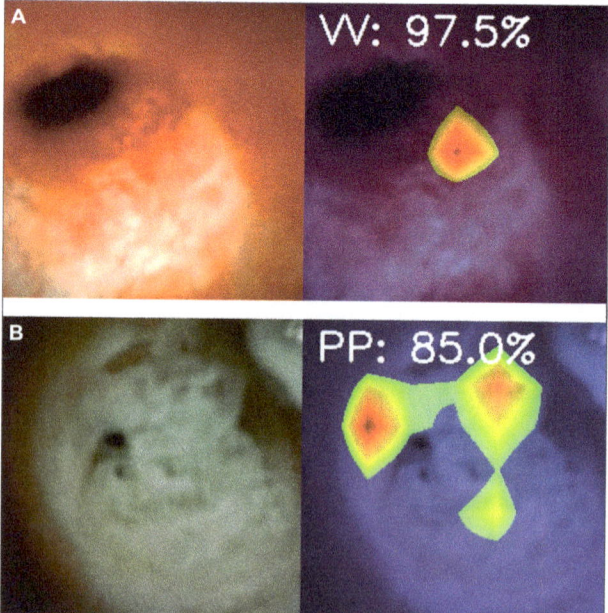

Figure 4. Heatmap analysis showing the prediction of the algorithm for the identification of tumor vessels (**A**) and papillary projections (PP), with the associated probability. (**A**)—Tumor vessels (VV); (**B**)—Papillary projections (PP).

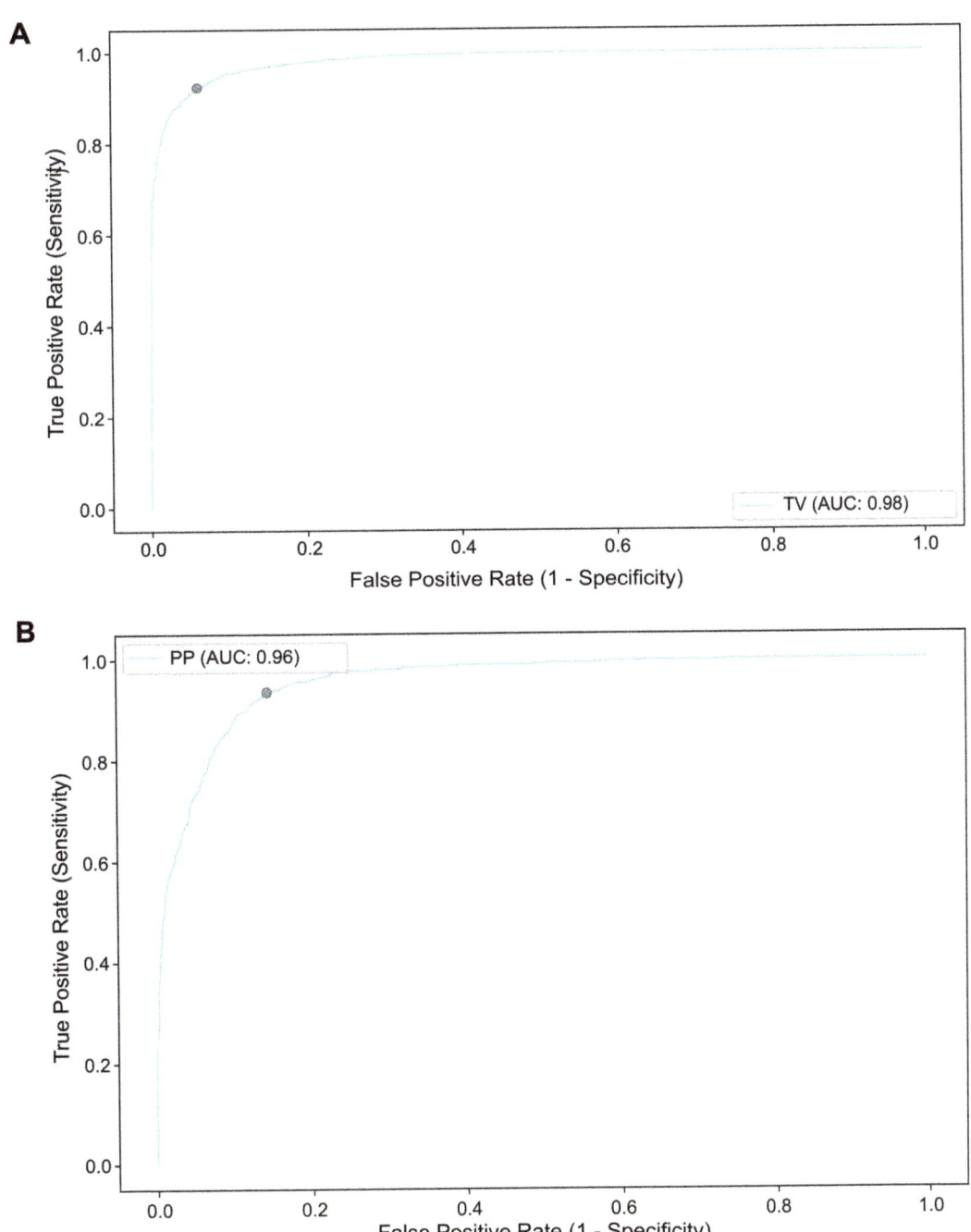

Figure 5. ROC analysis of the network's performance in the detection of morphological characteristics of malignancy. (**A**)—Tumor vessels (TV); (**B**)—Papillary projections (PP).

3.3. Computational Performance of the CNN

The CNN processed 4250 batches (each batch comprising of 128 frames) in 23 min and 16 s, which can be translated to an approximate reading rate of 390 frames per second.

4. Discussion

The utilization of AI tools in medical routines is experiencing rapid growth. Research in the field of deep learning systems in the field of gastrointestinal endoscopy has primarily concentrated on luminal endoscopy, while the research on hepatobiliary indications is significantly less robust [25]. Obtaining a conclusive diagnosis in patients with indeterminate bile duct strictures is crucial for tailoring treatments for each patient. Nonetheless, it is often challenging to attain a specific diagnosis due to frequently inconclusive tissue sampling. Recently, Gerges et al. demonstrated a higher sensitivity of D-SOC-guided biopsies compared to those obtained during ERCP procedures [9]. The sensitivity of D-SOC-guided biopsies was calculated at 74% in a recent meta-analysis [26]. Nevertheless, the introduction of D-SOC brought about a remarkable improvement, particularly evident in the accuracy of visually assessing significant biliary lesions. In a study conducted by Navaneethan et al., the estimated sensitivity for visual impression in diagnosing malignancy was reported to be an impressive 90% [27]. However, the diagnosis of malignancy through visual impression alone is hindered by suboptimal specificity and accuracy [14,28]. Currently, a universally accepted classification system for visually diagnosing malignancy during single-operator cholangioscopy is yet to be clinically established [12–14]. Furthermore, the utilization of existing classification systems has been linked to inadequate interobserver agreement, exacerbating the challenges in this field [14].

The primary objective in managing a biliary stricture is to effectively exclude malignancy. The advent of D-SOC has notably improved the diagnostic accuracy for indeterminate biliary strictures. Nonetheless, a missing rate as high as 10% has been reported for D-SOC with direct visualization or targeted biopsies [10], and a definite diagnosis of malignancy imperatively requires histologic confirmation. Considering these constraints, we firmly believe that integrating real-time AI technology into D-SOC has the potential to bridge this gap and address these challenges effectively. A recent systematic review and meta-analysis by Njei et al. suggested the application of AI systems as the most promising solution for the distinction between malignant and benign BSs [29]. Recently, significant interest has been devoted to AI algorithms for the identification of malignant biliary strictures. Robles-Medranda et al. developed a CNN-based model for the identification of biliary malignancy using pre-defined endoscopic classifications [30]. This algorithm has been shown to be highly accurate in the detection of tumor vessels. Moreover, the CNN outperformed non-expert endoscopists in the identification of malignant BSs. Nevertheless, this study has not performed explainability analysis, thus not allowing the full assessment of the predictions of the CNN. More recently, Zhang et al. have developed consecutive deep learning algorithms for the selection of quality D-SOC images for subsequent development of a CNN for the classification of biliary strictures [31]. Their deep learning algorithm achieved a sensitivity of 92% and a specificity of 88% for the detection of malignant strictures at a video level. This study simultaneously provided heatmap analysis to ascertain suspicious areas, which allowed the identification of areas contributing significantly for the predictions of the algorithm. The improvement in the accuracy of AI systems integrated in real-time into D-SOC systems may enhance the evaluation of visual features of biliary strictures. However, it is crucial to note that these systems are expected to assist instead of replacing conventional tissue sampling. Integrating visual features linked to a higher likelihood of malignancy (such as tumor vessels and papillary projections) into these models can facilitate the precise identification of areas where suspected malignant lesions are present. This, in turn, has the potential to enhance the diagnostic yield of existing D-SOC-guided tissue sampling. Further development of these algorithms, combined with ongoing efforts to improve staging and prognostication with the assistance of AI, will provide more personalized care to patients with suspected biliary malignancy, thus offering the potential to improve the prognosis of these patients [32–35].

The algorithm developed in this study had a dual purpose: to categorize biliary strictures as either malignant or benign and to identify the morphological features associated with an increased risk of malignancy, such as tumor vessels and papillary projections. To ensure a robust and diverse dataset, we included images from two large-volume centers, resulting in a comprehensive collection of nearly 85,000 biliary stricture images. The findings of our study revealed that this model demonstrated exceptional sensitivity, specificity and accuracy. Overall, our network achieved an AUC of 0.92 in distinguishing malignant from benign strictures. Additionally, our CNN exhibited outstanding performance in detecting tumor vessels and papillary projections, with AUC values of 0.98 and 0.96, respectively. Furthermore, our algorithm displayed remarkable image processing efficiency, with an approximate reading rate of 390 frames per second. Our results are in line with a recent study by Marya et al., which focused on the development of a CNN for the identification of malignant BSs, which showed an adequate performance in differentiating malignant from benign BSs, with an overall accuracy of 91% [36]. These results demonstrate the potential of these systems in advancing the field of biliary stricture diagnosis and management.

This study has several points of merit. First, the development of this deep learning algorithm included a large volume and variety of images obtained from D-SOC exams performed at two European high-volume referral centers. Second, we included a robust dataset of almost 85,000 images of patients with BSs, for whom the diagnosis of biliary malignancy required unequivocal histological proof. Third, we have built upon previously published work on the application of AI systems to D-SOC. In this study, we have expanded the evidence on the application of these algorithms for the detection of morphological features associated with an increased risk of biliary malignancy. Indeed, our system detected tumor vessels and papillary projections with an AUC of 0.98 and 0.96. The detection of these morphologic features is of paramount importance as they have been demonstrated to predict the presence of malignant BSs. Indeed, Robles-Medranda and coworkers have shown that the identification of tumor vessels predicted the presence of a malignant biliary stricture with a sensitivity of 94% and an overall accuracy of 86%. Nevertheless, the specificity of this finding was suboptimal (63%) [15]. The introduction of AI models may provide a solution in decreasing the problematic issues of both false negative and false positive results, which lead to inadequate treatments and morbidity. Indeed, our network achieved a sensitivity of 96% and a specificity of 87%. This is in line with previously published studies on the detection of tumor vessels in malignant BSs [30,37]. Besides the importance of classifying a BS as malignant or benign, real-time AI models accurately identifying the morphologic features associated with biliary malignancy may provide guidance to D-SOC-oriented tissue sampling, therefore increasing its yield.

This study has several limitations to be acknowledged. First, despite the large dataset for the context of a proof-of-concept study, clinical validation of this algorithm will require a much larger volume of data. Secondly, our deep learning model was developed and tested exclusively on a single D-SOC platform, which limits the generalizability of the algorithm to other cholangioscopy systems. Third, at this stage, we did not assess the use of deep learning with prior knowledge for the enhancement of the performance of our algorithm. Moreover, distinct deep learning models other than convolutional neural networks have been shown to be more efficient than CNNs [38], and their use should be assessed in further studies. Interoperability remains a significant concern in the development and application of AI technologies in the medical field, as the ability to generalize a given technology across multiple devices is a crucial requirement for its clinical applicability. Therefore, it is essential to develop and validate this deep learning model across different D-SOC devices. Thirdly, while efforts were made to mitigate the risk of overfitting, it cannot be eliminated. As other systems designed for pancreatobiliary endoscopy, the technological maturity of our algorithm remains unfit for clinical practice. Subsequent development of these algorithms on an adequate environment, as well as prototype validation in a real-life clinical setting should follow suite. Therefore, while the performance marks of this algorithm on a preclinical stage suggest that it would provide accurate predictions in a real-life setting, these results should be interpreted considering the stage of development of the algorithm. Subsequent development of these algorithms should include: the development of international multicentric studies, with the aim of increasing datasets, both in quantity as well as in variability; engaging with practitioners for the development of user-friendly prototypes, combining an increase in the accuracy provided by these software with the current standards of practice of expert centers, alerting the endoscopists for meaningful findings and preventing "noisy" overpredictions; finally, the ultimate application of these algorithms in clinical practice should be strictly regulated by competent agencies, and effective polices should be enforced to ensure the quality of these systems as well as their clinical benefit.

5. Conclusions

The influence of AI in everyday clinical practice is expected to continue growing in the near future. The potential impact of deep learning algorithms on the care of patients with suspected biliary malignancy is significant. This study aimed to evaluate the performance of a CNN in detecting and distinguishing between malignant and benign biliary disorders, utilizing a large dataset of D-SOC images from two experienced centers in this field. The favorable performance demonstrated by this model establishes a solid groundwork for further investigation of AI technologies in this specific patient subset, with the ultimate goal of enhancing the clinical outcomes for individuals suspected of having biliary malignancy.

Author Contributions: Conceptualization, M.M.S., T.R., P.P., F.V.B., M.G.-H., B.A.C. and G.M.; methodology, M.M.S., T.R., J.A., P.C., F.M. and M.M.; software, J.P.S.F.; validation, P.P., F.V.B., M.G.-H., B.A.C. and G.M.; formal analysis, M.M.S., T.R. and J.P.S.F.; investigation, M.M.S., T.R. and J.P.S.F.; resources, P.P., F.V.B., M.G.-H., B.A.C. and G.M.; data curation, J.P.S.F.; writing—original draft preparation, M.M.S. and T.R. with equal contribution; writing—review and editing, M.M.S., T.R., J.A., P.C., F.M. and M.M.; visualization, T.R., J.A., F.M. and M.M.; supervision, P.P., F.V.B. and G.M.; project administration, M.M.S.; funding acquisition, M.M.S. All authors have read and agreed to the published version of the manuscript.

Funding: The authors acknowledge NVIDIA for supporting our study by supplying graphic processing units.

Institutional Review Board Statement: This study was approved by the ethics committee of Centro Hospitalar Universitário de São João/Faculdade de Medicina da Universidade do Porto (CE 41/2021) e Hospital Universitario Puerta de Hierro Majadahonda (PI 153/22) and was conducted respecting the declaration of Helsinki. This study is retrospective and of a non-interventional nature. Any information deemed to potentially identify the subjects was omitted.

Informed Consent Statement: Not applicable.

Data Availability Statement: Not applicable.

Conflicts of Interest: João P.S. Ferreira is currently an employee of DigestAID—Digestive Artificial Intelligence Development.

References

1. Larghi, A.; Tringali, A.; Lecca, P.G.; Giordano, M.; Costamagna, G. Management of hilar biliary strictures. *Am. J. Gastroenterol.* **2008**, *103*, 458–473. [CrossRef]
2. Pimpinelli, M.; Makar, M.; Kahaleh, M. Endoscopic management of benign and malignant hilar stricture. *Dig. Endosc.* **2023**, *35*, 443–452. [CrossRef]
3. Tummala, P.; Munigala, S.; Eloubeidi, M.A.; Agarwal, B. Patients with obstructive jaundice and biliary stricture +/− mass lesion on imaging: Prevalence of malignancy and potential role of EUS-FNA. *J. Clin. Gastroenterol.* **2013**, *47*, 532–537. [CrossRef]
4. Paranandi, B.; Oppong, K.W. Biliary strictures: Endoscopic assessment and management. *Frontline Gastroenterol.* **2017**, *8*, 133–137. [CrossRef]
5. Singhi, A.D.; Slivka, A. Evaluation of indeterminate biliary strictures: Is there life on MARS? *Gastrointest. Endosc.* **2020**, *92*, 320–322. [CrossRef]

6. Burnett, A.S.; Calvert, T.J.; Chokshi, R.J. Sensitivity of endoscopic retrograde cholangiopancreatography standard cytology: 10-y review of the literature. *J. Surg. Res.* **2013**, *184*, 304–311. [CrossRef]
7. Navaneethan, U.; Njei, B.; Lourdusamy, V.; Konjeti, R.; Vargo, J.J.; Parsi, M.A. Comparative effectiveness of biliary brush cytology and intraductal biopsy for detection of malignant biliary strictures: A systematic review and meta-analysis. *Gastrointest. Endosc.* **2015**, *81*, 168–176. [CrossRef]
8. Pereira, P.; Vilas-Boas, F.; Peixoto, A.; Andrade, P.; Lopes, J.; Macedo, G. How SpyGlass May Impact Endoscopic Retrograde Cholangiopancreatography Practice and Patient Management. *GE Port. J. Gastroenterol.* **2018**, *25*, 132–137. [CrossRef]
9. Gerges, C.; Beyna, T.; Tang, R.S.Y.; Bahin, F.; Lau, J.Y.W.; van Geenen, E.; Neuhaus, H.; Reddy, D.N.; Ramchandani, M. Digital single-operator peroral cholangioscopy-guided biopsy sampling versus ERCP-guided brushing for indeterminate biliary strictures: A prospective, randomized, multicenter trial (with video). *Gastrointest. Endosc.* **2020**, *91*, 1105–1113. [CrossRef]
10. Jang, S.; Stevens, T.; Kou, L.; Vargo, J.J.; Parsi, M.A. Efficacy of digital single-operator cholangioscopy and factors affecting its accuracy in the evaluation of indeterminate biliary stricture. *Gastrointest. Endosc.* **2020**, *91*, 385–393.e1. [CrossRef]
11. Chen, Y.K.; Pleskow, D.K. SpyGlass single-operator peroral cholangiopancreatoscopy system for the diagnosis and therapy of bile-duct disorders: A clinical feasibility study (with video). *Gastrointest. Endosc.* **2007**, *65*, 832–841. [CrossRef] [PubMed]
12. Robles-Medranda, C.; Valero, M.; Soria-Alcivar, M.; Puga-Tejada, M.; Oleas, R.; Ospina-Arboleda, J.; Alvarado-Escobar, H.; Baquerizo-Burgos, J.; Robles-Jara, C.; Pitanga-Lukashok, H. Reliability and accuracy of a novel classification system using peroral cholangioscopy for the diagnosis of bile duct lesions. *Endoscopy* **2018**, *50*, 1059–1070. [CrossRef] [PubMed]
13. Fukasawa, Y.; Takano, S.; Fukasawa, M.; Maekawa, S.; Kadokura, M.; Shindo, H.; Takahashi, E.; Hirose, S.; Kawakami, S.; Hayakawa, H.; et al. Form-Vessel Classification of Cholangioscopy Findings to Diagnose Biliary Tract Carcinoma's Superficial Spread. *Int. J. Mol. Sci.* **2020**, *21*, 3311. [CrossRef] [PubMed]
14. Sethi, A.; Tyberg, A.; Slivka, A.; Adler, D.; Desai, A.; Sejpal, D.; Pleskow, D.; Bertani, H.; Gan, S.-I.; Shah, R.; et al. Digital Single-operator Cholangioscopy (DSOC) Improves Interobserver Agreement (IOA) and Accuracy for Evaluation of Indeterminate Biliary Strictures: The Monaco Classification. *J. Clin. Gastroenterol.* **2022**, *56*, e94–e97. [CrossRef] [PubMed]
15. Robles-Medranda, C.; Oleas, R.; Sánchez-Carriel, M.; Olmos, J.I.; Alcivar-Casquez, J.; Puga-Tejada, M.; Baquerizo-Burgos, J.; Icaza, I.; Pitanga-Lukashok, H. Vascularity can distinguish neoplastic from non-neoplastic bile duct lesions during digital single-operator cholangioscopy. *Gastrointest. Endosc.* **2021**, *93*, 935–941. [CrossRef]
16. Kahaleh, M.; Gaidhane, M.; Shahid, H.M.; Tyberg, A.; Sarkar, A.; Ardengh, J.C.; Kedia, P.; Andalib, I.; Gress, F.; Sethi, A.; et al. Digital single-operator cholangioscopy interobserver study using a new classification: The Mendoza Classification (with video). *Gastrointest. Endosc.* **2022**, *95*, 319–326. [CrossRef]
17. Sethi, A.; Doukides, T.; Sejpal, D.V.; Pleskow, D.K.; Slivka, A.; Adler, D.G.; Shah, R.J.; Edmundowics, S.A.; Itoi, T.; Petersen, B.T.; et al. Interobserver agreement for single operator choledochoscopy imaging: Can we do better? *Diagn. Ther. Endosc.* **2014**, *2014*, 730731. [CrossRef]
18. Gargeya, R.; Leng, T. Automated Identification of Diabetic Retinopathy Using Deep Learning. *Ophthalmology* **2017**, *124*, 962–969. [CrossRef]
19. Esteva, A.; Kuprel, B.; Novoa, R.A.; Ko, J.; Swetter, S.M.; Blau, H.M.; Thrun, S. Dermatologist-level classification of skin cancer with deep neural networks. *Nature* **2017**, *542*, 115–118. [CrossRef]
20. Hughes, J.W.; Olgin, J.E.; Avram, R.; Abreau, S.A.; Sittler, T.; Radia, K.; Hsia, H.; Walters, T.; Lee, B.; Gonzalez, J.E.; et al. Performance of a Convolutional Neural Network and Explainability Technique for 12-Lead Electrocardiogram Interpretation. *JAMA Cardiol.* **2021**, *6*, 1285–1295. [CrossRef]
21. Ding, Z.; Shi, H.; Zhang, H.; Meng, L.; Fan, M.; Han, C.; Zhang, K.; Ming, F.; Xie, X.; Liu, H.; et al. Gastroenterologist-Level Identification of Small-Bowel Diseases and Normal Variants by Capsule Endoscopy Using a Deep-Learning Model. *Gastroenterology* **2019**, *157*, 1044–1054.e5. [CrossRef]
22. Hassan, C.; Spadaccini, M.; Iannone, A.; Maselli, R.; Jovani, M.; Chandrasekar, V.T.; Antonelli, G.; Yu, H.; Areia, M.; Dinis-Riberio, M.; et al. Performance of artificial intelligence in colonoscopy for adenoma and polyp detection: A systematic review and meta-analysis. *Gastrointest. Endosc.* **2021**, *93*, 77–85.e6. [CrossRef] [PubMed]
23. Xia, J.; Xia, T.; Pan, J.; Gao, F.; Wang, S.; Qian, Y.-Y.; Wang, H.; Zhao, J.; Jiang, X.; Zou, W.-B.; et al. Use of artificial intelligence for detection of gastric lesions by magnetically controlled capsule endoscopy. *Gastrointest. Endosc.* **2021**, *93*, 133–139.e4. [CrossRef] [PubMed]
24. Pedregosa, F.; Varoquaux, G.; Michel, V.; Thirion, B.; Grisel, O.; Blondel, M.; Prettenhofer, P.; Weiss, R.; Dubourg, V.; Vanderplas, J.; et al. Scikit-learn: Machine Learning in Python. *J. Mach. Learn* **2011**, *12*, 2825.
25. Le Berre, C.; Sandborn, W.J.; Aridhi, S.; Devignes, M.-D.; Fournier, L.; Smail-Tabbone, M.; Danese, S.; Peyrin-Biroulet, L. Application of Artificial Intelligence to Gastroenterology and Hepatology. *Gastroenterology* **2020**, *158*, 76–94.e2. [CrossRef] [PubMed]
26. Wen, L.J.; Chen, J.H.; Xu, H.J.; Yu, Q.; Liu, R. Efficacy and Safety of Digital Single-Operator Cholangioscopy in the Diagnosis of Indeterminate Biliary Strictures by Targeted Biopsies: A Systematic Review and Meta-Analysis. *Diagnostics* **2020**, *10*, 666. [CrossRef] [PubMed]
27. Navaneethan, U.; Hasan, M.K.; Kommaraju, K.; Zhu, X.; Hebert-Magee, S.; Hawes, R.H.; Vargo, J.J.; Varadarajulu, S.; Parsi, M.A. Digital, single-operator cholangiopancreatoscopy in the diagnosis and management of pancreatobiliary disorders: A multicenter clinical experience (with video). *Gastrointest. Endosc.* **2016**, *84*, 649–655. [CrossRef]

28. Sun, X.; Zhou, Z.; Tian, J.; Wang, Z.; Huang, Q.; Fan, K.; Mao, Y.; Sun, G.; Yang, Y. Is single-operator peroral cholangioscopy a useful tool for the diagnosis of indeterminate biliary lesion? A systematic review and meta-analysis. *Gastrointest. Endosc.* **2015**, *82*, 79–87. [CrossRef] [PubMed]
29. Njei, B.; McCarty, T.R.; Mohan, B.P.; Fozo, L.; Navaneethan, U. Artificial intelligence in endoscopic imaging for detection of malignant biliary strictures and cholangiocarcinoma: A systematic review. *Ann. Gastroenterol.* **2023**, *36*, 223–230. [CrossRef]
30. Robles-Medranda, C.; Baquerizo-Burgos, J.; Alcivar-Vasquez, J.; Kahaleh, M.; Raijman, I.; Kunda, R.; Puga-Tejada, M.; Egas-Izquierdo, M.; Arevalo-Mora, M.; Mendez, J.C.; et al. Artificial intelligence for diagnosing neoplasia on digital cholangioscopy: Development and multicenter validation of a convolutional neural network model. *Endoscopy* **2023**, *55*, 719–727. [CrossRef]
31. Zhang, X.; Tang, D.; Zhou, J.D.; Ni, M.; Yan, P.; Zhang, Z.; Yu, T.; Zhan, Q.; Shen, Y.; Zhou, L.; et al. A real-time interpretable artificial intelligence model for the cholangioscopic diagnosis of malignant biliary stricture (with videos). *Gastrointest. Endosc.* **2023**, *98*, 199–210.e110. [CrossRef] [PubMed]
32. Jeong, S.; Ge, Y.; Chen, J.; Gao, Q.; Luo, G.; Zheng, B.; Sha, M.; Shen, F.; Cheng, Q.; Sui, C.; et al. Latent Risk Intrahepatic Cholangiocarcinoma Susceptible to Adjuvant Treatment After Resection: A Clinical Deep Learning Approach. *Front. Oncol.* **2020**, *10*, 143. [CrossRef] [PubMed]
33. Ji, G.W.; Zhang, Y.D.; Zhang, H.; Zhu, F.-P.; Wang, K.; Xia, Y.-X.; Zhang, Y.-D.; Jiang, W.-J.; Li, X.-C.; Wang, X.-H. Biliary Tract Cancer at CT: A Radiomics-based Model to Predict Lymph Node Metastasis and Survival Outcomes. *Radiology* **2019**, *290*, 90–98. [CrossRef] [PubMed]
34. Li, Z.; Yuan, L.; Zhang, C.; Sun, J.; Wang, Z.; Wang, Y.; Hao, X.; Gao, F.; Jiang, X. A Novel Prognostic Scoring System of Intrahepatic Cholangiocarcinoma With Machine Learning Basing on Real-World Data. *Front. Oncol.* **2020**, *10*, 576901. [CrossRef] [PubMed]
35. Shao, F.; Huang, Q.; Wang, C.; Qiu, L.; Hu, Y.G.; Zha, S.Y. Artificial Neural Networking Model for the Prediction of Early Occlusion of Bilateral Plastic Stent Placement for Inoperable Hilar Cholangiocarcinoma. *Surg. Laparosc. Endosc. Percutan. Tech.* **2018**, *28*, e54–e58. [CrossRef]
36. Marya, N.B.; Powers, P.D.; Petersen, B.T.; Law, R.; Storm, A.; Abusaleh, R.R.; Rau, P.; Stead, C.; Levy, M.J.; Martin, J.; et al. Identification of patients with malignant biliary strictures using a cholangioscopy-based deep learning artificial intelligence (with video). *Gastrointest. Endosc.* **2023**, *97*, 268–278.e1. [CrossRef]
37. Pereira, P.; Mascarenhas, M.; Ribeiro, T.; Alfonso, J.; Ferreira, J.P.S.; Vilas-Boas, F.; Parente, M.P.L.; Jorge, R.N.; Macedo, G. Automatic detection of tumor vessels in indeterminate biliary strictures in digital single-operator cholangioscopy. *Endosc. Int. Open* **2022**, *10*, E262–E268. [CrossRef]
38. Zhang, J.; Li, Y.; Xiao, W.; Zhang, Z. Non-iterative and Fast Deep Learning: Multilayer Extreme Learning Machines. *J. Frankl. Inst.* **2020**, *357*, 8925–8955. [CrossRef]

Disclaimer/Publisher's Note: The statements, opinions and data contained in all publications are solely those of the individual author(s) and contributor(s) and not of MDPI and/or the editor(s). MDPI and/or the editor(s) disclaim responsibility for any injury to people or property resulting from any ideas, methods, instructions or products referred to in the content.

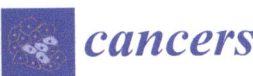

Article

Deep Transfer Learning with Enhanced Feature Fusion for Detection of Abnormalities in X-ray Images

Zaenab Alammar [1,2,*], Laith Alzubaidi [2,3,4,*], Jinglan Zhang [1,2], Yuefeng Li [1], Waail Lafta [5] and Yuantong Gu [3,4]

1. School of Computer Science, Queensland University of Technology, Brisbane, QLD 4000, Australia; jinglan.zhang@qut.edu.au (J.Z.); y2.li@qut.edu.au (Y.L.)
2. Centre for Data Science, Queensland University of Technology, Brisbane, QLD 4000, Australia
3. School of Mechanical, Medical and Process Engineering, Queensland University of Technology, Brisbane, QLD 4000, Australia; yuantong.gu@qut.edu.au
4. ARC Industrial Transformation Training Centre-Joint Biomechanics, Queensland University of Technology, Brisbane, QLD 4000, Australia
5. HMA Group, Brisbane, QLD 4172, Australia; wlafta@hmagroup.com.au
* Correspondence: zaenbkareemabood@hdr.qut.edu.au (Z.A.); l.alzubaidi@qut.edu.au (L.A.)

Simple Summary: In this paper, we introduce a new technique for enhancing medical image diagnosis through transfer learning (TL). The approach addresses the issue of limited labelled images by pre-training deep learning models on similar medical images and then refining them with a small set of annotated medical images. Our method demonstrated excellent results in classifying the humerus and wrist, surpassing previous methods, and showing greater robustness in various experiments. Furthermore, we demonstrate the adaptability of the approach with a CT case, which showed improvements in the results.

Abstract: Medical image classification poses significant challenges in real-world scenarios. One major obstacle is the scarcity of labelled training data, which hampers the performance of image-classification algorithms and generalisation. Gathering sufficient labelled data is often difficult and time-consuming in the medical domain, but deep learning (DL) has shown remarkable performance, although it typically requires a large amount of labelled data to achieve optimal results. Transfer learning (TL) has played a pivotal role in reducing the time, cost, and need for a large number of labelled images. This paper presents a novel TL approach that aims to overcome the limitations and disadvantages of TL that are characteristic of an ImageNet dataset, which belongs to a different domain. Our proposed TL approach involves training DL models on numerous medical images that are similar to the target dataset. These models were then fine-tuned using a small set of annotated medical images to leverage the knowledge gained from the pre-training phase. We specifically focused on medical X-ray imaging scenarios that involve the humerus and wrist from the musculoskeletal radiographs (MURA) dataset. Both of these tasks face significant challenges regarding accurate classification. The models trained with the proposed TL were used to extract features and were subsequently fused to train several machine learning (ML) classifiers. We combined these diverse features to represent various relevant characteristics in a comprehensive way. Through extensive evaluation, our proposed TL and feature-fusion approach using ML classifiers achieved remarkable results. For the classification of the humerus, we achieved an accuracy of 87.85%, an F1-score of 87.63%, and a Cohen's Kappa coefficient of 75.69%. For wrist classification, our approach achieved an accuracy of 85.58%, an F1-score of 82.70%, and a Cohen's Kappa coefficient of 70.46%. The results demonstrated that the models trained using our proposed TL approach outperformed those trained with ImageNet TL. We employed visualisation techniques to further validate these findings, including a gradient-based class activation heat map (Grad-CAM) and locally interpretable model-independent explanations (LIME). These visualisation tools provided additional evidence to support the superior accuracy of models trained with our proposed TL approach compared to those trained with ImageNet TL. Furthermore, our proposed TL approach exhibited greater robustness in various experiments compared to ImageNet TL. Importantly, the proposed TL approach and the feature-fusion technique are not limited to specific tasks. They can be applied to various medical

Citation: Alammar, Z.; Alzubaidi, L.; Zhang, J.; Li, Y.; Lafta, W.; Gu, Y. Deep Transfer Learning with Enhanced Feature Fusion for Detection of Abnormalities in X-ray Images. *Cancers* 2023, 15, 4007. https://doi.org/10.3390/cancers15154007

Academic Editor: Dania Cioni

Received: 16 June 2023
Revised: 29 July 2023
Accepted: 5 August 2023
Published: 7 August 2023

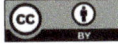

Copyright: © 2023 by the authors. Licensee MDPI, Basel, Switzerland. This article is an open access article distributed under the terms and conditions of the Creative Commons Attribution (CC BY) license (https://creativecommons.org/licenses/by/4.0/).

image applications, thus extending their utility and potential impact. To demonstrate the concept of reusability, a computed tomography (CT) case was adopted. The results obtained from the proposed method showed improvements.

Keywords: musculoskeletal X-ray; deep learning; transfer learning; data scarcity; convolution neural network (CNN); machine learning; feature fusion; gradient-based class activation heat map

1. Introduction

X-ray medical images are widely recognised as powerful tools for identifying abnormalities in bone classification. They provide valuable information on the structure and condition of bones, helping to diagnose and treat various skeletal disorders. However, one of the most-significant challenges faced in the use of artificial intelligence (AI) algorithms for medical image analysis is the scarcity of data available for training and validation [1].

The limited availability of labelled medical images poses a substantial obstacle to the development of accurate and reliable AI models for bone classification tasks. Obtaining a large and diverse medical image dataset is crucial to the effective training of AI algorithms because the performance and generalisation capabilities of AI models can be compromised without sufficient data.

Addressing the issue of data scarcity in medical imaging is essential to unlocking the full potential of AI to improve bone classification accuracy and aid clinical decision-making. Researchers and practitioners continue to explore methods such as active learning (AL), synthetic data generation [2], generative data augmentation [3], transfer learning (TL) [4], and collaboration between institutions to overcome the challenges posed by limited medical image datasets. By expanding the availability and quality of annotated medical images, the performance and robustness of AI algorithms for bone classification will be enhanced and ultimately improve patient care in the medical imaging domain [5].

Despite advancements in medical applications and the progress made in computer vision, detecting abnormalities in the humerus and wrist using X-ray images remains a challenge [6]. The complexity of bone structures, subtle variations in abnormalities, and the inherent limitations of X-ray imaging techniques contribute to this challenge. Ongoing research and development efforts focus on using AI and machine learning (ML) techniques to improve the accuracy and efficiency of humerus and wrist abnormality detection in X-ray images. ML models can be trained on large datasets of annotated X-ray images, which enables them to recognise patterns and detect subtle pathological indicators.

By integrating AI and ML technologies into the field of orthopaedics, medical professionals can benefit from improved accuracy and efficiency when diagnosing and treating patients with bone conditions. Deep learning (DL) is a branch of AI techniques that has demonstrated exceptional abilities in accurately, reliably, and rapidly classifying medical images into binary and multiclass categories [7,8]. DL has become the gold standard in medical image analysis and has demonstrated remarkable performance in various areas, such as radiology [9,10], dermatology [11], pathology [12], and ophthalmology [13,14]. These applications, which span different medical fields, are based on human experience, thus making DL a valuable tool in a competitive domain.

The requirement for large amounts of labelled data is a significant challenge to the development of high-performing DL models. However, the scarcity and imbalance of medical image datasets pose significant challenges due to the cost effectiveness and time consumption associated with DL approaches. Despite these challenges, DL models have consistently demonstrated impressive performance in classifying medical images. Krizhevsky et al. [15] introduced a model based on a convolutional neural network (CNN) architecture that represented a significant milestone in the history of DL and computer vision. Their developing work demonstrated the potential of deep CNNs in image-classification tasks, thus setting new standards for accuracy and inspiring further research and innovation in the

ImageNet Large Scale Visual Recognition Challenge (ILSVRC), a critical image classification competition. Several studies have successfully used TL techniques in DL models to address data scarcity. TL involves using models that were pre-trained on large-scale datasets and fine-tuning them on target medical image datasets [16]. This approach has been shown to be effective in improving the performance of DL models in various studies [1]. For example, Fang et al. [17] used fine-tuning and feature augmentation methods and an area under the curve (AUC) of 0.73. However, unbalanced data remain a limitation in certain studies [18]. Musculoskeletal radiographs (MURA) is a dataset designed specifically for musculoskeletal medical imaging, as it comprises a large collection of radiographs (X-rays). The dataset covers a diverse set of musculoskeletal abnormalities, as well as normal cases, which makes it a valuable resource for training and evaluating medical image classifiers [19]. The use of TL techniques for medical image classification has increased significantly, and this trend highlights the growing recognition of TL as a valuable strategy for handling data scarcity and improving the performance of DL models in the medical field.

CNNs have been widely used to classify input data as various states of disease [20]. CNNs' deep architecture feedforward neural networks serve as the basis for many deep neural network models (DNN) in the medical field [20]. In addition to CNNs, other types of neural networks have also been used, such as recurrent neural networks (RNNs) with variations such as long short-term memory (LSTM), transformers, and generative adversarial networks (GANs) [21]. CNNs have proven to be particularly effective for image-processing and -classification tasks. One of their key strengths lies in their ability to extract meaningful patterns and characteristics from images regardless of scaling, mirroring, rotation, or translation [22]. This property makes CNNs highly suitable for medical image analysis, where the accurate identification and classification of image characteristics are crucial for diagnosis and treatment.

Furthermore, it should be noted that most studies that focus on humerus and wrist abnormalities do not thoroughly evaluate the "black box" explanation [23]. However, the lack of model explainability associated with black box methods is considered a significant obstacle to clinical adoption and user confidence [24]. To identify biases and ensure the reliability of DL applications, it is essential to explain the decision-making processes of the models. The use of TL is specifically recommended to address the issue of data scarcity and inconsistency in the medical field. TL leverages pre-trained DL models by using source datasets and fine-tuning them for target tasks. TL has had a positive impact on the medical field, especially in scenarios where limited data are available. Given the challenges of gathering medical imaging data, TL has become a crucial tool in medical image analysis. The ImageNet Large Scale Visual Recognition Challenge (ILSVRC-2012) competition dataset is widely recognised and widely used to improve the performance of various image-processing tasks, including classification, segmentation, and detection [25–27]. Although ImageNet has improved model performance, it is essential to note that medical images differ significantly from the natural images represented in ImageNet. These differences encompass various aspects, such as shape, colour, resolution, and dimensionality.

Models pre-trained on ImageNet are limited in terms of performance enhancement when dealing with medical images due to domain mismatch. Several authors have explained how TL using the same domain improved the performance of DL models in medical imaging applications [16,28,29].

Alternatively, the fusion technique could be used as an effective way to merge the features extracted by various CNN models for further enhancement. However, supporting the models' results using the appropriate tools is necessary in order to trust the DL outcome [30].

The trade-off lies in the ability of DL models to leverage large amounts of data and learn complex patterns, whereas traditional techniques may have been more suitable for cases with limited data availability [31].

This paper aims to address the problem of data scarcity and the mismatch features of TL. Furthermore, it also addresses feature generalisation in training ML classifiers. Therefore, in this paper:

1. We propose a new TL approach to address the issue of data scarcity and the drawbacks of previous TL methods in medical imaging applications.
2. An improved feature fusion is proposed to increase trust in the final decision.
3. We employed two pre-trained ImageNet models for experimenting with two X-ray tasks to detect abnormalities in the humerus and wrist.
4. We applied a feature fusion strategy to train multiple ML classifiers in two different training scenarios.
5. We achieved an accuracy of 87.85%, an F1-score of 87.63%, and a Cohen's Kappa coefficient of 75.69% in humerus classification. For wrist classification, our approach achieved an accuracy of 85.58%, an F1-score of 82.70%, and a Cohen's Kappa coefficient of 70.46%.
6. We briefly review the most-recent DL techniques from the MURA dataset.
7. We explain how the decision was made to adopt two visualisation tools, i.e., gradient-weighted class activation mapping (Grad-CAM) and local printable model-agnostic explanations (LIME), to verify the robustness of the proposed method.
8. We show that the proposed TL approach and feature-fusion technique can be applied to various medical image applications, thus expanding their utility and potential impact, as demonstrated by adopting a computed tomography (CT) case that showed significant improvements in the results.

2. Related Work

This section provides an overview of the latest techniques used in the field. One such technique is the use of CNNs, which have demonstrated remarkable success in computer vision tasks and have become crucial for image classification. As mentioned above, the availability of large datasets and the time-consuming nature of training classifiers pose significant challenges to achieving optimal training results. Various techniques have been proposed to increase the size of the datasets, and one such strategy is active learning (AL). AL involves iteratively selecting the most-informative samples from an unlabelled dataset for annotation and model training. The primary goal of AL is to maximise the model's performance while minimising the amount of labelled data required for training. This is particularly beneficial in scenarios where obtaining labelled data can be costly or time-consuming. The AL process relies on initially training the model on a small labelled dataset and then using a query strategy to determine which unlabelled samples should be selected for labelling. The query strategy is crucial, as it selects samples based on their potential impact on the model's performance. There are several common query strategies used, including uncertainty sampling, query-by-committee, and information-density-based methods. After selecting and labelling these informative samples, the samples are incorporated into the training set to update the model using the newly labelled data. The training process for AL is often repeated over time until the model reaches a desired performance level or satisfies other specific criteria relevant to the desired application. This iterative approach helps the model learn from diverse and informative examples, which gradually improves its performance with fewer labelled samples. A key limitation of AL algorithms is that they are based on labelling one sample at a time. This means that, after each sample is labelled, the model needs to be retrained, which can be computationally expensive and time-consuming [32]. Researchers have thus been working on optimising this process to reduce the retraining burden.

For example, Wen et al. [33] conducted a study on using AL for nucleus segmentation in pathology images in which they investigated how AL performance improves for three different algorithm families: support vector machines (SVMs), random forest (RF), and CNNs. By employing AL, the researchers aimed to enhance the efficiency and accuracy of nucleus segmentation in medical imaging. Moreover, synthetic data generation is a powerful technique used to address data scarcity or privacy concerns by creating additional data artificially. In various domains, obtaining a sufficient amount of labelled data to train ML models can be challenging. Synthetic data generation offers a solution by generating new data points that are similar to the existing data, but are not direct replicas, thus expanding the dataset [3]. GANs have emerged as highly successful and versatile approaches that can find applications across various domains, including image generation, text generation, and video synthesis. GANs possess the remarkable ability to generate high-quality, diverse, and realistic synthetic data, making them invaluable for a wide range of tasks, including data augmentation, data synthesis, and creative applications [34]. Adar et al. [35] demonstrated the successful application of GANs for enhancing the classification performance for liver lesion classification by employing data augmentation techniques. In their study, conducted in 2018, the authors used GANs to increase the amount and diversity of training data, specifically for liver lesion classification. The authors observed a significant improvement in sensitivity and specificity compared to using traditional data-augmentation methods. Specifically, the classification performance increased from 78.6% sensitivity and 88.4% specificity (when using traditional enhancements) to 85.7% sensitivity and 92.4% specificity (when using GAN-generated data). This improvement can be attributed to the GAN's ability to provide a more-diverse and -representative training dataset, allowing the classifier to better generalise and make more-accurate predictions on real-world liver lesion data.

Furthermore, Yi et al. [36] extensively explored and discussed the application of GAN image synthesis in various critical medical imaging domains. They highlighted the significant impact of GANs on improving medical image generation, analysis, and diagnostics across a range of applications. In the domain of brain magnetic resonance imaging (MRI), GANs have proven to be particularly valuable. Calimeri et al. [37] and Bermudez et al. [38] successfully used GAN-based image synthesis to generate realistic brain MRI scans. This synthetic data augmentation has led to the improved training of brain image analysis models and better performance in tasks such as segmentation and disease classification. For lung cancer diagnostics, Chuquicusma et al. [39] demonstrated the effectiveness of GANs in generating synthetic lung nodules and lesions. This data synthesis enabled the development and validation of robust and accurate lung-cancer-detection models, even when dealing with limited real-world data. High-resolution skin imaging is another domain where GANs have shown promise. Baur et al. [40] used GANs to synthesise high-resolution melanoma images. This approach enhanced the quality and diversity of the dataset used for training skin-cancer-detection models, leading to improved diagnostic accuracy and the early detection of skin cancer. While data augmentation is a powerful tool for improving model performance, its lack of interpretability can be a concern, especially in sensitive or critical applications. Ensuring transparency and explainability is essential for building trust and confidence in AI models, enabling users to comprehend why certain augmentations lead to improved performance. By incorporating human-understandable augmentation strategies and leveraging model interpretability techniques, researchers and practitioners can strike a balance between performance enhancement and interpretability, thereby making AI systems more trustworthy and responsible [41].

Additionally, Tahmina et al. [42] applied data augmentation in their study to detect humerus fractures. They used preprocessed images to increase the quality of the dataset, and the performance of their study was 78%.

Despite the promise of data augmentation, there are challenges that must be considered. Selecting appropriate augmentation techniques and parameters requires careful consideration. In addition, achieving the correct balance between augmenting and maintaining the integrity of the medical data is crucial to ensuring that the synthetic examples remain consistent with the real-world distribution of medical images. In this context, TL and pre-training are two alternative strategies for learning the low-level properties in CNNs. TL has proven to be an effective technique to train CNNs with limited data, thus improving the performance of DL models. TL enables one to leverage the knowledge and features learned from pre-existing models and apply them to new tasks or domains, thus reducing the need for extensive data collection and training time. By capitalising on pre-trained models, TL enables the efficient and effective training of CNNs even with smaller datasets. CNNs have been effectively trained using TL techniques in which the weights of pre-trained CNNs are used to classify other target images [20]. TL can be broadly categorised into two types: fine-tuned TL and feature extraction TL. The feature extraction TL approach employs a well-trained CNN model that was trained on a large dataset. The convolutional layers of the pre-trained model are frozen, whereas the fully connected layers are discarded. The frozen convolutional layers act as fixed feature extractors, which capture meaningful representations from the input images. These extracted features are then fed into a new classifier, which can be implemented using new fully connected layers or a supervised ML approach. During this type of TL, only the parameters of the new classifier are trained using the pre-learned features of the pre-trained CNN model [43].

This approach transfers knowledge from the pre-trained CNN model, which has learned rich representations from a large dataset, to the new medical task at hand. By using the extracted features and training only the classifier, feature-extracting TL enables efficient training with limited data, thus reducing the need for extensive computational resources and training time.

In contrast, the fine-tuning TL approach involves replacing the classifier layers while using the pre-trained CNN model that was trained on a large dataset as a base. In this approach, the convolutional and classifier layers are fine-tuned during the training process. The weights of the convolutional layers are initialised with the pre-trained weights from the CNN model, while the classifier layers start with random weights. The entire network is trained through this training process, allowing it to adapt and learn task-specific representations [44].

The fine-tuning TL approach is beneficial when the target task requires more-specialised knowledge and the available target dataset is more extensive. The model can learn task-specific features and improve its performance by updating the weights of the convolutional and classifier layers.

Both feature-extracting TL and fine-tuning TL have their advantages and are, thus, used based on the specific requirements of the task at hand. Feature-extracting TL is particularly useful when limited training data are available, as it leverages the pre-trained model's learned features. Fine-tuning TL, however, can enhance performance by allowing the model to learn task-specific representations by updating both the convolutional and classifier layers. For this reason, this study used the fine-tuning TL type.

Various studies applied DL models to detect abnormalities in X-ray images, such as Ortiz et al. [45], who investigated three AI models to detect pneumonia in chest X-ray images; the authors used the feature-extraction technique with three different ML classifiers, and the accuracy of this study was 83.00% and with an 89% sensitivity for radiomics, an accuracy of 89.9% with a 93.6% sensitivity for fractal dimension, and 91.3% accuracy with a 90.5% sensitivity for superpixel-based histon. Moreover, Canayaz et al. [46] implemented feature fusion by combining AlexNet and VGG19 models to classify COVID-19, pneumonia, and normal X-ray images; the authors' approach achieved 99.38% accuracy. In addition, Rajinikanth et al. [47] used InceptionV3, which was pre-trained, to detect pneumonia in chest X-ray images. The authors used deep feature extraction and feature reduction with the Firefly Algorithm and multi-class classification using five-fold cross-validation; the results of the K-nearest neighbour (KNN) classifier demonstrated an accuracy of 85.18%. Furthermore, Rajinikanth et al. [48] also applied one-fold and two-fold training by using UNet lung section segmentation.

Indeed, DL models have been implemented in various studies to improve the detection of abnormalities in musculoskeletal images. Rajpurkar et al. [19] conducted a study using a dataset called MURA, consisting of 40,005 musculoskeletal images. Their research employed a DenseNet169 CNN architecture, as described in Huang et al. [49], whereby each layer was linked to all other layers in a feedforward fashion, thus achieving a deep network design. The model classified the images as abnormal if the prediction probability was greater than 0.5. The performance of the model was evaluated using two metrics: sensitivity and specificity. The sensitivity, which measures the ability of the model to identify true positives correctly, was 81.5%. The specificity, which measures the model's ability to identify true negatives correctly, was 88.7%. These metrics indicate the model's ability to detect normal and abnormal cases accurately. The model's overall performance was also assessed using the area under the receiver operator characteristic (AUROC) metric, which considers the trade-off between sensitivity and specificity. The model achieved an AUROC of 92.9%, indicating its solid discriminative power. When diagnosing abnormalities in fingers and wrists, the model's performance was roughly equivalent to that of the best radiologists. Despite the model's agreement with the gold standard being similar to that of other radiologists, it was still relatively low. However, when diagnosing abnormalities in elbows, forearms, hands, humerus, and shoulders, the model's performance was worse than that of the best radiologists [19].

To investigate this, Chada [50] conducted a study to evaluate the performance of three state-of-the-art CNN architectures, namely DenseNet169, DenseNet201, and InceptionResNetV2, on the MURA dataset. The researchers fine-tuned these CNN models using the Adam optimiser with a learning rate of 0.001. The evaluation was performed separately for humerus and finger images.

For the humerus task, the best performance was observed with the DenseNet201 model, which achieved a Cohen's Kappa score of 76.4%. This indicated a substantial agreement between the predictions of the model and the ground-truth labels. For the images of fingers, however, the InceptionResNetV2 model demonstrated the best performance, obtaining a Cohen's Kappa score (which assesses the agreement between the model's predictions and the ground-truth beyond chance) of 55.5%. These results highlight the effectiveness of these CNN architectures in detecting abnormalities in musculoskeletal images, with performance variations depending on the specific anatomical areas. However, the performance of finger X-rays was less promising, undoubtedly due to the limitations of high inter-radiologist variation.

Another study focused on classifying proximal humerus fractures using the Neer classification system [51]. The researchers used a pre-trained ResNet-152 classifier that was fine-tuned for the specific task of classifying fractures. This approach leveraged the pre-trained weights of the ResNet-152 model and trained the classifier layers on the target dataset. Using this TL technique, the model accurately classified 86% of the proximal humerus fractures according to the Neer classification system. Despite the fact that the Neer classification is the most-regularly used technique for proximal humerus fracture classification, the reliability of this study needs to improve. The author in [51] assessed the diagnostic performance of CNNs with a cropped single-shoulder X-ray image, but this might not be applicable to the relative clinical scenario.

Furthermore, Lindsey et al. [52] investigated the detection of wrist fractures, comparing the performance of radiologists with and without the assistance of CNN models. The study aimed to assess how the use of CNN models affected radiologists' diagnostic capabilities. The results indicated a marked increase in radiological performance when aided by CNN models, highlighting the potential of DL models as supportive tools in the field of fracture detection. However, the study had a number of drawbacks, such as the fact that the experiment was a review of the data performed through the web interface that simulated an image archiving and communication system (PACS) used by medical professionals for medical imaging. Furthermore, the accuracy of the physicians' and the model's diagnoses in this study was restricted to the determination of what is visible inside a radiograph. Finally, the diagnosed condition's improvement or deterioration was influenced by factors other than DL accuracy in diagnosis.

Saif et al. [53] proposed a capsule-network-based approach to classify abnormalities in the musculoskeletal system. They conducted experiments by training their network on images of different sizes, specifically images of 64×64, 128×128, and 224×224 px. The goal was to determine the optimal image size to achieve an accurate classification, and the results indicated that, when using 224 × 224 px images, the network achieved the highest training accuracy (96%) for wrist radiography images. However, it is possible that the network's performance in some studies was influenced by overfitting, a situation where the model becomes excessively tailored to the training data, which leads to the poor generalisation for unseen data.

However, in 2019, Varma et al. [54] introduced the MURA dataset, which included a private dataset of 93,455 lower-extremity radiographs with images of the foot, ankle, knee, and hip. This dataset was explicitly curated for abnormality detection using less-adequate extremity radiographs. To evaluate the performance of different CNN architectures, Varma et al. trained ResNet-50, DenseNet-161, and ResNet-101 on a subset of their private dataset. Despite the structural differences between these architectures, the authors found that performance did not vary significantly. However, the authors then proposed a comparison explicitly focused on the DenseNet-161 architecture, which was trained on both the ImageNet and MURA datasets, to assess the impact of TL on model performance. This comparison aimed to investigate the effect of TL, where a CNN model is initially pre-trained on a large-scale dataset (such as ImageNet) and then fine-tuned on a specific task or domain (in this case, the MURA dataset). Using pre-trained weights and pre-learned representations from the large-scale dataset, TL can potentially improve the performance of CNN models for the target task. However, the limitation of this study comes from the fact that it reviewed data with datasets from a single institution; thus, the performance of the authors' models may differ in the real world when different images are used.

Furthermore, Kandel et al. [55] conducted a study using the MURA dataset to examine the performance of six CNN architectures, namely, VGG, Xception, ResNet, GoogLeNet, InceptionResNet, and DenseNet, to detect bone abnormalities. They compared models trained from scratch with pre-trained models using ImageNet and then fine-tuned them on the MURA dataset. The study's results highlighted that TL has the potential to enhance model performance while reducing the susceptibility to overfitting. Among the five state-of-the-art CNNs evaluated for the MURA dataset, the humerus datasets achieved the highest precision (81.66%). Although the authors used the TL approach, the training-from-scratch approach's poor performance could have been due to the number of images in the dataset, as well as the hyperparameter selection. The CNNs considered are distinguished by their incorporation of a significant number of trainable parameters (such as weights), and the number of images used to train these networks is insufficient to develop an effective model. Hyperparameters indicate the significance of the learning rate. Although the authors used a lower value of the learning rate in the fine-tuning technique to avoid significantly modifying the original weights of the designs, the training-from-scratch strategy may demand a higher value of the learning rate.

Feature fusion of DL techniques also was implemented by Bhan et al. [56] to classify fracture or non-fracture in the MURA dataset; the five pre-trained models were DenseNet-169, MobileNetV2 ResNet-50, ResNeXt-50 and VGG16, and then, these pre-trained models were combined in this study. The results of the feature-fusion approach were that the humerus achieved an 87.85% accuracy and a 75.72% Cohen's Kappa, while the accuracy was 83.13% and a 66.25% Cohen's Kappa for the shoulder. In the same study, the performance of the wrist classification was 86.65% accuracy and a 72.59% Cohen's Kappa.

This literature review focused on the significant challenge caused by the limited availability of annotated data in the medical domain. The scarcity of annotated medical datasets prevents the full potential and effectiveness of DL algorithms. This challenge has motivated the main objective of this article, which was to explore strategies that can achieve greater performance with minimal data in the field of medical DL.

3. Materials and Methods

3.1. Dataset

The dataset used in this study is called MURA. It consists of X-ray images that represent seven different skeletal bones, namely the elbow, finger, forearm, hand, humerus, shoulder, and wrist. Each bone category is divided into two subclasses: positive (abnormal) and negative (standard). In total, the dataset contains 40,561 images. The dataset was partitioned into separate training and test sets, the details of which are presented in Table 1 below [19].

Table 1. Number of images in the MURA dataset.

Class	Training		Testing	
-	Negative	Positive	Negative	Positive
Elbow	2925	2006	234	230
Finger	3138	1968	214	247
Hand	4059	1484	271	189
Humerus	673	599	148	140
Forearm	1164	661	150	151
Shoulder	4211	4168	285	278
Wrist	5765	3987	364	295

Two main categories were created from the dataset:

1. Target dataset: As shown in Figure 1, the categories of the humerus and wrist were specifically chosen as the target datasets for analysis and classification. These categories represent anatomical regions within the musculoskeletal system that are particularly interesting for medical image processing.
2. Source of TL: The source of TL is an important consideration in DL applications. In the context of TL, the source refers to the pre-trained models or datasets that are used as a starting point for training a new model on a target dataset. The rest of the MURA dataset was used as a source of TL, including the elbow, finger, forearm, hand and shoulder.

3.2. Proposed TL Technique

A large dataset was used in the TL stage to leverage the knowledge gained from this dataset and apply it to a smaller target dataset. One commonly used source for TL is pre-trained models that were trained on the ImageNet dataset. The ImageNet dataset comprises a vast collection of images categorised into 1000 classes, including various natural objects, people, plants, and animals. The pre-trained models derived from the ImageNet dataset have been widely used in multiple applications to address the challenge of limited data availability [57]. These models have demonstrated remarkable performance in object-detection and agriculture tasks, where the dataset encompasses diverse visual characteristics and requires robust feature-extraction capabilities. When the target task dataset shares relevant features with the ImageNet dataset, TL that uses pre-trained models becomes particularly valuable. However, it is essential to note that the ImageNet dataset consists primarily of colour images, which may not directly enhance the functionality of grayscale medical imaging. This distinction between colour and grayscale images highlights the need for careful consideration and customisation when applying TL techniques to medical imaging tasks, which often involve specific imaging modalities and grayscale representations [16].

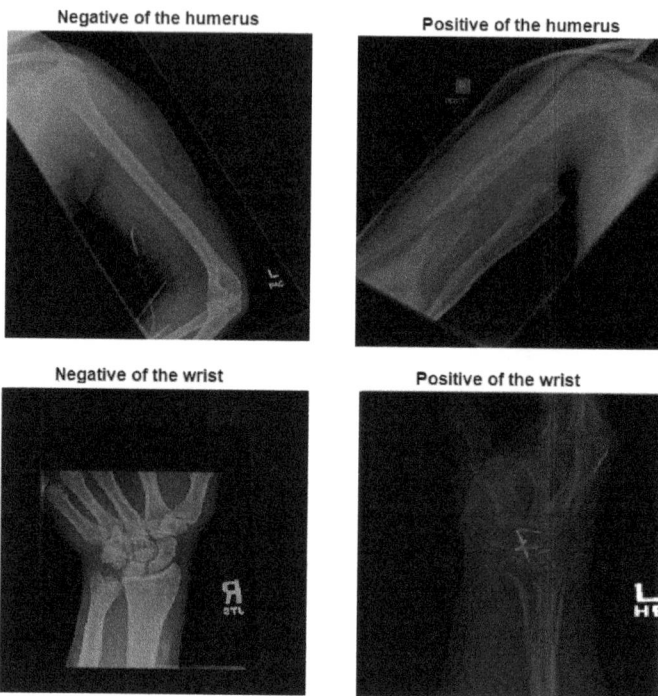

Figure 1. Four samples of the two tasks: the humerus and the wrist.

This work presents a new approach to TL and is called TL domain adaptation. This approach aims to address the challenge of limited annotated data and improve the performance of pre-trained ImageNet models in specific domains. The proposed method involves updating the features of the pre-trained models by incorporating in-domain images (source of TL) before fine-tuning the models on the target dataset (see Figure 2). This approach aims to leverage the knowledge and features learned from a wide range of musculoskeletal images to enhance the performance of the models. By incorporating various classes from the MURA dataset, the models can capture a greater understanding of musculoskeletal abnormalities and potentially generalise better to the target tasks of humerus and wrist abnormalities. One notable advantage of using the same image modality (X-ray) and having a common goal of detecting abnormalities across the MURA dataset and the humerus/wrist tasks is the similarities in the image characteristics and diagnostic objectives. These similarities enable a more-effective transfer of knowledge and features from TL source classes to the target humerus and wrist tasks. They also allow the models to capture relevant patterns, structures, and consistent abnormalities in different musculoskeletal areas. This approach improves the ability of the models to extract meaningful features and make predictions for abnormalities of the humerus and wrist, thereby improving performance and diagnostic precision. Figure 2 shows the workflow of the proposed method, which is as follows:

1. Step 1: Train the models on the source of TL (all MURA classes, except the target dataset).
2. Step 2: Load the pre-trained models.
3. Step 3: Replace the final layers (fully connected layer and classification layer).
4. Step 4: Train the model on the target (humerus or wrist) by freezing 70% of the layer of the model, and then, train the rest.
5. Step 5: Predict and assess the performance of the trained model in the target's test images (humerus or wrist).

6. Step 6: Deploy the results.

This proposed TL eliminates the need for a large number of annotated images specific to the target task. This is beneficial when labelled data are scarce for the target task because valuable time and resources are saved. This study used two pre-trained models, both with and without the proposed TL approach. These models were chosen based on their strong performance on the ImageNet dataset, a benchmark for various computer vision tasks. The selection of diverse models allows for a comprehensive investigation of the effectiveness of the proposed TL technique. Table 2 presents the key characteristics of the selected models, including their sizes, depths, and image input sizes. By considering models with different architectures and specifications, this study aimed to assess the impact of TL in a variety of model configurations. This diversity allows a thorough evaluation of the effectiveness of the proposed TL technique and its potential application in various CNN models.

The limitation of this proposed TL is its need for a source of training, which requires time and computational resources. However, the ImageNet (S1) models have already been trained.

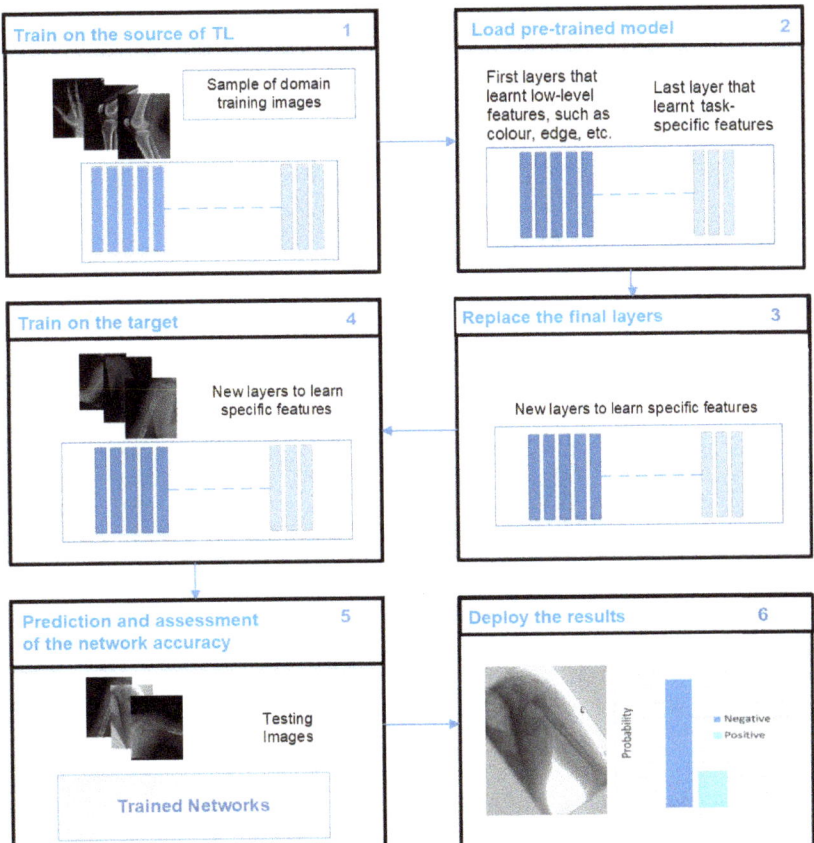

Figure 2. The proposed TL solution.

Table 2. Selected models of pre-trained deep neural networks.

Model	Input Size	Parameters 10^6	Depth
InceptionResNetV2	299 × 299 × 3	55.9	164
Xception	299 × 299 × 3	22.9	71

3.3. Training Scenarios

Three groups were created from the dataset: training, validation, and testing. The training scenarios used in this study were calculated and conducted in the following ways (see Figure 3):

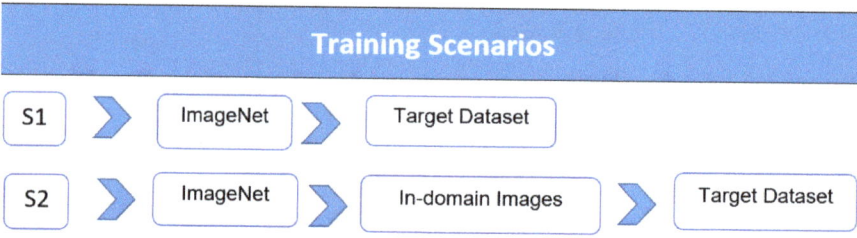

Figure 3. The two training scenarios.

1. Scenario 1 (S1): TL from the ImageNet dataset was used to train the target dataset in the DL models.
2. Scenario 2 (S2): ImageNet (S1) models were trained with the TL source collection (in-domain images), and then, the models were trained on the target dataset. The training parameters included Adam optimisation, a minibatch size of 15, a maximum of 100 epochs, a shuffle for each epoch, and a starting learning rate of 0.001. An Intel (R) Core i7/32 GB/1 TB/Nvidia RTX A3000 12 GB were the GPU specifications used in the experiment. Matlab 2022a was used for the tests.

3.4. Deep Feature Fusion

The feature-fusion approach is used to improve overall performance by combining features from different DL models. It aims to capture and combine complementary information from multiple models to improve the representation of the features.

The first layers of each model learn basic features, such as colours, edges, and shapes, while the last layers learn all the features of the object. Therefore, we extracted the features from the last layers. Moreover, each DL model has its own structure and different filter sizes to learn the features, and combining them provides a better representation of the features. The two deep CNNs were trained and evaluated, and once trained, the models extracted the relevant features from the input data. These extracted features were then used to train the ML classifiers. In this process, the features extracted from both CNN models were combined into a single feature space. ML classifiers were trained to categorise and classify the abnormalities of the humerus or effectively classify the abnormalities of the humerus. The combination of the features of the two models allows for a more-comprehensive representation of the underlying patterns and characteristics present in the data.

The combination of the features of multiple models offers several advantages in ML classifiers. Combining the features extracted from various models makes a more-diverse and -comprehensive set of information available for classifiers to learn from. This approach allows ML classifiers to take advantage of the strengths and unique characteristics of each CNN model, resulting in a more-holistic understanding of the target tasks. The combination of trained models and the pooling of their features provides the final ML classifiers with the collective knowledge and discriminative power acquired from each model. This integration of features from multiple sources aims to improve the accuracy and robustness of the classification process. By considering a wider range of characteristics and capturing different aspects of the input data, classifiers can better capture the underlying patterns and nuances of abnormalities of the humerus and wrist.

This study adopted various ML classifiers to use fused features. These classifiers included linear discriminant analysis, neural networks, coarse KNN, cubic SVM, the boosted tree, and the coarse tree. By applying multiple classifiers, each with its own strengths and characteristics, this study explored different approaches and identified the most-effective classifier for the given task, as shown in Figure 4.

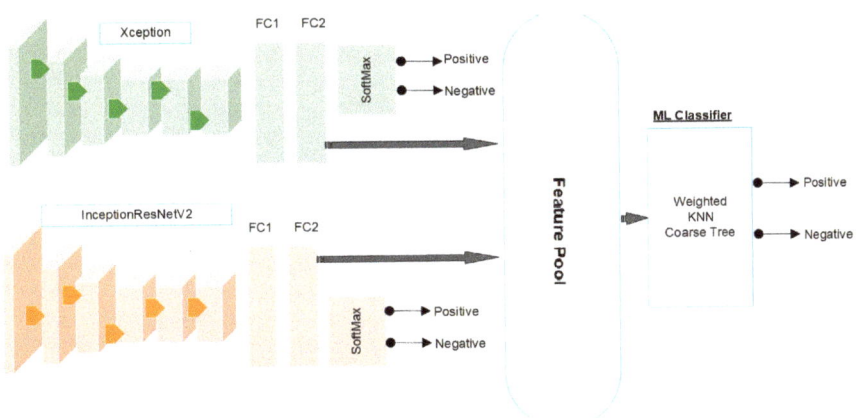

Figure 4. The feature-fusion process.

3.5. Visualisation Techniques for Explainable Deep Learning Models

DL models are often referred to as "black boxes" due to the challenge of understanding why a model makes specific decisions. Gaining insight into their decision-making processes is essential to ensure confidence in DL models throughout the research and implementation stages. The methodologies used in this study have a wide range of applications, including model selection, debugging, learning, and bias assessment. One technique used to shed light on the predictions made by a network trained on image data is the use of test images, as depicted in Figure 5. These test images are used to clarify and understand the model predictions, and they also ensure that the models focus on the relevant regions of interest (ROIs) when making decisions. The gradient-weighted class activation mapping (Grad-CAM) visualisation technique, as well as local interpretable model-agnostic explanations (LIME) are interpretability techniques that explain the predictions of any ML model in an interpretable and understandable manner. Unlike Grad-CAM, however, which focuses on visualising important image regions, LIME can be applied to any input data type, including text and tabular data.

These techniques take advantage of the gradient by highlighting areas of the image that contribute significantly to the decision-making process of the model. The heat map is generated by computing the gradients of the target class score with respect to the feature maps in the final layer of the CNN.

Gradients involve taking partial derivatives of the loss function with respect to each parameter in the network. By iteratively computing and applying the gradients to update the parameters, the model learns to adjust its predictions and improve its performance on the given task. Gradients are then globally averaged together to obtain the importance weights for each feature map. A heat map is created by linearly combining the feature maps with their corresponding weights, which indicate the regions of the image that strongly influence the classification decision [58].

The visualisation techniques such as Grad-CAM and LIME aim to address the "black box" nature of DL models and enhance their interpretability and transparency. These techniques provide valuable information on the features of the image that the model considers crucial for decision-making. By analysing and understanding these critical regions, researchers can gain a deeper understanding of the model's reasoning process and validate that the regions of influence align with the expectations. This helps to build confidence in the prediction of the model, especially in medical-image-analysis and diagnostic tasks.

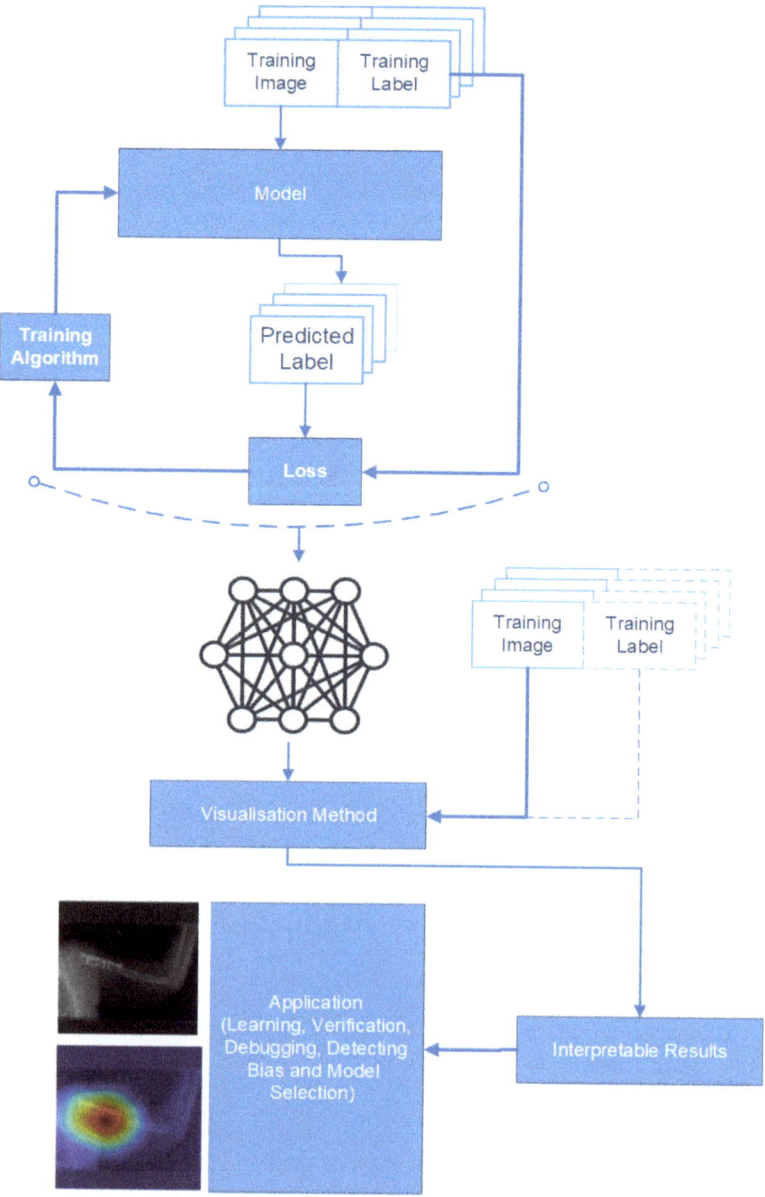

Figure 5. Workflow of visualisation techniques.

4. Experimental Evaluation

This section focuses on the experimental assessment of the proposed TL method (S2) to detect any abnormalities in the humerus and wrist.

4.1. Evaluation Metrics

All models were evaluated based on various training scenarios, which used a comprehensive set of evaluation metrics, including accuracy, specificity, recall, precision, the F1-score, and Cohen's Kappa. These metrics provide a comprehensive assessment of the model's performance and ability to classify instances accurately. The evaluation metrics were calculated based on the values of the true negatives (TNs), true positives (TPs), false negatives (FNs), and false positives (FPs). The TN and TP values represent the correct classification of negative and positive examples, respectively, while the FP and FN values represent the incorrect classification of positive and negative examples, respectively.

These evaluation metrics collectively provide a comprehensive understanding of the performance of the model, thereby allowing an in-depth analysis of its strengths and weaknesses. By examining these metrics, researchers can assess the model's capability to classify instances accurately and make informed decisions about its effectiveness in solving the target tasks. Each evaluation metric is presented as follows:

$$\text{Accuracy} = \frac{TP + TN}{TP + TN + FP + FN} \tag{1}$$

$$\text{Recall} = \frac{\sum \frac{TP}{TP+FP}}{num - classes} \tag{2}$$

$$\text{Specificity} = \frac{TN}{FP + TN} \tag{3}$$

$$\text{Precision} = \frac{TP}{TP + FP} \tag{4}$$

$$F1 - score = 2 \times \frac{Precision * Recall}{Precision + Recall} \tag{5}$$

Cohen's Kappa equation:

$$Ko = \frac{TP + TN}{TP + TN + FP + FN} \tag{6}$$

$$Kpositive = \frac{(TP + FP)(TP + FN)}{(TP + TN + FP + FN)^2} \tag{7}$$

$$Knegative = \frac{(FN + TN)(FP + TN)}{(TP + TN + FP + FN)^2} \tag{8}$$

$$Ke = Kpositive + Knegative \tag{9}$$

Cohen's Kappa score=

$$\frac{Ko - Ke}{1 - Ke} \tag{10}$$

4.2. Experimental Evaluation of End-to-End DL Models

Two DL models were tested with the help of two training scenarios, as shown in Tables 3 and 4.

Table 3. The results of the DL models on the test set of the MURA dataset for the humerus task on Xception and InceptionResNetV2.

Evaluation Metric (%)	Xception	
-	S1	S2
Accuracy	69.10	84.72
Recall	64.29	89.29
Precision	69.77	81.17
Specificity	73.65	80.41
F1-score	66.91	85.03
Cohen's Kappa	38.02	69.83
	InceptionResNetV2	
Accuracy	80.21	86.11
Recall	74.29	85.00
Precision	83.81	86.23
Specificity	85.81	87.16
F1-score	78.49	85.61
Cohen's Kappa	60.27	72.20

Table 4. The results of the DL models on the test set of the MURA dataset for the wrist task on Xception and InceptionResNetV2.

Evaluation Metric (%)	Xception	
-	S1	S2
Accuracy	69.10	84.07
Recall	64.29	73.56
Precision	69.77	88.93
Specificity	73.65	92.58
F1-score	66.91	80.52
Cohen's Kappa	38.02	68.11
	InceptionResNetV2	
Accuracy	80.21	82.85
Recall	74.29	67.80
Precision	83.81	91.74
Specificity	85.81	95.05
F1-score	78.49	77.97
Cohen's Kappa	60.27	64.45

1. Humerus task: As shown in Figures 6 and 7, the confusion matrix was initially calculated for all training cases. The assessment metrics were derived from the confusion matrix values, which provided a detailed breakdown of the model classifications. The data demonstrated the performance of the different scenarios, with S2 achieving the best overall results. S2 obtained an accuracy of 84.72%, and the recall, also known as the true positive rate, was 89.29%. The precision, which measures the accuracy of positive predictions, was 81.17%, while the specificity, which represents the true negative rate, was 80.41%. The F1-score, which balances precision and recall, was 85.03%, providing an overall measure of the performance of the model, and Cohen's Kappa,

which assesses the agreement between the model predictions and the ground-truth beyond chance, was 69.83% with the Xception DL model. S2 with the InceptionresNetV2 model had an accuracy of 86.11%, a recall of 85.00%, a precision of 86.23%, a specificity of 87.16%, an F1-score of 85.61%, and a Cohen's Kappa of 72.20%. In comparison, S1 with the Xception model achieved a precision of 69.10%, indicating a lower general accuracy of the predictions. The recall, precision, specificity, and F1-score for S1 were 64.29%, 69.77%, 73.65%, and 66.91%, respectively. Cohen's Kappa for S1 was 38.02%. In contrast, S1 with the InceptioiresNetV2 model achieved an accuracy of 80.21%. Meanwhile, the recall, precision, specificity, F1-score, and Cohen's Kappa for S1 were 74.29%, 83.81%, 85.81%, 78.49%, and 60.27%, respectively.

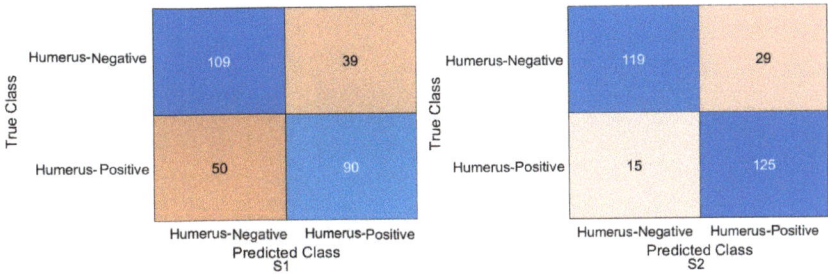

Figure 6. Confusion matrix of the Xception model on the test set with two different training scenarios of the humerus task.

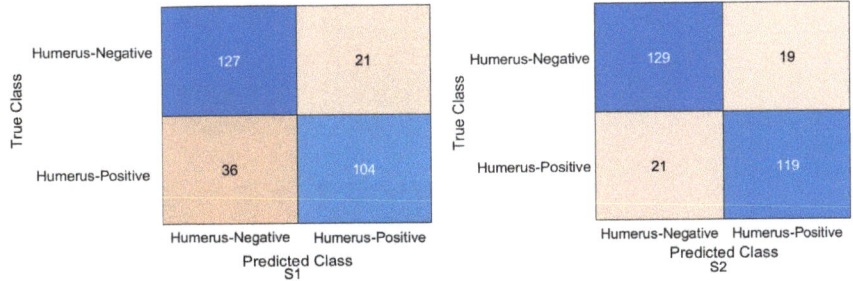

Figure 7. Confusion matrix of the InceptionResNetV2 model on the test set with two different training scenarios of the humerus task.

The Grad-CAM visualisation technique was used to explain the black box nature of the DL models for the two training scenarios. In this section, we used trained models with the test images to calculate the confidence value for Grad-CAM, and two examples are presented to illustrate the performance of the models. The first example is shown in Figure 8, which includes three situations with positive samples. The heat maps reveal the behaviour of the S1 and S2 models when identifying the test samples and focussing on the region of interest (ROI). For S1, the misusing model, the heat map indicates that the model identified the test sample, but concentrated on areas outside the ROI. This suggests that S1 may not accurately capture the essential features within the ROI. However, the proposed TL (S2) method accurately identified the sample with a high confidence value, and the associated heat map focuses on the ROI. This demonstrates the effectiveness of S2 in capturing the relevant information within the ROI. The second example shown in Figure 9 presents negative samples and exhibits the same comparison of S1 and S2. In this case, S2 successfully identifies the samples with a high confidence value, and the heat map targets the ROI. Although it has a low confidence value, S2 still correctly identifies the samples, indicating its robustness. In contrast, the heat map produced by S1 reveals that it focuses on regions outside the ROI, which suggests that it is unable to capture important features within the intended area. These two examples highlight how the proposed TL (S2) method significantly improves the results compared to the misusing model. Although S1 may demonstrate accurate predictions, its low confidence level and lack of an ROI-focused approach make it unreliable. On the contrary, S2 achieves accurate predictions with high confidence values and effectively focuses on the ROI, thus showcasing the enhancement provided by the proposed method (S2).

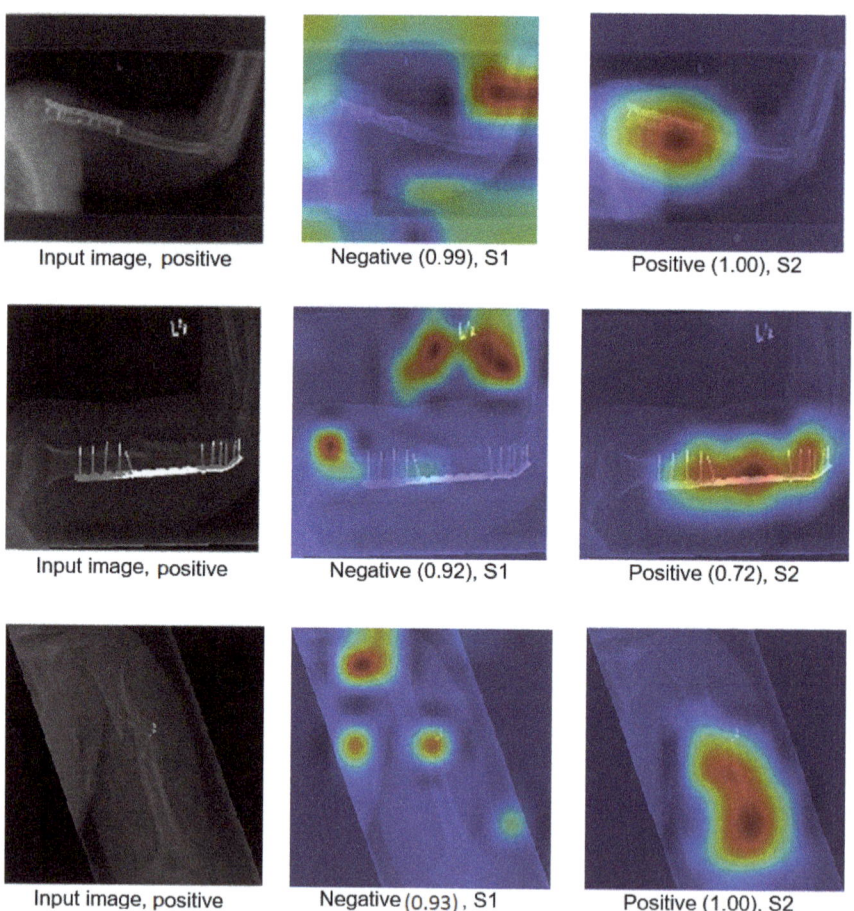

Figure 8. Grad-CAM and score Grad-CAM for the humerus X-ray images. The correct classification is positive.

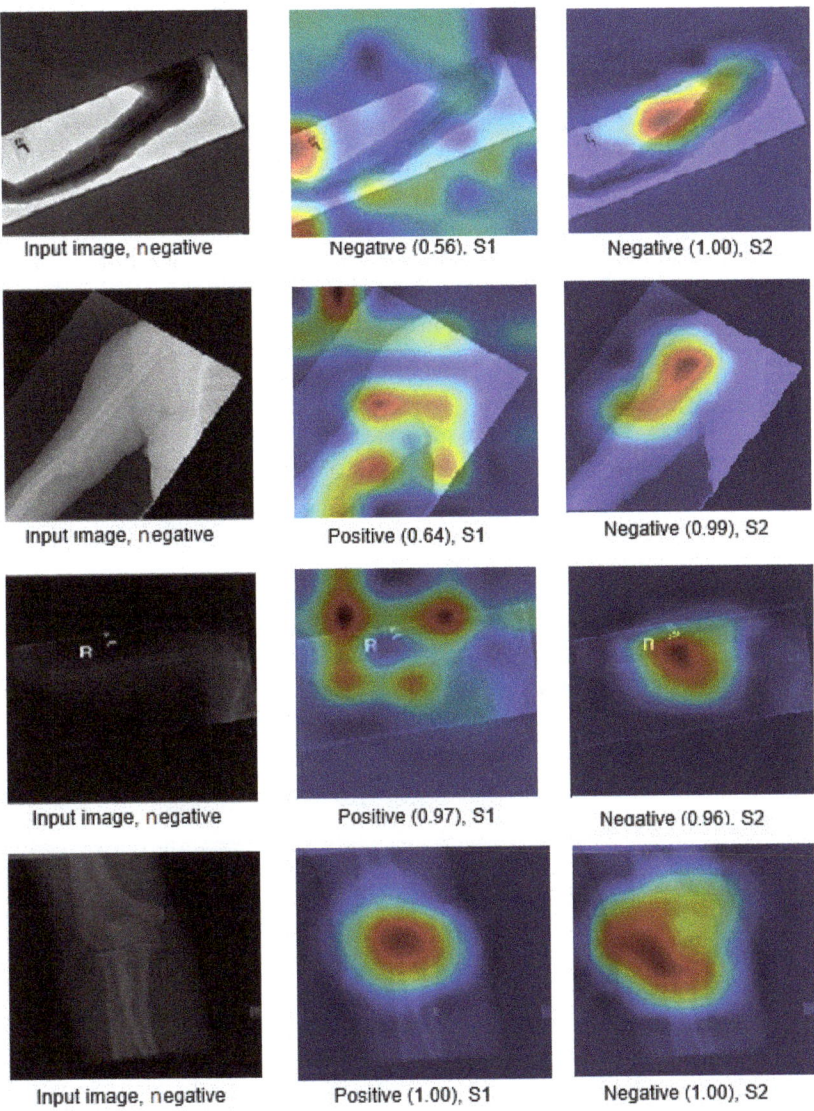

Figure 9. Grad-CAM and score Grad-CAM for the humerus X-ray images. The correct classification is negative.

2. Wrist task: The confusion matrix was calculated for all training cases in both models of DL, and the results are shown in Figures 10 and 11. Using the values of the confusion matrix, various assessment measures were derived. The results demonstrate that S2 outperforms the other model with the Xception DL model, and S2 achieves the highest performance. Specifically, S2 achieves an accuracy of 84.07%, a recall of 73.56%, a precision of 88.93%, a specificity of 92.58%, an F1-score of 80.52%, and a Cohen's Kappa of 68.11%. In contrast, S1 achieves an accuracy of 69.10%, a recall of 64.29%, a precision of 69.77%, a specificity of 73.65%, an F1-score of 66.91%, and a Cohen's Kappa of 38.02%.

As in the InceptionresNetV2 DL model, the results demonstrate that S2 achieves an accuracy of 82.85%, a recall of 67.80%, a precision of 91.74%, a specificity of 95.05%, an F1-score of 77.97%, and a Cohen's Kappa of 64.45%. S1 achieves an accuracy, recall, and precision of 80.21%, 74.29%, and 83.81%, respectively. Meanwhile, the different performance metrics obtain a specificity of 85.81%, an F1-score of 78.49%, and a Cohen's Kappa of 60.27%.

These results highlight the superior performance of S2 compared to S1. S2 shows superior precision, recall, specificity, and F1-score, highlighting its classification ability. The higher Cohen's Kappa value suggests better agreement between the predicted and true labels. On the contrary, S1 exhibits lower performance in all assessment measures, indicating its limitations in accurately classifying data.

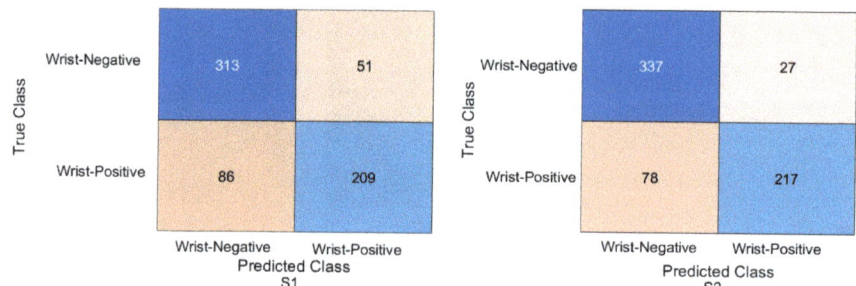

Figure 10. Confusion matrix of the Xception model on the test set with two different training scenarios of the wrist task.

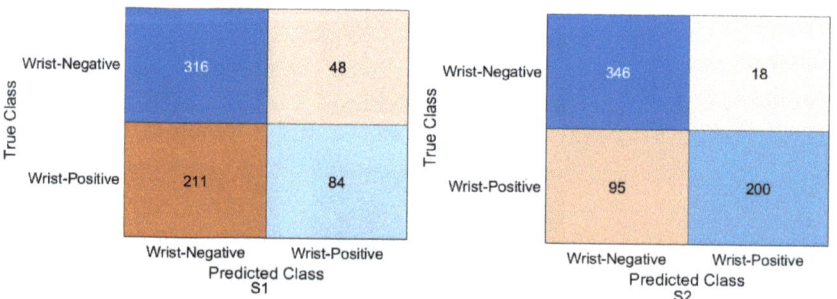

Figure 11. Confusion matrix of the InceptionResNetV2 model on the test set with two different training scenarios of the wrist task.

Figure 12 illustrates how S2 confirms the proposed method (S2) for the wrist task, as well as with Grade-CAM.

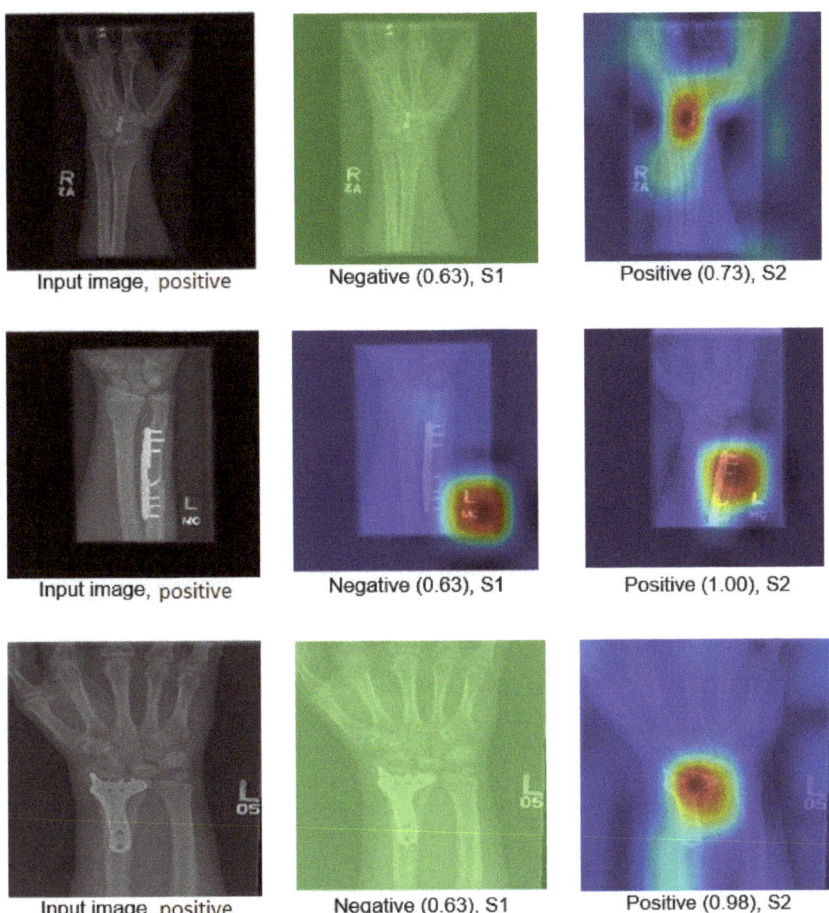

Figure 12. Grad-CAM and score Grad-CAM for the wrist X-ray images. The correct classification is positive.

In terms of LIME and score LIME, Figure 13 provides a comparison between S1 and S2. For S1, the figure illustrates that the model mispredicts the test sample, where the high-intensity area is outside the ROI. This misprediction is evident from the LIME visualisation, highlighting the incorrect area as having maximum intensity. The confidence level of the model in this prediction is not specified. In contrast, S2 shows a significant improvement in accuracy. The model predicts the input sample confidently with a confidence level of 100%. The LIME visualisation confirms that the model correctly identifies the ROI, as the maximum intensity value is assigned to the relevant area. This example serves as a demonstration of the effectiveness of the proposed TL (S2) method. By incorporating the proposed approach, the model prediction is transformed from an incorrect prediction (as observed in S1) to an accurate prediction (as demonstrated in S2). The visualisation provided by LIME further supports this improvement by highlighting the crucial regions that contribute to the correct prediction. In general, the comparison of S1 and S2 using LIME and score LIME emphasises the efficacy of the proposed TL (S2) method in improving the accuracy and reliability of the prediction of the model, particularly by ensuring that the ROI is correctly identified and considered during the decision-making process.

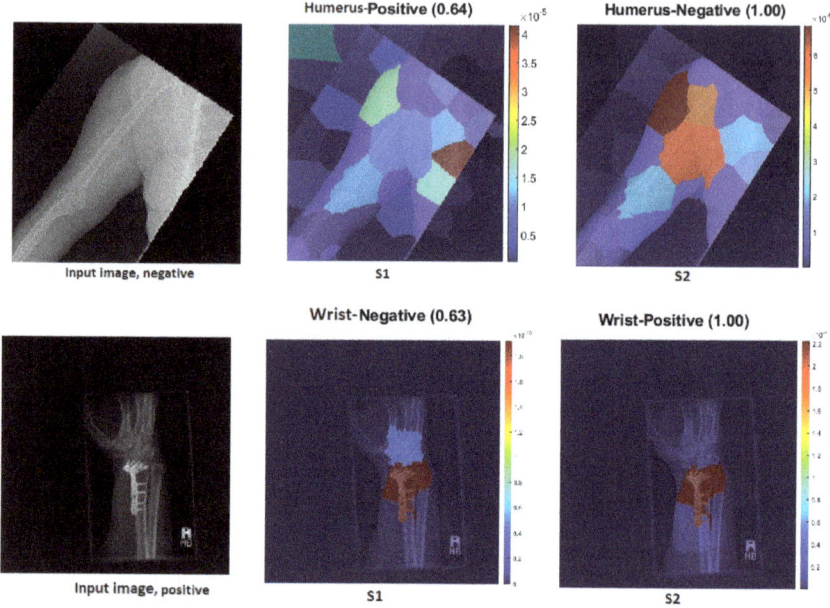

Figure 13. LIME and score LIME for the humerus and wrist X-ray images. The correct classification is negative for the humerus and positive for the wrist.

4.3. Experimental Evaluation of Deep Feature Fusion for the Humerus Task

Several ML classifiers were trained using features extracted from two models, such as the decision tree, linear discriminant analysis, naive Bayes, support vector machine (SVM), coarse KNN, K-nearest neighbour, logistic regression, and neural networks.

Interestingly, the coarse KNN classifier exhibited excellent performance in both scenarios. Figure 14 illustrates the confusion matrix using the cotoNN classifier for each scenario. However, the results presented in Table 5 show that both S1 and S2 significantly improved the results compared to the baseline. Specifically, S2 achieved an accuracy rate of 87.85%, a recall of 88.57%, a precision of 86.71%, a specificity of 87.16%, an F1-score of 87.63%, and a Cohen's Kappa of 75.69%. These metrics indicate a high level of performance and reliability for S2. On the contrary, S1, which was trained using the same coarse KNN classifier, achieved an accuracy of 84.03%, a recall of 80.71%, a precision of 85.61%, a specificity of 87.16%, an F1-score of 83.09%, and a Cohen's Kappa of 67.98%. Although slightly lower than S2, these results nevertheless demonstrated the effectiveness of S1 in improving overall performance compared to the baseline. The comparison between S1 and S2 using the coarse KNN classifier emphasised the superior performance of the proposed method (S2). Both scenarios significantly improved the accuracy, recall, precision, specificity, F1-score and Cohen's Kappa. These results highlighted the effectiveness of the proposed TL (S2) method in enhancing the overall performance of classifiers.

In comparison with another ML classifier, Table 6 displays the result for the humerus task with the Gaussian naive Bayes ML classifier, and Figure 15 confirms the result with the confusion matrix.

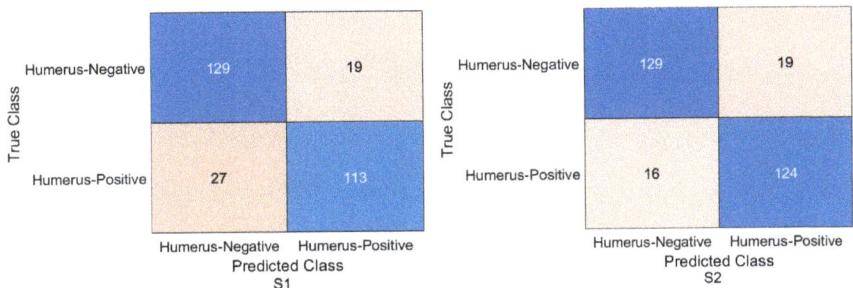

Figure 14. Confusion matrix of the two models and the coarse KNN classifier on the test set with two different training scenarios of the humerus task.

Table 5. The results of feature fusion with the coarse KNN classifier on a test set of the MURA dataset for the humerus task.

Evaluation Metric (%)	Two Models and the Coarse KNN Classifier	
-	S1	S2
Accuracy	84.03	87.85
Recall	80.71	88.57
Precision	85.61	86.71
Specificity	87.16	87.16
F1-score	83.09	87.63
Cohen's Kappa	67.98	75.69

Table 6. The results of feature fusion with the Gaussian naive Bayes classifier on a test set of the MURA dataset for the humerus task.

Evaluation Metric (%)	Two Models and the Gaussian Naive Bayes Classifier	
-	S1	S2
Accuracy	80.60	86.80
Recall	80.50	86.90
Precision	80.60	86.90
Specificity	80.50	86.90
F1-score	80.50	86.90
Cohen's Kappa	61.05	73.64

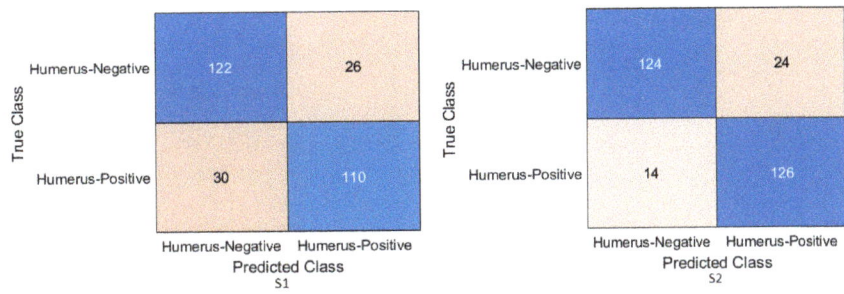

Figure 15. Confusion matrix of the two models and Gaussian naive Bayes classifier on the test set with two different training scenarios of the humerus task.

4.4. Experimental Evaluation of Deep Feature Fusion for Wrist Task

The features extracted from the two models for the wrist task were used to train various ML classifiers, including the decision trees, linear discriminants, naive Bayes, support vector machine (SVM), coarse KNN, K-nearest neighbour, logistic regression, and neural networks. The features were obtained from the two training scenarios, and the outcomes of the classifiers showed a similar pattern. In particular, the coarse KNN classifier exhibited exceptional performance in both scenarios. The confusion matrix was initially constructed using the coarse KNN classifier for each situation, as shown in Figure 16. However, the results presented in Table 7 reveal that both S1 and S2 significantly outperformed the baseline in terms of improving the overall results.

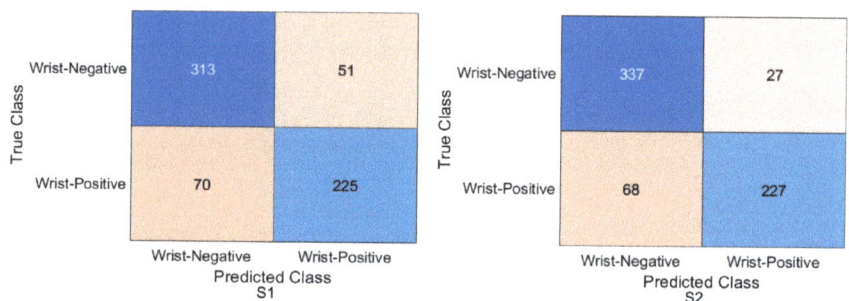

Figure 16. Confusion matrix of the two models and coarse KNN classifier on the test set with two different training scenarios of the wrist task.

Table 7. The results of feature fusion with the coarse KNN Classifier on a test set of the MURA dataset for the wrist task.

Evaluation Metric (%)	Two Models and the Coarse KNN Classifier	
-	S1	S2
Accuracy	81.64	85.58
Recall	76.27	76.95
Precision	81.52	89.37
Specificity	85.99	92.58
F1-score	78.81	82.70
Cohen's Kappa	62.64	70.46

Specifically, S2 achieved an accuracy of 85.58%, a recall of 76.95%, a precision of 89.37%, a specificity of 92.58%, an F1-score of 82.70%, and a Cohen's Kappa of 70.46%. These metrics indicated high precision and performance for S2 on the wrist task. In comparison, S1, which was trained using the same coarse KNN classifier, achieved an accuracy of 81.64%, a recall of 76.27%, a precision of 81.52%, a specificity of 85.99%, an F1-score of 78.81%, and a Cohen's Kappa of 62.64%. Although slightly lower than S2, these results demonstrated the effectiveness of S1 in improving the overall performance compared to the baseline.

The comparison between S1 and S2 using the coarse KNN classifier emphasised the superior performance of the proposed TL (S2) method. Both scenarios significantly improved the accuracy, recall, precision, specificity, F1-score, and Cohen's Kappa. These results highlighted the effectiveness of the proposed approach in improving the overall performance of ML classifiers in the wrist task.

Table 8 shows the result for the feature fusion for the wrist task with the linearSVM ML classifier on the test MURA dataset for the wrist task, and Figure 17 confirms the result with the confusion matrix.

Table 8. The results of feature fusion with the linearSVM classifier on a test set of the MURA dataset for the wrist task.

Evaluation Metric (%)	Two Models and the LinearSVM Classifier	
-	S1	S2
Accuracy	81.20	85.00
Recall	80.40	84.20
Precision	80.40	85.50
Specificity	80.40	84.20
F1-score	81.00	84.90
Cohen's Kappa	61.48	69.26

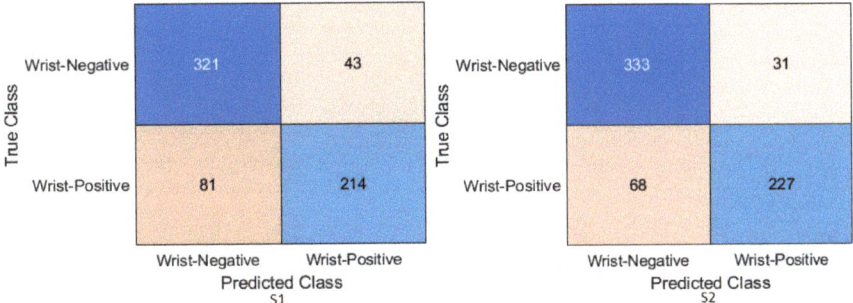

Figure 17. Confusion matrix of the two models and the linearSVM classifier on the test set with two different training scenarios of the wrist task.

Tables 5 and 7 provide some key conclusions:

1. The results obtained from both the humerus and wrist tasks demonstrated that, in Scenario 1 (S1), the performance was inferior compared to Scenario 2 (S2), despite the employment of feature-fusion techniques in both cases. However, it is worth noting that the application of feature fusion without addressing the underlying problem of data scarcity might have weakened the fusion process due to inadequate feature representation.
2. Significantly, it should be noted that, in Scenario 2 (S2), the fusion process exhibited remarkable improvement once the data scarcity problem was addressed. This enhancement can be attributed to the use of the high-quality features extracted by the models. The introduction of sufficient and diverse data allowed for a more-robust and -comprehensive representation of the underlying information, resulting in improved fusion performance.
3. By integrating features from different models or sources, feature fusion plays a crucial role in diversifying the representation of a model, thus reducing the risk of overfitting. This process involves incorporating diverse information, which allows the model to learn from multiple perspectives and reduces its dependence on specific features or patterns in the training data. Consequently, the model becomes more flexible and capable of effectively generalising its knowledge to unseen data instances. Moreover, feature fusion contributes significantly to the achievement of high generalisation performance. Generalisation refers to the model's ability to perform well on data samples that lie beyond the training set.

4.5. Comparison Against the State-of-the-Art Methods

Our proposed method (S2) obtained good results compared to many studies, as shown in Tables 9 and 10.

Table 9. Comparison against the state-of-the-art methods considering the test set of the MURA dataset for the humerus detection task.

Authors	Accuracy	Recall	Precision	Specificity	F1-Score	Cohen's Kappa
Ibrahem et al. [59]	82.08%	81.01%	80.60%	83.21%	80.80%	64.17%
Huynh et al. [60]	68.40%	64.00%	68.70%	72.20%	70.40%	-
Olczak et al. [61]	83.00%	-	-	-	-	-
Luong et al. [62]	84.00%	-	-	-	-	-
This Study	87.85%	88.57%	86.71%	87.16%	87.63%	75.69%

Table 10. Comparison against the state-of-the-art methods considering the test set of the MURA dataset for the wrist detection task.

Authors	Accuracy	Recall	Precision	Specificity	F1 Score	Cohen's Kappa
Ibrahem et al. [59]	82.79%	89.89%	87.38%	71.80%	88.60%	64.60%
Mall et al. [63]	62.00%	35.40%	60.50%	82.30%	44.70%	-
Karam et al. [64]	74.91%	61.98%	72.11%	-	66.66%	-
Saadawy et al. [65]	73.42%	-	-	-	-	-
Nazim et al. [66]	78.10%	-	-	-	-	-
Dang et al. [67]	79.00%	-	-	-	-	-
This Study	85.58%	76.95%	89.37%	92.58%	82.70%	70.46%

4.6. Robustness of Our Proposal

This section demonstrates the robustness of our methodology in the following ways:

1. Improvement of results:

    Figures 18 and 19 demonstrate the comparison between S1 and S2 and visually depict the significant contrast in the prediction outcomes, highlighting the remarkable improvement achieved by S2 over S1. S2 successfully transformed incorrect predictions into correct predictions and did so with a high confidence value.

    The two figures provide concrete evidence of how the proposed TL (S2) method substantially improved the performance of the model by accurately identifying the ROI. In the visualisations, it is evident that S2 precisely identified the crucial areas within the image that influenced the correct prediction. This focus on the ROI was instrumental in achieving the improved accuracy and reliability in the model predictions. The comparison between S1 and S2 is compelling proof of the effectiveness of the proposed TL (S2) method. It demonstrated the significant impact that the consideration of the ROI and the implementation of appropriate techniques can have on enhancing prediction outcomes. The improved performance of S2, along with the high confidence value associated with the correct predictions, highlighted the success of the proposed TL (S2) method in improving both the accuracy and the reliability of the model.

    In particular, Grad-CAM and score Grad-CAM in Figure 18 display a negative case of the humerus as an input image. It is obvious in the S1 of ImageNet that the model incorrectly classified. However, the TL approach (S2) correctly classified with a confidence of 98.00%. On the other hand, Figure 19 displays how our approach TL

(S2) correctly classified the input images in both cases (humerus and wrist), while ImageNet (S1) misclassified them.

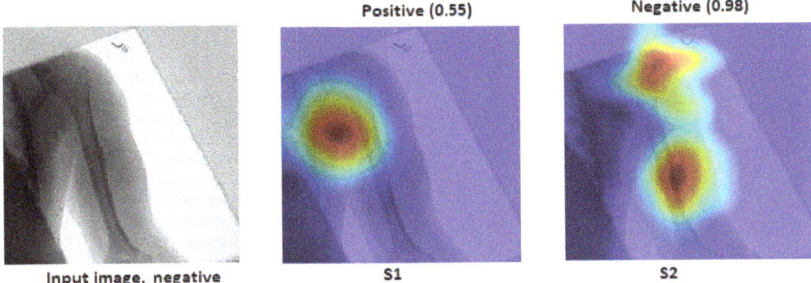

Figure 18. Grad-CAM and score Grad-CAM for the humerus X-ray images. The correct classification is negative.

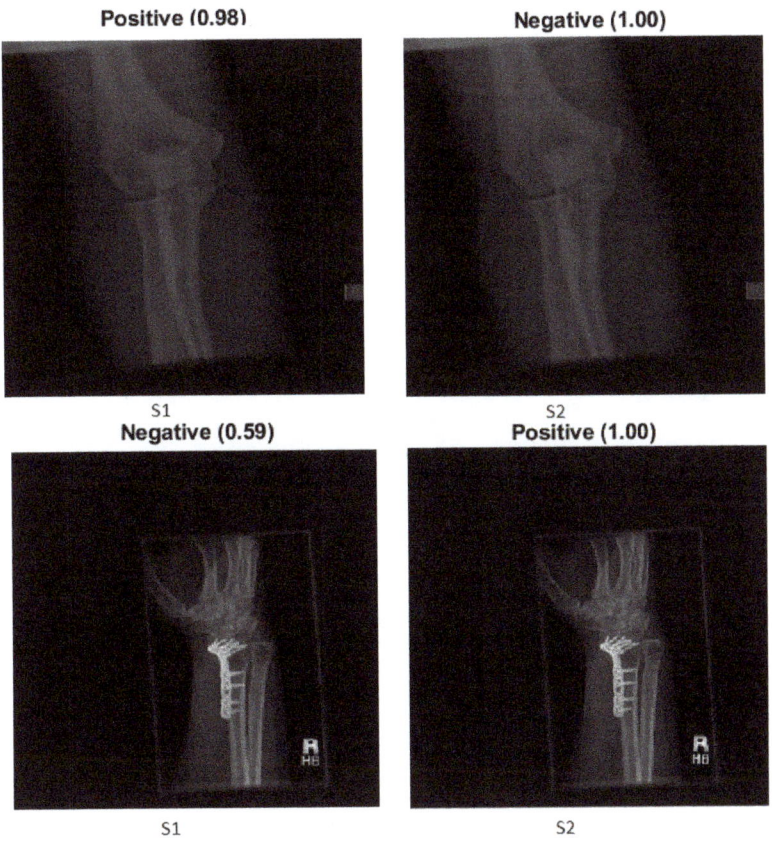

Figure 19. Comparison of S1 and S2, where S1 misclassified the samples and S2 correctly classified them.

2. Changes to sensitivity:
   To demonstrate the robustness of our technique (S2), S2 was tested against various alterations. Figures 20 and 21 show how a small adjustment, such as removing the printed letters from the red circle, can affect the performance of S1. The estimate

was made outside of the ROI and went from being accurate to erroneous before and after being adjusted. However, S2 demonstrated consistent performance by correctly predicting the samples with a high prediction and correctly identifying the ROI.

Figures 20 and 21 illustrate that, despite removing the letter from both tasks (humerus and wrist), TL (S2) was not affected by these changes. However, ImageNet (S1) was affected by these changes and changed the classification from positive (0.86) to negative (0.99) in the humerus task when the input image was positive and from negative (0.75) to positive (0.89) in the wrist task, despite the input image being negative.

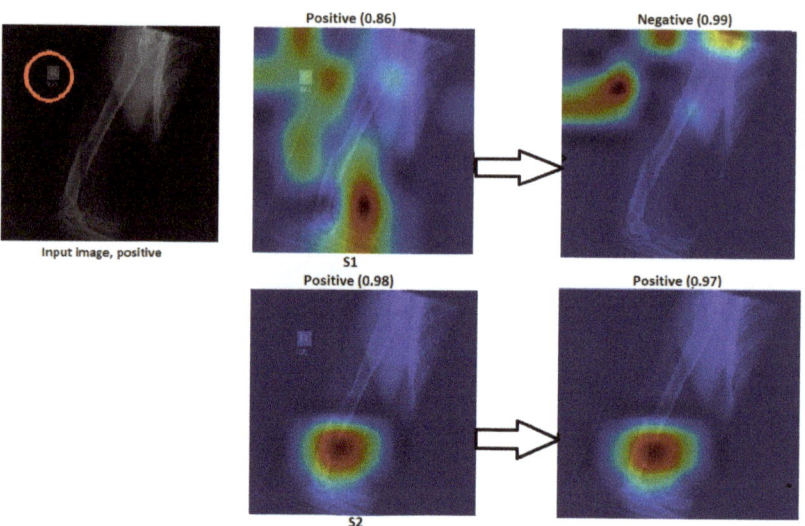

Figure 20. The effect of certain modifications made by eliminating the letters in the red circle. Positive is the correct classification in the humerus task.

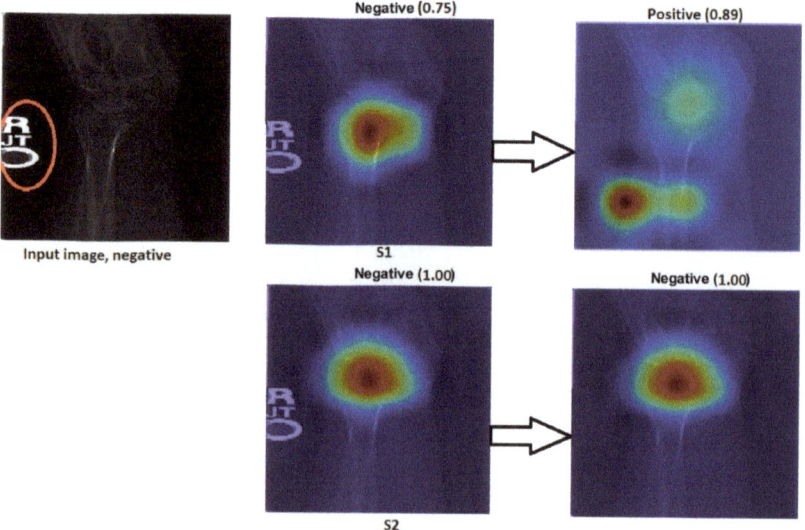

Figure 21. The effect of certain modifications made by eliminating the letters in the red circle. Negative is the correct classification in the wrist task.

3. Assessment of confidence:
   - S1 had a high score with high confidence and correctly recognised the sample in Figure 22 despite not being focused on the ROI, which is interesting. Although the confidence level was high, S1 cannot be relied upon because the Grad-CAM visualisation suggested the opposite to be true. The sample was incorrectly classified with a high confidence value by eliminating the background.
   To approve our approach of TL (S2) by removing the background in Figure 22, TL (S2) still had more confidence with 100% accuracy with the background and without rather than ImageNet (S1), which failed when the background was removed and directly changed from (0.87) positive to (0.77) negative with the positive input image.

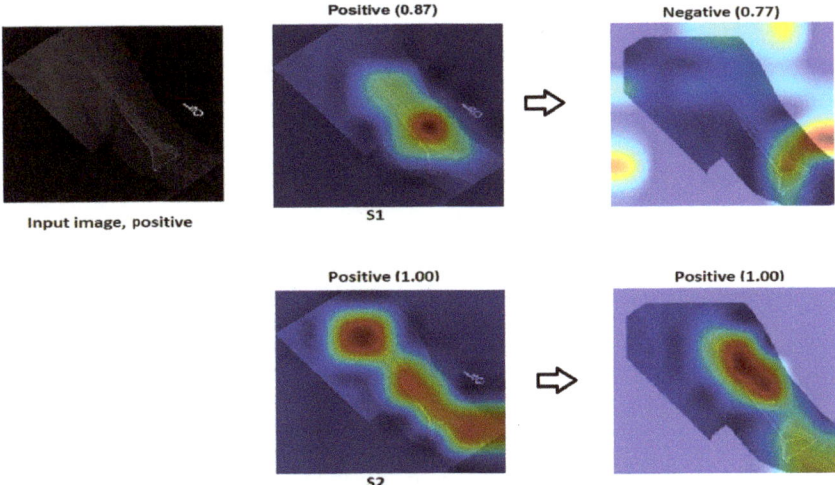

Figure 22. Comparison of S1 and S2. The right classification is positive.

   - Low score: Several test samples are shown in Figure 23, where S1 and S2 successfully identified them. S1 anticipated the samples with low confidence values, but these samples were unreliable because the model did not guarantee them, particularly the samples with confidence values in the 0.50 range. However, S2 displayed a high confidence score that corresponded to the confidence expectation.
   In Figure 23, we can see the obvious difference in the score of classification between ImageNet (S1) and TL (S2); TL (S2) correctly classified with 100% confidence. Meanwhile, ImageNet (S1) correctly classified some images with a low score of confidence.

4. Better feature representation:
   - Fusing two or three DL models enhances the feature representation for ML classifiers and improves the overall performance. Figure 24 shows that one model missed the classification and made incorrect feature selections, while the other model correctly classified the sample. Employing the feature-fusion technique can significantly reduce the chances of misclassification.
   Figure 24 confirms the feature-fusion technique, with the positive humerus and positive wrist that InceptionResNetV2 correctly classified in the TL (S2). However, the same model (InceptionResNetV2) incorrectly classified them (humerus and wrist) with ImageNet (S1).

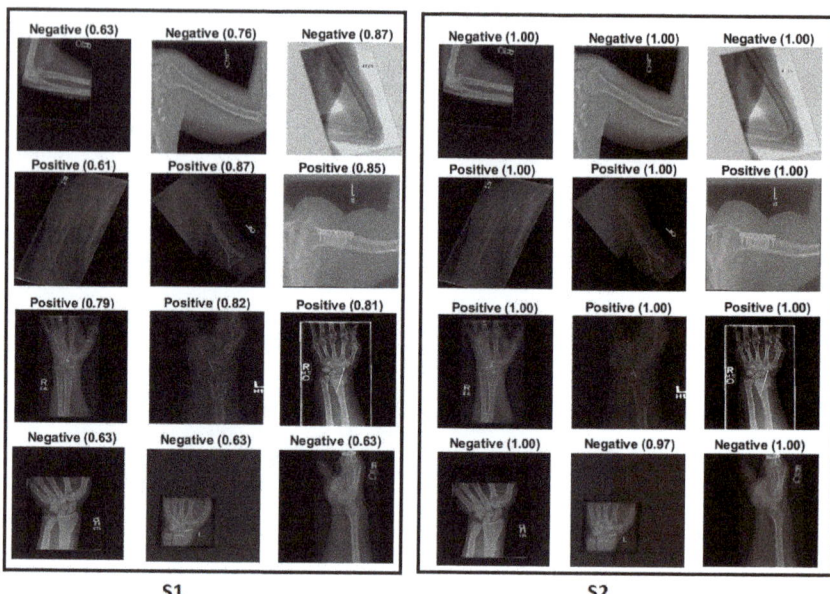

Figure 23. Comparison of S1 and S2, where S1 and S2 correctly predicted the samples, but had varying confidence scores.

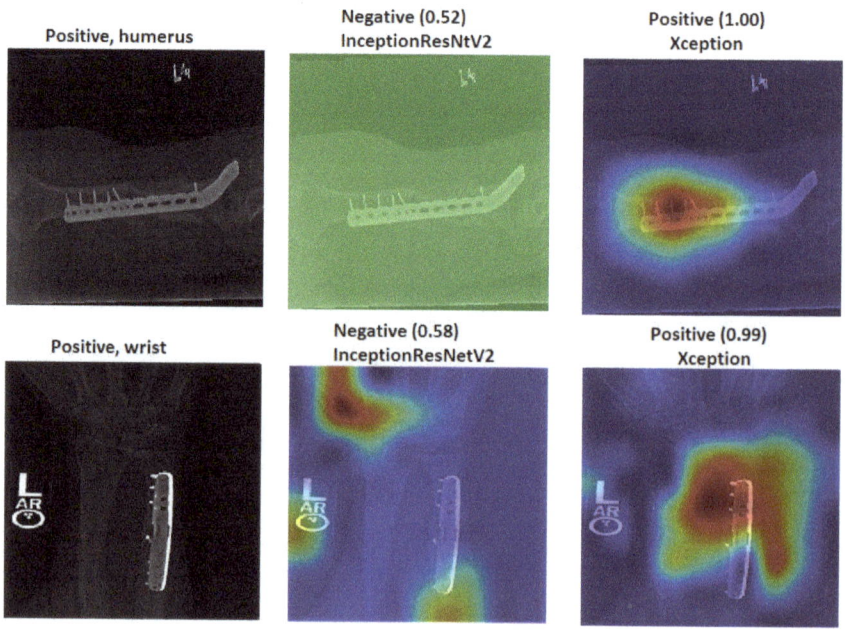

Figure 24. Comparison of InceptionResNetV2 and Xception. The correct classification is positive.

5. Reusability of the Proposed Solution

To approve our TL (S2) approach, we applied our proposed method (S2) to another dataset (chest CT scan), which includes two classes (normal and squamous.cell.carcinoma-left). First, we trained the dataset with Xception and InceptionResNetV2 from scratch to generate S1. Next, we used our source of X-rays without any images of new data (chest CT scan). Table 11 demonstrates the performance for both scenarios in the two models. Figures 25 and 26 display the confusion matrix for both DL models (Xception and InceptionResNetV2) on a test of the chest CT scan dataset.

Table 11. The results of the DL models on the test dataset of chest CT scan on Xception and InceptionResNetV2.

Evaluation Metric (%)	Xception	
-	S1	S2
Accuracy	96.65	99.30
Recall	95.30	99.40
Precision	97.40	99.20
Specificity	95.30	99.40
F1-score	96.30	99.30
Cohen's Kappa	92.34	98.57
Evaluation Metric (%)	InceptionResNetV2	
-	S1	S2
Accuracy	96.65	98.50
Recall	95.30	98.20
Precision	97.40	98.60
Specificity	95.30	98.20
F1-score	96.30	98.40
Cohen's Kappa	92.34	96.77

Figure 25 displays that the Xception model with ImageNet (S1) misclassified (21) images of a normal class, when with the TL (S2), only (1) of the normal class and (3) of the squamous.cell.carcinoma-left were misclassified. Meanwhile, Figure 26 clarifies that the InceptionResNetV2 model misclassified (21) images of the normal class in the ImageNet (S1), and our approach with TL (S2) misclassified (7) images of the normal class and (2) images of the squamous.cell.carcinoma-left.

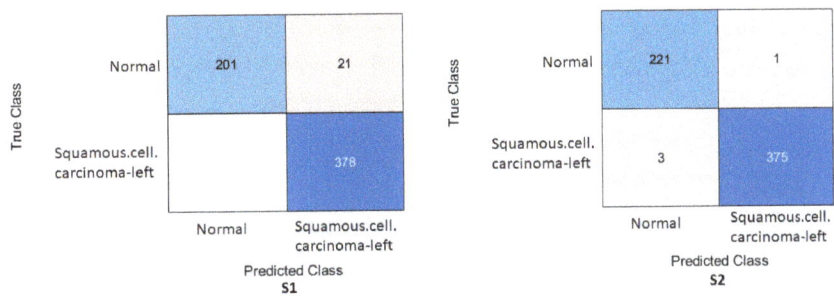

Figure 25. Confusion matrix of the Xception model on the test set with two different chests CT scan task training scenarios.

Furthermore, the Grad-CAM and LIME tools were applied to the CT scan dataset to confirm our proposed method of TL (S2), as shown in Figure 27.

Specifically, the model in Figure 27 demonstrates that ImageNet (S1) incorrectly classified the squamous.cell.carcinoma-left as the input image. Meanwhile, our approach of TL

(S2) confirmed the squamous.cell.carcinoma-left images with a confidence of 100% using the Grad-CAM and LIME tools of the visualisation technique.

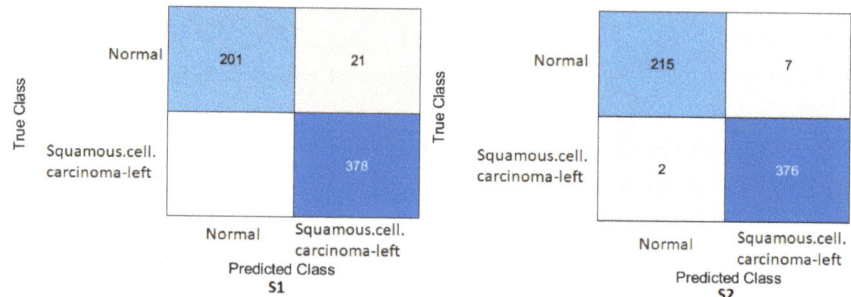

Figure 26. Confusion matrix of the InceptionResNetV2 model on the test set with two different chest CT scan task training scenarios.

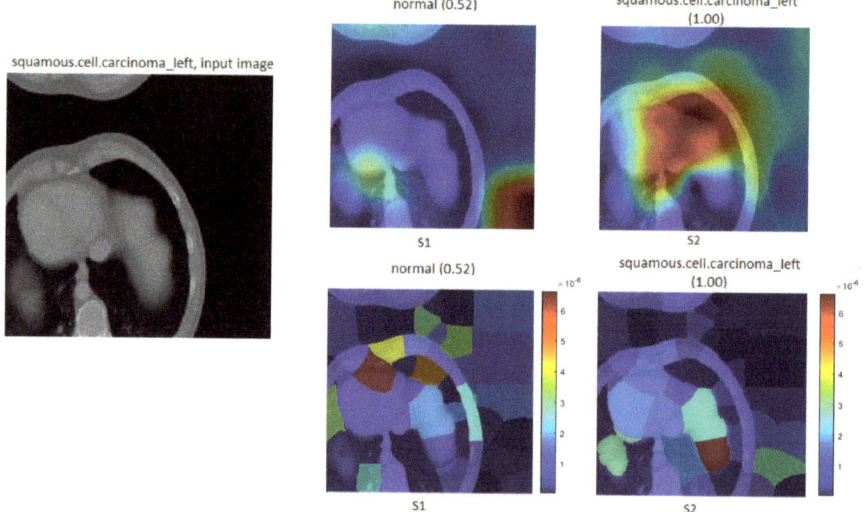

Figure 27. Grad-CAM in the first row and LIME in the second row for chest CT scan images. The correct classification is squamous.cell.carcinoma-left.

6. Conclusions and Future Work

In this paper, a robust technique was introduced for identifying abnormalities in X-ray images of the humerus and wrist. The technique addresses the challenge of domain mismatch between coloured natural images and grayscale X-ray images by training two pre-trained models from ImageNet (S1) on in-domain X-ray images specifically related to the elbow, finger, forearm, hand, humerus, and wrist. These models were then fine-tuned using a dataset specific to the tasks of the humerus and wrist.

The proposed method (S2) was compared with two other training conditions. The first condition (S1) involved using ImageNet (S1) directly on the intended dataset without addressing the domain mismatch. The second condition consisted of training multiple ML classifiers using the fused features extracted from the two models obtained in each scenario.

By overcoming the domain mismatch and training the models on in-domain X-ray images, the proposed method (S2) aimed to improve the accuracy and effectiveness of anomaly detection in humerus and wrist X-ray images. A comparison against other training conditions provided information on the benefits of the proposed approach (S2) in capturing relevant features and improving anomaly detection performance. From this research, we concluded the following:

1. The test dataset consisted of pure MURA images without any preprocessing applied. It is worth noting that many state-of-the-art studies use various preprocessing techniques to enhance image quality and improve their results. However, our approach outperformed these state-of-the-art methods despite not employing preprocessing techniques on the test dataset. By demonstrating superior performance without preprocessing, our approach highlights the effectiveness of the proposed methodology (S2) in accurately detecting anomalies in MURA images. It suggests that our models' robust feature extraction and classification capabilities can capture the relevant information directly from the raw MURA dataset.
2. The results obtained from S2 demonstrate the effectiveness of the proposed TL approach (S2) in reducing the mismatch between the two domains. By training the models on in-domain X-ray images and then fine-tuning them on the humerus and wrist tasks datasets, the TL method effectively bridged the gap between the coloured natural images and the grayscale X-ray images. The reduced mismatch in the domain is reflected in the improved performance of S2 compared to S1 and other training conditions. The models trained using S2 exhibited enhanced prediction accuracy and demonstrated the ability to correctly identify the ROIs in the X-ray images. This reduction in domain mismatch can be attributed to the transfer of knowledge and features from the pre-trained ImageNet (S1) models to the specific tasks of humerus and wrist anomaly detection.
3. For some models of ImageNet (S1), despite specific models showing comparable or higher performance in the evaluation metrics, the visual confirmations provided by Grad-CAM and LIME emphasised the superiority of S2 in accurately detecting and focusing on the relevant ROI. These visualisation techniques added a layer of confidence to the outcomes obtained by S2.
4. The proposed approach (S2) is not limited to the specific dataset used in this study; it has the potential to be applied to a wide range of tasks and applications. The flexibility and adaptability of the proposed TL (S2) method allow exploration and investigation of various domains, as validated through the significant improvements observed in the CT case.

The next step is to include most grayscale medical modalities (MRI, CT, and ultrasound) in the source of TL to cover most grayscale medical applications. Thus, this type of TL will offer a better generalisation of features and will be able to be used for any grayscale medical modalities.

Author Contributions: Conceptualisation: Z.A., L.A. and J.Z.; methodology: Z.A.; software: Z.A., L.A. and J.Z.; validation: Z.A., L.A., J.Z., Y.L., W.L. and Y.G.; formal analysis: Z.A., L.A., J.Z., Y.L., W.L. and Y.G.; investigation: Z.A., L.A., J.Z., Y.L., W.L. and Y.G.; resources: Z.A., L.A., J.Z., Y.L., W.L. and Y.G.; data curation: Z.A., L.A., J.Z., Y.L., W.L. and Y.G.; writing—original draft preparation: Z.A.; writing—review and editing: Z.A., L.A., J.Z., Y.L., W.L. and Y.G.; visualisation: Z.A., L.A., J.Z., Y.L., W.L. and Y.G.; supervision: L.A., J.Z., and Y.L.; project administration: Z.A., L.A., J.Z., Y.L., W.L. and Y.G.; funding acquisition: Z.A., L.A., J.Z., Y.L. and Y.G. All authors have read and agreed to the published version of the manuscript.

Funding: Y.G. and L.A. would like to acknowledge the support received through the following funding schemes of the Australian Government: The Australian Research Council (ARC) and the Industrial Transformation Training Centre (ITTC) for Joint Biomechanics under Grant IC190100020.

Institutional Review Board Statement: Not applicable.

Informed Consent Statement: Not applicable.

Data Availability Statement: https://stanfordmlgroup.github.io/competitions/mura/ (accessed on 23 March 2023).

Conflicts of Interest: The authors declare no conflict of interest.

Reference

1. Alzubaidi, L.; Al-Amidie, M.; Al-Asadi, A.; Humaidi, A.J.; Al-Shamma, O.; Fadhel, M.A.; Zhang, J.; Santamaría, J.; Duan, Y. Novel transfer learning approach for medical imaging with limited labeled data. *Cancers* 2021, *13*, 1590. [CrossRef] [PubMed]
2. Alzubaidi, L.; Bai, J.; Al-Sabaawi, A.; Santamaría, J.; Albahri, A.S.; Al-dabbagh, B.S.N.; Fadhel, M.A.; Manoufali, M.; Zhang, J.; Al-Timemy, A.H.; et al. A survey on deep learning tools dealing with data scarcity: Definitions, challenges, solutions, tips, and applications. *J. Big Data* 2023, *10*, 1.
3. Dahmen, J.; Cook, D. SynSys: A synthetic data generation system for healthcare applications. *Sensors* 2019, *19*, 1181. [CrossRef] [PubMed]
4. Torrey, L.; Shavlik, J. Transfer learning. In *Handbook of Research on Machine Learning Applications and Trends: Algorithms, Methods, and Techniques*; IGI Global: Hershey, PA, USA, 2010; pp. 242–264.
5. Mandal, S.; Greenblatt, A.B.; An, J. Imaging intelligence: AI is transforming medical imaging across the imaging spectrum. *IEEE Pulse* 2018, *9*, 16–24. [CrossRef] [PubMed]
6. Zhou, G.; Hu, C.; Zhang, Y.; Jiang, J. An unsupervised deep clustering for Bone X-ray classification and anomaly detection. *medRxiv* 2023. [CrossRef]
7. Millán Arias, P.; Alipour, F.; Hill, K.A.; Kari, L. DeLUCS: Deep learning for unsupervised clustering of DNA sequences. *PLoS ONE* 2022, *17*, e0261531. [CrossRef]
8. Teoh, L.; Ihalage, A.A.; Harp, S.; F. Al-Khateeb, Z.; Michael-Titus, A.T.; Tremoleda, J.L.; Hao, Y. Deep learning for behaviour classification in a preclinical brain injury model. *PLoS ONE* 2022, *17*, e0268962. [CrossRef] [PubMed]
9. Rajpurkar, P.; Irvin, J.; Zhu, K.; Yang, B.; Mehta, H.; Duan, T.; Ding, D.; Bagul, A.; Langlotz, C.; Shpanskaya, K.; et al. Chexnet: Radiologist-level pneumonia detection on chest x-rays with deep learning. *arXiv* 2017, arXiv:1711.05225.
10. Hamamoto, R.; Suvarna, K.; Yamada, M.; Kobayashi, K.; Shinkai, N.; Miyake, M.; Takahashi, M.; Jinnai, S.; Shimoyama, R.; Sakai, A.; et al. Application of artificial intelligence technology in oncology: Towards the establishment of precision medicine. *Cancers* 2020, *12*, 3532. [CrossRef]
11. Liu, Y.; Jain, A.; Eng, C.; Way, D.H.; Lee, K.; Bui, P.; Kanada, K.; de Oliveira Marinho, G.; Gallegos, J.; Gabriele, S.; et al. A deep learning system for differential diagnosis of skin diseases. *Nat. Med.* 2020, *26*, 900–908. [CrossRef]
12. Valieris, R.; Amaro, L.; Osório, C.A.B.d.T.; Bueno, A.P.; Rosales Mitrowsky, R.A.; Carraro, D.M.; Nunes, D.N.; Dias-Neto, E.; Silva, I.T.d. Deep learning predicts underlying features on pathology images with therapeutic relevance for breast and gastric cancer. *Cancers* 2020, *12*, 3687. [CrossRef]
13. Nazir, T.; Irtaza, A.; Javed, A.; Malik, H.; Hussain, D.; Naqvi, R.A. Retinal image analysis for diabetes-based eye disease detection using deep learning. *Appl. Sci.* 2020, *10*, 6185. [CrossRef]
14. Gulshan, V.; Peng, L.; Coram, M.; Stumpe, M.C.; Wu, D.; Narayanaswamy, A.; Venugopalan, S.; Widner, K.; Madams, T.; Cuadros, J.; et al. Development and validation of a deep learning algorithm for detection of diabetic retinopathy in retinal fundus photographs. *JAMA* 2016, *316*, 2402–2410. [CrossRef]
15. Krizhevsky, A.; Sutskever, I.; Hinton, G.E. Imagenet classification with deep convolutional neural networks. *Commun. ACM* 2017, *60*, 84–90. [CrossRef]
16. Alzubaidi, L.; Fadhel, M.A.; Al-Shamma, O.; Zhang, J.; Santamaría, J.; Duan, Y.; R. Oleiwi, S. Towards a better understanding of transfer learning for medical imaging: A case study. *Appl. Sci.* 2020, *10*, 4523. [CrossRef]
17. Fang, L.; Jin, Y.; Huang, L.; Guo, S.; Zhao, G.; Chen, X. Iterative fusion convolutional neural networks for classification of optical coherence tomography images. *J. Vis. Commun. Image Represent.* 2019, *59*, 327–333. [CrossRef]
18. Buda, M.; Maki, A.; Mazurowski, M.A. A systematic study of the class imbalance problem in convolutional neural networks. *Neural Netw.* 2018, *106*, 249–259. [CrossRef] [PubMed]
19. Rajpurkar, P.; Irvin, J.; Bagul, A.; Ding, D.; Duan, T.; Mehta, H.; Yang, B.; Zhu, K.; Laird, D.; Ball, R.L.; et al. Mura: Large dataset for abnormality detection in musculoskeletal radiographs. *arXiv* 2017, arXiv:1712.06957.
20. Alzubaidi, L.; Zhang, J.; Humaidi, A.J.; Al-Dujaili, A.; Duan, Y.; Al-Shamma, O.; Santamaría, J.; Fadhel, M.A.; Al-Amidie, M.; Farhan, L. Review of deep learning: Concepts, CNN architectures, challenges, applications, future directions. *J. Big Data* 2021, *8*, 1–74.
21. Mao, S.; Sejdić, E. A review of recurrent neural network-based methods in computational physiology. *IEEE Trans. Neural Netw. Learn. Syst.* 2022 . [CrossRef] [PubMed]
22. Fraiwan, M.; Audat, Z.; Fraiwan, L.; Manasreh, T. Using deep transfer learning to detect scoliosis and spondylolisthesis from X-ray images. *PLoS ONE* 2022, *17*, e0267851. [CrossRef]
23. Mesejo, P.; Martos, R.; Ibáñez, Ó.; Novo, J.; Ortega, M. A survey on artificial intelligence techniques for biomedical image analysis in skeleton-based forensic human identification. *Appl. Sci.* 2020, *10*, 4703. [CrossRef]
24. Liang, W.; Tadesse, G.A.; Ho, D.; Fei-Fei, L.; Zaharia, M.; Zhang, C.; Zou, J. Advances, challenges and opportunities in creating data for trustworthy AI. *Nat. Mach. Intell.* 2022, *4*, 669–677. [CrossRef]
25. Girshick, R.; Donahue, J.; Darrell, T.; Malik, J. Rich feature hierarchies for accurate object detection and semantic segmentation. In Proceedings of the IEEE Conference on Computer Vision and Pattern Recognition, Columbus, OH, USA, 23–28 June 2014; pp. 580–587.

26. Al-Timemy, A.H.; Alzubaidi, L.; Mosa, Z.M.; Abdelmotaal, H.; Ghaeb, N.H.; Lavric, A.; Hazarbassanov, R.M.; Takahashi, H.; Gu, Y.; Yousefi, S. A Deep Feature Fusion of Improved Suspected Keratoconus Detection with Deep Learning. *Diagnostics* **2023**, *13*, 1689. [CrossRef] [PubMed]
27. Jeon, H.; Edwin, J.; Kim, S.; Yang, C. Sea Fog Classification from GOCI Images using CNN Transfer Learning Models. *IEICE Tech. Rep. IEICE Tech. Rep.* **2019**, *119*, 87–90.
28. Alzubaidi, L.; Al-Shamma, O.; Fadhel, M.A.; Farhan, L.; Zhang, J.; Duan, Y. Optimizing the performance of breast cancer classification by employing the same domain transfer learning from hybrid deep convolutional neural network model. *Electronics* **2020**, *9*, 445. [CrossRef]
29. Azizi, S.; Culp, L.; Freyberg, J.; Mustafa, B.; Baur, S.; Kornblith, S.; Chen, T.; Tomasev, N.; Mitrović, J.; Strachan, P.; et al. Robust and data-efficient generalization of self-supervised machine learning for diagnostic imaging. *Nat. Biomed. Eng.* **2023**, *7*, 756–779. [CrossRef] [PubMed]
30. Albahri, A.; Duhaim, A.M.; Fadhel, M.A.; Alnoor, A.; Baqer, N.S.; Alzubaidi, L.; Albahri, O.; Alamoodi, A.; Bai, J.; Salhi, A.; et al. A systematic review of trustworthy and explainable artificial intelligence in healthcare: Assessment of quality, bias risk, and data fusion. *Inf. Fusion* **2023**, *96*, 156–191. [CrossRef]
31. Alammar, Z.; Alzubaidi, L.; Zhang, J.; Santamaréa, J.; Li, Y. A concise review on deep learning for musculoskeletal X-ray images. In Proceedings of the 2022 International Conference on Digital Image Computing: Techniques and Applications (DICTA), Sydney, Australia, 30 November–2 December 2022; pp. 1–8.
32. Hoi, S.C.; Jin, R.; Zhu, J.; Lyu, M.R. Batch mode active learning and its application to medical image classification. In Proceedings of the 23rd International Conference on Machine Learning, Pittsburgh, PA, USA, 25–29 June 2006; pp. 417–424.
33. Wen, S.; Kurc, T.M.; Hou, L.; Saltz, J.H.; Gupta, R.R.; Batiste, R.; Zhao, T.; Nguyen, V.; Samaras, D.; Zhu, W. Comparison of different classifiers with active learning to support quality control in nucleus segmentation in pathology images. *AMIA Summits Transl. Sci. Proc.* **2018**, *2018*, 227.
34. Zhao, A.; Balakrishnan, G.; Durand, F.; Guttag, J.V.; Dalca, A.V. Data augmentation using learned transformations for one-shot medical image segmentation. In Proceedings of the IEEE/CVF Conference on Computer Vision and Pattern Recognition, Long Beach, CA, USA, 15–20 June 2019; pp. 8543–8553.
35. Frid-Adar, M.; Klang, E.; Amitai, M.; Goldberger, J.; Greenspan, H. Synthetic data augmentation using GAN for improved liver lesion classification. In Proceedings of the 2018 IEEE 15th International Symposium on Biomedical Imaging (ISBI 2018), Washington, DC, USA, 4–7 April 2018; pp. 289–293.
36. Yi, X.; Walia, E.; Babyn, P. Generative adversarial network in medical imaging: A review. *Med. Image Anal.* **2019**, *58*, 101552. [CrossRef]
37. Calimeri, F.; Marzullo, A.; Stamile, C.; Terracina, G. Biomedical data augmentation using generative adversarial neural networks. In Proceedings of the International Conference on Artificial Neural Networks, Alghero, Italy, 11–14 September 2017; pp. 626–634.
38. Bermudez, C.; Plassard, A.J.; Davis, L.T.; Newton, A.T.; Resnick, S.M.; Landman, B.A. Learning implicit brain MRI manifolds with deep learning. In *Medical Imaging 2018: Image Processing*; SPIE: Washington, DC, USA, 2018; Volume 10574, pp. 408–414.
39. Chuquicusma, M.J.; Hussein, S.; Burt, J.; Bagci, U. How to fool radiologists with generative adversarial networks? A visual turing test for lung cancer diagnosis. In Proceedings of the 2018 IEEE 15th International Symposium on Biomedical Imaging (ISBI 2018), Washington, DC, USA, 4–7 April 2018; pp. 240–244.
40. Baur, C.; Albarqouni, S.; Navab, N. MelanoGANs: High resolution skin lesion synthesis with GANs. *arXiv* **2018**, arXiv:1804.04338.
41. Shorten, C.; Khoshgoftaar, T.M. A survey on image data augmentation for deep learning. *J. Big Data* **2019**, *6*, 1–48. [CrossRef]
42. Sumi, T.A.; Basnin, N.; Hossain, M.S.; Andersson, K.; Hoassain, M.S. Classifying Humerus Fracture Using X-ray Images. In *The Fourth Industrial Revolution and Beyond: Select Proceedings of IC4IR+*; Springer: Berlin/Heidelberg, Germany, 2023; pp. 527–538.
43. Cheplygina, V.; de Bruijne, M.; Pluim, J. Not-so-supervised: A survey of semi-supervised, multi-instance, and transfer learning in medical image analysis. *arXiv* **2018**, arXiv:1804.06353.
44. Kensert, A.; Harrison, P.J.; Spjuth, O. Transfer learning with deep convolutional neural networks for classifying cellular morphological changes. *SLAS Discov. Adv. Life Sci. R&D* **2019**, *24*, 466–475. [CrossRef] [PubMed]
45. Ortiz-Toro, C.; Garcia-Pedrero, A.; Lillo-Saavedra, M.; Gonzalo-Martin, C. Automatic detection of pneumonia in chest X-ray images using textural features. *Comput. Biol. Med.* **2022**, *145*, 105466. [CrossRef] [PubMed]
46. Canayaz, M. MH-COVIDNet: Diagnosis of COVID-19 using deep neural networks and meta-heuristic-based feature selection on X-ray images. *Biomed. Signal Process. Control* **2021**, *64*, 102257. [CrossRef]
47. Rajinikanth, V.; Kadry, S.; Damaševičius, R.; Pandeeswaran, C.; Mohammed, M.A.; Devadhas, G.G. Pneumonia detection in chest X-ray using inceptionV3 and multi-class classification. In Proceedings of the 2022 Third International Conference on Intelligent Computing Instrumentation and Control Technologies (ICICICT), Kannur, India, 11–12 August 2022; pp. 972–976.
48. Rajinikanth, V.; Kadry, S.; Damaševičius, R.; Gnanasoundharam, J.; Mohammed, M.A.; Devadhas, G.G. UNet with two-fold training for effective segmentation of lung section in chest X-ray. In Proceedings of the 2022 Third International Conference on Intelligent Computing Instrumentation and Control Technologies (ICICICT), Kannur, India, 11–12 August 2022; pp. 977–981.
49. Huang, G.; Liu, Z.; Van Der Maaten, L.; Weinberger, K.Q. Densely connected convolutional networks. In Proceedings of the IEEE Conference on Computer Vision and Pattern Recognition, Honolulu, HI, USA, 21–26 July 2017; pp. 4700–4708.
50. Chada, G. Machine learning models for abnormality detection in musculoskeletal radiographs. *Reports* **2019**, *2*, 26. [CrossRef]

51. Chung, S.W.; Han, S.S.; Lee, J.W.; Oh, K.S.; Kim, N.R.; Yoon, J.P.; Kim, J.Y.; Moon, S.H.; Kwon, J.; Lee, H.J.; et al. Automated detection and classification of the proximal humerus fracture by using deep learning algorithm. *Acta Orthop.* **2018**, *89*, 468–473. [CrossRef]
52. Lindsey, R.; Daluiski, A.; Chopra, S.; Lachapelle, A.; Mozer, M.; Sicular, S.; Hanel, D.; Gardner, M.; Gupta, A.; Hotchkiss, R.; et al. Deep neural network improves fracture detection by clinicians. *Proc. Natl. Acad. Sci. USA* **2018**, *115*, 11591–11596. [CrossRef] [PubMed]
53. Saif, A.; Shahnaz, C.; Zhu, W.P.; Ahmad, M.O. Abnormality detection in musculoskeletal radiographs using capsule network. *IEEE Access* **2019**, *7*, 81494–81503. [CrossRef]
54. Varma, M.; Lu, M.; Gardner, R.; Dunnmon, J.; Khandwala, N.; Rajpurkar, P.; Long, J.; Beaulieu, C.; Shpanskaya, K.; Fei-Fei, L.; et al. Automated abnormality detection in lower extremity radiographs using deep learning. *Nat. Mach. Intell.* **2019**, *1*, 578–583. [CrossRef]
55. Kandel, I.; Castelli, M.; Popovič, A. Musculoskeletal images classification for detection of fractures using transfer learning. *J. Imaging* **2020**, *6*, 127. [CrossRef] [PubMed]
56. Bhan, A.; Singh, S.; Vats, S.; Mehra, A. Ensemble Model based Osteoporosis Detection in Musculoskeletal Radiographs. In Proceedings of the 2023 13th International Conference on Cloud Computing, Data Science & Engineering (Confluence), Noida, India, 19–20 January 2023; pp. 523–528.
57. Alzubaidi, L.; Duan, Y.; Al-Dujaili, A.; Ibraheem, I.K.; Alkenani, A.H.; Santamaría, J.; Fadhel, M.A.; Al-Shamma, O.; Zhang, J. Deepening into the suitability of using pre-trained models of ImageNet against a lightweight convolutional neural network in medical imaging: An experimental study. *PeerJ Comput. Sci.* **2021**, *7*, e715. [CrossRef]
58. Selvaraju, R.R.; Cogswell, M.; Das, A.; Vedantam, R.; Parikh, D.; Batra, D. Grad-cam: Visual explanations from deep networks via gradient-based localization. In Proceedings of the IEEE International Conference on Computer Vision, Venice, Italy, 22–29 October 2017; pp. 618–626.
59. Kandel, I.; Castelli, M.; Popovič, A. Comparing stacking ensemble techniques to improve musculoskeletal fracture image classification. *J. Imaging* **2021**, *7*, 100. [CrossRef]
60. Huynh, H.X.; Nguyen, H.B.T.; Phan, C.A.; Nguyen, H.T. Abnormality Bone Detection in X-Ray Images Using Convolutional Neural Network. In Proceedings of the International Conference on Context-Aware Systems and Applications, International Conference on Nature of Computation and Communication, Online, 28–29 October 2021; pp. 31–43.
61. Olczak, J.; Fahlberg, N.; Maki, A.; Razavian, A.S.; Jilert, A.; Stark, A.; Sköldenberg, O.; Gordon, M. Artificial intelligence for analyzing orthopedic trauma radiographs: deep learning algorithms—Are they on par with humans for diagnosing fractures? *Acta Orthop.* **2017**, *88*, 581–586. [CrossRef]
62. Luong, H.H.; Le, L.T.T.; Nguyen, H.T.; Hua, V.Q.; Nguyen, K.V.; Bach, T.N.P.; Nguyen, T.N.A.; Nguyen, H.T.Q. Transfer Learning with Fine-Tuning on MobileNet and GRAD-CAM for Bones Abnormalities Diagnosis. In *Complex, Intelligent and Software Intensive Systems, Proceedings of the 16th International Conference on Complex, Intelligent and Software Intensive Systems (CISIS-2022), Kitakyushu, Japan, 29 June–1 July 2022*; Springer: Berlin/Heidelberg, Germany, 2022; pp. 171–179.
63. Mall, P.K.; Singh, P.K.; Yadav, D. Glcm based feature extraction and medical x-ray image classification using machine learning techniques. In Proceedings of the 2019 IEEE Conference on Information and Communication Technology, Jeju, Republic of Korea, 16–18 October 2019; pp. 1–6.
64. Karam, C.; Zini, J.E.; Awad, M.; Saade, C.; Naffaa, L.; Amine, M.E. A Progressive and Cross-Domain Deep Transfer Learning Framework for Wrist Fracture Detection. *J. Artif. Intell. Soft Comput. Res.* **2021**, *12*, 101–120. [CrossRef]
65. El-Saadawy, H.; Tantawi, M.; Shedeed, H.A.; Tolba, M.F. A two-stage method for bone X-rays abnormality detection using mobileNet network. In Proceedings of the International Conference on Artificial Intelligence and Computer Vision (AICV2020), Cairo, Egypt, 8–10 April 2020; pp. 372–380.
66. Nazim, S.; Hussain, S.; Moinuddin, M.; Zubair, M.; Ahmad, J. A neoteric ensemble deep learning network for musculoskeletal disorder classification. *Neural Netw. World* **2021**, *31*, 377. [CrossRef]
67. Dang, T.; Martin, K.; Patel, M.; Thompson, A.; Leishman, L.; Wiratunga, N. Assessing the clinicians' pathway to embed artificial intelligence for assisted diagnostics of fracture detection. In Proceedings of the CEUR Workshop Proceedings, Bologna, Italy, 14–16 September 2020.

Disclaimer/Publisher's Note: The statements, opinions and data contained in all publications are solely those of the individual author(s) and contributor(s) and not of MDPI and/or the editor(s). MDPI and/or the editor(s) disclaim responsibility for any injury to people or property resulting from any ideas, methods, instructions or products referred to in the content.

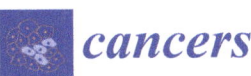

Article

Explainable CAD System for Classification of Acute Lymphoblastic Leukemia Based on a Robust White Blood Cell Segmentation

Jose Luis Diaz Resendiz [1], Volodymyr Ponomaryov [1,*], Rogelio Reyes Reyes [1] and Sergiy Sadovnychiy [2]

1. Instituto Politecnico Nacional, Escuela Superior de Ingenieria Mecanica y Electrica–Culhuacan, Av. Sta. Ana 1000, Mexico City 04440, Mexico; jdiazr2100@alumno.ipn.mx (J.L.D.R.); rreyesre@ipn.mx (R.R.R.)
2. Instituto Mexicano del Petroleo, Eje Central Lazaro Cardenas Norte 152, Mexico City 07730, Mexico; ssadovny@imp.mx
* Correspondence: vponomar@ipn.mx; Tel.: +52-555-729-6000 (ext. 73263)

Citation: Diaz Resendiz, J.L.; Ponomaryov, V.; Reyes Reyes, R.; Sadovnychiy, S. Explainable CAD System for Classification of Acute Lymphoblastic Leukemia Based on a Robust White Blood Cell Segmentation. *Cancers* **2023**, *15*, 3376. https://doi.org/10.3390/cancers15133376

Academic Editors: Marcin Woźniak and Muhammad Fazal Ijaz

Received: 6 May 2023
Revised: 25 June 2023
Accepted: 26 June 2023
Published: 27 June 2023

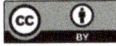

Copyright: © 2023 by the authors. Licensee MDPI, Basel, Switzerland. This article is an open access article distributed under the terms and conditions of the Creative Commons Attribution (CC BY) license (https://creativecommons.org/licenses/by/4.0/).

Simple Summary: Leukemia is a type of cancer that affects white blood cells and can lead to serious health problems and death. Diagnosing leukemia is currently performed through a combination of morphological and molecular criteria, which can be time-consuming and, in some cases, unreliable. Computer-aided diagnosis (CAD) systems based on deep-learning methods have shown promise in improving diagnosis efficiency and accuracy. However, these systems suffer from the "black box problem," which can lead to incorrect classifications. This research proposes a novel deep-learning approach with visual explainability for ALL diagnoses based on robust white blood cell nuclei segmentation to provide a highly reliable and interpretable classification. The aim is to develop a CAD system that can assist physicians in diagnosing leukemia more efficiently, potentially improving patient outcomes. The findings of this research may impact the research community by providing a more reliable and explainable deep-learning-based approach to blood disorder diagnosis.

Abstract: Leukemia is a significant health challenge, with high incidence and mortality rates. Computer-aided diagnosis (CAD) has emerged as a promising approach. However, deep-learning methods suffer from the "black box problem", leading to unreliable diagnoses. This research proposes an Explainable AI (XAI) Leukemia classification method that addresses this issue by incorporating a robust White Blood Cell (WBC) nuclei segmentation as a hard attention mechanism. The segmentation of WBC is achieved by combining image processing and U-Net techniques, resulting in improved overall performance. The segmented images are fed into modified ResNet-50 models, where the MLP classifier, activation functions, and training scheme have been tested for leukemia subtype classification. Additionally, we add visual explainability and feature space analysis techniques to offer an interpretable classification. Our segmentation algorithm achieves an Intersection over Union (IoU) of 0.91, in six databases. Furthermore, the deep-learning classifier achieves an accuracy of 99.9% on testing. The Grad CAM methods and clustering space analysis confirm improved network focus when classifying segmented images compared to non-segmented images. Overall, the proposed visual explainable CAD system has the potential to assist physicians in diagnosing leukemia and improving patient outcomes.

Keywords: acute lymphoblastic leukemia; deep-learning; XAI; nuclei segmentation; leukemia classification

1. Introduction

Blood disorders are among the most challenging problems in medical diagnosis and image processing, where blood samples can be used to analyze a person's state of health and diagnose various diseases such as allergies, infections, or cancer. Specifically, one of the most lethal cancers with the highest incidence rate is Leukemia, where malformation of the white blood cells causes serious health problems that can lead to death. Although WBCs are involved in protecting the human body, they are also susceptible to illness. The most critical pathological conditions of the white blood cells are blood cancers. As a consequence of malignant mutations in the lymphoid or myeloid cells, there is an uncontrolled proliferation of malformed cells that do not function correctly in the organism, causing a decrease in the patient's health and even death. This process of malformation and uncontrolled reproduction of white blood cells is called Leukemia [1,2].

Leukemia can be classified according to the type of malignant cell, either lymphoid or myeloid, or the speed of symptoms development, chronic or acute. Acute Lymphoblastic Leukemia (ALL) is the most common during childhood, and due to genetic factors, the most affected ethnicity worldwide by ALL is the Hispanic population [2]. Currently, the way to diagnose Leukemia is based on a mixture of morphological and molecular criteria. The morphological classification relies on the FAB (French-American-British) medical criteria, established on recognizing characteristics or patterns such as the number of white blood cells, shape, and size, among others, where it is possible to differentiate between the types [2,3].

One major disadvantage of this procedure is the time consumption for the specialist in the analysis of each sample and the reliability of the diagnosis [4]. In addition, in low-income countries where health systems are overwhelmed, the time to find an appointment for the performance of these tests is high, which can result in a late diagnosis. Computer Aided Diagnostic (CAD) systems assist physicians in routine tasks to diagnose more efficiently, accurately, and with shorter diagnostic times, providing a better outcome for the patient.

In particular, CAD systems based on Deep Learning methods have recently gained relevance due to the good metrics obtained in research articles. However, as Loddo and Putzu [5] stipulate, many of the systems based on Deep Learning, specifically segmentation and classification systems of blood smear images, need a deeper analysis of the results beyond the metrics and learning curves. One major challenge associated with Deep Learning models is the "Black box problem," where the lack of semantic associations between input data and predicted classes hinders interpretability. This means that although a Deep Learning model may achieve excellent metrics and accurately classify results, the underlying associations made by the model might be incorrect. This conveys a significant risk when applying these systems to different databases or integrating them into routine clinical practice.

The growing spectrum of diseases and the potential of Computer Diagnosis have sparked intense research into white blood cell (WBC) segmentation and leukemia classification. Propelled by progress in computer vision and Deep Learning, considerable strides have been taken in addressing the challenges intrinsic to WBC nuclei segmentation and leukemia classification [6,7].

Recent research has shown the positive impact of appropriate pre-segmentation on deep-learning classification in medical imaging. The research of Mahbod et al. [8] highlighted improved performance with the correct use of segmentation masks on dermoscopic images, however, when segmentation was applied inaccurately, it resulted in a decrease in model performance. Similarly, Al-masni et al. [9] found that feeding segmented skin lesions into an integrated computer-aided diagnosis (CAD) system resulted in more effective diagnostic classification.

In the context of WBC segmentation, one of the most relevant studies was carried out by Vogado et al. [10], where color space transformations from RGB to CMYK and Lab* were applied, followed by contrast adjustment and median filtering to enhance the image. Leukocytes were highlighted by subtracting the B channel from the M channel. K-means clustering and morphological operations were subsequently employed. Alternatively, Makem and Tiedeu [11] introduced a WBC nucleus segmentation method by leveraging color space transformations, arithmetical operations, and adaptive PCA fusion. Their approach demonstrated excellent performance with Dice Coefficients of 94.75%, 97.06%, and 90.79% on the BloodSeg, CellaVision, and JTSC databases, respectively, validating its effectiveness across diverse datasets. Meanwhile, Mousavi et al. [12] addressed the WBC nucleus segmentation problem by employing a color balancing method based on the color channels means, converting the image to CMYK and extracting the Magenta channel and then segmenting the image. This approach was trained and tested with 985 and 250 images from the Raabin WBC, respectively, obtaining a Dice Coefficient of 95.42%. After, Tavakoli et al. [13] developed a three-step method for WBC nucleus segmentation. Applying color balancing, RGB to HSL and CMYK conversions, and arithmetic operations to enhance nuclei visibility, followed by Otsu filtering for binarization. The method achieved a Dice Coefficient of 96.75% on a subset of 250 images from the Raabin WBC dataset.

Makem et al. [14] proposed a robust WBC segmentation method based on arithmetic operations and the Fourier transform. They segment the WBC using RGB space operations and Otsu thresholding, followed by Fourier-based image enhancement. The K-means algorithm is then applied for nuclei grouping and segmentation. The method achieved high segmentation accuracy on five databases, with Dice Coefficient results ranging from 86.02% to 97.35%. In comparison, Mayala and Haugsøen. [15] proposed a WBC segmentation method based on finding the minima between two local peaks in the image histogram analysis.

Ochoa-Montiel et al. [16] proposed an intermediate approach between handcrafted and deep-learning methods for WBC segmentation and ALL classification. They employ RGB to HSI transformation, Otsu's segmentation method, and handcrafted feature extraction techniques. Classification is performed using handcrafted approaches and deep-learning methods based on Alexnet and LeNet architectures.

In contrast, a few WBC segmentation schemes are based entirely on the Deep Learning approach. For example, Haider et al. [17] proposed a Deep Learning approach for WBC segmentation, specifically nucleus and cytoplasm segmentation. They introduced two networks, LDS-NET and LDAS-NET, which are modifications of U-NET with additional features such as residual connections. The combination of these features helps retain information and improve accuracy. The approach of Garcia-Lamont et al. [18] proposes six methods for WBC nucleus segmentation: CPNNHSV, CPNRGB (neural network-based), SOMHSV, SOMRGB (Self Organized Maps-based), and VarHSV, VarRGB (based on chromatic variance). This approach has been tested using three different databases with 660 images.

Zhou et al. [19] applied a modified version of U-Net, a well-known Deep Learning method used for segmentation. U-Net++ architecture modifies the plain skip connections for nested and dense skip connections to combine the high-resolution map feature. This algorithm was trained and tested with 989 and 250 images of the Raabin WBC database, respectively, reaching a Dice Coefficient of 97.19%. Similarly, Oktay et al. [20] proposed a new U-Net-based model with attention. This attention gate allows for highlighting relevant features and removing irrelevant ones resulting in better segmentation. The algorithm was implemented with the Raabin WBC dataset, trained and tested with 989 and 250 images, respectively, resulting in a Dice Coefficient of 96.33%. Finally, He et al. [21] enhanced the Faster R-CNN approach with the Mask R-CNN architecture for WBC segmentation. The method improves the segmentation results by introducing a connection between the convolutional feature maps and generating a masked ROI as an attention module.

The review of the state-of-the-art shows that WBC segmentation and Leukemia classification remains an active and evolving research area. In recent years, the significance of model interpretability and explainability has garnered increasing attention in medical diagnosis. Current methodologies encounter challenges regarding robustness and the elucidation of the underlying rationale behind model predictions. Traditional Handcraft approaches often involve intricate and non-intuitive segmentation steps and typically perform worse than AI models. Deep Learning methods, while achieving impressive performance, frequently suffer from the "Black box problem," difficulting in the reliability of the diagnosis. Thus, there is a pressing need to explore novel techniques prioritizing model interpretability and explainability. In addition, in assisted medical diagnosis systems, the doctor must understand the reasons that lead to a particular Deep Learning classification so that the physician can implement an accurate and reliable hybrid diagnosis.

In this article, we introduce a novel method for leukemia classification using Explainable Artificial Intelligence (XAI) and segmentation techniques. The unique feature of our approach lies in its use of segmentation as a form of 'hard attention' mechanism, which enhances the classifier's accuracy and interpretability by targeting the nucleus of white blood cells (WBCs). We demonstrate the robustness of our segmentation method by testing it across multiple databases. To make the network associations more tangible, we use gradient attention maps that visualize the relevance of various regions, considering both the intensity and location of the 'attention' within the Region of Interest (ROI). By focusing on the WBC nuclei before classification, our proposed method significantly improves the quantitative and qualitative criteria, outperforming classifiers that do not use segmentation. We also compare Deep Learning approaches and demonstrate the superior efficacy of the Mish activation function over the commonly used Rectified Linear Unit (ReLU). Through these findings, we hope to advance the field of leukemia classification by offering an approach that is not only more accurate but also more explainable.

Furthermore, this research has four main sections; Section 2 shows the datasets and the metrics used for evaluation; Section 3 presents the proposed methodology; Section 4 exhibits results as well as the discussion; finally Section 5 summarized scientific contributions of this research.

2. Materials

2.1. Datasets

This research used six databases with digitalized images of blood or bone marrow samples. A total of 2823 different images were used to test the developed method. The databases employed have different characteristics concerning each other, such as the number and size of white blood cells, image color, saturation, illumination, etc.

- Leukemia Dataset [16] is formed by 651 classified images of Acute Lymphoblastic Leukemia according to FAB classification (217-ALL1, 217-ALL2, 217-ALL3), with dimensions of 256×320 pixels. This dataset is the only one in the state-of-the-art that labels the different types of Acute Lymphoblastic Leukemia with reliability through cytogenetic tests.
- CellaVision [22] is made up of 100 blood samples, and each image has dimensions of 300×300 pixels and a bit depth of 24 bits. This dataset usually consists of a single cell, and the core color is violet, while the background has pinkish and yellowish tints.
- JTSC [22] is made by the Jiangxi Telecom Science Corporation in China. This dataset consists of 300 images of 120×120 pixels containing the GT of the nucleus and cytoplasm for comparative analysis. It contains a wide variability among its samples since there are cells in which the nucleus has a highly saturated coloration, while in others, the nucleus is almost translucent. Furthermore, the image's background varies from an intense yellow to a pinkish white.
- SMC_ID (Blood_Seg) [23] is composed of 367 images of WBC with a size of 640×480 pixels. Each sample characterizes by the GT of the nucleus, which facilitates its analysis. Commonly, the images that integrate this dataset have a cell nucleus with low color saturation. Additionally, the WBC is located in diverse positions over the image.
- Raabin_WBC [24]. It provides 1145 images of blood samples, with dimensions of 545×545 pixels, where white blood cells are subdivided into 242 lymphocytes, 242 monocytes, 242 neutrophils, 201 eosinophils, and 218 basophils. Each of these 1145 samples also contains a ground truth, both whole cell and nucleus. This is one of the best databases by now, as it has numerous samples of different cell types classified and annotated with ground truth for analysis and comparison of results.

- ALL_IDB2 [25]. It consists of 260 images of 257 × 257 pixels. This dataset derives from the ALL-IDB1 dataset, where individual cells have been cropped to obtain the region of interest.

Examples of the datasets used in the research are shown in Figure 1.

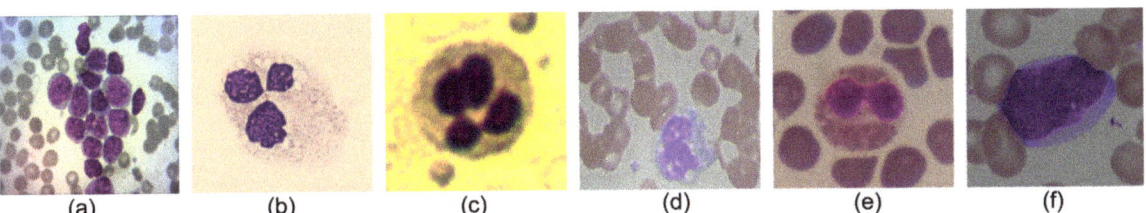

Figure 1. Used dataset images: Leukemia Dataset (**a**), CellaVision (**b**); JTSC (**c**); BloodSeg (**d**); Raabin_WBC (**e**); ALL_IDB2 (**f**).

2.2. Metrics

For evaluating the proposed segmentation and classification method, seven of the most widely used metrics were employed [26]:

- **Accuracy** value measures the appropriate classification over the total elements.

$$Acc = \frac{T_P + T_N}{T_P + T_N + F_P + F_N}. \qquad (1)$$

- **Precision** metric estimates the number of elements correctly classified among all the positive elements to evaluate.

$$Pre = \frac{T_P}{T_P + F_P}. \qquad (2)$$

- **Recall** also known as sensitivity, is used to denote the number of positive elements that are correctly classified.

$$Rec = \frac{T_P}{T_P + F_N}. \qquad (3)$$

- **Specificity** measures the proportion of true negatives that are successfully identified by the model.

$$Spec = \frac{T_N}{T_N + F_P}. \qquad (4)$$

- **Dice Similarity Coefficient** or DSC can be considered to be a harmonic mean of precision and recall. Furthermore, known as F1-Score.

$$DSC = 2 * \frac{Precision * Recall}{Precision + Recall}. \qquad (5)$$

- **Intersection over Union** also known as Jaccard Index is the most important metric in image segmentation tasks since it measures the magnitude of overlap between the GT and the segmented image.

$$IoU = \frac{T_P}{T_P + F_P + F_N}. \qquad (6)$$

were **TP** represents true positives, **TN** true negatives, **FP** false positives and **FN** false negatives.

3. Proposed Method

In this work, a novel CAD system for Acute Lymphoblastic Leukemia classification was developed. The novel approach relies on an ensemble state of art white blood cell segmentation that acts as a hard attention mechanism for the network, increasing diagnostic accuracy and reliability. Furthermore, a visual Grad CAM interpretation with four gradient activations maps (GradCAM, GRADCAM++, Hi-Res-CAM, Xgrad-CAM) and a clustering space analysis increase the reliability of the method. The proposed system diagram is shown in Figure 2. Below, each of the three phases of the method is presented.

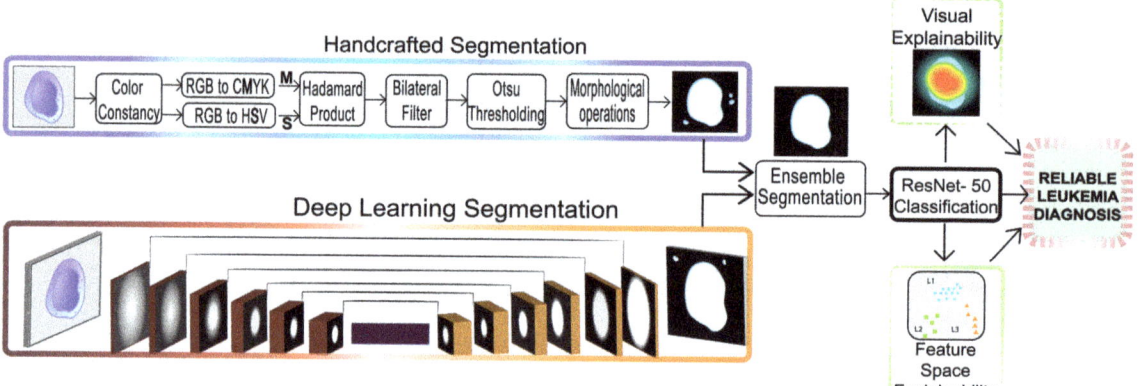

Figure 2. Proposed Method.

3.1. Handcrafted WBC Nuclei Segmentation

This research proposes a new robust and consistent segmentation method for differentiating the WBC nucleus from the rest of the sample. To address the issue of color variations between blood samples, caused by factors such as illumination, microscope type, and staining, a method proposed by Hedge et al. [27] is employed. This method involves multiplying the original RGB channels by a weight calculated based on the ratio between the average grayscale intensity and the average intensity of the respective channel (Red, Green, and Blue), as can be seen below in Equation (7). By applying this approach, the colors in the samples are homogenized, enhancing the tonal consistency across different datasets and improving the method's applicability and robustness.

$$CC_{Channel} = ChannelIntensity \left(\frac{mean\ Grayscale}{mean\ ChannelIntensity} \right). \quad (7)$$

We enhance the WBC nucleus by matching image tonalities and employing color space transformations (RGB to CMYK and HSV). Guided by purple tonalities and high saturation in the ROI region, the Saturation and Magenta channels are combined using the Hadamard product to highlight nuclei and remove unwanted elements. The bilateral filter [28] is employed after the Hadamard product to refine the segmentation process further to eliminate image noise and blur the WBC nucleus. This step ensures that any regions potentially lost during the Hadamard product operation are recovered while maintaining the original shape and integrity of the cell edges. The grayscale image is then transformed to a binary image via the adaptive Otsu Thresholding [29], resulting in an image where the WBC nuclei are highlighted in white and the other components of the image in black.

Since areas with holes could be found in the nucleus of the binarized image, the morphological transformations of closing and filling holes are applied to improve the segmentation process. The closing eliminates the small black regions, filling holes operation dilates the white regions within the WBC nucleus. Finally, a filter by ROI pixel area removes small spurious elements that remain, where the elements with a smaller area of pixels than those established by the threshold are eliminated from the image. All the presented steps of the WBC nuclei segmentation method can be summarized in Algorithm 1.

Algorithm 1 Proposed Handcrafted WBC Nuclei Segmentation.

1: Read RGB image
2: $CC\_RGB \leftarrow Apply\ Color\ Constancy\ to\ RGB\ image$
3: $CMYK_{Image} \leftarrow Transform\ CC\_RGB\ to\ CMYK$
4: $M \leftarrow split(CMYK_{Image})$
5: $HSV_{Image} \leftarrow Transform\ CC\_RGB\ to\ HSV$
6: $S \leftarrow split(HSV_{Image})$
7: $Mult_{Image} \leftarrow M \odot S\ (Hadamard\ Product)$
8: $Bilateral_{Image} \leftarrow BilateralFilter(Mult_{Image})$
9: $Binarized_{Image} \leftarrow Th\_Otsu(Bilateral_{Image})$
10: $Binarized_{Image} \leftarrow Closing(Binarized_{Image})$
11: $Binarized_{Image} \leftarrow Fill\_Holes(Binarized_{Image})$
12: $AreaFilter_{Image} \leftarrow Binarized_{Image} >= pixel\ number$
13: $Segmented_{Image} \leftarrow Mask(AreaFilter_{Image}, RGB\ Image)$

3.2. Deep Learning WBC Nuclei Segmentation

The encoder-decoder architecture, U-Net [30], was implemented for the Deep Learning segmentation phase. The encoder downsamples the input image and extracts high-level features, while the decoder upsamples the features to reconstruct the original image size and generate a segmentation map. The skip connections between the encoder and decoder help to preserve spatial information and enable precise segmentation of objects. Our implementation of the UNet model has the following structure: Designed for 2-dimensional spatial inputs, begins with an input of 3 channels. The model progresses through five distinct levels, each corresponding to a different size of the channel, expanding from 32 to 512. At each level, the model performs downsampling using strided convolutions, with strides of 1 at the first level, and 2 at subsequent levels. The model employs Instance Normalization, includes a dropout rate of 0.5 for regularization, and uses the Mish activation function for non-linearity [31] (see Equation (8))

$$Mish(x) = x * tanh(ln((1 + e^x)) \,. \tag{8}$$

Furthermore, we used the state-of-the-art Unified Focal Loss function [32] as a loss function for our UNet-based model, which can improve the segmentation due to its better handling of class imbalance and the combination of Focal Loss, Equation (9), (distribution-based loss) and Tversky Loss, Equation (10), (region-based loss).

$$\mathcal{L}_{mFocalLoss} = \delta(1-p)^{1-\gamma} * \mathcal{L}_{BinaryCrossEntropy} \,. \tag{9}$$

$$\mathcal{L}_{mFocalTverskyLoss} = \sum_{c=1}^{C}(1-mTI)^{\gamma} \,. \tag{10}$$

$$\mathcal{L}_{Unified\ Focal\ Loss} = \lambda\mathcal{L}_{mFocalLoss} + (1-\lambda)\mathcal{L}_{mFocalTverskyLoss} \,. \tag{11}$$

For Unified Focal Loss, see Equation (11), the three tuning parameters are defined as: δ controls the relative weighting of positive and negative classes, γ manages the suppression of background classes and the attention of rare classes, and lastly, λ handles the weights between the distribution-based loss and the region-based loss.

3.3. Ensemble Segmentation

Ensemble segmentation is a technique for improving the accuracy and robustness of image segmentation using multiple segmentation models. Combining the predictions of several models can improve the overall performance of the segmentation. The novel method employs a Hybrid ensemble segmentation technique. By combining the proposed Handcrafted and Deep Learning segmentations, we can overcome the limitations of individual approaches and produce more reliable segmentation results. Since the biggest problem in both segmentation methods was the false positives, the logical AND operation was used to merge both masks, significantly reducing the number of false positives and increasing the stability of the ensemble segmentation. For instance, when one of the two methods does not correctly remove a non-ROI region and the other does, this non-ROI region is removed from the Ensemble segmentation mask. After the fusion technique, we applied an area opening as a post-processing operation.

$$Ensemble\ Mask = Handcrafted Mask \wedge Deep Learning Mask . \quad (12)$$

3.4. ALL Classification

In this study, the proposed classifier is based on ResNet-50 [33], which through their residual connections, allows a better back-propagated gradient flow through the network, contributing simultaneously to assembling more layers in a CNN network while improving the network's learning. Since the ResNet-50 architecture forms a vector of 2048 features in the Fully Connected layer, and the proposed method attempts to classify three classes of Leukemia, it is necessary to modify the MLP classifier layer. It has been proposed two different configurations: One going from 2048 to 1024-512-3 (Medium) and the other from 2048 to 3 (Linear). The objective behind the different classifiers configurations is based on the assumption that adding more hidden layers is needed to approximate the feature function of each class, leading to a classification improvement.

To find the best classifier for this problem, eight models were trained based on ResNet-50, changing the activation function, the number of hidden layers and neurons in the MLP classifier, and the input images, Segmented and NoSegmented, as is shown in Table 1:

Table 1. Summary of the different modifications in the developed models.

	Input Image
Segmented	Train the model with the previously Segmented Images
NoSegmented (Ablation)	Train the model with the original images (No Segmented Images) (Traditional manner)
	MLP Classifier
Linear	Modify the MLP classifier from 2048 to 3 neurons
Medium	Modify the MLP classifier from 2048 to 1024-512-3 neurons
	Activation Function
Mish	Change all the activation functions of the model to Mish, including MLP classifier
ReLU	Change all the activation functions of the model to ReLU, including MLP classifier

3.5. Visual Explainability

A crucial component of our proposed method is the integration of a visual explainability stage, which aims to provide insights into the network's learning process and ensure that the regions of interest (ROIs) are accurately identified during Deep Learning classification. This step enhances the method's overall effectiveness and enables clinicians to interpret the results generated by the network. Since, in the field of Deep Learning interpretability, there is currently no consensus on the best metrics-based approach for activation map generation, and it is known that each method could highlight different regions. Therefore, we perform a comprehensive analysis of four gradient-based methods, namely GRAD-CAM [34],

Grad CAM++ [35], HiRes-CAM [36], and XGrad-CAM [37]. By examining these methods' outputs, we ensure a robust evaluation of the network's attention and activation patterns. This approach enables us to better understand the network's decision-making process and further strengthens the interpretability of our proposed method.

3.6. Clustering Space Analysis

We introduced a clustering space analysis to visualize class predictions in the proposed method to enhance reliability and robustness. By obtaining the logits of each sample in the test set and their corresponding true targets, a 3-dimensional map was generated where the coordinates represented class predictions (L1, L2, and L3). Principal Component Analysis (PCA) was applied to reduce dimensionality and visualize clusters. This visualization technique allowed us to observe how the network grouped classes in the logits space, aiming to maximize inter-class variance and minimize intra-class variance. The analysis included calculating the Euclidean distance between cluster centroids to measure inter-class variance and using the standard deviation of "PC1" and "PC2" within each cluster to quantify intra-class variance. Recognizing the significance of inter-cluster distance in class prediction, we introduced the Dist/SD Ratio, a weighted ratio of 3-1 Distance/SD intra-class. We think that models amplifying this ratio may exhibit superior robustness when clustering-classifying new data, reflecting better class separability and tighter intra-class clustering for enhanced generalization performance, as is shown in Figure 3.

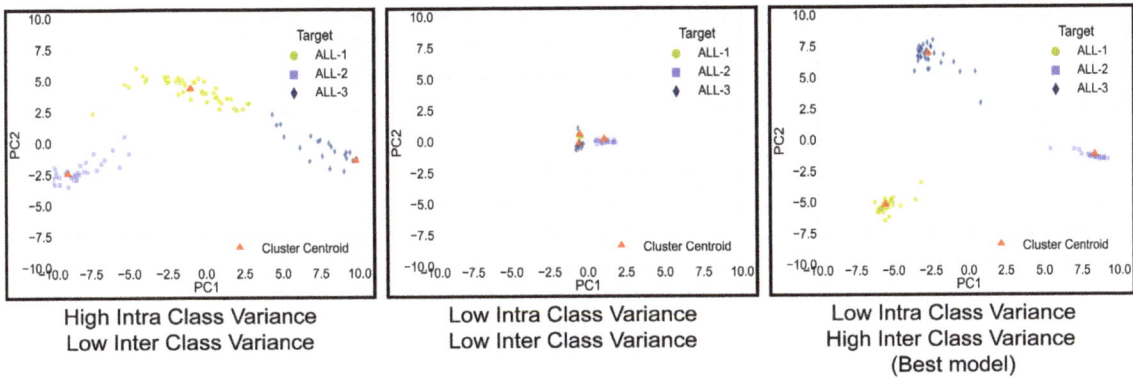

Figure 3. Model clustering space comparison. Where the best model is the one that enhances inter-class distance and reduces intra-class separability.

4. Results and Discussion

4.1. Segmentation Results

The handcrafted segmentation method was implemented using a PC, with an Intel Core i7-4510U processor, 8 GB RAM, the operating system Windows 64-bit, using Python version 3.9.7 and the libraries Scikit-image[38] and OpenCV [39]. The deep-learning segmentation was made in a Google Colab environment, using a Tesla T4 GPU, Pytorch v1.12.1 [40], Scikit-learn [41] and Monai [42]. A 10-fold cross-validation was used to assess the predictive performance of the proposed model. The dataset was randomly shuffled and divided into 10 equal parts or folds. During each iteration, nine of these folds were used for training the model, while the remaining fold was reserved for testing. This process was repeated 10 times, with each fold as the test set once. The model's performance was evaluated on diverse data by rotating the test set across different folds improving reliability, [43,44]. Furthermore, we applied data augmentation techniques on the fly [45], such as VerticalFlip, HorizontalFlip, RandomRotate90, Transpose with a probability of $p = 0.5$ and RandomGamma, CLAHE, GaussNoise with $p = 0.2$ and a Resize (256,256) with $p = 1$. General hyperparameters were: Adam optimizer, unified focal loss, and ReduceLROnPlateau. Specific hyperparameters, for each UNet such as lambda, delta, gamma, learning rate, dropout probability, and weight decay, can be seen in Table A2.

The proposed WBC nuclei segmentation method was evaluated in Leukemia Dataset, CellaVision, JTSC, SMC_IDB, Raabin_WBC, and ALL_IDB2 datasets. Figure 4 compares the three proposed methods on two images, one of JTSC and one from the Leukemia dataset. It can be seen that the combination of both methods, Handcraft and Deep, results in improved segmentation, even with the color differences or cell numbers in the images.

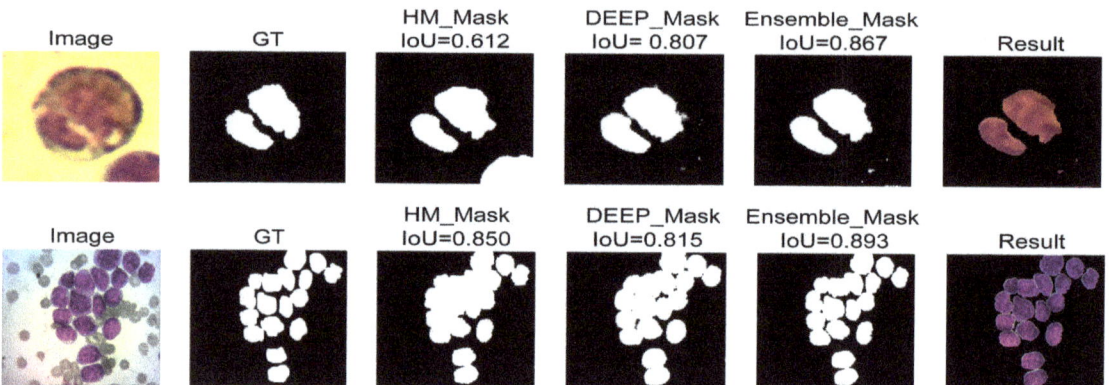

Figure 4. Comparison between HM, DEEP, and Ensemble results.

Further perceptual results of the Ensemble method are shown in Figure 5, where a cyan border surrounds the segmented WBC nuclei. From the figure, one can perceive the overall accuracy of the segmentation method, despite the differences in saturation, color, transparency of the cells, etc.

Meanwhile, the quantitative results were obtained by comparing segmented images against their GT. Seven different quality metrics were used to assess the performance of the proposed methods. In Table 2, it can be seen that the proposed method obtains competitive results for all the databases and all the proposed quality metrics. These high-performance results confirm the robustness of the proposed segmentation system, where this system appears to demonstrate minimal variability in the output results despite changes in the input.

Table 2. Results of the proposed Ensemble method for the WBC datasets.

Dataset	Acc (%)	Pre (%)	Rec (%)	Spec (%)	DSC (%)	IoU
Leukemia Dataset	98.50	88.32	95.03	98.59	91.16	0.840
CellaVision	99.32	97.08	97.88	99.57	97.40	0.951
JTSC	99.03	96.38	96.09	99.50	96.10	0.926
SMC_IDB	99.62	95.57	96.30	99.81	95.78	0.920
Raabin_WBC	98.99	97.38	94.71	99.65	94.83	0.923
ALL_IDB2	98.51	93.45	97.14	98.60	95.14	0.910
AVERAGE	**99.00**	**94.77**	**96.19**	**99.28**	**95.69**	**0.917**

Moreover to general results, the proposed system is explicitly compared using each of the databases and against recent state-of-the-art methods. The results derived from these comparisons can be seen in Tables 3 and 4.

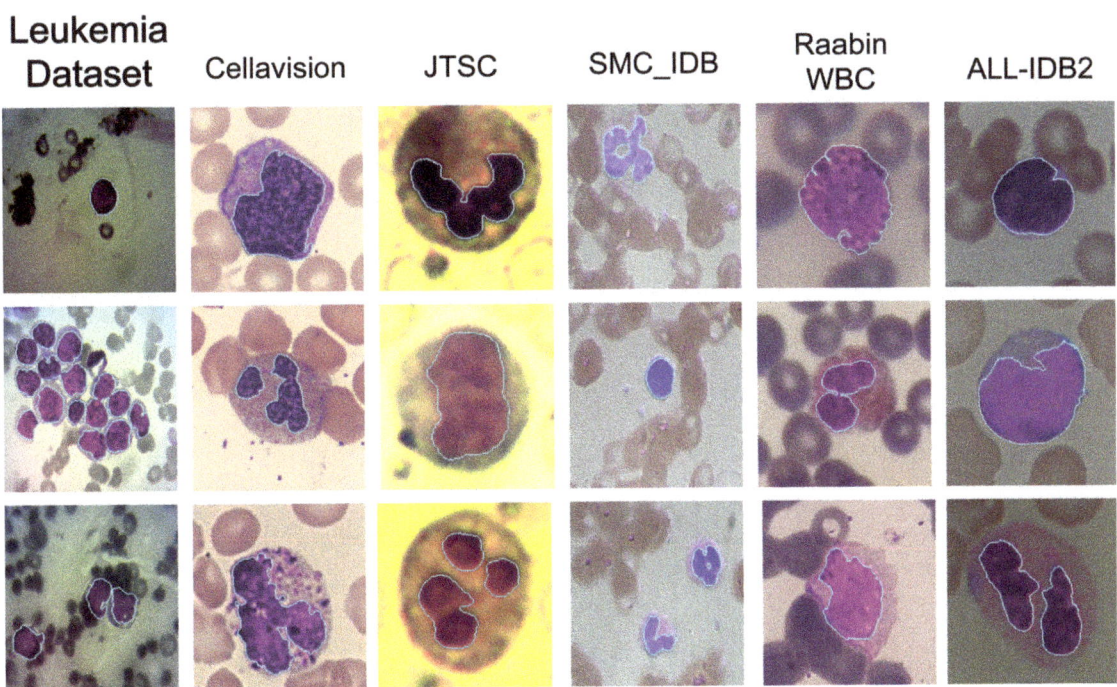

Figure 5. Qualitative results of the ensemble segmentation method on the six datasets. Cyan color borders the segmented nuclei.

Table 3. Leukemia Dataset WBC nuclei segmentation results. The best results are in bold, and the second best is underlined.

	Leukemia Dataset					
Method	Acc (%)	Pre (%)	Rec (%)	Spec (%)	DSC (%)	IoU
Proposed HM	97.96	82.43	**97.63**	97.70	89.01	0.806
Proposed DEEP	<u>98.30</u>	<u>85.82</u>	95.81	<u>98.30</u>	<u>90.02</u>	<u>0.823</u>
Proposed Ensemble	**98.50**	**88.32**	<u>95.03</u>	**98.59**	**91.16**	**0.840**

The training and validation plots for each fold were obtained for evaluating the adequate training of each U-Net model, as shown in Figure 6. From these graphs, it is possible to observe the correct network learning for Cellavision and the other databases. The rest of the curves can be found in Figure A1.

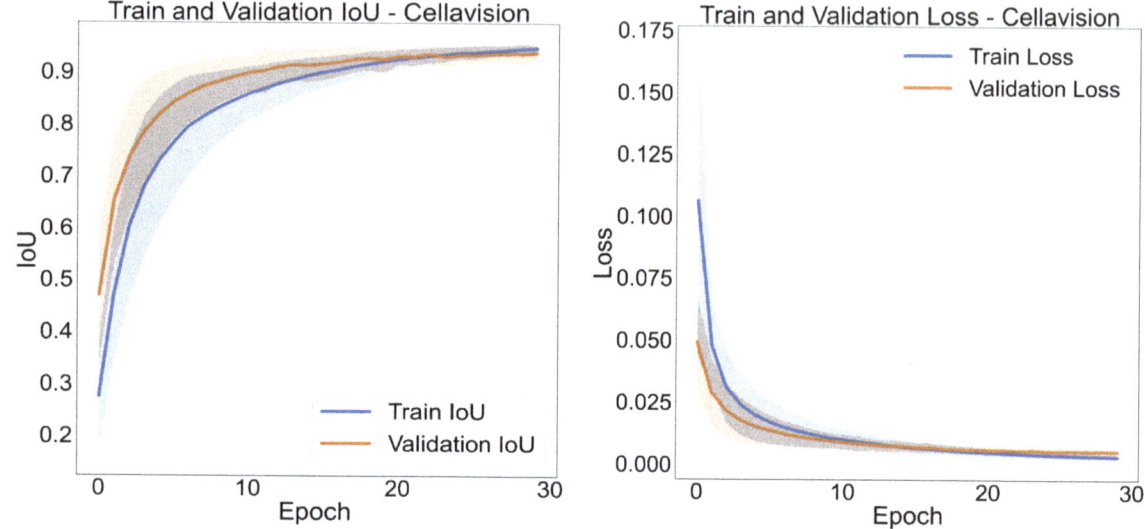

Figure 6. Training and Validation Intersection Over Union and Loss curves for the 10 folds.

Table 4. WBC nuclei segmentation comparison. The best results are in bold, and the second best is underlined.

			Cellavision				
Method	Acc (%)	Pre (%)	Rec (%)	Spec (%)	DSC (%)	IoU	# Test Images
Vogado et al. [10]	98.77	97.88	**99.75**	89.39	93.22	0.873	100
Makem & Tiedeu [11]	<u>99.37</u>	97.37	96.97	-	97.06	0.945	100
CPNNHSV [18]	99.2	94.86	97.31	99.41	96.31	0.929	100
Makem et al. [14]	**99.43**	97.31	97.60	**99.61**	97.35	0.950	100
LDS-NET [17]	-	<u>98.48</u>	95.91	-	97.18	0.945	20
LDAS-NET [17]	-	**99.09**	97.11	-	**98.09**	**0.963**	20
Proposed Ensemble	99.32	97.08	97.88	<u>99.57</u>	97.40	<u>0.951</u>	100
			JTSC				
Method	Acc (%)	Pre (%)	Rec (%)	Spec (%)	DSC (%)	IoU	# Test Images
Vogado et al. [10]	97.13	93.55	**98.99**	83.18	87.68	0.781	300
Makem & Tiedeu [11]	97.29	91.01	93.12	-	90.79	0.843	300
VarRGB [18]	<u>98.38</u>	91.10	96.29	98.68	93.88	0.885	300
Makem et al. [14]	97.79	93.64	97.60	98.43	93.17	0.884	300
Mayala & Haugsøen [15]	-	94.89	95.30	<u>99.31</u>	94.81	0.903	300
LDS-NET [17]	-	<u>98.85</u>	92.39	-	95.56	0.917	60
LDAS-NET [17]	-	94.42	<u>98.36</u>	-	**96.35**	**0.931**	60
Proposed Ensemble	**99.03**	96.38	96.09	**99.50**	96.10	<u>0.926</u>	300
			SMC_IDB (BloodSeg)				
Method	Acc (%)	Pre (%)	Rec (%)	Spec (%)	DSC (%)	IoU	# Test Images
Vogado et al. [10]	99.15	80.51	94.51	<u>99.30</u>	86.46	0.761	367
Makem & Tiedeu. [11]	**99.63**	**92.99**	**97.06**	-	94.75	0.902	367
Makem et al. [14]	97.67	91.27	<u>96.93</u>	97.82	93.48	0.883	367
Proposed Ensemble	<u>99.62</u>	**95.57**	96.30	**99.81**	**95.78**	**0.920**	367

Table 4. Cont.

Method	Acc (%)	Pre (%)	Rec (%)	Spec (%)	DSC (%)	IoU	# Test Images
			Raabin				
U-Net ++ [19]	-	95.98	98.73	-	97.19	0.945	250
Attention U-Net [20]	-	94.78	98.50	-	96.33	0.929	250
Mask R-CNN [21]	-	8.59	96.80	-	91.98	0.852	250
Mousavi et al. [12].	-	93.62	98.27	-	95.42	0.912	250
Tavakoli et al. [13].	-	**99.72**	95.26	-	96.75	0.936	250
Proposed Ensemble	**98.99**	97.38	94.71	**99.65**	94.83	0.923	1145

Method	Acc (%)	Pre (%)	Rec (%)	Spec (%)	DSC (%)	IoU	# Test Images
			ALL_IDB2				
Vogado et al. [10]	**98.59**	91.24	**98.09**	98.62	94.17	0.890	300
CPNNHSV.[18]	98.32	91.59	96.11	**98.66**	93.42	0.877	300
Proposed Ensemble	98.51	**93.45**	97.14	98.60	**95.14**	**0.910**	300

4.2. Leukemia Classification

For the classification stage of the method, previously segmented images from the Leukemia Dataset were used for the **Segmented** Models and Original Images for the **Non-Segmented** Models. Both datasets were divided into a 90% Train-Validation split and a 10% Test split. A stratified K-fold with 10 folds was then applied to the Train-Validation Split. Each model was trained for 30 epochs during each K-fold. For each training set in the K-fold, 'on the fly' data augmentation operations were applied, including Vertical Flip, Horizontal Flip, RandomRotate90, Random Gamma, CLAHE, Transpose, and Gaussian Noise, each with a probability of $p = 0.5$. Finally, all the images were transformed with Resize (232), CenterCrop (224), and Normalize (mean = (0.485, 0.456, 0.406), std = (0.229, 0.224, 0.225)). The hyperparameters of the ResNet-50 models included a batch size of 8, a learning rate of 1×10^{-5}, an Adam optimizer with a weight decay of 1×10^{-4}, cross-entropy loss, and the ReduceLROnPlateau learning rate scheduler.

The top four results from the ten K-fold validations across the eight models are presented in Table 5, while the corresponding training and validation plots can be found in Figure A2. These results provide evidence for the accuracy of the proposed classifier.

Table 5. Best results for the train-validation 10 K-fold.

Model	Acc (%)
Segmented Mish Medium	99.99
NoSegmented ReLU Medium	99.97
Segmented Mish Linear	99.97
No Segmented ReLU Linear	99.97

Comparing our method with six classifiers used by Ochoa-Montiel et al. for the Leukemia Dataset reveals that deep-learning-based methods, such as LeNet, AlexNet, and our proposed method, yield superior results in contrast to handcrafted methods such as MLP and Random Forest (see Table 6). Our study presents methods that are competitive within this landscape. However, as outlined in the Related Work (Section 1) and Methods (Section 3) sections, we go a step further by extending our analysis beyond conventional metrics. We incorporate Explainable AI (XAI) and clustering space analysis to affirm the robustness and reliability of our model [5,7].

Table 6. Performance Comparison for ALL Classification. The best results are in bold, and the second best is underlined.

Method	Validation Accuracy (%)
Random_Forest Set_Full. [16]	97.08
LeNet. [16]	98.36
AlexNet. [16]	<u>99.98</u>
Proposed Method	**99.99**

4.3. Clustering Space Analysis Results

In this phase, 10% of the hold-out datasets were used to test the robustness of the model. Transformations commonly found in real environments [46], such as MotionBlur (blur_limit = 5), MultiplicativeNoise, GaussNoise (var_limit = 10, mean = 0), were applied to each image, in addition to the transformations mentioned in Section 4.2. Table 7 demonstrates that the two most robust models, yielding the best metrics, are those trained on segmented images, specifically with the Mish and ReLU activations, respectively. In contrast, the models most sensitive to daily noise are those trained on raw, non-segmented images.

Table 7. Best and worst models in Test Dataset. The best results are in bold, and the second best is underlined.

	Test Dataset			
Architecture	Acc (%)	Pre (%)	Rec (%)	F1 (%)
Segmented Mish Medium	**100**	**100**	**100**	**100**
<u>Segmented ReLU Medium</u>	<u>98.50</u>	<u>98.60</u>	<u>98.50</u>	<u>98.50</u>
No Segmented ReLU Linear	89.40	89.70	89.40	89.40
No Segmented Mish Medium	80.30	87.60	80.30	80.30

On the other hand, the results of the clustering analysis, shown in Table 8, indicate that the two best models, those that improve inter-class separability and decrease intra-class separability, are the segmented models with Mish and ReLU activations. In contrast, the models with the poorest clustering results are the unsegmented ones. The visual results from the aforementioned tables are presented in Figure 7. Here, the 'Segmented Mish Medium' model, shown in Figure 7a, performs the best in clustering and achieves higher separability, suggesting that it is learning features that better differentiate the classes. Conversely, the 'NoSegmented' model, shown in Figure 7b, has lower intra-class separability, making classification more difficult. This leads to the classification results that can be appreciated at their respective confusion matrix.

Table 8. Prediction Cluster Analysis on the test dataset. The best separability results are bold, and the second best is underlined.

	Dist L1–L2	Dist L2–L3	Dist L1–L3	Dist Total	SD Cluster L1	SD Cluster L2	SD Cluster L3	SD Total	Ratio Dist/SD
SegmentedMish Medium	**10.12**	**8.22**	**7.31**	**25.65**	2.05	0.68	2.06	2.99	**25.78**
<u>Segmented ReLU Medium</u>	<u>6.60</u>	<u>5.17</u>	<u>3.65</u>	<u>15.41</u>	1.09	1.43	<u>0.66</u>	1.92	<u>24.12</u>
NoSegmented ReLU Linear	3.94	3.34	2.99	10.27	1.32	1.60	1.33	2.46	12.52
NoSegmented Mish Linear	3.15	2.08	1.88	7.11	**0.94**	1.49	**0.50**	**1.83**	11.63

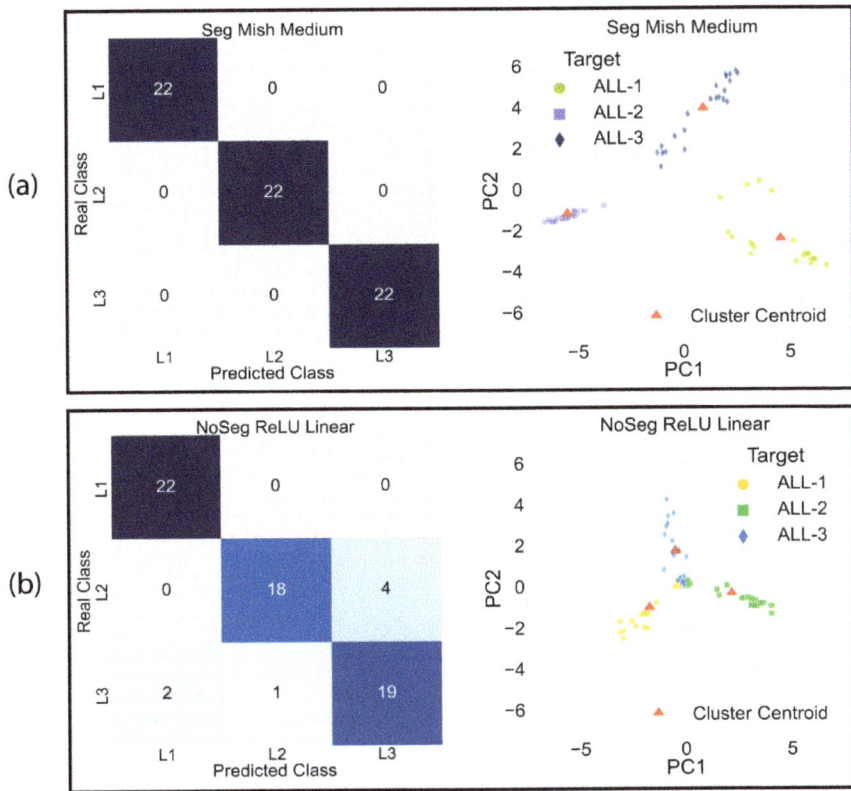

Figure 7. Clustering comparison between the best model Segmented Mish Medium in (**a**) and the worst model in No Segmented ReLU Linear (**b**).

4.4. Class Activation Maps

The class activation maps for the 'Segmented Mish Medium' and 'NoSegmented ReLU Linear' models are shown in Figure 8. From these, it is apparent that applying segmentation to the WBC images, as shown in Figure 8a, allows the network to focus precisely where the WBC kernels are located. Conversely, in Figure 8b, the network is easily distracted due to the shared similarities between the WBC and blood cell characteristics.

By employing various activation maps, we can discern the semantic connections inferred by the network for classification. This is illustrated in Figure 9, where the network makes two distinct semantic associations from the same images in the Test Dataset, both leading to correct classifications. The segmented image model accurately classifies L3 with a high confidence level of 0.999, attributable to the model's focus on the WBC. On the other hand, the 'NoSegmented' model also correctly classifies L3 but with a reduced confidence level of 0.734, indicating that the model may be making associations atypical to L3. For additional results, see Table A3.

Finally, based on the previous results, the 'Segmented Mish Medium' model emerged as the best overall for classification, as it improves both classification performance and explainability. Summary results from our proposed method can be found in Figure 10.

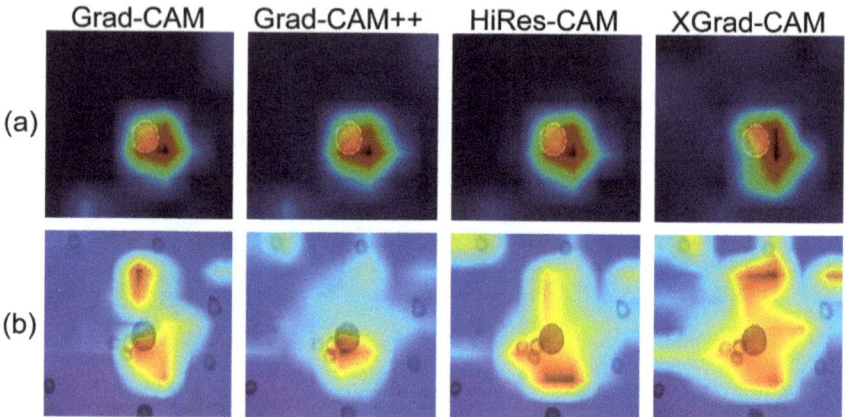

Figure 8. Comparison of Gradient Class Activation Maps between Segmented Mish Medium in (**a**) and NoSegmented ReLU Linear in (**b**). Red highlighted areas indicate more attention, while deep blue areas mean null attention.

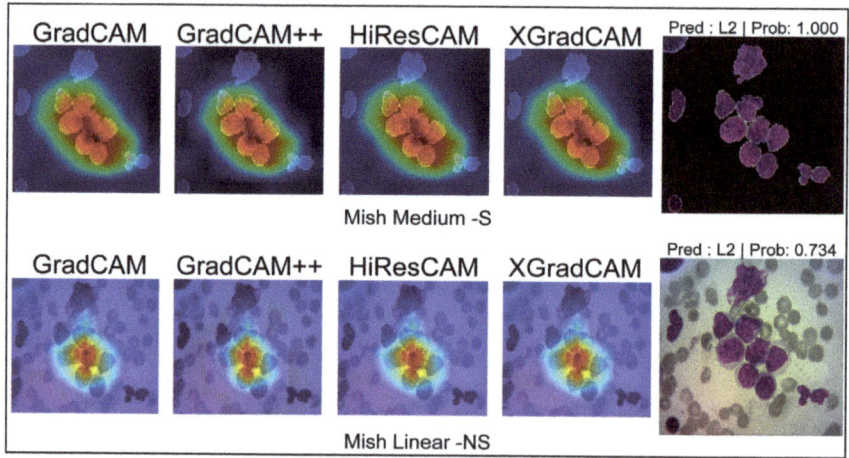

Figure 9. Comparison of Gradient Class Activation Maps between Segmented Model Mish Medium and NoSegmented Mish Linear. Red highlighted areas indicate more attention, while deep blue areas mean null attention.

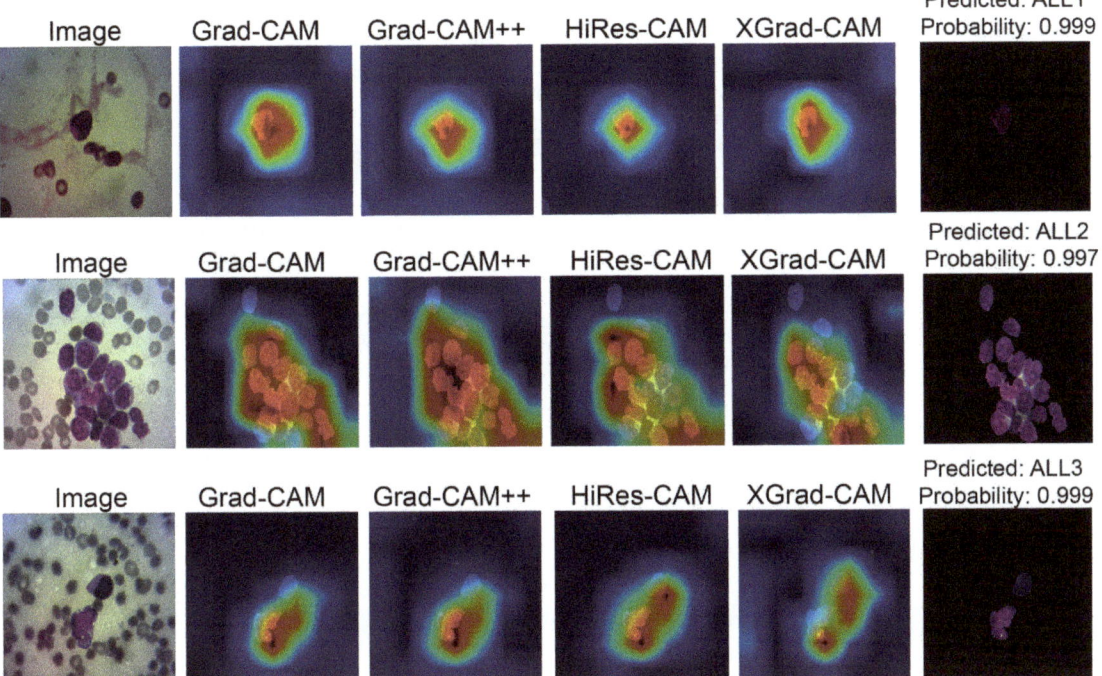

Figure 10. Visual explainability and classification results. The input image is segmented to enhance ResNet-50 attention; then, the image is classified with high accuracy. Red highlighted areas indicate more attention, while deep blue areas mean null attention.

4.5. Discussion

Our experimental results underscore the advantages of integrating a highly accurate handcrafted segmentation algorithm with deep-learning-based segmentation. This combination has proven to significantly enhance the classification process. Employing a pre-segmentation approach as a hard attention mechanism prior to the classification of a Leukemia Dataset not only improves the quantitative outcomes but also enhances the model's explainability. Furthermore, segmented models have demonstrated the capability to direct greater attention to the Region of Interest (ROI) for white blood cells (WBCs). The fusion of these methodologies significantly boosts model interpretability and reliability through the attention mechanism and visual explanation. It also paves the way for analyzing the logit space generated by the models through cluster space analysis. This could provide measures of class separability and indirectly assess the model's ability to extract high-quality deep features that enhance classification.

This integrated segmentation approach could help to improve the segmentation and differentiation of cytoplasm in various cells and could be a valuable preprocessing step for classifying other malignancies.

Despite the promising results produced by our methodology, there is room for further enhancement. The need for labeled images, while necessary, is time-consuming and prone to errors. Future research could address these challenges by exploring unsupervised or deep reinforcement learning. Additionally, the incorporation of modern diagnostic techniques, such as Flow cytometric immunophenotyping, into morphology-based studies could lead to a more comprehensive and robust diagnostic tool by combining genetic and morphological characteristics.

5. Conclusions

In this research, we developed a novel Computer-Aided Diagnosis (CAD) system for Acute Lymphoblastic Leukemia (ALL) classification. This innovative system utilizes an ensemble of state-of-the-art white blood cell segmentation techniques, functioning as a hard attention mechanism, and has achieved a remarkable Intersection over Union (IoU) of 0.91 across six databases. Our ResNet-50 model, equipped with the hard attention mechanism provided by the white blood cell segmentation, demonstrated enhanced performance. Furthermore, we ensured greater transparency by incorporating visual Grad CAM interpretation and clustering analysis. The developed CAD system represents a significant step forward in improving the accuracy of ALL diagnoses, potentially leading to better patient outcomes.

In terms of future work, we plan to expand our model to classify various types of white blood cells and synergize image and genetic data to create a more powerful ensemble classifier.

Author Contributions: J.L.D.R.: Conceptualization, Methodology, Software, Validation, Formal Analysis, Investigation, Resources, Writing—Original Draft; V.P.: Conceptualization, Methodology, Formal analysis, Writing—Review & Editing, Supervision, Project Administration, Funding acquisition; R.R.R.: Conceptualization, Methodology, Resources, Data Curation, Supervision, Project administration; S.S.: Conceptualization, Methodology, Formal analysis, Supervision. All authors have read and agreed to the published version of the manuscript.

Funding: This research received no external funding.

Institutional Review Board Statement: Not applicable.

Informed Consent Statement: Not applicable.

Data Availability Statement: The code presented in this study shall be made available upon reasonable request to the corresponding author for academic purposes.

Acknowledgments: The authors would like to thank Instituto Politecnico Nacional (IPN) (Mexico), Comision de Operacion y Fomento de Actividades Economicas (COFAA) of IPN, and the Consejo Nacional de Humanidades, Ciencias y Tecnologias (Mexico) for their support in this work.

Conflicts of Interest: The authors declare no conflict of interest.

Appendix A. Segmentation and Classification Parameter's and Extra Results

Appendix A.1. WBC Nuclei Segmentation

The parameters for each technique that makes up the handcraft segmentation method are presented in Table A1.

Table A1. Handcrafted segmentation parameters.

Technique	Parameter
Bilateral Filter (Kernel size)	9
Bilateral Filter (radial, spatial sigma)	50
Closing Kernel	3
Area Filter	150
Dilation	2
Dilation (Raabin-Basophil)	4

Appendix A.2. WBC Deep Learning Segmentation

The hyperparameters for each employed U-Net that conformed the Deep Learning segmentation phase are listed in Table A2.

Table A2. U-Net Train Parameters for each dataset.

Dataset	U-Net Train Parameters					
	Lambda	Delta	Gamma	Learning Rate	Dropout	Weight Decay
Cellavision	0.4	0.7	1.0	1×10^{-4}	0.1	1×10^{-3}
JTSC	0.5	0.8	1.0	1×10^{-4}	0.05	1×10^{-4}
SMC_IDB	0.6	0.7	1.0	1×10^{-4}	0.05	1×10^{-3}
Raabin_WBC	0.4	0.7	1.0	1×10^{-4}	0.5	1×10^{-2}
ALL-IDB2	0.4	0.7	1.0	1×10^{-4}	0.1	1×10^{-4}
Dataset Leukemia	0.4	0.4	1.0	1×10^{-4}	0.05	1×10^{-5}

Learning curves for the deep-learning segmentation procedure with a 10 K-Fold. Left column shows the IoU and at the right column the loss curve.

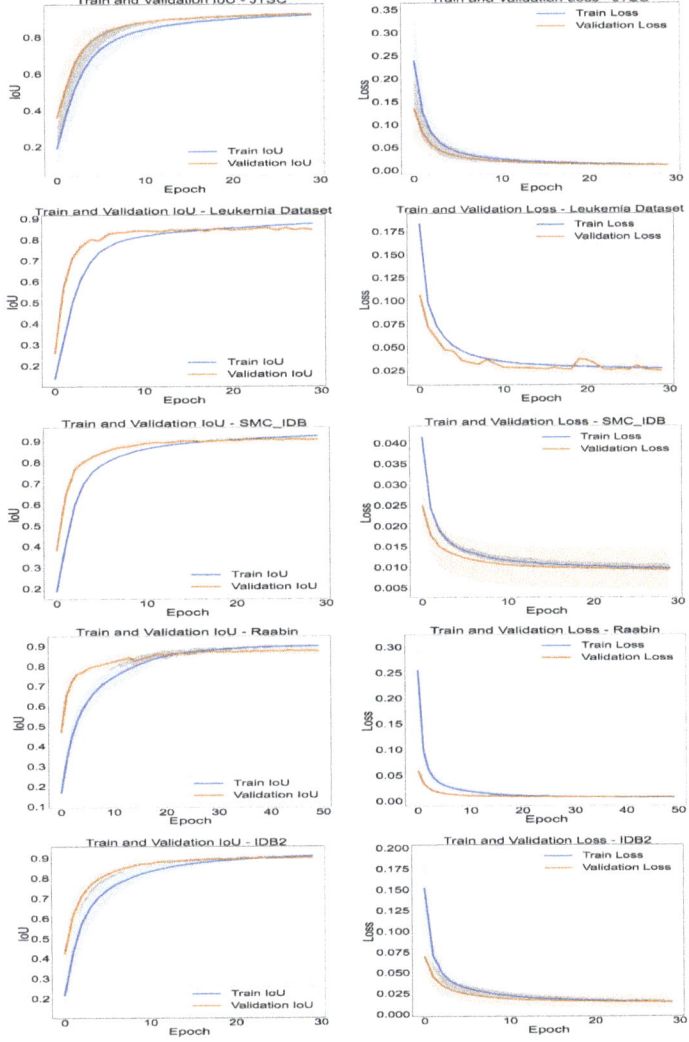

Figure A1. Intersection Over Union and Loss curves over 30 epochs and for each of the 10 folds.

Appendix A.3. Deep Learning Classification

Deep-learning classification curves for the eight proposed models are presented in Figure A2. On the left column, Train and Validation Accuracy over epochs, and on the right column, Train and Validation Loss.

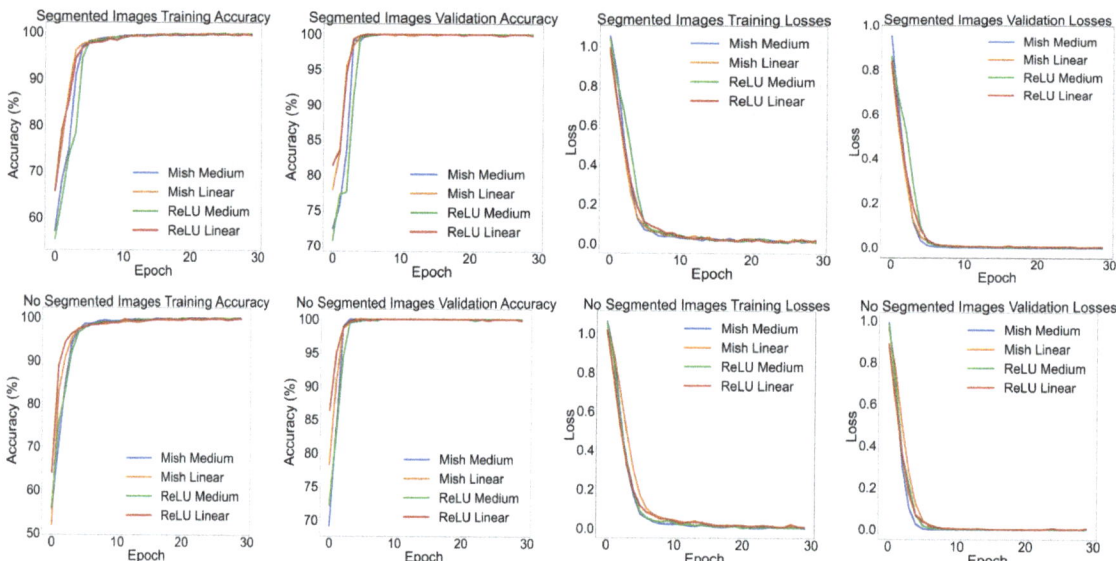

Figure A2. Average accuracy and loss curves for the eight proposed models with 10 K-fold.

Table A3 shows the nine results of "accurate" classification from ALL with four models. Although all the images were correctly classified, the classification certainty differs between them.

Table A3. Leukemia class prediction probabilities of nine correct diagnoses. Most reliable results are in bold and second best results are underlined.

		Class Prediction Probability			
	Image	Mish Linear-S	Mish Linear-NS	Mish Medium-S	Mish Medium-NS
ALL-1	1_1_7	0.998	0.426	**1.000**	0.945
	1_3_132	0.992	0.430	**0.999**	0.993
	1_3_158	0.998	0.464	**1.000**	0.993
ALL-2	2_1_33	0.998	0.750	**1.000**	0.991
	2_2_127	0.999	0.734	**1.000**	0.990
	2_3_202	0.999	0.778	**1.000**	0.970
ALL-3	3_1_3	0.973	0.570	**0.997**	0.846
	3_1_32	0.993	0.439	**0.999**	0.806
	3_2_11	0.998	0.492	**1.000**	0.838
Average		0.994	0.565	**0.999**	0.930

References

1. Guyton A.C.; Hall, J.E. Resistencia del organismo a la infección: I. Leucocitos, granulocitos, sistema monocitomacrofágico e inflamación. In *Tratado de Fisiología Médica*, 12th ed.; Elsevier: Barcelona, Spain, 2011; Chapter 34, pp. 1118–1139.
2. Kumar, V.; Abul, A.; Jon, C. Hematopoietic and Lymphoid Systems. In *Robins Basic Pathology*; Elsevier: Amsterdam, The Netherlands, 2018; Chapter 12, pp. 459–467.

3. Secretaria de Salud de México. *Diagnóstico Oportuno de la Leucemia Aguda en Pediatría en Primer y Segundo Nivel de Atención*; Technical Report; Secretaria de Salud: Ciudad de México, Mexico, 2017.
4. Brereton, M.; De La Salle, B.; Ardern, J.; Hyde, K.; Burthem, J. Do We Know Why We Make Errors in Morphological Diagnosis? An Analysis of Approach and Decision-Making in Haematological Morphology. *EBioMedicine* **2015**, *2*, 1224–1234. [CrossRef] [PubMed]
5. Loddo, A.; Putzu, L. On the Reliability of CNNs in Clinical Practice: A Computer-Aided Diagnosis System Case Study. *Appl. Sci.* **2022**, *12*, 3269. [CrossRef]
6. Andrade, A.R.; Vogado, L.H.; Veras, R.d.M.; Silva, R.R.; Araujo, F.H.; Medeiros, F.N. Recent computational methods for white blood cell nuclei segmentation: A comparative study. *Comput. Methods Programs Biomed.* **2019**, *173*, 1–14. [CrossRef]
7. Loddo, A.; Putzu, L. On the Effectiveness of Leukocytes Classification Methods in a Real Application Scenario. *Ai* **2021**, *2*, 394–412. [CrossRef]
8. Mahbod, A.; Tschandl, P.; Langs, G.; Ecker, R.; Ellinger, I. The effects of skin lesion segmentation on the performance of dermatoscopic image classification. *Comput. Methods Programs Biomed.* **2020**, *197*, 105725.
9. Al-masni, M.A.; Kim, D.H.; Kim, T.S. Multiple skin lesions diagnostics via integrated deep convolutional networks for segmentation and classification. *Comput. Methods Programs Biomed.* **2020**, *190*, 105351. [CrossRef]
10. Vogado, L.H.; Veras, R.D.M.; Andrade, A.R.; De Araujo, F.H.; E Silva, R.R.; De Medeiros, F.N. Unsupervised leukemia cells segmentation based on multi-scale color channels. In Proceedings of the 2016 IEEE International Symposium on Multimedia, ISM 2016, San Jose, CA, USA, 11–13 December 2016; pp. 451–456. [CrossRef]
11. Makem, M.; Tiedeu, A. An efficient algorithm for detection of white blood cell nuclei using adaptive three stage PCA-based fusion. *Inform. Med. Unlocked* **2020**, *20*, 100416. [CrossRef]
12. Mousavi, K.; Tavakoli, S.; Alipanah, A. Easy-GT: Open-Source Software to Facilitate Making the Ground Truth for White Blood Cells' Nucleus. *arXiv* **2021**. [CrossRef]
13. Tavakoli, S.; Ghaffari, A.; Kouzehkanan, Z.M.; Hosseini, R. New segmentation and feature extraction algorithm for classification of white blood cells in peripheral smear images. *Sci. Rep.* **2021**, *11*, 19428. [CrossRef]
14. Makem, M.; Tiedeu, A.; Kom, G.; Nkandeu, Y.P.K. A robust algorithm for white blood cell nuclei segmentation. *Multimed. Tools Appl.* **2022**, *81*, 17849–17874. [CrossRef]
15. Mayala, S.; Haugsøen, J.B. Threshold estimation based on local minima for nucleus and cytoplasm segmentation. *BMC Med. Imaging* **2022**, *22*, 77.
16. Ochoa-montiel, R.; Ibarra, L.M.; Sossa, H.; Olague, G.; Polit, I. Handcraft and Automatic Approaches for the Recognition of Leukemia Images. *Res. Comput. Sci.* **2020**, *149*, 271–280.
17. Haider, A.; Arsalan, M.; Lee, Y.W.; Park, K.R. Deep features aggregation-based joint segmentation of cytoplasm and nuclei in white blood cells. *IEEE J. Biomed. Health Inform.* **2022**, *26*, 3685–3696. [CrossRef]
18. García-Lamont, F.; Alvarado, M.; López-Chau, A.; Cervantes, J. Efficient nucleus segmentation of white blood cells mimicking the human perception of color. *Color Res. Appl.* **2022**, *47*, 657–675. [CrossRef]
19. Zhou, Z.; Siddiquee, M.R.; Tajbakhsh, N. UNet++ : A Nested U-Net Architecture. In *Lecture Notes in Computer Science (Including Subseries Lecture Notes in Artificial Intelligence and Lecture Notes in Bioinformatics)*; Springer International Publishing: Berlin/Heidelberg, Germany, 2018; pp. 3–11. [CrossRef]
20. Oktay, O.; Schlemper, J.; Folgoc, L.L.; Lee, M.; Heinrich, M.; Misawa, K.; Mori, K.; McDonagh, S.; Hammerla, N.Y.; Kainz, B.; et al. Attention U-Net: Learning Where to Look for the Pancreas. *arXiv* **2018**. [CrossRef]
21. He, K.; Gkioxari, G.; Dollár, P.; Girshick, R. Mask R-CNN. *IEEE Trans. Pattern Anal. Mach. Intell.* **2020**, *42*, 386–397.
22. Zheng, X.; Wang, Y.; Wang, G.; Liu, J. Fast and robust segmentation of white blood cell images by self-supervised learning. *Micron* **2018**, *107*, 55–71. [CrossRef]
23. Mohamed, M.; Far, B.; Guaily, A. An efficient technique for white blood cells nuclei automatic segmentation. In Proceedings of the IEEE International Conference on Systems, Man and Cybernetics, Seoul, Republic of Korea, 14–17 October 2012; pp. 220–225. [CrossRef]
24. Kouzehkanan, Z.M.; Saghari, S.; Tavakoli, S.; Rostami, P.; Abaszadeh, M.; Mirzadeh, F.; Satlsar, E.S.; Gheidishahran, M.; Gorgi, F.; Mohammadi, S.; et al. A large dataset of white blood cells containing cell locations and types, along with segmented nuclei and cytoplasm. *Sci. Rep.* **2022**, *12*, 1123. . [CrossRef]
25. Ruggero Donida Labati, Vincenzo Piuri, F.S. All-IDB: The Acute Lymphoblastic Leukemia Image Database for Image Processing. In Proceedings of the IEEE International Conference On Image Processing, Brussels, Belgium, 11–14 September 2011; pp. 2089–2092.
26. Müller, D.; Soto-Rey, I.; Kramer, F. Towards a guideline for evaluation metrics in medical image segmentation. *BMC Res. Notes* **2022**, *15*, 1–7.
27. Hegde, R.B.; Prasad, K.; Hebbar, H.; Singh, B.M.K. Comparison of traditional image processing and deep learning approaches for classification of white blood cells in peripheral blood smear images. *Biocybern. Biomed. Eng.* **2019**, *39*, 382–392. [CrossRef]
28. Paris, S.; Kornprobst, P.; Tumblin, J.; Durand, F. Bilateral filtering: Theory and applications. *Found. Trends Comput. Graph. Vis.* **2009**, *4*, 1–73. [CrossRef]
29. Otsu, N. A Threshold Selection Method from Gray-Level Histograms. *IEEE Trans. Syst. Man Cybern.* **1979**, *20*, 62–66. [CrossRef]

30. Ronneberger, O.; Fischer, P.; Brox, T. U-Net: Convolutional Networks for Biomedical Image Segmentation. In Proceedings of the Medical Image Computing and Computer-Assisted Intervention—MICCAI 2015, Munich, Germany, 5–9 October 2015; Navab, N., Hornegger, J., Wells, W.M., Frangi, A.F., Eds.; Springer International Publishing: Cham, Switzerland, 2015; pp. 234–241.
31. Misra, D. Mish: A Self Regularized Non-Monotonic Activation Function. *arXiv* **2019**.
32. Yeung, M.; Sala, E.; Schönlieb, C.B.; Rundo, L. Unified Focal loss: Generalising Dice and cross entropy-based losses to handle class imbalanced medical image segmentation. *Comput. Med. Imaging Graph.* **2022**, *95*, 102026.
33. He, K.; Zhang, X.; Ren, S.; Sun, J. Deep residual learning for image recognition. In Proceedings of the IEEE Computer Society Conference on Computer Vision and Pattern Recognition, Las Vegas, NV, USA, 27–30 June 2016; pp. 770–778.
34. Selvaraju, R.R.; Cogswell, M.; Das, A.; Vedantam, R.; Parikh, D.; Batra, D. Grad-CAM: Visual Explanations from Deep Networks via Gradient-Based Localization. *Int. J. Comput. Vis.* **2020**, *128*, 336–359.
35. Chattopadhay, A.; Sarkar, A.; Howlader, P.; Balasubramanian, V.N. Grad-CAM++: Generalized gradient-based visual explanations for deep convolutional networks. In Proceedings of the 2018 IEEE Winter Conference on Applications of Computer Vision, WACV 2018, Lake Tahoe, NV, USA, 12–15 March 2018; pp. 839–847.
36. Draelos, R.L.; Carin, L. Use HiResCAM instead of Grad-CAM for faithful explanations of convolutional neural networks. *arXiv* **2020**, arXiv:2011.08891.
37. Fu, R.; Hu, Q.; Dong, X.; Guo, Y.; Gao, Y.; Li, B. Axiom-based Grad-CAM: Towards Accurate Visualization and Explanation of CNNs. *arXiv* **2020**, arXiv:2008.02312.
38. Van der Walt, S.; Schönberger, J.L.; Nunez-Iglesias, J.; Boulogne, F.; Warner, J.D.; Yager, N.; Gouillart, E.; Yu, T. scikit-image: Image processing in Python. *PeerJ* **2014**, *2*, e453. [CrossRef] [PubMed]
39. Bradski, G. The OpenCV Library. *Dr. Dobb'S J. Softw. Tools* **2000**, *11*, 120–123.
40. Paszke, A.; Gross, S.; Massa, F.; Lerer, A.; Bradbury, J.; Chanan, G.; Killeen, T.; Lin, Z.; Gimelshein, N.; Antiga, L.; et al. PyTorch: An Imperative Style, High-Performance Deep Learning Library. In *Advances in Neural Information Processing Systems 32*; Curran Associates, Inc.: Red Hook, NY, USA, 2019; pp. 8024–8035.
41. Pedregosa, F.; Varoquaux, G.; Gramfort, A.; Michel, V.; Thirion, B.; Grisel, O.; Blondel, M.; Prettenhofer, P.; Weiss, R.; Dubourg, V.; et al. Scikit-learn: Machine Learning in Python. *J. Mach. Learn. Res.* **2011**, *12*, 2825–2830.
42. Cardoso, M.J.; Li, W.; Brown, R.; Ma, N.; Kerfoot, E.; Wang, Y.; Murrey, B.; Myronenko, A.; Zhao, C.; Yang, D.; et al. MONAI: An open-source framework for deep learning in healthcare. *arXiv* **2022**, arXiv:cs.LG/2211.02701.
43. Szeghalmy, S.; Fazekas, A. A Comparative Study of the Use of Stratified Cross-Validation and Distribution-Balanced Stratified Cross-Validation in Imbalanced Learning. *Sensors* **2023**, *23*, 2333. [CrossRef] [PubMed]
44. Vakharia, V.; Shah, M.; Suthar, V.; Patel, V.K.; Solanki, A. Hybrid perovskites thin films morphology identification by adapting multiscale-SinGAN architecture, heat transfer search optimized feature selection and machine learning algorithms. *Phys. Scr.* **2023**, *98*, 025203. [CrossRef]
45. Buslaev, A.A. Parinov, E.K.V.I.I.; Kalinin, A.A. Albumentations: Fast and flexible image augmentations. *arXiv* **2018**, arXiv:1809.06839.
46. Motlagh, M.H.; Science, C. *Automatic Segmentation and Classification of Red and White Blood Cells in Thin Blood*; Concordia University: Montreal, QC, USA, 2015.

Disclaimer/Publisher's Note: The statements, opinions and data contained in all publications are solely those of the individual author(s) and contributor(s) and not of MDPI and/or the editor(s). MDPI and/or the editor(s) disclaim responsibility for any injury to people or property resulting from any ideas, methods, instructions or products referred to in the content.

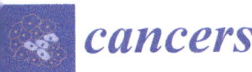

Article

Performing Automatic Identification and Staging of Urothelial Carcinoma in Bladder Cancer Patients Using a Hybrid Deep-Machine Learning Approach

Suryadipto Sarkar [1,*], Kong Min [2], Waleed Ikram [3], Ryan W. Tatton [3], Irbaz B. Riaz [3], Alvin C. Silva [2], Alan H. Bryce [3], Cassandra Moore [4], Thai H. Ho [3], Guru Sonpavde [4], Haidar M. Abdul-Muhsin [5], Parminder Singh [3] and Teresa Wu [6]

1. Department Artificial Intelligence in Biomedical Engineering, Friedrich-Alexander-Universität Erlangen-Nürnberg, 91054 Erlangen, Germany
2. Department of Radiology, Mayo Clinic, Phoenix, AZ 85054, USA
3. Division of Hematology and Oncology, Mayo Clinic, Phoenix, AZ 85054, USA
4. Dana Farber Cancer Institute, Harvard Medical School, Boston, MA 02215, USA
5. Department of Internal Medicine, Mayo Clinic, Phoenix, AZ 85054, USA
6. ASU-Mayo Center for Innovative Imaging, School of Computing and Augmented Intelligence, Arizona State University, Tempe, AZ 85281, USA
* Correspondence: suryadipto.sarkar@fau.de

Simple Summary: Early and accurate bladder cancer staging is important as it determines the mode of initial treatment. Non-muscle invasive bladder cancer (NMIBC) can be treated with transurethral resection whereas muscle invasive bladder cancer (MIBC) requires neoadjuvant chemotherapy with subsequent cystectomy as indicated. Our hybrid machine/deep learning model demonstrates improved accuracy of bladder cancer staging by CECT using a hybrid machine/deep learning model which will facilitate appropriate clinical management of the patients with bladder cancer, ultimately improving patient outcome.

Abstract: Accurate clinical staging of bladder cancer aids in optimizing the process of clinical decision-making, thereby tailoring the effective treatment and management of patients. While several radiomics approaches have been developed to facilitate the process of clinical diagnosis and staging of bladder cancer using grayscale computed tomography (CT) scans, the performances of these models have been low, with little validation and no clear consensus on specific imaging signatures. We propose a hybrid framework comprising pre-trained deep neural networks for feature extraction, in combination with statistical machine learning techniques for classification, which is capable of performing the following classification tasks: (1) bladder cancer tissue vs. normal tissue, (2) muscle-invasive bladder cancer (MIBC) vs. non-muscle-invasive bladder cancer (NMIBC), and (3) post-treatment changes (PTC) vs. MIBC.

Keywords: bladder cancer; urothelial carcinoma; lymph node metastasis; deep learning; computed tomography (CT) imaging; machine learning

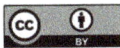

1. Introduction

Bladder cancer imaging can be misleading. Findings such as perivesical fat stranding, hydronephrosis, focal bladder wall thickening, or a small bladder lesion may be wrongly perceived as a more advanced stage of bladder cancer. It is common to see small lymph nodes in the pelvis post transurethral resection of bladder tumor (TURBT) [1–3] or at the time of diagnosis [4]. These otherwise non-significant lymph nodes may harbor metastasis, which in turn might be difficult to decipher relying solely on visual inspection from CT scans [5,6]. Furthermore, bladder cancer is a heterogeneous disease with an extremely varied range of case-specific diagnoses [7,8]. From low-grade tumors such as T_a (noninvasive papillary carcinoma) and T_{is} (tumor in situ or "flat lesion"), which require TURBT or less aggressive endoscopic intervention [8], to high-grade muscle-invasive tumors, which require chemotherapy [9,10], bladder cancer diagnosis is highly dependent on the type and stage of the tumor [4,6,11].

Radiomics can provide tools to significantly improve the accuracy of clinical staging by analyzing multiple qualitative features, including but not restricted to texture analysis, raw digital data and deep model-generated embeddings.

Texture analysis helps capture local patterns in images from the intensity information contained within them. Such features are very effective in identifying tissue types from grayscale medical scans. The texture-based features generally used in medical imaging can be broadly categorized into two subdivisions, namely statistical approaches and transformation-based approaches.

First, we will review some of the most commonly used statistical texture features for bladder cancer detection and staging from medical scans. Ref. [12] utilized a set of functional, second-order statistical and morphological features to perform staging between T1 and T2 types of bladder cancer from MRI scans. The second-order statistical feature extraction approach included a total of 25 GLCM features and 16 gray level run length matrix (GLRLM) features obtained from 42 bladder MRIs (21 T1, 21 T2) post ROI segmentation, yielding an accuracy, sensitivity and specificity of 95.24% and an AUC of 98.64%. Furthermore, the authors also performed an extensive comparison between their proposed model and two state-of-the-art approaches, namely [13,14]. Ref. [15] makes use of LBP and GLCM features to perform primary tumor staging of bladder cancer into two groups: (1) tumor stage and primary tumor located completely within the bladder; (2) tumor stage and primary tumor extending outside the bladder. The SVM classifier, which was trained on T2-weighted MRI scans from 65 bladder cancer patients all with stage 1, reported an AUC of 80.60%. Ref. [16] performs prediction of recurrence and progression of urothelial carcinoma from a dataset of 42 patients—13 without recurrence, 14 with recurrence but not progression, and 15 with progression. Features extracted using LBP and local variance, after classification using the RUSBoost classifier, provided an accuracy of 70% and sensitivity of 84%. Ref. [17] utilizes LBP and GLCM features to classify the invasiveness of bladder cancer. The dataset comprised T2-weighted MRI scans from 65 preoperative bladder cancer patients followed by radical cystectomy. The proposed model reported a patient-level sensitivity of 74.20%, specificity of 82.40%, accuracy of 78.50% and AUC of 80.60%. Ref. [18] performed survival prediction of bladder urothelial carcinoma (BLCA) from CECT scans by utilizing LBP, wavelet and GLCM features. The dataset comprised scans from 62 bladder cancer patients with stages of urothelial carcinoma. The radiomics features extracted from the CECTs were used in combination with RNA-seq data for a complete radiogenomics signature, which in turn helped predict the survival of the patients. This study exhibits the applicability of radiomics and transcriptomics data in predicting BLCA survival. However, owing to the sheer small size of the dataset, the authors think that the model needs to be validated on a larger set of samples for a more foolproof analysis. The literature exhibits that statistical texture analysis is not only fast and easy to implement but also very effective in performing classification, staging and segmentation of bladder cancer from medical images.

Transformation-based approaches such as Fourier and Gabor wavelet transform are very effective in learning textural patterns from images and are therefore a popular option among medical imaging researchers. Ref. [19] utilized Gabor features to perform carcinoma cell classification from biopsy images associated with 14 distinct cancer types, scanned from 14 different patients. An SVM classifier with a radial basis function (RBF) kernel was subsequently trained on these features. The SVM classifier provides the highest cross-validation accuracy of 99.20% with a Gabor window size of 400 pixels and an image magnification of 10. Ref. [20] makes use of 2D Fourier-based features to identify cancer from 182 optical coherence tomography (OCT) scans obtained from 21 patients who were identified as high risk of having transitional cell carcinoma (TCC) and from 68 different areas of the bladder. The task was two-fold: (1) to perform classification between non-cancerous, dysplasia, carcinoma in situ (CIS), and papillary lesions; (2) to predict the invasiveness of the lesion. Other than 2D Fourier transform, the authors also extracted four different statistical feature extraction approaches, resulting in a total of 74 features obtained from the raw OCT images. A simple cross-correlation-based filter with a correlation threshold of 0.85 was employed for feature selection, which resulted in a final set of nine selected features. The decision tree classifier was utilized to finally perform classification on the selected feature set. The authors reported a non-cancerous versus cancerous classification sensitivity of 92.00% and specificity of 62.00%. Ref. [21], which has been summarized earlier, reports that GLCM and GLDM perform better than Fourier transform-based feature extractors in differentiating between tumors and peritumoral fat tissues.

From the literature reviewed above, it is evident that texture analysis is an effective approach when performing classification tasks on medical imaging, in general, and histologic analysis in particular.

Recently, deep learning-based models have emerged and gained popularity among researchers owing to their automatic feature extraction capabilities. Convolutional neural networks (CNNs) are the most commonly used type of deep models and a very popular framework when performing classification tasks on imaging-based applications, in general, and radiological data in particular. The authors of [22] designed a set of nine CNN-based models for the classification of MIBC and NMIBC from contrast-enhanced CT (CECT) images. The dataset comprised 1200 CT scans obtained from 369 patients undergoing radical cystectomy. A total of 249 out of these patients had NMIBC, while the remaining 120 had MIBC. The CNN model was pre-trained on the ImageNet dataset in order to improve classification performance. The model with the highest AUC on the test set was obtained using the VGG16 algorithm—with an AUC of 99.70%, accuracy of 93.90%, sensitivity of 88.90%, specificity of 98.90%, precision of 98.80% and negative predictive value of 89.90%. In contrast, the authors of [13] made use of Haralick features, which are a variant of GLCM, to identify muscular invasiveness in MRI scans containing a total of 118 volumes of interest (VOI) obtained from 68 patients—34 volumes labeled non-muscle-invasive bladder cancer (NMIBC), and 84 labeled muscle-invasive bladder cancer (MIBC). The final SVM classifier obtained an AUC of 86.10% and Youden index of 71.92%.

Ref. [21] performs classification between bladder cancers with and without response to chemotherapy from a set of CT scans obtained before and after treatment. The authors have reviewed three different models and their capabilities in performing classification: (1) a deep learning-convolutional neural network-based model (DL-CNN); (2) a more deterministic radiomics feature-based classifier (RF-SL); (3) an intermediate model that extracts radiomics features from image patterns (RF-ROI). The training dataset comprised 82 patients having 87 bladder cancers, scanned pre- and post-chemotherapy. The test set comprised 41 patients with 43 cancers. The radiomics feature-based model (RF-SL) performed the best with an AUC of 77.00%, while the two radiologists reported AUCs of 76.00% and 77.00%, respectively.

Ref. [23] proposed a CNN-based model for performing classification between low- and high-stage bladder cancer. The training dataset comprised 84 bladder cancer CR urography (CTU) images obtained from 76 patients (43 CTUs contained low-stage cancer, while 41 contained high-stage cancer). The test set consisted of 90 bladder CTUs obtained from 86 patients. The CNN classifier had a test set prediction accuracy of 91.00%, which the authors claim is higher as compared to texture-based classification using SVM on the same dataset (which had a prediction accuracy of 88.00%). In comparison, ref. [21] extracted GLCM- and histogram-based features from apparent diffusion coefficient (ADC) and diffusion-weighted images (DWI) to perform bladder cancer grading. A total of 61 patients were scanned for this study, 32 out of whom were in low-grade and the remaining 29 in high-grade classes. A combination of 102 GLCM and histogram features were initially extracted, out of which 47 were finally selected using the Mann–Whitney U-test, and an

SVM classifier was used to perform classification between high- and low-grade bladder cancer with an accuracy of 82.90%. Ref. [21] extracted histogram and GLCM features to perform classification between high-grade and low-grade bladder cancer scans from a set of diffusion-based MRIs obtained from 61 bladder cancer patients (32 of them having low-grade and 29 having high-grade bladder cancer), yielding an accuracy of 82.90% and area under the curve (AUC) of 86.10%. Ref. [24] made use of GLCM, wavelet filter and Laplacian of Gaussian filter to extract features from a small dataset of 145 patients to perform grading on bladder cancer CT scans. Out of these 145 scans, 108 were used to train the model, and the remaining 37 were used to perform validation. The model provided an accuracy of 83.80% on the validation set.

From the literature reviewed above, it is evident that neural network-based classifiers are more effective than texture analysis when performing identification and staging of bladder cancer from medical imaging alone.

The authors of [25] claim that feature extraction when governed by domain knowledge performs better than CNN-based classifiers that are capable of automatic feature generation. The task in this case was to classify two early stages of bladder cancer that are histologically difficult to differentiate, namely Ta (non-invasive) and T1 (superficially invasive). The dataset comprised a total of 1177 bladder scans—460 non-invasive, 717 superficially invasive. CNN classifiers achieved the highest accuracy of 84.00%, performing considerably poorer than supervised machine learning classifiers that were trained on manually extracted features. The aforementioned literature on CNNs comprises end-to-end models, where both training and testing are performed on the same dataset. The problem with such an approach is that deep neural networks require large quantities of training data in order to avoid the pervasive issue of over-fitting. As a substitute to end-to-end deep models, researchers make use of a concept called "transfer learning", where the neural network is first pre-trained on a large dataset such as ImageNet, and the learned weights are subsequently fine-tuned on the small target data. Since we were using a small dataset of 200 CT scans for this study, we decided to make use of transfer learning to improve classification results and alleviate overfitting. A 71-layer ResNet-18 model pre-trained on the publicly available ImageNet dataset was utilized to extract features from the bladder scans. The extracted features, after feature selection using a combination of supervised and unsupervised techniques, were finally used to perform classification by five different machine learning classifiers, namely k-nearest neighbor (KNN), support vector machine (SVM), linear discriminant analysis (LDA), decision tree (DT) and naive Bayes (NB).

2. Materials and Methods

Figure 1 provides a pictorial depiction of the entire workflow, starting from the raw bladder scans to the prediction labels obtained after classification. The proposed methodology comprises feature extraction, feature selection, and finally classification. In this hybrid approach, we extract feature vectors from the images using the trained model weights from the last pooling layer of the five most widely used pre-trained deep models, namely AlexNet, GoogleNet, InceptionV3, ResNet-50 and XceptionNet. We subsequently employ our feature selection algorithm on this feature vector. Finally, we use five machine learning classification algorithms on the selected feature set, namely k-nearest neighbor (KNN), naive Bayes (NB), support vector machine (SVM), linear discriminant analysis (LDA) and decision tree (DT).

2.1. Feature Extraction Using Pre-Trained Deep Models

Five popular neural network-based deep models, namely AlexNet, GoogleNet, InceptionV3, ResNet-50 and XceptionNet, all pre-trained on the ImageNet dataset [26], were trained using our bladder CT scan data to fine-tune the model parameters. The trained weights from the last pooling layer of each of these models were extracted and subsequently used as feature descriptors. Table 1 provides a comprehensive description of each of these models—including information regarding the pooling layer and the size of the extracted feature vector.

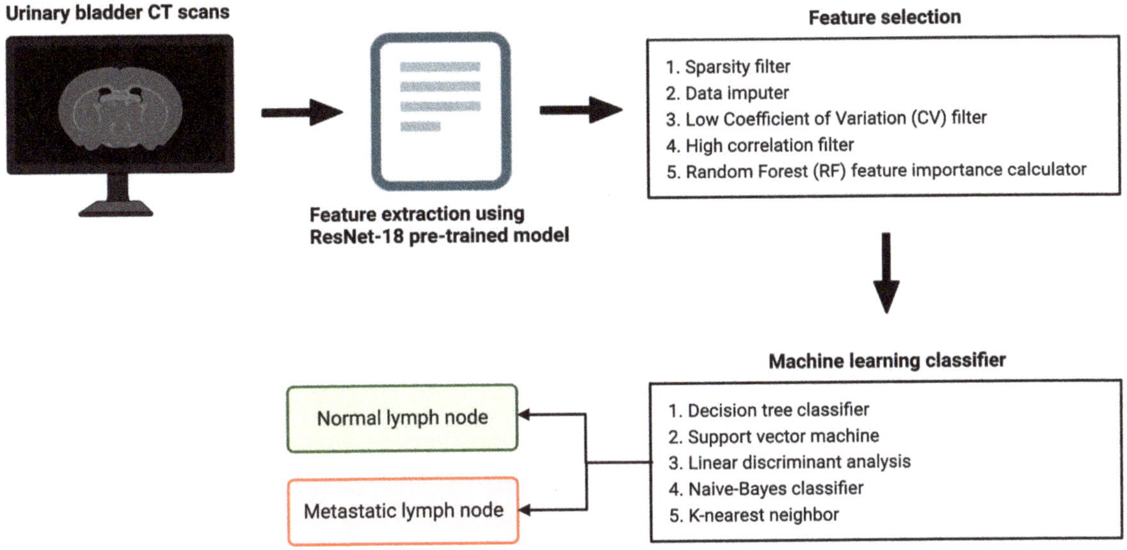

Figure 1. A schematic representation of the overall workflow.

Table 1. A description of the five pre-trained models used for feature extraction from the bladder scans, namely AlexNet, GoogleNet, InceptionV3, ResNet-50 and XceptionNet. The table contains the total number of layers per model; the last pooling layer from which features were being extracted; the layer number of the last pooling layer; and the length of the extracted feature vector.

Pre-Trained Model	Total No. of Layers in the Network	Last Pooling Layer	Layer No. of the Last Pooling Layer	Feature Vector Length
AlexNet	25	Max Pooling	16	9216
GoogleNet	144	Global Average Pooling	140	1024
InceptionV3	315	Global Average Pooling	312	2048
ResNet-50	177	Global Average Pooling	174	2048
XceptionNet	170	Global Average Pooling	167	2048

2.2. Feature Selection Mechanism

An ensemble feature selection technique was used to select the most important features from the originally extracted feature vector—which was obtained using five different pre-trained models, namely AlexNet, GoogleNet, Inception V3, ResNet-50 and XceptionNet, for performing the classification of normal vs. metastatic lymph nodes. First, we make use of a "sparsity filter" to remove the features that were not updated by the deep model. Through this step, we not only exclude features that have low variance but also automatically remove those that are less likely to have an impact on the classification process. Next, we utilize the "data imputer" to impute the unchanged values of the remaining columns by the mean value of the respective column. Subsequently, we made use of the "low coefficient of variation (CV) filter" to drop features with a CV value of less than 0.1. CV, or standard deviation normalized by mean, is a measure of information content; a lower CV indicates features with a lower normalized variance. Furthermore, in the next step, a correlation matrix was generated, which contains information regarding the cross-correlation values between every pair of features. For each pair with >95% correlation, the one with a lower correlation to the output is dropped. Finally, we employed random forest, a boosted decision tree algorithm, to train the remaining columns and target variables for feature importance score generation. The number of trees was set to a default value of 100, and the Gini index was used as the metric for calculating feature importance. The first four steps were unsupervised (statistical approaches used to perform selection on features alone, not labels); the last feature importance calculation step was supervised (relationship between dependent and independent variables critical in determining feature selection). Figure 2 provides a schematic depiction of the feature selection algorithm.

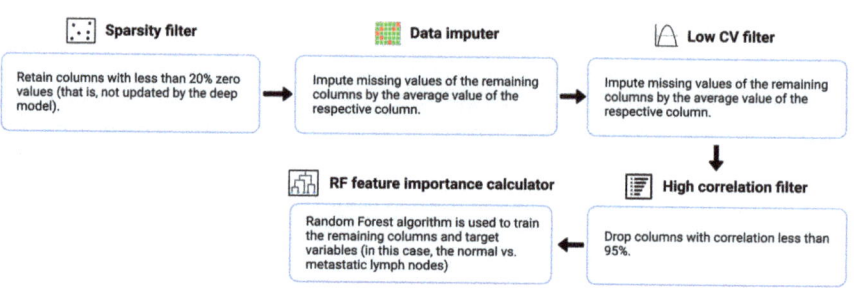

Figure 2. A pictorial representation of the feature selection procedure.

2.3. Machine Learning-Based Classification

The important features obtained using the feature selection algorithm were used as inputs into the machine learning classifier. The three classification tasks that were performed were: (1) normal vs. bladder cancer, (2) NMIBC vs. MIBC, (3) post-treatment changes (PTC) vs. MIBC. A 10-fold cross-validation was utilized to evaluate the prediction performance of the proposed model. The samples were randomly re-arranged, then the dataset was split into 10 equal divisions. Nine of these divisions, at every iteration, were used for training; and the remaining was one used for testing. This process was repeated for 10 iterations, each time the test set being a different group. The prediction evaluation metrics calculated across the ten iterations were averaged and reported. Classification was performed using five different machine learning classifiers, namely k-nearest neighbor (KNN), naive Bayes (NB), support vector machine (SVM), linear discriminant analysis (LDA) and decision tree (DT).

2.4. Evaluation Metrics

In order to evaluate the efficacy of the classification model, the following five metrics were used:

$$Accuracy = \frac{TP + TN}{TP + TN + FP + FN} \quad (1)$$

$$Sensitivity = \frac{TP}{TP + FN} \quad (2)$$

$$Specificity = \frac{TN}{TN + FP} \quad (3)$$

$$Precision = \frac{TP}{TP + FP} \quad (4)$$

$$F1 = \frac{2 \times Precision \times Sensitivity}{Precision + Sensitivity} \quad (5)$$

where *TP* is the # of true positives, *TN* is the # of true negatives, *FP* is the # of false positives and *FN* is the # of false negatives.

Since our dataset is small and highly imbalanced, accuracy, precision and recall are not ideal in representing the classification performance of the models. Therefore, the F1-score was used to determine the overall effectiveness of the classifiers. While accuracy represents the overall percentage of correctly classified samples, precision represents the percentage of identified samples where the condition actually exists, and recall represents the proportion of samples with the condition that have been correctly diagnosed, none of them corrects for data imbalance. The F1-score, which is the harmonic mean of precision and recall, has been employed to rank classifiers in terms of diagnostic performance for this particular study.

3. Software and Tools

MATLAB version R2021b (developed by MathWorks, Massachussets USA) was used for the purpose of feature extraction and machine learning-based classification (The Deep Learning Toolbox was used to train the five pre-trained deep models, namely AlexNet, GoogleNet, InceptionV3, ResNet50 and XceptionNet. The Statistics and Machine Learning Toolbox was used to train the four machine learning-based classifiers, namely naive Bayes, support vector machine, linear discriminant analysis and decision tree).

ImageJ (developed by National Institutes of Health, Maryland USA) and RadiAnt Dicom Viewer (open source application) were used to analyze the CT images. BioRender was used to generate all the illustrations in the paper (Figures 1–4).

Python 3 (open source programming language) was used to program the feature selection workflow and generate the plots containing the F1-scores per model per classifier (Figures 5–7).

4. Dataset

A urothelial carcinoma dataset was provided by Mayo Clinic, Arizona. The dataset contained de-identified grayscale CT scans obtained from patients who were imaged before radical cystectomy and pelvic lymph node dissection as part of a trial. The location of each bladder mass was confirmed, and labels of the preoperative CT data were generated. The labels were "cancer" (meaning malignant cells) and "normal" (normal bladder wall).

There were a total of 100 CT scans of the pelvis with intravenous contrast images visualizing the bladder, obtained from 100 patients (one image captured per patient). Each scan had 2 masks (normal bladder wall and bladder cancer) manually annotated by encompassing both the entire region of biopsy-proven malignancy and the normal-appearing bladder by two radiologists familiar with bladder imaging, which were used to extract the respective regions of interest (ROI)—therefore resulting in 200 ROIs (100 normal tissue and 100 abnormal tissue). These ROIs were used as input for classification instead of the entire image. The patients were distributed across seven bladder cancer stages, namely T_a, T_{is}, T_0, T_1, T_2, T_3 and T_4. Figure 3 provides an axial CT scan with IV contrast, along with its corresponding region of interest (ROI) on the bladder wall, pertaining to each of the seven stages. T_0 represents a stage where the tissue of interest shows no evidence of malignancy, possibly but not necessarily following tumor resection and/or chemotherapy. This indicates carcinoma in situ, where the malignant cells only involves the innermost lining of the bladder wall. T_1 represents a stage where malignant cells involve the connective tissue beyond the innermost lining without involvement of the bladder muscle. T_2 represents the malignant spread of tumor involving the bladder muscle. T_3 represents a stage where malignant mass spreads outside the confines of bladder muscle with involvement of the perivesical fat. T_4 stage indicates the spread of tumor beyond the bladder with involvement of abdominal/pelvic wall and/or nearby organs. T_a, T_{is} and T_1 stages are classified as non-muscle-invasive bladder cancer (NMIBC); T_2, T_3 and T_4 stages are classified as muscle-invasive bladder cancer (MIBC) [4,27]. Figure 4 is a pictorial depiction of the different stages of bladder cancer. As is evident from Figure 3, the stages are difficult to distinguish on visual inspection—thereby making it suitable for classification using AI-based models. Table 2 provides a summary of the number of patients per stage.

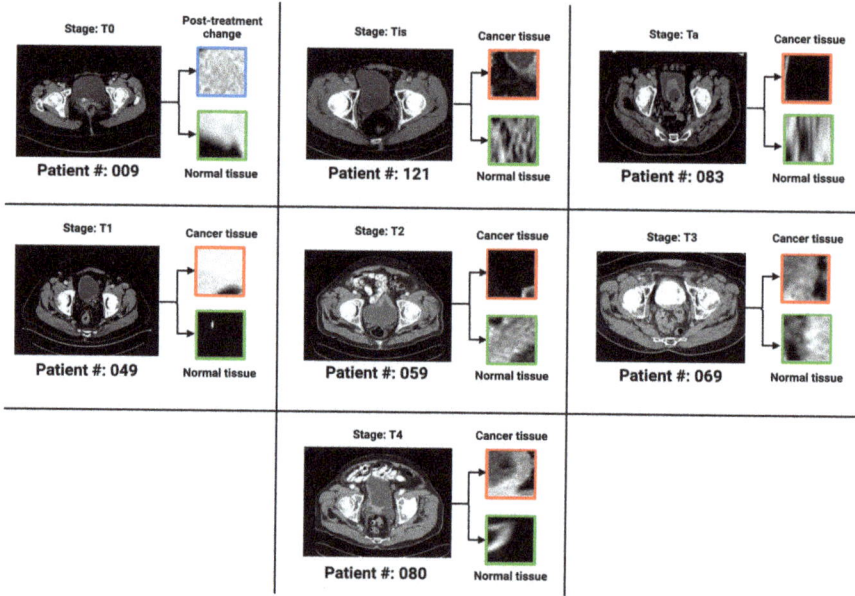

Figure 3. One bladder CT scan per stage (along with the corresponding regions of interest that were used in the various classification tasks) have been provided. The 7 stages of urothelial carcinoma analyzed in the study are: T_a, T_{is}, T_0, T_1, T_2, T_3 and T_4 (T_0 has not been shown in the figure because T_0 represents a stage where the tissue of interest shows no evidence of malignancy).

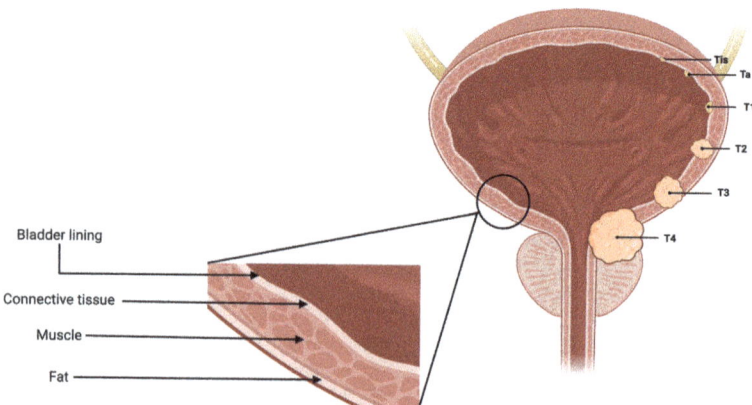

Figure 4. A pictorial representation of the 7 stages of urothelial carcinoma analyzed in the study (T_0 has not been shown in the figure because T_0 represents a stage where the tissue of interest shows no evidence of malignancy).

Table 2. A summary of the number of patients per stage.

T_a	T_{is}	T_0	T_1	T_2	T_3	T_4
6	9	35	9	13	24	4

5. Results

The proposed model was used to perform three different classification tasks during the course of this study: (1) normal vs. bladder cancer; (2) NMIBC vs. MIBC; (3) post-treatment changes (PTC) vs. MIBC. In this section, for each of the three tasks, the best classification performances corresponding to each of the five pre-trained deep model-based features have been presented. The class-wise number of ROIs used for each of the individual tasks has also been summarized.

5.1. Normal vs. Cancer

Normal vs. cancer classification was performed with 10-fold cross-validation on a dataset of 165 ROIs (100 normal, 65 cancer)—35 T0 images were not relevant because they represent post-treatment changes (PTC) and not cancer. The LDA classifier on XceptionNet-based features provides the best performance with an accuracy of 86.07%, sensitivity of 96.75%, specificity of 69.65%, precision of 83.07% and F1-score of 89.39%. Table 3 summarizes the classification performances of the 10-fold machine learning classifiers on features extracted from each of the five pre-trained deep models (results visualized on the associated Figure 5 bar plot).

Table 3. Classification performances of the 10-fold machine learning classifiers on features extracted from each of the five pre-trained deep models.

Feature Extractor	Classifier	Accuracy	Sensitivity	Specificity	Precision	F1-Score
AlexNet	NB	0.8053 ± 0.0029	0.8936 ± 0.004	0.6694 ± 0.0054	0.8062 ± 0.0025	0.8476 ± 0.0024
	SVM	0.7835 ± 0.0058	0.8944 ± 0.0056	0.6128 ± 0.0122	0.7805 ± 0.0055	0.8335 ± 0.0043
	LDA	0.7987 ± 0.0037	0.9307 ± 0.0027	0.5957 ± 0.0078	0.7799 ± 0.0034	0.8486 ± 0.0026
	DT	0.7373 ± 0.0113	0.8043 ± 0.0120	0.6342 ± 0.0231	0.7724 ± 0.0114	0.7877 ± 0.0089
GoogleNet	NB	0.7642 ± 0.0049	0.8674 ± 0.0058	0.6054 ± 0.0085	0.7718 ± 0.0040	0.8168 ± 0.0039
	SVM	0.7661 ± 0.0053	0.8921 ± 0.0068	0.5722 ± 0.0084	0.7624 ± 0.0038	0.8221 ± 0.0043
	LDA	0.7899 ± 0.0036	0.9368 ± 0.0038	0.5640 ± 0.0061	0.7678 ± 0.0027	0.8439 ± 0.0027
	DT	0.7562 ± 0.0136	0.8056 ± 0.0167	0.6803 ± 0.0231	0.7954 ± 0.0123	0.8001 ± 0.0116
InceptionV3	NB	0.7988 ± 0.0031	0.9016 ± 0.0042	0.6406 ± 0.0052	0.7942 ± 0.0024	0.8445 ± 0.0025
	SVM	0.7740 ± 0.0042	0.9036 ± 0.0041	0.5746 ± 0.0080	0.7657 ± 0.0036	0.8290 ± 0.0031
	LDA	0.7935 ± 0.0012	0.9096 ± 0.0010	0.6148 ± 0.0019	0.7841 ± 0.0009	0.8422 ± 0.0009
	DT	0.7295 ± 0.0127	0.7690 ± 0.0155	0.6686 ± 0.0211	0.7816 ± 0.0114	0.7749 ± 0.0110
ResNet50	NB	0.8248 ± 0.0039	0.9290 ± 0.0045	0.6646 ± 0.0073	0.8100 ± 0.0034	0.8654 ± 0.0030
	SVM	0.7771 ± 0.0051	0.9092 ± 0.0065	0.5738 ± 0.0081	0.7665 ± 0.0036	0.8317 ± 0.0040
	LDA	0.7862 ± 0.0028	0.9224 ± 0.0043	0.5766 ± 0.0056	0.7702 ± 0.0022	0.8395 ± 0.0022
	DT	0.8079 ± 0.0111	0.8418 ± 0.0135	0.7558 ± 0.0256	0.8424 ± 0.0135	0.8416 ± 0.0089
XceptionNet	NB	0.8395 ± 0.0035	0.8866 ± 0.0048	0.7671 ± 0.0058	0.8542 ± 0.0031	0.8701 ± 0.0030
	SVM	0.8322 ± 0.0047	0.9614 ± 0.0034	0.6335 ± 0.0100	0.8015 ± 0.0045	0.8742 ± 0.0033
	LDA	0.8607 ± 0.0038	0.9675 ± 0.0027	0.6965 ± 0.0094	0.8307 ± 0.0042	0.8939 ± 0.0026
	DT	0.8145 ± 0.0099	0.8453 ± 0.0134	0.7672 ± 0.0173	0.8486 ± 0.0095	0.8466 ± 0.0086

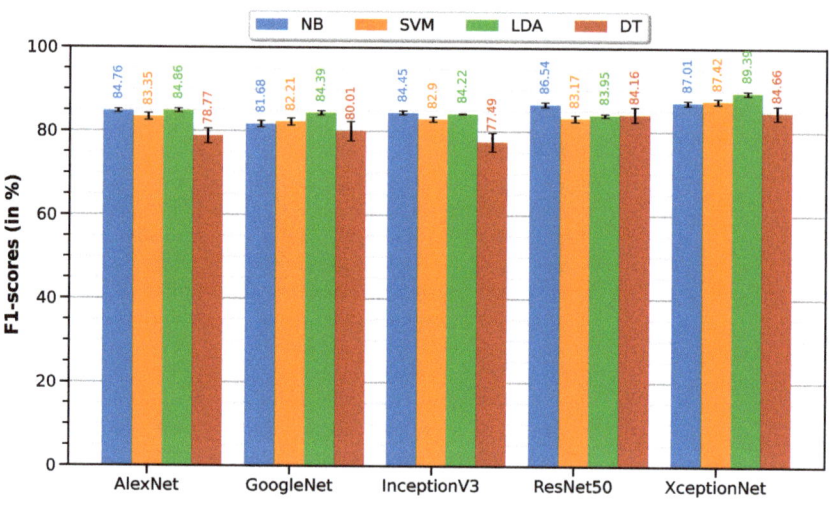

Figure 5. F1-scores of the 10-fold machine learning classifiers on features extracted from each of the five pre-trained deep models.

5.2. NMIBC vs. MIBC

NMIBC vs. MIBC classification was performed with 10-fold cross-validation on a dataset of 65 ROIs (24 NMIBC, 41 MIBC). The LDA classifier on XceptionNet-based features provides the best performance with an accuracy of 79.72%, sensitivity of 66.62%, specificity of 87.39%, precision of 75.58% and F1-score of 70.81%. Table 4 summarizes the classification performances of the 10-fold machine learning classifiers on features extracted from each of the five pre-trained deep models (results visualized on the associated Figure 6 bar plot).

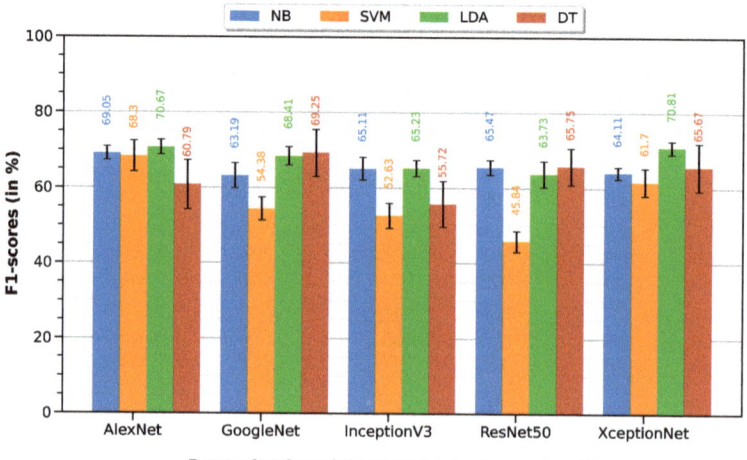

Figure 6. F1-scores of the 10-fold machine learning classifiers on features extracted from each of the five pre-trained deep models.

Table 4. Classification performances of the 10-fold machine learning classifiers on features extracted from each of the five pre-trained deep models.

Feature Extractor	Classifier	Accuracy	Sensitivity	Specificity	Precision	F1-Score
AlexNet	NB	0.7768 ± 0.0067	0.6746 ± 0.0117	0.8366 ± 0.0089	0.7079 ± 0.0112	0.6905 ± 0.0090
	SVM	0.7709 ± 0.0143	0.6692 ± 0.0244	0.8305 ± 0.0147	0.6989 ± 0.0214	0.6830 ± 0.0203
	LDA	0.7963 ± 0.0065	0.6650 ± 0.0125	0.8732 ± 0.0076	0.7547 ± 0.0114	0.7067 ± 0.0097
	DT	0.7160 ± 0.0215	0.6008 ± 0.0445	0.7834 ± 0.0286	0.6223 ± 0.0329	0.6079 ± 0.0324
GoogleNet	NB	0.7480 ± 0.0108	0.5867 ± 0.0202	0.8424 ± 0.0124	0.6864 ± 0.0178	0.6319 ± 0.0166
	SVM	0.7238 ± 0.0088	0.4462 ± 0.0158	0.8863 ± 0.0107	0.6984 ± 0.0215	0.5438 ± 0.0154
	LDA	0.7758 ± 0.0069	0.6583 ± 0.0157	0.8446 ± 0.0064	0.7127 ± 0.0099	0.6841 ± 0.0120
	DT	0.7740 ± 0.0220	0.6925 ± 0.0408	0.8217 ± 0.0239	0.6968 ± 0.0312	0.6925 ± 0.0310
InceptionV3	NB	0.7575 ± 0.009	0.6137 ± 0.0194	0.8417 ± 0.0093	0.6945 ± 0.0139	0.6511 ± 0.0149
	SVM	0.7242 ± 0.0069	0.4163 ± 0.0179	0.9044 ± 0.0033	0.7174 ± 0.0114	0.5263 ± 0.0167
	LDA	0.7698 ± 0.0060	0.5854 ± 0.0134	0.8778 ± 0.0056	0.7373 ± 0.0098	0.6523 ± 0.0105
	DT	0.6909 ± 0.0210	0.5300 ± 0.0409	0.7851 ± 0.0306	0.5963 ± 0.0353	0.5572 ± 0.0306
ResNet50	NB	0.6878 ± 0.0103	0.8013 ± 0.0135	0.6215 ± 0.0149	0.5539 ± 0.0105	0.6547 ± 0.0098
	SVM	0.7240 ± 0.0065	0.3167 ± 0.0115	0.9624 ± 0.0074	0.8343 ± 0.0279	0.4584 ± 0.0138
	LDA	0.7748 ± 0.0098	0.5375 ± 0.0221	0.9137 ± 0.0130	0.7874 ± 0.0220	0.6373 ± 0.0173
	DT	0.7665 ± 0.0159	0.6088 ± 0.0300	0.8588 ± 0.0189	0.7190 ± 0.0287	0.6575 ± 0.0242
XceptionNet	NB	0.7240 ± 0.0094	0.6667 ± 0.0001	0.7576 ± 0.0149	0.6182 ± 0.0146	0.6411 ± 0.0079
	SVM	0.7597 ± 0.0094	0.5258 ± 0.0219	0.8966 ± 0.0085	0.7489 ± 0.0167	0.6170 ± 0.0182
	LDA	0.7972 ± 0.0058	0.6662 ± 0.0100	0.8739 ± 0.0058	0.7558 ± 0.0094	0.7081 ± 0.0086
	DT	0.7403 ± 0.0243	0.6733 ± 0.0379	0.7795 ± 0.0286	0.6446 ± 0.0344	0.6567 ± 0.0313

5.3. Post-Treatment Changes (PTC) vs. MIBC

PTC vs. MIBC classification was performed with a 10-fold cross-validation on a dataset of 76 ROIs (35 PTC, 41 MIBC). LDA classifier on XceptionNet-based features provided the best performance with an accuracy of 74.96%, sensitivity of 80.51%, specificity of 70.22%, precision of 69.78% and F1-score of 74.73%. Table 5 summarizes the classification performances of the 10-fold machine learning classifiers, on features extracted from each of the five pre-trained deep models (results visualized on associated Figure 7 bar plot).

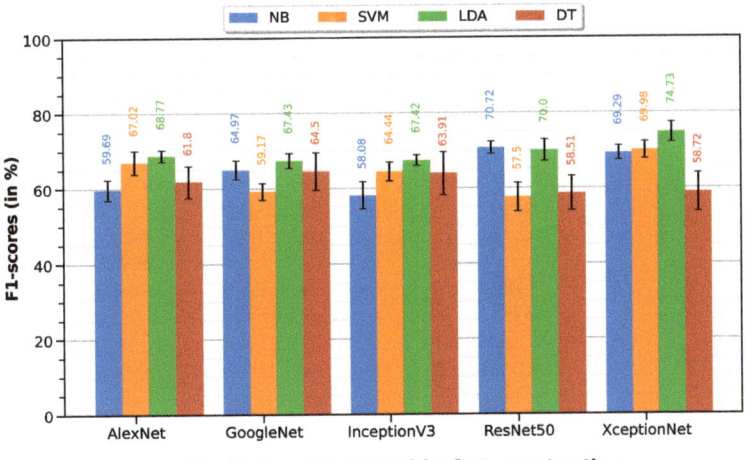

Figure 7. F1-scores of the 10-fold machine learning classifiers on features extracted from each of the five pre-trained deep models.

Table 5. Classification performances of the 10-fold machine learning classifiers on features extracted from each of the five pre-trained deep models.

Feature Extractor	Classifier	Accuracy	Sensitivity	Specificity	Precision	F1-Score
AlexNet	NB	0.6695 ± 0.0097	0.5323 ± 0.0172	0.7866 ± 0.0114	0.6806 ± 0.0133	0.5969 ± 0.0139
	SVM	0.6880 ± 0.0139	0.6894 ± 0.0216	0.6868 ± 0.0168	0.6530 ± 0.0145	0.6702 ± 0.0157
	LDA	0.7100 ± 0.0070	0.6934 ± 0.0116	0.7241 ± 0.0121	0.6826 ± 0.0091	0.6877 ± 0.0076
	DT	0.6503 ± 0.0187	0.6160 ± 0.0290	0.6795 ± 0.0270	0.6226 ± 0.0215	0.6180 ± 0.0214
GoogleNet	NB	0.7176 ± 0.0101	0.5689 ± 0.0139	0.8446 ± 0.0149	0.7589 ± 0.0180	0.6497 ± 0.0124
	SVM	0.6592 ± 0.0085	0.5366 ± 0.0128	0.7639 ± 0.0111	0.6602 ± 0.0122	0.5917 ± 0.0110
	LDA	0.7276 ± 0.0072	0.6129 ± 0.0126	0.8256 ± 0.0082	0.7502 ± 0.0094	0.6743 ± 0.0097
	DT	0.6725 ± 0.0237	0.6471 ± 0.0321	0.6941 ± 0.0345	0.6464 ± 0.0288	0.6450 ± 0.0252
InceptionV3	NB	0.6495 ± 0.0150	0.5280 ± 0.0207	0.7532 ± 0.0205	0.6475 ± 0.0214	0.5808 ± 0.0182
	SVM	0.6907 ± 0.0100	0.6094 ± 0.0169	0.7600 ± 0.0121	0.6846 ± 0.0122	0.6444 ± 0.0129
	LDA	0.7083 ± 0.0068	0.6554 ± 0.0086	0.7534 ± 0.0109	0.6945 ± 0.0096	0.6742 ± 0.0070
	DT	0.6589 ± 0.0260	0.6583 ± 0.0383	0.6595 ± 0.0327	0.6238 ± 0.0270	0.6391 ± 0.0287
ResNet50	NB	0.6688 ± 0.0085	0.8689 ± 0.0138	0.4980 ± 0.0125	0.5965 ± 0.0066	0.7072 ± 0.0079
	SVM	0.6197 ± 0.0157	0.5600 ± 0.0251	0.6707 ± 0.0232	0.5930 ± 0.0186	0.5750 ± 0.0189
	LDA	0.6895 ± 0.0094	0.7903 ± 0.0306	0.6034 ± 0.0169	0.6298 ± 0.0069	0.7000 ± 0.0144
	DT	0.6161 ± 0.0207	0.5891 ± 0.0298	0.6390 ± 0.0313	0.5838 ± 0.0239	0.5851 ± 0.0229
XceptionNet	NB	0.6849 ± 0.0087	0.7726 ± 0.0142	0.6100 ± 0.0094	0.6284 ± 0.0075	0.6929 ± 0.0094
	SVM	0.6868 ± 0.0105	0.7931 ± 0.0170	0.5961 ± 0.0102	0.6263 ± 0.0085	0.6998 ± 0.0112
	LDA	0.7496 ± 0.0119	0.8051 ± 0.0193	0.7022 ± 0.0133	0.6978 ± 0.0113	0.7473 ± 0.0131
	DT	0.6253 ± 0.0219	0.5806 ± 0.0320	0.6634 ± 0.0298	0.5967 ± 0.0251	0.5872 ± 0.0254

6. Discussion

Optimal management of bladder cancer requires a multidisciplinary approach, with tumor staging an important prognostic factor that determines the mode of initial treatment. Cystoscopy examination, together with a biopsy, remains the primary mode of tumor detection and clinical staging in patients with suspected bladder cancer. CT is often the first exam modality for bladder cancer detection due to its wide availability and minimal associated complication. However, the CT findings are nonspecific with limited accuracy. At least one article [28] reported the accuracy of CT evaluation for bladder cancer as low as 49%.

Differentiating non-muscle-invasive bladder cancer (NMIBC), consisting of Ta, Tis, and T1 stages, from muscle-invasive bladder cancer (MBIC), consisting of T_2-$T_4$4 stages, is important as MIBC is more likely to spread to lymph nodes and other organs requiring radical cystectomy with or without systemic chemotherapy [29]. In contrast, NMBIC has low risk of recurrent disease but can be effectively treated with intravesical chemotherapy, immunotherapy, and transurethral resection of bladder tumor (TURBT) [30]. Early differentiation of two bladder cancer stages is critical for the appropriate utilization of medical resources and optimization of targeted treatment. Therefore, accurate initial staging on the CT exam is crucial for therapeutic decision-making [31].

While histopathologic cancer detection using pre-trained neural network-based models is mainstream, in this project, we were faced with the additional issues of imbalanced data and limited sample size. In comparison to [32], where the number of image samples was 1350, and the number of classification categories was 2 (1200 bladder cancer tissues, 1150 normal tissues), we had a total of only 100 tissue scans distributed across 7 stages of urothelial carcinoma (6 T_a, 9 $T_i s$, 35 T_0, 9 T_1, 13 T_2, 24 T_3, 4 T_4). The issue of class-imbalanced samples could not be solved using SMOTE because the sheer lack of samples in some of the categories (especially T_a and T_4) meant that the synthetically generated samples were very similar to the few original ones, and contributed towards decreased variance in the training dataset—therefore resulting in overfitting. Next, the issue of overfitting, which we faced while performing end-to-end classification using pre-trained networks, was tackled by:

(1) making use of a combined deep learning-machine learning approach where the trained weights from the pre-trained neural network were then classified using statistical machine learning approaches. (2) An ensemble statistical- and supervised learning-based feature selection approach that helped remove features that were unimportant. Ref. [32], which focused on bladder cancer detection from cytoscopic images alone, reported an accuracy of 86.36% with deep learning-based classifiers and 84.09% with human surgical experts; however, no significant difference was found between the two (p-value greater than 0.05).

The LDA classifier on XceptionNet performed best in terms of the F1-score for all three experiments in our study—namely, normal vs. cancer, NMIBC vs. MIBC and PTC vs. MIBC. For normal vs. cancer classification, LDA on XceptionNet had an F1-score of (89.39 ± 0.26)%, which will facilitate clinicians in better detection of lesions because, for histopathologic images in general, and bladder scans in particular, flat and subtle lesions are often missed on visual inspection. For NMIBC vs. MIBC classification, LDA on XceptionNet had an F1-score of (70.81 ± 0.86). For PTC vs. MIBC classification, LDA on XceptionNet had an F1-score of (74.73 ± 1.31)%, which is especially encouraging because there is an unmet demand to develop new non-invasive techniques to assess accurate prediction of recurrence and response to chemotherapy. Currently, patients with bladder cancer require repeat cystoscopies and biopsies of the bladder to assess the response and recurrence of the disease. This procedure is very costly and invasive, with several associated complications, including bladder perforation.

Our study has certain limitations. It is a retrospective design based on a single-center small dataset that may overestimate the diagnostic performance of our model. Therefore, our next step is to extend the diagnostic model on prospective, multi-center datasets with external validation.

7. Conclusions

Our model showed a high F1-score, which means that our model indicated a high value for both recall and precision. We used the F1-score to compare our classifiers. We opted for the ResNet-50, whose F1-score was higher among others and ResNet-50 showed the best classification based on the F1-score for all three experiments.

Radiomics-assisted interpretation of CT by radiologists may help more accurately diagnose bladder cancer. This can allow the timely utilization of medical resources and consultation with oncologists and urologists, ultimately improving patients' clinical outcomes.

Author Contributions: Conceptualization, S.S., K.M., W.I., A.C.S., P.S. and T.W.; methodology, S.S., T.W. and A.C.S.; software, S.S.; validation, S.S. and K.M.; formal analysis, S.S.; investigation, S.S.; resources, T.W., A.C.S. and P.S.; data curation, K.M., R.W.T., I.B.R., A.C.S., A.H.B., C.M., T.H.H., G.S., H.M.A.-M. and P.S.; writing—original draft preparation, S.S. and W.I.; writing—review and editing, S.S., K.M., W.I., T.W., A.C.S. and P.S.; visualization, S.S.; supervision, T.W., P.S. and A.C.S.; project administration, T.W., P.S. and A.C.S. All authors have read and agreed to the published version of the manuscript.

Funding: This research received no external funding.

Institutional Review Board Statement: The study was conducted according to the guidelines of the Declaration of Helsinki, and approved by the Institutional Review Board (or Ethics Committee) of Mayo Clinic Arizona (protocol code 20-012296 and date of approval 15 December 2020).

Informed Consent Statement: Informed consent was obtained from all subjects involved in the study. Furthermore, all data used in the study have been de-identified of any personal information.

Data Availability Statement: Data will be made available under reasonable request.

Conflicts of Interest: The authors declare no conflict of interest.

References

1. Kim, L.H.; Patel, M.I. Transurethral resection of bladder tumour (TURBT). *Transl. Androl. Urol.* **2020**, *9*, 3056. [CrossRef]
2. Furuse, H.; Ozono, S. Transurethral resection of the bladder tumour (TURBT) for non-muscle invasive bladder cancer: Basic skills. *Int. J. Urol.* **2010**, *17*, 698–699. [CrossRef] [PubMed]
3. Richterstetter, M.; Wullich, B.; Amann, K.; Haeberle, L.; Engehausen, D.G.; Goebell, P.J.; Krause, F.S. The value of extended transurethral resection of bladder tumour (TURBT) in the treatment of bladder cancer. *BJU Int.* **2012**, *110*, E76–E79. [CrossRef] [PubMed]
4. Sanli, O.; Dobruch, J.; Knowles, M.A.; Burger, M.; Alemozaffar, M.; Nielsen, M.E.; Lotan, Y. Bladder cancer. *Nat. Rev. Dis. Primers* **2017**, *3*, 1–19. [CrossRef] [PubMed]
5. Bostrom, P.J.; Van Rhijn, B.W.; Fleshner, N.; Finelli, A.; Jewett, M.; Thoms, J.; Hanna, S.; Kuk, C.; Zlotta, A.R. Staging and staging errors in bladder cancer. *Eur. Urol. Suppl.* **2010**, *9*, 2–9. [CrossRef]
6. Colombel, M.; Soloway, M.; Akaza, H.; Böhle, A.; Palou, J.; Buckley, R.; Lamm, D.; Brausi, M.; Witjes, J.A.; Persad, R. Epidemiology, staging, grading, and risk stratification of bladder cancer. *Eur. Urol. Suppl.* **2008**, *7*, 618–626. [CrossRef]
7. Kaufman, D.S.; Shipley, W.U.; Feldman, A.S. Bladder cancer. *Lancet* **2009**, *374*, 239–249. [CrossRef]
8. Kirkali, Z.; Chan, T.; Manoharan, M.; Algaba, F.; Busch, C.; Cheng, L.; Kiemeney, L.; Kriegmair, M.; Montironi, R.; Murphy, W.M.; et al. Bladder cancer: Epidemiology, staging and grading, and diagnosis. *Urology* **2005**, *66*, 4–34. [CrossRef]
9. Sharma, S.; Ksheersagar, P.; Sharma, P. Diagnosis and treatment of bladder cancer. *Am. Fam. Physician* **2009**, *80*, 717–723.
10. Gofrit, O.; Shapiro, A.; Pode, D.; Sidi, A.; Nativ, O.; Leib, Z.; Witjes, J.; Van Der Heijden, A.; Naspro, R.; Colombo, R. Combined local bladder hyperthermia and intravesical chemotherapy for the treatment of high-grade superficial bladder cancer. *Urology* **2004**, *63*, 466–471. [CrossRef]
11. Sun, M.; Trinh, Q.D. Diagnosis and staging of bladder cancer. *Hematol./Oncol. Clin.* **2015**, *29*, 205–218. [CrossRef]
12. Hammouda, K.; Khalifa, F.; Soliman, A.; Ghazal, M.; Abou El-Ghar, M.; Badawy, M.A.; Darwish, H.E.; Khelifi, A.; El-Baz, A. A multiparametric MRI-based CAD system for accurate diagnosis of bladder cancer staging. *Comput. Med. Imaging Graph.* **2021**, *90*, 101911. [CrossRef]
13. Xu, X.; Liu, Y.; Zhang, X.; Tian, Q.; Wu, Y.; Zhang, G.; Meng, J.; Yang, Z.; Lu, H. Preoperative prediction of muscular invasiveness of bladder cancer with radiomic features on conventional MRI and its high-order derivative maps. *Abdom. Radiol.* **2017**, *42*, 1896–1905. [CrossRef]
14. He, K.; Zhang, X.; Ren, S.; Sun, J. Deep residual learning for image recognition. In Proceedings of the IEEE Conference on Computer Vision and Pattern Recognition, Las Vegas, NV, USA, 27–30 June 2016; pp. 770–778.
15. Wang, C.; Udupa, J.K.; Tong, Y.; Chen, J.; Venigalla, S.; Odhner, D.; Guzzo, T.J.; Christodouleas, J.; Torigian, D.A. Urinary bladder cancer T-staging from T2-weighted MR images using an optimal biomarker approach. In *Medical Imaging 2018: Computer-Aided Diagnosis*; SPIE: Bellingham, WA, USA, 2018; Volume 10575, pp. 526–531.
16. Urdal, J.; Engan, K.; Kvikstad, V.; Janssen, E.A. Prognostic prediction of histopathological images by local binary patterns and RUSBoost. In Proceedings of the 2017 25th European Signal Processing Conference (EUSIPCO), Kos Island, Greece, 28 August–2 September 2017; IEEE: Piscataway, NJ, USA, 2017; pp. 2349–2353.
17. Tong, Y.; Udupa, J.K.; Wang, C.; Chen, J.; Venigalla, S.; Guzzo, T.J.; Mamtani, R.; Baumann, B.C.; Christodouleas, J.P.; Torigian, D.A. Radiomics-guided therapy for bladder cancer: Using an optimal biomarker approach to determine extent of bladder cancer invasion from t2-weighted magnetic resonance images. *Adv. Radiat. Oncol.* **2018**, *3*, 331–338. [CrossRef]
18. Lin, P.; Wen, D.Y.; Chen, L.; Li, X.; Li, S.h.; Yan, H.B.; He, R.Q.; Chen, G.; He, Y.; Yang, H. A radiogenomics signature for predicting the clinical outcome of bladder urothelial carcinoma. *Eur. Radiol.* **2020**, *30*, 547–557. [CrossRef]
19. Çinar, U.; Çetin, Y.Y.; Çetin-Atalay, R.; Çetin, E. Classification of human carcinoma cells using multispectral imagery. In *Medical Imaging 2016: Digital Pathology*; SPIE: Bellingham, WA, USA, 2016; Volume 9791, pp. 341–346.
20. Lingley-Papadopoulos, C.A.; Loew, M.H.; Manyak, M.J.; Zara, J.M. Computer recognition of cancer in the urinary bladder using optical coherence tomography and texture analysis. *J. Biomed. Opt.* **2008**, *13*, 024003. [CrossRef]
21. Zhang, X.; Xu, X.; Tian, Q.; Li, B.; Wu, Y.; Yang, Z.; Liang, Z.; Liu, Y.; Cui, G.; Lu, H. Radiomics assessment of bladder cancer grade using texture features from diffusion-weighted imaging. *J. Magn. Reson. Imaging* **2017**, *46*, 1281–1288. [CrossRef]
22. Yang, Y.; Zou, X.; Wang, Y.; Ma, X. Application of deep learning as a noninvasive tool to differentiate muscle-invasive bladder cancer and non–muscle-invasive bladder cancer with CT. *Eur. J. Radiol.* **2021**, *139*, 109666. [CrossRef]
23. Chapman-Sung, D.H.; Hadjiiski, L.; Gandikota, D.; Chan, H.P.; Samala, R.; Caoili, E.M.; Cohan, R.H.; Weizer, A.; Alva, A.; Zhou, C. Convolutional neural network-based decision support system for bladder cancer staging in CT urography: Decision threshold estimation and validation. In *Medical Imaging 2020: Computer-Aided Diagnosis*; SPIE: Bellingham, WA, USA, 2020; Volume 11314, pp. 424–429.
24. Zhang, G.; Xu, L.; Zhao, L.; Mao, L.; Li, X.; Jin, Z.; Sun, H. CT-based radiomics to predict the pathological grade of bladder cancer. *Eur. Radiol.* **2020**, *30*, 6749–6756. [CrossRef]
25. Yin, P.N.; Kc, K.; Wei, S.; Yu, Q.; Li, R.; Haake, A.R.; Miyamoto, H.; Cui, F. Histopathological distinction of non-invasive and invasive bladder cancers using machine learning approaches. *BMC Med. Inform. Decis. Mak.* **2020**, *20*, 1–11. [CrossRef]
26. Deng, J.; Dong, W.; Socher, R.; Li, L.J.; Li, K.; Fei-Fei, L. ImageNet: A Large-Scale Hierarchical Image Database. In Proceedings of the 2009 IEEE Conference on Computer Vision and Pattern Recognition, Miami, FL, USA, 20–25 June 2009; pp. 248–255.

27. Magers, M.J.; Lopez-Beltran, A.; Montironi, R.; Williamson, S.R.; Kaimakliotis, H.Z.; Cheng, L. Staging of bladder cancer. *Histopathology* **2019**, *74*, 112–134. [CrossRef] [PubMed]
28. Tritschler, S.; Mosler, C.; Straub, J.; Buchner, A.; Karl, A.; Graser, A.; Stief, C.; Tilki, D. Staging of muscle-invasive bladder cancer: Can computerized tomography help us to decide on local treatment? *World J. Urol.* **2012**, *30*, 827–831. [CrossRef] [PubMed]
29. Chang, S.S.; Bochner, B.H.; Chou, R.; Dreicer, R.; Kamat, A.M.; Lerner, S.P.; Lotan, Y.; Meeks, J.J.; Michalski, J.M.; Morgan, T.M.; et al. Treatment of non-metastatic muscle-invasive bladder cancer: AUA/ASCO/ASTRO/SUO guideline. *J. Urol.* **2017**, *198*, 552–559. [CrossRef]
30. Chang, S.S.; Boorjian, S.A.; Chou, R.; Clark, P.E.; Daneshmand, S.; Konety, B.R.; Pruthi, R.; Quale, D.Z.; Ritch, C.R.; Seigne, J.D.; et al. Diagnosis and treatment of non-muscle invasive bladder cancer: AUA/SUO guideline. *J. Urol.* **2016**, *196*, 1021–1029. [CrossRef]
31. Brierley, J.D.; Gospodarowicz, M.K.; Wittekind, C. *TNM Classification of Malignant Tumours*; John Wiley & Sons: Hoboken, NJ, USA, 2017.
32. Yang, R.; Du, Y.; Weng, X.; Chen, Z.; Wang, S.; Liu, X. Automatic recognition of bladder tumours using deep learning technology and its clinical application. *Int. J. Med. Robot. Comput. Assist. Surg.* **2021**, *17*, e2194. [CrossRef] [PubMed]

Disclaimer/Publisher's Note: The statements, opinions and data contained in all publications are solely those of the individual author(s) and contributor(s) and not of MDPI and/or the editor(s). MDPI and/or the editor(s) disclaim responsibility for any injury to people or property resulting from any ideas, methods, instructions or products referred to in the content.

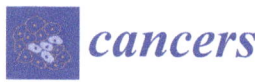

Article

Adaptive Aquila Optimizer with Explainable Artificial Intelligence-Enabled Cancer Diagnosis on Medical Imaging

Salem Alkhalaf [1,*], Fahad Alturise [1], Adel Aboud Bahaddad [2], Bushra M. Elamin Elnaim [3], Samah Shabana [4], Sayed Abdel-Khalek [5] and Romany F. Mansour [6]

[1] Department of Computer, College of Science and Arts in Ar Rass, Qassim University, Ar Rass 58892, Saudi Arabia
[2] Department of Information Systems, Faculty of Computing and Information Technology, King Abdulaziz University, Jeddah 21589, Saudi Arabia
[3] Department of Computer Science, College of Science and Humanities in Al-Sulail, Prince Sattam Bin Abdulaziz University, Al-Kharj 16278, Saudi Arabia
[4] Pharmacognosy Department, Faculty of Pharmaceutical Sciences and Drug Manufacturing, Misr University for Science and Technology (MUST), Giza 3236101, Egypt
[5] Department of Mathematics, College of Science, Taif University, Taif 21944, Saudi Arabia
[6] Department of Mathematics, Faculty of Science, New Valley University, El-Kharga 1064188, Egypt
* Correspondence: s.alkhalaf@qu.edu.sa

Simple Summary: For automated cancer diagnosis on medical imaging, explainable artificial intelligence technology uses advanced image analysis methods like deep learning to make a diagnosis and analyze medical images, as well as provide a clear explanation for how it arrived at its diagnosis. The objective of XAI is to provide patients and doctors with a better understanding of the system's decision-making process and to increase transparency and trust in the diagnosis method. The manual classification of cancer using medical images is a tedious and tiresome process, which necessitates the design of automated tools for the decision-making process. In this study, we explored the significant application of explainable artificial intelligence and an ensemble of deep-learning models for automated cancer diagnosis. To demonstrate the enhanced performance of the proposed model, a widespread comparison study is made with recent models, and the results exhibit the significance of the proposed model on benchmark test images. Therefore, the proposed model has the potential as an automated, accurate, and rapid tool for supporting the detection and classification process of cancer.

Citation: Alkhalaf, S.; Alturise, F.; Bahaddad, A.A.; Elnaim, B.M.E.; Shabana, S.; Abdel-Khalek, S.; Mansour, R.F. Adaptive Aquila Optimizer with Explainable Artificial Intelligence-Enabled Cancer Diagnosis on Medical Imaging. *Cancers* 2023, 15, 1492. https://doi.org/10.3390/cancers15051492

Academic Editors: Marcin Woźniak and Muhammad Fazal Ijaz

Received: 28 January 2023
Revised: 19 February 2023
Accepted: 20 February 2023
Published: 27 February 2023

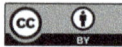

Copyright: © 2023 by the authors. Licensee MDPI, Basel, Switzerland. This article is an open access article distributed under the terms and conditions of the Creative Commons Attribution (CC BY) license (https://creativecommons.org/licenses/by/4.0/).

Abstract: Explainable Artificial Intelligence (XAI) is a branch of AI that mainly focuses on developing systems that provide understandable and clear explanations for their decisions. In the context of cancer diagnoses on medical imaging, an XAI technology uses advanced image analysis methods like deep learning (DL) to make a diagnosis and analyze medical images, as well as provide a clear explanation for how it arrived at its diagnoses. This includes highlighting specific areas of the image that the system recognized as indicative of cancer while also providing data on the fundamental AI algorithm and decision-making process used. The objective of XAI is to provide patients and doctors with a better understanding of the system's decision-making process and to increase transparency and trust in the diagnosis method. Therefore, this study develops an Adaptive Aquila Optimizer with Explainable Artificial Intelligence Enabled Cancer Diagnosis (AAOXAI-CD) technique on Medical Imaging. The proposed AAOXAI-CD technique intends to accomplish the effectual colorectal and osteosarcoma cancer classification process. To achieve this, the AAOXAI-CD technique initially employs the Faster SqueezeNet model for feature vector generation. As well, the hyperparameter tuning of the Faster SqueezeNet model takes place with the use of the AAO algorithm. For cancer classification, the majority weighted voting ensemble model with three DL classifiers, namely recurrent neural network (RNN), gated recurrent unit (GRU), and bidirectional long short-term memory (BiLSTM). Furthermore, the AAOXAI-CD technique combines the XAI approach LIME for better understanding and explainability of the black-box method for accurate cancer detection. The simulation evaluation of the AAOXAI-CD methodology can be tested on medical cancer imaging databases, and the outcomes ensured the auspicious outcome of the AAOXAI-CD methodology than other current approaches.

Keywords: cancer diagnosis; explainable artificial intelligence; ensemble learning; Adaptive Aquila Optimizer; deep learning

1. Introduction

Diagnosis of cancer is an indispensable problem in the medical sector. Initial identification of cancer is vital for better chances of treatment and the best course of action [1]. Therefore, cancer can be considered as one major topic where numerous authors carried out various research to attain higher performance in treatment prevention and diagnosis. Initial identification of tumors can increase treatment options and chances of survival of patients. Medical images like Magnetic Resonance Imaging, mammograms, microscopic images, and ultrasound were the typical technique for diagnosing cancer [2].

In recent times, computer-aided diagnosis (CAD) mechanism was utilized to help doctors in diagnosing tumors so that the accuracy level of diagnosis gets enhanced. CAD helps in reducing missed cancer lesions because of medical practitioner fatigue, minimizing data overloading and work pressure, and reducing the variability of intra-and-inter readers of imageries [3]. Problems like technical reasons are relevant to imaging quality, and errors caused by humans have augmented the misdiagnosis of breast cancer in the interpretation of radiologists. To solve these limitations, CAD mechanisms were advanced to automate breast cancer diagnosis and categorize malignant and benign lesions [4]. The CAD mechanism enhances the performance of radiologists in discriminating and finding abnormal and normal tissues. Such a process can be executed only as a double reader, but decisions are made by radiologists [5]. Figure 1 represents the structure of explainable artificial intelligence.

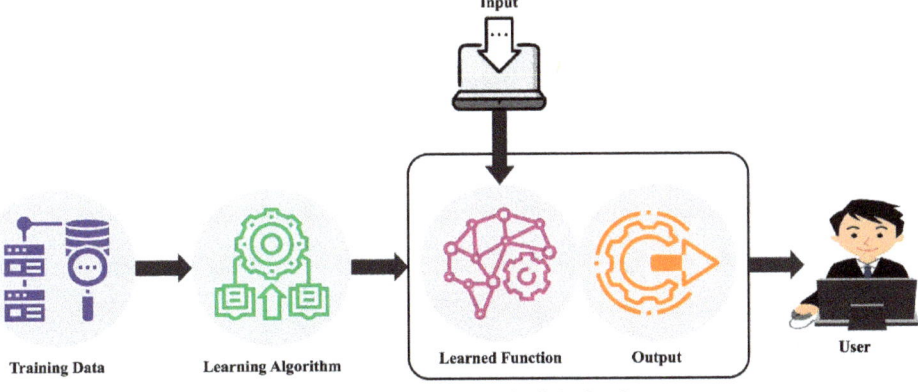

Figure 1. Structure of XAI.

Recent advancements in the resolution of medical imaging modalities have enhanced diagnostic accuracy [6]. Effective use of imaging data for enhancing the diagnosis becomes significant. Currently, computer-aided diagnosis systems (CAD) have advanced a novel context in radiology to make use of data that should be implemented in the diagnosis of different diseases and different imaging modalities [7–10]. The efficacy of radiologists' analysis can be enhanced in the context of consistency and accuracy in diagnosis or detection, while production can be enhanced by minimizing the hours needed to read the imageries. The results can be extracted through several methods in computer vision (CV) for presenting certain important variables like the likelihood of malignancy and the location of suspicious lesions of the detected lesions [11]. Then, DL technology has now significantly advanced, increasing expectations for the likelihood of computer software relevant to tumor screening again. Deep learning (DL) is a type of neural network (NNs). This NN has an output layer, an input layer, and a hidden layer. DL can be a NN with a lot of hidden layers. In the past, DL had more achievements, i.e., incredible performance improvements, particularly in speech recognition and image classification [12]. Recently, DL has been utilized in various areas. As they can solve complicated issues, DNNs are now common in the healthcare field. However, decision-making by these methods was fundamentally a black-box procedure making it problematic for doctors to determine whether choices were dependable. The usage of explainable artificial intelligence (XAI) can be recommended as the key to this issue [13].

1.1. Related Works

Van der Velden et al. [14] presented an outline of explainable AI (XAI) utilized in DL-related medical image analysis. A structure of XAI criteria can be presented for classifying DL-related medical image analysis techniques. As per the structure and anatomical location, studies on the XAI mechanism in medical image analysis were categorized and surveyed. Esmaeili et al. [15] intend to assess the performance of selective DL methods on localizing cancer lesions and differentiating lesions from healthier areas in MRI contrasts. Despite an important correlation between lesion localization accuracy and classification, the familiar AI techniques inspected in this study categorize certain cancer brains dependent upon other non-related attributes. The outcomes advocate that the abovementioned AI methods can formulate an intuition for method interpretability and play a significant role in the performance assessment of DL methods.

In [16], a new automatic classification system by merging several DL methods was devised for identifying prostate cancer from MRI and ultrasound (US) imageries. To enrich the performance of the model, particularly on the MRI data, the fusion model can be advanced by integrating the optimal pretrained method as feature extractors with shallow ML techniques (e.g., K-NN, SVM, RF, and Adaboost). At last, the fusion model can be inspected by explainable AI to identify the fact why it finds samples as Malignant or Benign Stage in prostate tumors. Kobylińska et al. [17] modeled selective techniques from the XAI domain in the instance of methods implemented for assessing lung cancer risk in the screening process of lung cancer using low-dose CT. The usage of such methods offers a good understanding of differences and similarities among the three typically used methods in screening lung cancer they are LCART, BACH, and PLCOm2012.

In [18], an explainable AI (XAI) structure was devised in this study for presenting the local and global analysis of auxiliary identification of hepatitis while maintaining good predictive outcomes. Firstly, a public hepatitis classifier benchmark from UCI was utilized for testing the structure feasibility. Afterward, the transparent and black-box ML methods were used to predict the deterioration of hepatitis. Transparent methods like KNN, LR, and DT were selected. While the black-box method like the RF, XGBoost, and SVM were selected. Watson and Al Moubayed [19] devised a method agnostic explainability-related technique for the precise identification of adversarial instances on two datasets with various properties and complexity: chest X-ray (CXR) data and Electronic Health Record (EHR). In [20], the XAI tool can be applied to the breast cancer (BC) dataset and offers a graphical analysis. The medical implication and molecular processes behind circulating adiponectin, HOMA, leptin, and BC resistance were sightseen, and XAI techniques were utilized for constructing methods for the diagnosis of new BC biomarkers.

1.2. Paper Contributions

This study develops an Adaptive Aquila Optimizer with Explainable Artificial Intelligence Enabled Cancer Diagnosis (AAOXAI-CD) technique on Medical Imaging. The proposed AAOXAI-CD technique uses the Faster SqueezeNet model for feature vector generation. As well as the execution of hyperparameter tuning of the Faster SqueezeNet model done with the AAO algorithm. For cancer classification, the majority weighted voting ensemble model with three DL classifiers, namely recurrent neural network (RNN), gated recurrent unit (GRU), and bidirectional long short-term memory (BiLSTM). Furthermore, the AAOXAI-CD technique combines the XAI approach LIME for better understanding and explainability of the black-box method for accurate cancer detection. The simulation evaluation of the AAOXAI-CD technique is tested on medical cancer imaging databases.

2. Materials and Methods

In this article, we have developed an automated cancer diagnosis approach using the AAOXAI-CD approach on medical images. The proposed AAOXAI-CD system attained the effectual colorectal and osteosarcoma cancer classification process. It encompasses Faster SqueezeNet-based feature vector generation, AAO-based parameter tuning, ensemble classification, and XAI modeling. Figure 2 defines the overall flow of the AAOXAI-CD approach. The overall process involved in the proposed model is given in Algorithm 1.

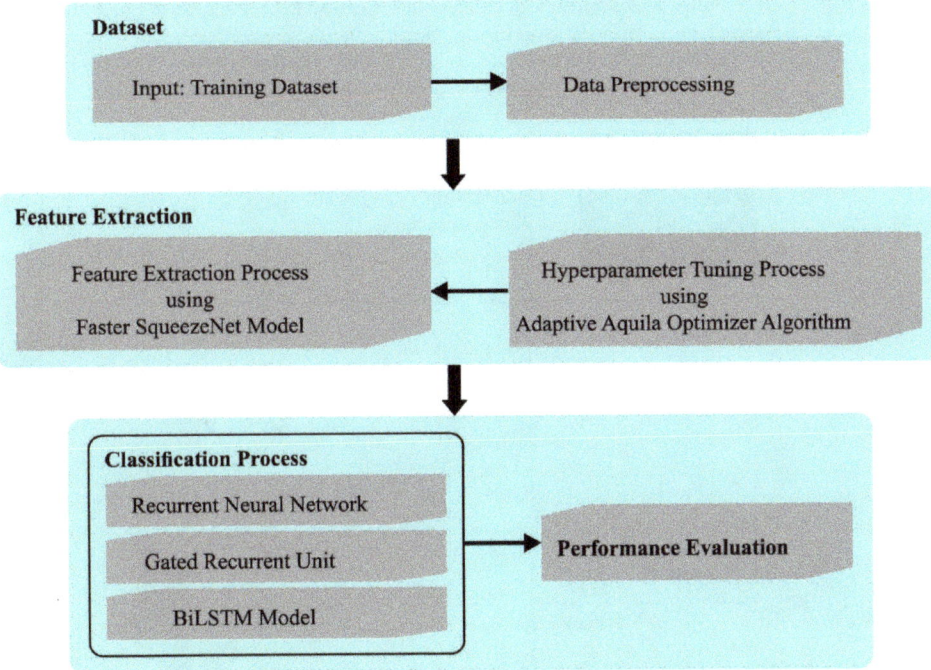

Figure 2. The overall flow of AAOXAI-CD approach.

Algorithm 1: Process Involved in AAOXAI-CD Technique

Step 1: Input Dataset (Training Images)
Step 2: Image Pre-Processing
Step 3: Feature Extraction Using Faster SqueezeNet Model
Step 4: Parameter Tuning Process
    Step 4.1: Initialize the Population and Its Parameters
    Step 4.2: Calculate the Fitness Values
    Step 4.3: Exploration Process and Exploitation Process
    Step 4.4: Update the Fitness Values
    Step 4.5: Obtain Best Solution
Step 5: Ensemble of Classifier (RNN, GRU, and Bi-LSTM)
Step 6: Classification Output

2.1. Feature Extraction Using Faster SqueezeNet

Primarily, the AAOXAI-CD technique employed the Faster SqueezeNet method for feature vector generation. Fast SqueezeNet was proposed to enrich the real-time performance and accuracy of cancer classification [21]. We added BatchNorm and residual structure to prevent overfitting. Simultaneously, like DenseNet, concat is employed to interconnect dissimilar layers to increase the expressiveness of the first few layers in the network. Figure 3 represents the architecture of the Faster SqueezeNet method.

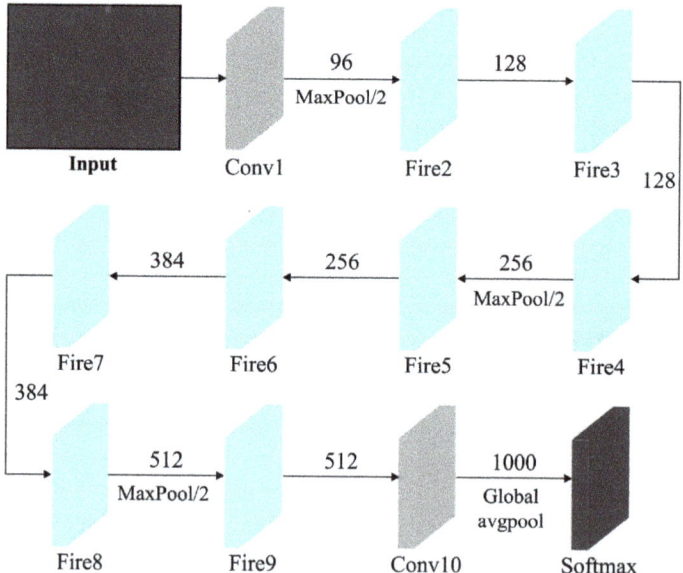

Figure 3. Architecture of Faster SqueezeNet.

Fast SqueezeNet comprises a global average pooling layer, 1 BatchNorm layer, 3 block layers, and 4 convolutional layers. In the following ways, Fast SqueezeNet can be improved:

(1) To further enrich the information flow among layers DenseNet is imitated, and a distinct connection mode is devised. This covers a fire module and pooling layer, and lastly, 2 concat layers are interconnected to the following convolution layer.

The present layer receives each feature map of the previous layer, and we apply $x_0, \ldots, x_{l-1}$ as input; then, x_l is expressed as

$$x_l = H_l([x_0, x_1, \ldots, x_{l-1}]), \tag{1}$$

where $[x_0, x_1, \ldots, x_{l-1}]$ represent the connection of feature graphs produced in layers 0, 1, ..., $l-1$ and $H_l(\cdot)$ concatenated more than one input data. Now, characterizes the max pooling layer, x_1 designates Fire layers, and x_l indicates the concat layer.

Initially, the performance of the network is improved without excessively raising the number of network variables, and simultaneously, any two-layer network could directly transmit data.

(2) We learned from the ResNet structure and suggested constituent elements, which comprise a fire module and pooling layer, to ensure improved network convergence. Lastly, afterward, two layers were summed, and it was interconnected to the next convolution layers.

In ResNet, shortcut connection employs identity mapping that implies input of a convolutional stack will be added directly to the resultant of the convolutional stack. Formally, the underlying mapping can be represented as $H(x)$, considering the stacked non-linear layer fits another mapping of $F(x) := H(x) - x$. The original mapping is rewritten into $F(x) + x$. $F(x) + x$ is comprehended by the structure named shortcut connection in the encrypting process.

In this work, the hyperparameter tuning of the Faster SqueezeNet method occurs by employing the AAO algorithm. This abovementioned algorithm is based on the distinct hunting strategies of Aquila for different prey [22]. For faster-moving prey, the Aquila needs to obtain the prey in a precise and faster manner, where the global exploration capability of the model was reflected. The optimizer technique was characterized by mimicking 4 behaviors of Aquila hunting. Firstly, the population needs to arbitrarily generate in-between the lower bound (LB) and upper bound (UB) dependent upon the problem, as given in Equation (2). The approximate optimum solution at the time of the iteration can be defined as the optimum solution. The present set of candidate solutions X was made at random by using the following expression:

$$X = \begin{bmatrix} x_{1,1} & \cdots & x_{1,D} \\ \vdots & \ddots & \vdots \\ x_{n,1} & \cdots & x_{n,D} \end{bmatrix} \quad (2)$$

$$X_{i,j} = rand \times (UB_j - LB_j) + LB_j, \ i = 1, 2, \ldots, N j = 1, 2, \ldots D \quad (3)$$

where n signifies the overall amount of candidate solutions, D indicates the dimensionality of problems, and $x_{n,D}$ represents the location of n-th solutions in d dimensional space. Rand denotes a randomly generated value, and UB_j and LB_j signify the j-th dimensional upper and lower boundary of the problem.

Initially, choose search spaces by hovering above in vertical bends. Aquila hovers above to identify the prey area and rapidly choose the better prey region as follows:

$$X_1(t+1) = X_{best}(t) \times \left(1 - \frac{t}{T}\right) + (X_M(t) - X_{best}(t)) \times rand \quad (4)$$

$$X_M(t) = \frac{1}{N} \sum_{i=1}^{N} X_i(t), \forall j = 1, 2, \ldots, D \quad (5)$$

where $X_1(t+1)$ symbolizes the location of the individual at $t+1$ time, $X_{best}(t+1)$ signifies the present global optimum site at the t-th iteration, T and t symbolize the maximal amount of iterations and the present amount of iterations, correspondingly, $X(t)$ represents the average location of the individual at the existing iteration, and $Rand$ represents the randomly generated value within $[0, 1]$ in Gaussian distribution. The next strategy was a short gliding attack in isometric flight. Aquila flies over the targeted prey to prepare for assault while they find prey region from a higher altitude. This can be formulated as

$$X_2(t+1) = X_{best}(t) \times levy(D) + X_R(t) + (y - x) \times rand \quad (6)$$

$$levy\ (D) = s \times \frac{u \times \sigma}{|v|^{\frac{1}{\beta}}} \tag{7}$$

$$\sigma = \left(\frac{\Gamma(1+\beta) \times \sin\left(\frac{\pi\beta}{2}\right)}{\Gamma\left(\frac{1+\beta}{2}\right) \times \beta \times 2^{\left(\frac{\beta-1}{2}\right)}}\right) \tag{8}$$

where $X_2(t+1)$ denotes the new solution for the following iteration of t, D means spatial dimensions, $levy\ (D)$ denotes Lévy flight distribution functions, $X(t)$ indicates the arbitrary location of Aquila in $[1, N]$, s take the values of 1.5, y and χ presents the spiral situations in search region as follows:

$$y = r \times \cos(\theta) \tag{9}$$

$$x = r \times \sin(\theta) \tag{10}$$

$$r = r_1 + 0.00565 \times D_1 \tag{11}$$

$$\theta = -0.005 \times D_1 + \frac{3 \times \pi}{2} \tag{12}$$

where r_1 takes the fixed index between 1 and 20, D_1 denotes the integers from 1 to the length of the search region. The third strategy was a slow-descent attack and low-flying. The Aquila locks onto a hunting target in the hunting region and, with attack ready, makes the initial attacks in the vertical descent, thereby testing prey response. These behaviors are given as follows:

$$X_3(t+1) = (X_{besi}(t) - X_M(t)) \times \alpha - rand + ((UB - LB) \times rand + LB) \times \delta \tag{13}$$

where $X_3(t+1)$ denotes the solution of the following iteration of t, δ, and α denotes the mining adjustment parameter within $(0, 1)$, LB and UB represent the lower and upper boundaries of the issue. The fourth strategy was grabbing and walking prey. Once the Aquila approaches the prey, it starts to attack prey based on arbitrary movements of prey. These behaviors can be described as follows

$$X_4(t+1) = QF \times X_{best}(t) - (G_1 \times X(t) \times rand) - G_2 \times levy(D) \tag{14}$$

$$QF(t) = t^{\frac{2 \times rand - 1}{(1-T)^2}} \tag{15}$$

$$G_1 = 2 \times rand - 1 \tag{16}$$

$$G_1 = 2 \times \left(1 - \frac{t}{T}\right) \tag{17}$$

where $X_4(t+1)$ denotes the new solution for the following iteration of t, QF represents the mass function leveraged for balancing the search process, and $F \in (0, 1)$ G_1 represents various strategies utilized by the Aquila for prey escape; G_2 signifies slope value from the initial location to the final location at the chase time of Aquila's prey, which takes values from 2 to 0, · Rand denotes the random number within [0,1] in Gaussian distribution; and T and t denotes the maximal amount of iterations and existing amount of iterations, correspondingly. Niche thought is from biology in which microhabitats represent roles or functions of the organization in a specific environment, and organizations with general features are named species. In the AAO algorithm, Niche thought is used, which applies a sharing model for comparing the distance among individuals in a habitat. A specific threshold was set to increase the fitness of an individual with the highest fitness, ensuring that the individual state is optimal. For an individual with the lowest fitness, a penalty was presented to make them update and further find the optimum value in another region to guarantee the diversity of the population at the iteration and attain the optimum solution.

Here, the distance among individuals of the smallest habitat population was evaluated as follows:

$$d_{ij} = |X_i - X_j| \qquad (18)$$

The data exchange function among X_i and X_j individuals is given below

$$sh(d_{ij}) = \begin{cases} 1 - \frac{d_{ji}}{\rho}, d_{ij} < \rho \\ 0, \; d_{ij} > \rho \end{cases} \qquad (19)$$

where ρ denotes the radius of data sharing in microhabitats and $d_{ij} < \rho$ guarantees that individuals live in the microhabitat environments. After sharing the data, the optimum adaptation can be adjusted in time, as follows.

$$F_{i\_best} = \frac{F_i}{sh}, i = 1, 2, \ldots, N \qquad (20)$$

where F_i means optimum adaptation after sharing, and F_j denotes original adaptation.

The AAO method not only derived a fitness function from attaining superior classification performance as well describes positive values to symbolize the enhanced outcome of the candidate solutions. The reduction of classification error rates was treated as the fitness function.

$$\begin{aligned} fitness(x_i) &= Classifier Error Rate(x_i) \\ &= \frac{number\ of\ misclassified\ samples}{Total\ number\ of\ samples} \times 100 \end{aligned} \qquad (21)$$

2.2. Ensemble Learning-Based Classification

In this work, the DL paradigm is integrated, and the best outcome is selected by the weighted voting method. Assumed the D base classification model and amount of classes as n for voting, predictive class c_k of weighted voting for every instance as follows

$$c_k = \arg\max_{j} \sum_{i=1}^{D} (\Delta_{ji} \times w_i), \qquad (22)$$

where Δ_{ji} signifies binary parameter. As soon as ith base classification classifies the k instances into jth classes, then $\Delta_{ji} = 1$; or else, $\Delta_{ji} = 0$. w_i represents the weight of ith base classification in the ensemble.

$$Acc = \frac{\sum_k \{1|c_k \text{ is the true class of instance } k\}}{Size\ of\ test\ instances} \times 100\%. \qquad (23)$$

2.2.1. RNN Model

Initially, Elman recommended the recurrent unit as its essential block (1990). If they are used to exceedingly long sequences, the elementary RNN cell has common problems of expanding gradient and disappearing gradient [23]. It is a fact that the elementary RNN cell could not hold long-term dependence eventually. Hence it demonstrates that this cell has shortcomings. The backpropagated gradient tends to reduce once the sequence is particularly long, which prevents the effective updating of the weight. However, once the gradient is substantial, they might explode across a longer sequence, which renders the weight matrix unstable. The above two difficulties stem from the intractable nature of the gradient, which has made it more difficult for RNN cells to identify and be accountable for a long-term relationship. Equations (24) and (25) demonstrate the mathematical expression for RNN architecture.

$$h_{t-1} = \sigma(P_h \times h_{t-1} + P_x \times x_t + B_a) \qquad (24)$$

$$y_t = \tanh(P_o \times h_t + B_o) \qquad (25)$$

where h_t denotes the hidden state, and it was the only type of memory in the RNN cell. P_h and P_x epitomize the weight matrix for the hidden state and P_o bias vector for cell output correspondingly, x_t and y_t characterize the inputs and outputs of the cell at the t time step, correspondingly, B_a and B_o represent the bias vector for the hidden state and cell outputs, correspondingly.

The latter hidden state is conditioned on the hidden state of the previous time step and the existing inputs. The cellular feedback loop connects the current state to the succeeding one. This bond is crucial to consider prior data while adjusting the present cell state. In such cases, the hyperbolic tangent function, represented by Tanh, turned on the overt state, and the sigmoid function was applied, represented by, to turn on the latent state.

2.2.2. GRU Model

The RNN is a kind of ANN model with a cyclic structure and is appropriate for data processing in sequence. The gradient is lost, and learning ability is greatly reduced once the time interval is large [24]. Hochreiter and Schmidhuber resolved these problems and developed the LSTM. The LSTM was extensively applied in time-series data, and its basic concept is that the cell state was interconnected as a conveyor belt. In that regard, the gradient propagates although distance among the states rises. In LSTM cells, the cell state can be controlled by using three gating functions forget, input, and output gates. In 2014, the GRU was developed as a network that enhanced the learning accuracy of LSTM by adjusting the LSTM model. Different from LSTM, the GRU has a fast-learning speed and is encompassed two gating functions. Furthermore, parameters are smaller than LSTM since the hidden and cell states are incorporated into a single hidden state. Accordingly, the GRU shows outstanding performance for long-term dependency in time-series data processing and takes lesser computational time when compared to the LSTM. The GRU equations to determine the hidden state are shown below:

$$r_t = \sigma(W_r x_t + U_r h_{t-1} + b_r) \tag{26}$$

$$z_t = \sigma(W_z x_t + U_z h_{t-1} + b_z) \tag{27}$$

$$h_t = (1 - z_t) \odot h_{t-1} + z_t \odot \tanh(W_h x_t + U_h(r_t E \odot h_{t-1}) + b_h) \tag{28}$$

From the expression, r_t denotes the reset gate and z_t indicates the update gate at time t. x_t represents input value at t time, W and U indicate weights, and b refers to bias. h_t denotes the hidden state at time t. $\odot$ shows the component-wise (Hadamard) multiplication.

2.2.3. BiLSTM Model

RNN has the structural feature of the node connected in a loop, making them appropriate for data processing; however, it is frequently confronted with the problem of vanishing gradient [25]. The GRU and long and short-term memory (LSTM) improved on RNN by adding several threshold gates to mitigate gradient vanishing problems and enhance classification accuracy. Meanwhile, the LSTM method has a memory unit that prevents the network from facing gradient vanishing problems.

The LSTM could enhance the deficiencies of RNN; generally, the resultant of the present time was relevant to the state information of the past time, as well as state information of future time. The Bi-LSTM network was established concerning the problem that was integrating historical and future data by interconnecting two LSTMs. The architecture of the BiLSTM network comprises the back-to-forth and front-to-back LSTM layers. The forward and backward layers calculate the input dataset, and lastly, the architecture of two layers is integrated to obtain the output of the BiLSTM network as follows:

$$o_t = g(\omega_1 i_t + \omega_2 0_{t-1}) o'_t = g\left(\omega_3 i_t + \omega_5 0'_{t-1}\right), y_t = f(\omega_4 0_t + \omega_6 0_t) \tag{29}$$

In Equation (29), ω denotes weighted parameters in the BiLSTM network, i_t shows input at t time, 0_t indicates the results of the forward hidden layer at t time, $0'_t$ represents the output of the backward hidden layer at t time and y_t represents the last resultant of the network.

2.3. Modeling of XAI Using LIMA Approach

The AAOXAI-CD technique combines the XAI approach LIME for a better understanding and explainability of the black-box method for accurate cancer detection [26]. Local interpretable model-agnostic explanation (LIME) describes various ML approaches for regression prediction, using the featured value change of the data sample to transform the featured values into the contribution of the predictor. The explainer gives a local interpretation of the data samples. For example, the interpretable model in LIME often uses linear regression (LR) or decision trees (DTs) and are trained by the smaller perturbation (removing specific words, hiding part of the image, and adding random noise) in the model. The quality of these models seems to be increasing and was used to resolve the best part of the business victimization dataset. Similarly, there were persistent tradeoffs between model accuracy and interpretability. Generally, the performance can be improved and enhanced by applying sophisticated techniques such as call trees, random forest, material, boosting, and SVM, which are "blackbox" techniques. The LIME provides a clear explanation of the problems with the blackbox classifiers. The LIME is a way of understanding an ML BlackBox method by perturbing the input dataset and seeing how prediction changes. The LIME is used for any ML black-box models. The fundamental steps are shown as follows:

A TabularExplainer is initialized by the data used for the data training about the features and various class names.

In the class explain_instance, a technique called explain_instance accepts the reference to the instance where the explanation is essential, plus the number of features to be added in the explanation and the trained model's prediction technique.

3. Results and Discussion

The proposed model is simulated using Python 3.6.5 tool on PC i5-8600k, GeForce 1050 Ti 4 GB, 16 GB RAM, 250 GB SSD, and 1 TB HDD. The parameter settings are given as follows: learning rate: 0.01, dropout: 0.5, batch size: 5, epoch count: 50, and activation: ReLU. In this section, the simulation values of the AAOXAI-CD technique can be tested utilizing dual datasets: the colorectal cancer dataset (dataset 1) and the osteosarcoma dataset (dataset 2). Figure 4 defines the sample images of Colorectal Cancer. For experimental validation, 70:30 and 80:20 of the training set (TRS) and testing set (TSS) is used. Dataset 1 (Warwick-QU dataset) [27] comprises 165 images with 91 malignant tumors and 74 benign tumor images. The data were collected using the Zeiss MIRAX MIDI Scanner by implementing an image data weight range of 1.187 kilobytes, 716 kilobytes, and an image data resolution range of 567 × 430 pixels to 775 × 522 pixels with all pixels having a distance of 0.6 µm from the actual distance. Next, dataset 2 [28] contains 1144 images under 3 classes. It covers 536 images under Non-Tumor (NT) class, 345 images under viable tumor (VT), and 263 images under non-Viable Tumor (NVT). Figure 5 defines the sample images of osteosarcoma.

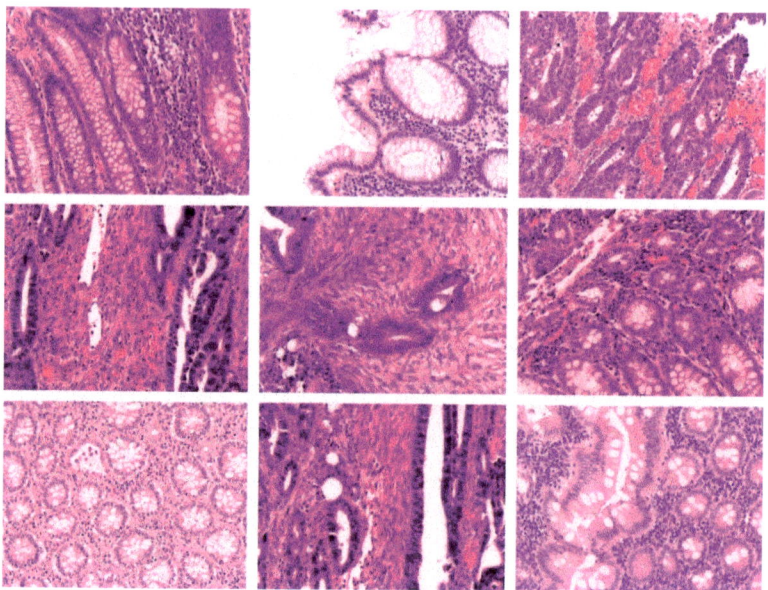

Figure 4. Sample Images of Colorectal Cancer.

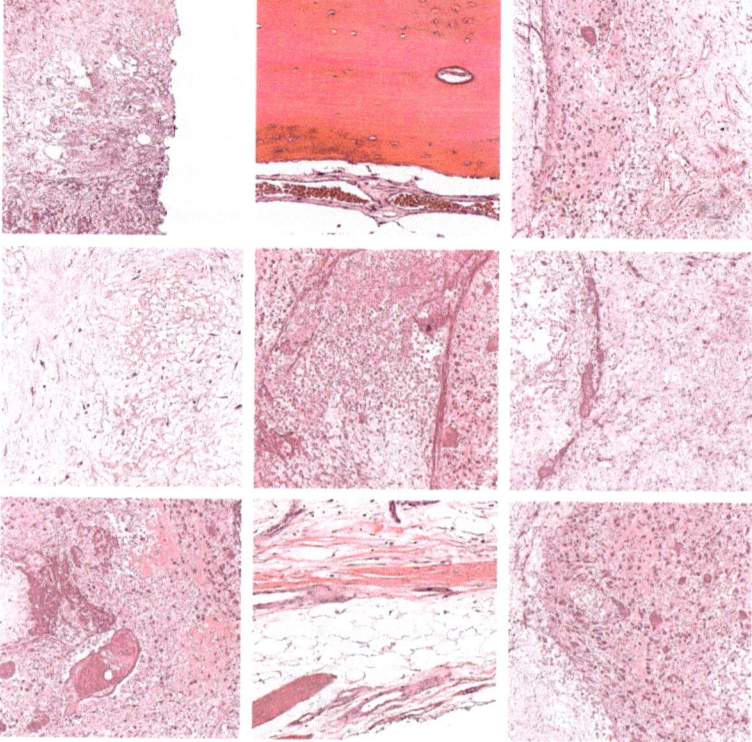

Figure 5. Sample images of osteosarcoma.

In Figure 6, the cancer classifier outcomes of the AAOXAI-CD method in terms of classification performance under dataset-1. The outcomes demonstrate that the AAOXAI-CD system has identified benign and malignant samples.

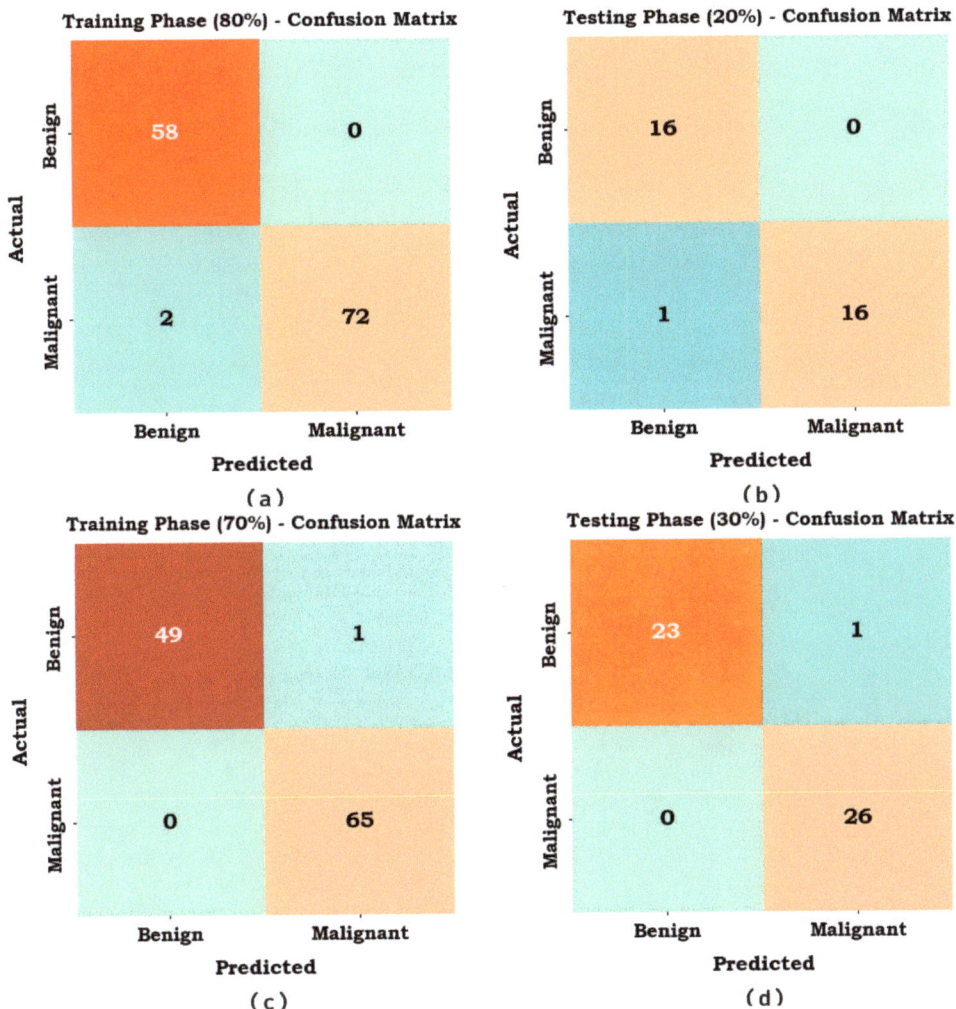

Figure 6. Confusion matrices of the AAOXAI-CD system on dataset-1 (**a**,**b**) TRS/TSS of 80:20 and (**c**,**d**) TRS/TSS of 70:30.

In Table 1, the overall classifier results of the AAOXAI-CD method on dataset-1. The results demonstrate that the AAOXAI-CD method has identified benign and malignant samples. For instance, with 80% of TRS, the AAOXAI-CD technique reaches an average $accu_y$ of 98.65%, $prec_n$ of 98.33%, $reca_l$ of 98.65%, $spec_y$ of 98.65%, F_{score} of 98.47%, and MCC of 96.98%. Meanwhile, with 20% of TSS, the AAOXAI-CD system reaches an average $accu_y$ of 97.06%, $prec_n$ of 97.06%, $reca_l$ of 97.06%, $spec_y$ of 97.06%, F_{score} of 96.97%, and MCC of 94.12%. Furthermore, with 70% of TRS, the AAOXAI-CD algorithm reaches an average $accu_y$ of 99%, $prec_n$ of 99.24%, $reca_l$ of 99%, $spec_y$ of 99%, F_{score} of 99.11%, and MCC of 98.24%.

Table 1. Classifier outcome of the AAOXAI-CD approach on dataset-1.

Classes	$Accu_y$	$Prec_n$	$Reca_l$	$Spec_y$	F_{score}	MCC
Training Phase (80%)						
Benign	100.00	96.67	100.00	97.30	98.31	96.98
Malignant	97.30	100.00	97.30	100.00	98.63	96.98
Average	98.65	98.33	98.65	98.65	98.47	96.98
Testing Phase (20%)						
Benign	100.00	94.12	100.00	94.12	96.97	94.12
Malignant	94.12	100.00	94.12	100.00	96.97	94.12
Average	97.06	97.06	97.06	97.06	96.97	94.12
Classes	Accuracy	Precision	Recall	Specificity	F-Score	MCC
Training Phase (70%)						
Benign	98.00	100.00	98.00	100.00	98.99	98.24
Malignant	100.00	98.48	100.00	98.00	99.24	98.24
Average	99.00	99.24	99.00	99.00	99.11	98.24
Testing Phase (30%)						
Benign	95.83	100.00	95.83	100.00	97.87	96.06
Malignant	100.00	96.30	100.00	95.83	98.11	96.06
Average	97.92	98.15	97.92	97.92	97.99	96.06

The TACY and VACY of the AAOXAI-CD model on dataset-1 are defined in Figure 7. The figure exhibited that the AAOXAI-CD method has improvised performance with augmented values of TACY and VACY. Visibly, the AAOXAI-CD model has maximum TACY outcomes.

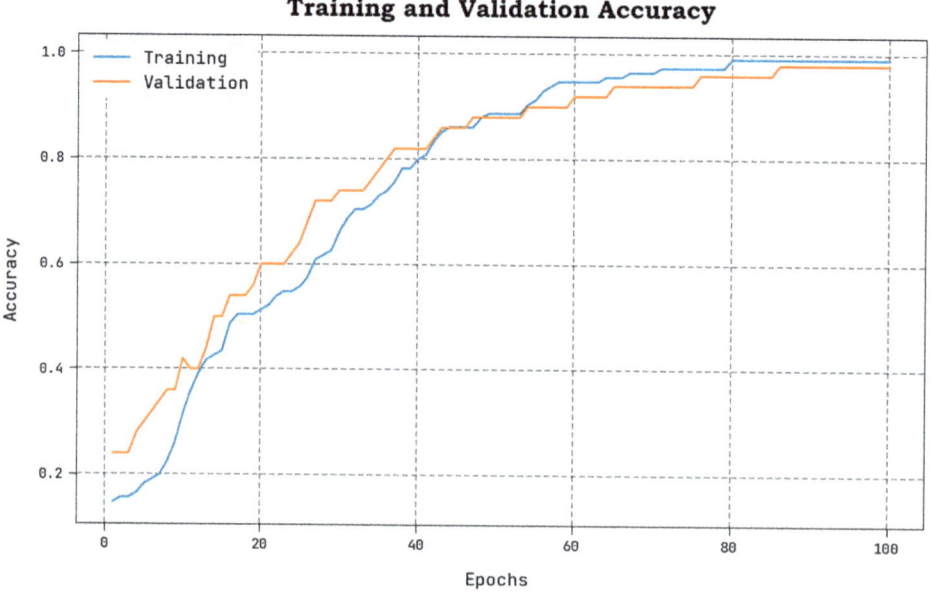

Figure 7. TACY and VACY analysis of the AAOXAI-CD approach on dataset-1.

The TLOS and VLOS of the AAOXAI-CD model on dataset-1 are defined in Figure 8. The figure inferred that the AAOXAI-CD approach has superior performance with minimal values of TLOS and VLOS. Notably, the AAOXAI-CD model has minimal VLOS outcomes.

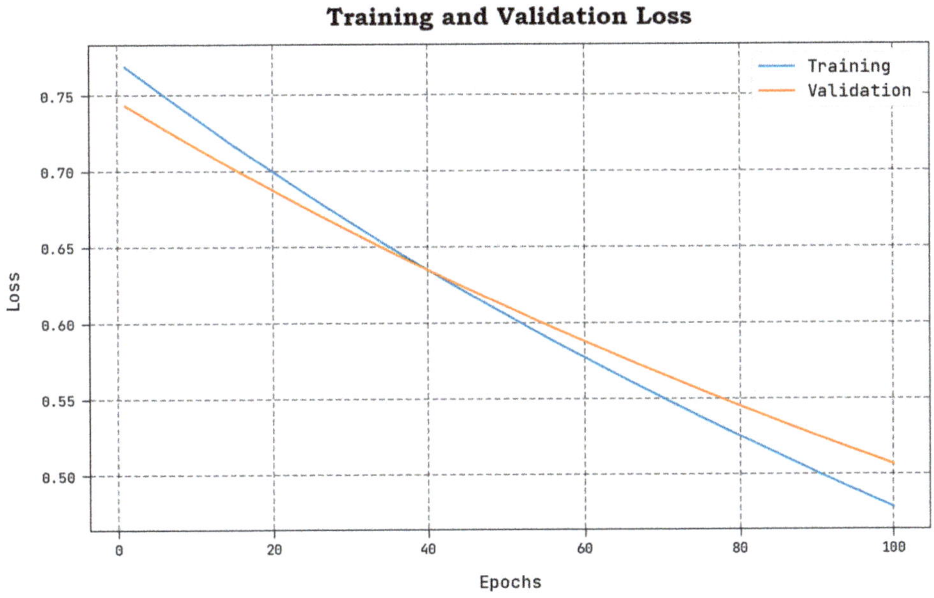

Figure 8. TLOS and VLOS analysis of AAOXAI-CD approach on dataset-1.

In Table 2 and Figure 9, the comparative interpretation of the AAOXAI-CD system with recent methods on dataset-1 [29–31]. The figures represented that the ResNet-18(60–40), ResNet-50 (60–40), and CP-CNN models resulted in the least performance. Although the AAI-CCDC technique results in moderately improved outcomes, the AAOXAI-CD technique accomplishes maximum performance with $prec_n$ of 99.24%, $reca_l$ of 99%, and $accu_y$ of 99%.

Table 2. Analysis outcome of AAOXAI-CD method with other systems on dataset-1.

Methods	Precision	Recall	Accuracy
ResNet-18 (60–40)	82.00	63.00	72.00
ResNet-18 (80–20)	86.00	82.00	84.00
ResNet-50 (60–40)	91.00	59.00	76.00
ResNet-50 (80–20)	82.00	92.00	87.00
SC-CNN Model	80.00	82.00	81.00
CP-CNN Model	71.00	68.00	69.00
AAI-CCDC Model	96.00	98.00	97.00
AAOXAI-CD	99.24	99.00	99.00

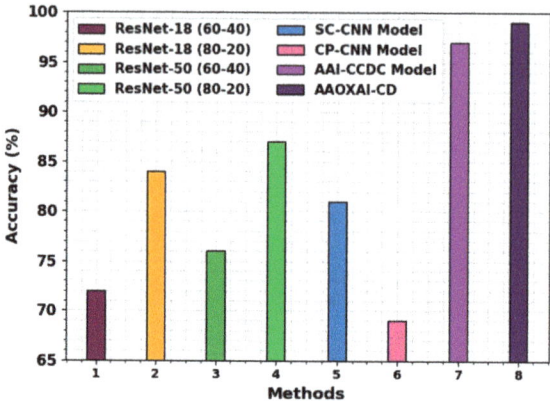

Figure 9. Comparative analysis of the AAOXAI-CD approach on dataset-1.

In Figure 10, the cancer classification outcomes of the AAOXAI-CD system in terms of classification performance under dataset-2. The results demonstrate that the AAOXAI-CD technique has identified benign and malignant samples.

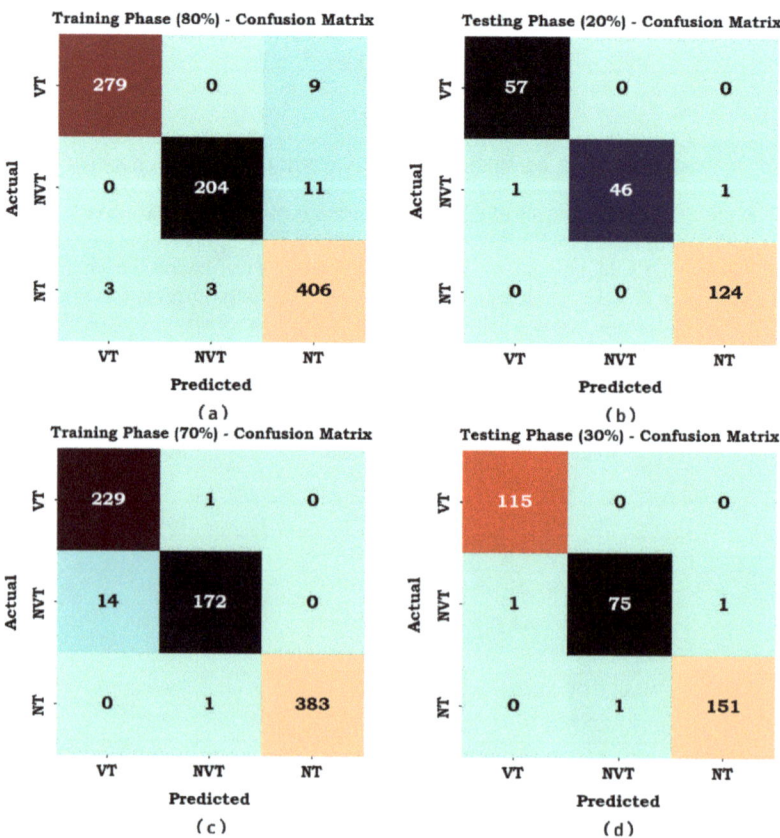

Figure 10. Confusion matrices of AAOXAI-CD system on dataset-2 (**a**,**b**) TRS/TSS of 80:20 and (**c**,**d**) TRS/TSS of 70:30.

In Table 3, the overall classifier results of the AAOXAI-CD system on dataset-2. The results demonstrate that the AAOXAI-CD method has identified benign and malignant samples. For instance, with 80% of TRS, the AAOXAI-CD technique reaches an average $accu_y$ of 98.11%, $prec_n$ of 97.60%, $reca_l$ of 96.77%, $spec_y$ of 98.37%, F_{score} of 97.16%, and MCC of 95.66%. Meanwhile, with 20% of TSS, the AAOXAI-CD algorithm reaches an average $accu_y$ of 99.42%, $prec_n$ of 99.16%, $reca_l$ of 98.61%, $spec_y$ of 99.49%, F_{score} of 98.87%, and MCC of 98.44%. Furthermore, with 70% of TRS, the AAOXAI-CD technique reaches an average $accu_y$ of 98.67%, $prec_n$ of 97.70%, $reca_l$ of 97.26%, $spec_y$ of 99.07%, F_{score} of 97.42%, and MCC of 96.56%.

Table 3. Classifier outcome of AAOXAI-CD approach on dataset-2.

Classes	$Accu_y$	$Prec_n$	$Reca_l$	$Spec_y$	F_{score}	MCC
Training Phase (80%)						
VT	98.69	98.94	96.88	99.52	97.89	96.95
NVT	98.47	98.55	94.88	99.57	96.68	95.72
NT	97.16	95.31	98.54	96.02	96.90	94.32
Average	98.11	97.60	96.77	98.37	97.16	95.66
Testing Phase (20%)						
VT	99.56	98.28	100.00	99.42	99.13	98.85
NVT	99.13	100.00	95.83	100.00	97.87	97.36
NT	99.56	99.20	100.00	99.05	99.60	99.12
Average	99.42	99.16	98.61	99.49	98.87	98.44
Classes	$Accu_y$	$Prec_n$	$Reca_l$	$Spec_y$	F_{score}	MCC
Training Phase (70%)						
VT	98.12	94.24	99.57	97.54	96.83	95.57
NVT	98.00	98.85	92.47	99.67	95.56	94.35
NT	99.88	100.00	99.74	100.00	99.87	99.75
Average	98.67	97.70	97.26	99.07	97.42	96.56
Testing Phase (30%)						
VT	99.71	99.14	100.00	99.56	99.57	99.35
NVT	99.13	98.68	97.40	99.63	98.04	97.48
NT	99.42	99.34	99.34	99.48	99.34	98.82
Average	99.42	99.05	98.91	99.56	98.98	98.55

The TACY and VACY of the AAOXAI-CD model on dataset-2 are defined in Figure 11. The figure highlighted that the AAOXAI-CD method has performance with increased values of TACY and VACY. Remarkably, the AAOXAI-CD model has higher TACY outcomes.

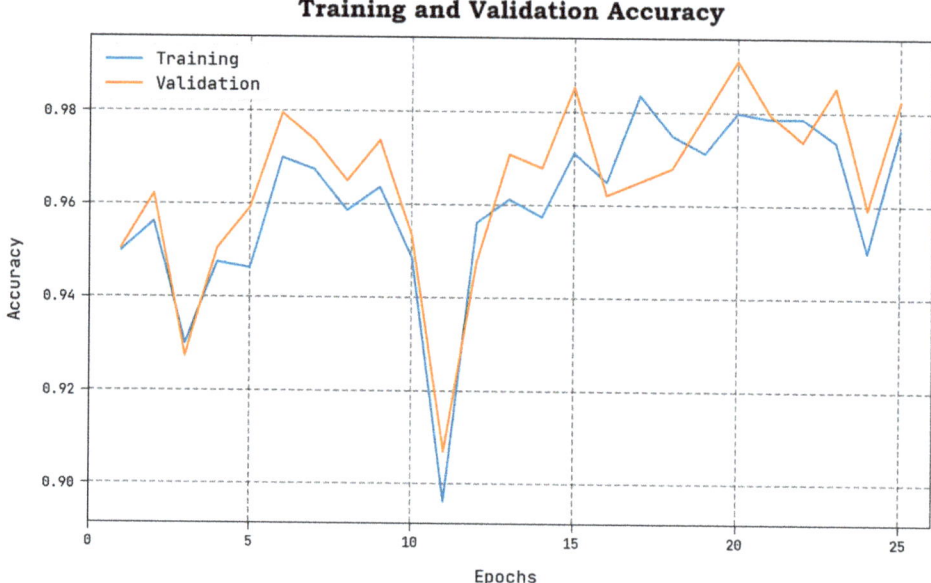

Figure 11. TACY and VACY analysis of AAOXAI-CD approach on dataset-2.

The TLOS and VLOS of the AAOXAI-CD model on dataset-2 are defined in Figure 12. The figure inferred the AAOXAI-CD system has better outcomes having minimal values of TLOS and VLOS. Visibly the AAOXAI-CD model has minimal VLOS outcomes.

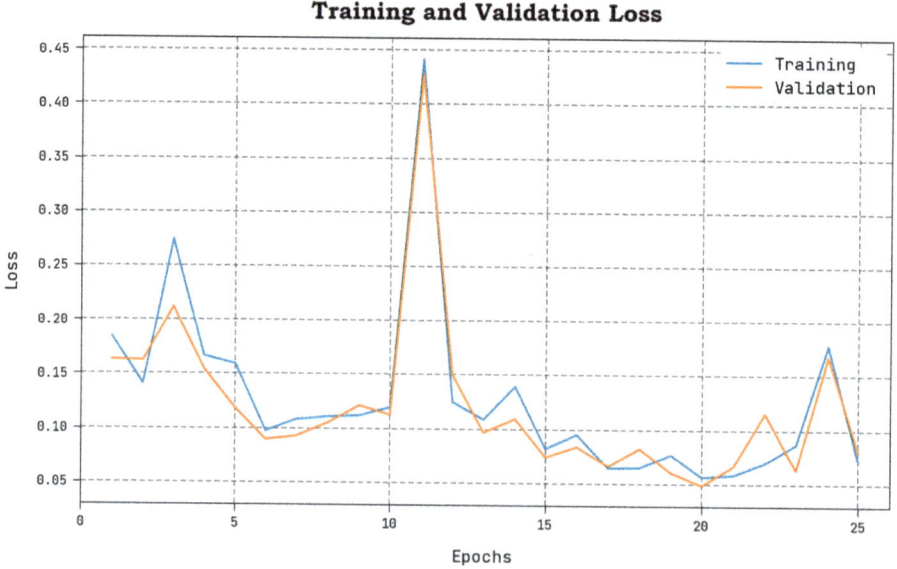

Figure 12. TLOS and VLOS analysis of AAOXAI-CD method on dataset-2.

Table 4 and Figure 13 show a brief study of the AAOXAI-CD method with the recent method on dataset-2 [32,33]. The experimental values represented that the CNN-Xception, CNN-EfficientNet, CNN-ResNet-50, and CNN-MobileNet-V2 models resulted in the least performance. Although the WDODTL-ODC and HBODL-AOC techniques result in moderately improved outcomes, the AAOXAI-CD technique accomplishes maximum performance with of $prec_n$ 99.05%, of $reca_l$ 98.91%, and $accu_y$ of 99.42%.

Table 4. Comparative analysis of AAOXAI-CD approach with other systems on dataset-2.

Methods	Precision	Recall	Accuracy
AAOXAI-CD	99.05	98.91	99.42
HBODL-AOC	98.94	98.12	98.43
WDODTL-ODC	98.76	97.65	98.17
CNN-EfficientNet	97.00	97.00	97.00
CNN-Xception	94.00	96.00	96.00
CNN-ResNet-50	98.00	94.00	97.00
CNN-MobileNet-V2	98.00	98.00	98.00

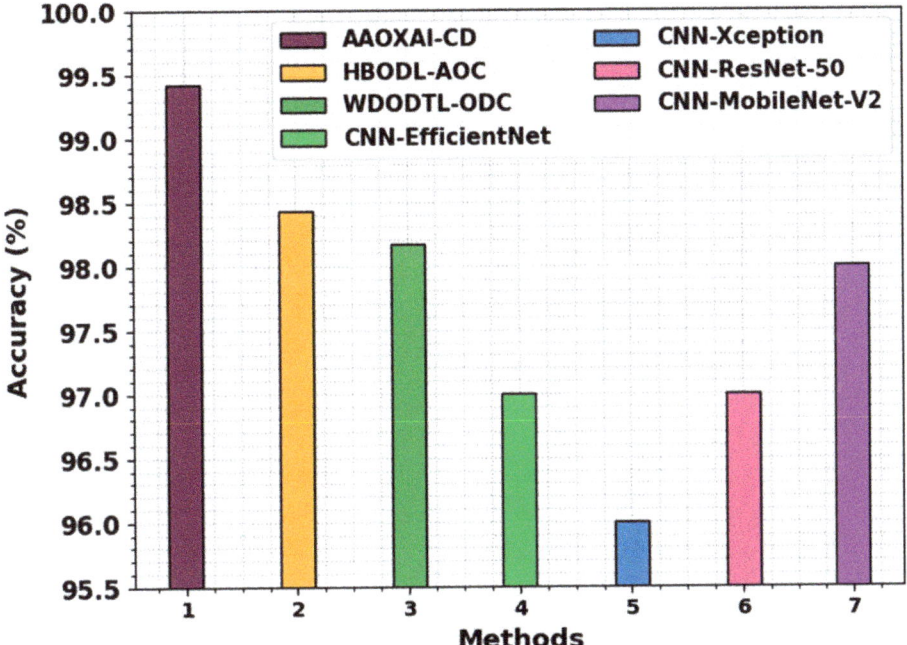

Figure 13. Comparative analysis of the AAOXAI-CD approach on dataset-2.

From the above-mentioned results, it is assured that the proposed model achieves effectual classification performance over other DL models. The enhanced performance of the proposed model is due to the inclusion of AAO-based hyperparameter tuning and ensemble classification processes. In addition, the use of LIME helps to build an effective predictive modeling technique in cancer diagnosis. Without transparency, it is hard to gain the trust of healthcare professionals and employ predictive approaches in their daily operations. XAI has received considerable interest in recent times. It enables the clients to generate instances and comprehend how the classification model accomplishes the results. Healthcare institutions are keenly designing predictive models for supporting operations. The XAI can be combined to improve the transparency of healthcare predictive modeling.

The interactions between healthcare professionals and the AI system are important for transferring knowledge and adopting models in healthcare operations.

4. Conclusions

In this study, we have developed an automated cancer diagnosis method using the AAOXAI-CD technique on medical images. The proposed AAOXAI-CD system attained the effectual colorectal and osteosarcoma cancer classification process. Primarily, the AAOXAI-CD technique utilized the Faster SqueezeNet model for feature vector generation. Moreover, the hyperparameter tuning of the Faster SqueezeNet model takes place with the AAO algorithm. For cancer classification, the majority-weighted voting ensemble model with three DL classifiers, namely RNN, GRU, and BiLSTM. Furthermore, the AAOXAI-CD technique combines the XAI approach LIME for better understanding and explainability of the black-box method for accurate cancer detection. The experimental evaluation of the AAOXAI-CD approach was tested on medical cancer imaging databases, and the outcomes ensured the promising outcome of the AAOXAI-CD method over other recent methods. In the future, a feature fusion-based classification model can be designed to boost the performance of the AAOXAI-CD technique.

Author Contributions: Conceptualization, S.A.-K.; Methodology, S.A. and R.F.M.; Validation, F.A. and B.M.E.E.; Formal analysis, R.F.M.; Investigation, S.S.; Resources, A.A.B. and B.M.E.E.; Data curation, F.A. and A.A.B.; Writing—original draft, S.A.-K.; Writing—review & editing, S.A.; Supervision, S.A. and S.A.-K. All authors have read and agreed to the published version of the manuscript.

Funding: This research received no external funding.

Institutional Review Board Statement: This article does not contain any studies with human participants performed by any of the authors.

Informed Consent Statement: Not applicable.

Data Availability Statement: Data sharing is not applicable to this article as no datasets were generated during the current study.

Acknowledgments: Researchers would like to thank the Deanship of Scientific Research, Qassim University for funding publication of this project.

Conflicts of Interest: The authors declare that they have no conflict of interest.

References

1. Cordova, C.; Muñoz, R.; Olivares, R.; Minonzio, J.G.; Lozano, C.; Gonzalez, P.; Marchant, I.; González-Arriagada, W.; Olivero, P. HER2 classification in breast cancer cells: A new explainable machine learning application for immunohistochemistry. *Oncol. Lett.* **2023**, *25*, 44. [CrossRef] [PubMed]
2. Hauser, K.; Kurz, A.; Haggenmüller, S.; Maron, R.C.; von Kalle, C.; Utikal, J.S.; Meier, F.; Hobelsberger, S.; Gellrich, F.F.; Sergon, M.; et al. Explainable artificial intelligence in skin cancer recognition: A systematic review. *Eur. J. Cancer* **2022**, *167*, 54–69. [CrossRef] [PubMed]
3. Farmani, A.; Soroosh, M.; Mozaffari, M.H.; Daghooghi, T. Optical nanosensors for cancer and virus detections. In *Nanosensors for Smart Cities*; Elsevier: Amsterdam, The Netherlands, 2020; pp. 419–432.
4. Salehnezhad, Z.; Soroosh, M.; Farmani, A. Design and numerical simulation of a sensitive plasmonic-based nanosensor utilizing MoS2 monolayer and graphene. *Diam. Relat. Mater.* **2023**, *131*, 109594. [CrossRef]
5. Amoroso, N.; Pomarico, D.; Fanizzi, A.; Didonna, V.; Giotta, F.; La Forgia, D.; Latorre, A.; Monaco, A.; Pantaleo, E.; Petruzzellis, N.; et al. A roadmap towards breast cancer therapies supported by explainable artificial intelligence. *Appl. Sci.* **2021**, *11*, 4881. [CrossRef]
6. Eminaga, O.; Loening, A.; Lu, A.; Brooks, J.D.; Rubin, D. Detection of prostate cancer and determination of its significance using explainable artificial intelligence. *J. Clin. Oncol.* **2020**, *38*, 5555. [CrossRef]
7. Sakai, A.; Komatsu, M.; Komatsu, R.; Matsuoka, R.; Yasutomi, S.; Dozen, A.; Shozu, K.; Arakaki, T.; Machino, H.; Asada, K.; et al. Medical professional enhancement using explainable artificial intelligence in fetal cardiac ultrasound screening. *Biomedicines* **2022**, *10*, 551. [CrossRef]
8. Ragab, M.; Albukhari, A.; Alyami, J.; Mansour, R.F. Ensemble deep-learning-enabled clinical decision support system for breast cancer diagnosis and classification on ultrasound images. *Biology* **2022**, *11*, 439. [CrossRef]

9. Escorcia-Gutierrez, J.; Mansour, R.F.; Beleño, K.; Jiménez-Cabas, J.; Pérez, M.; Madera, N.; Velasquez, K. Automated deep learning empowered breast cancer diagnosis using biomedical mammogram images. *Comput. Mater. Contin.* 2022, *71*, 3–4221. [CrossRef]
10. Mansour, R.F.; Alfar, N.M.; Abdel-Khalek, S.; Abdelhaq, M.; Saeed, R.A.; Alsaqour, R. Optimal deep learning based fusion model for biomedical image classification. *Expert Syst.* 2022, *39*, e12764. [CrossRef]
11. Davagdorj, K.; Bae, J.W.; Pham, V.H.; Theera-Umpon, N.; Ryu, K.H. Explainable artificial intelligence based framework for non-communicable diseases prediction. *IEEE Access* 2021, *9*, 123672–123688. [CrossRef]
12. Severn, C.; Suresh, K.; Görg, C.; Choi, Y.S.; Jain, R.; Ghosh, D. A Pipeline for the Implementation and Visualization of Explainable Machine Learning for Medical Imaging Using Radiomics Features. *Sensors* 2022, *22*, 5205. [CrossRef] [PubMed]
13. Pintelas, E.; Liaskos, M.; Livieris, I.E.; Kotsiantis, S.; Pintelas, P. Explainable machine learning framework for image classification problems: Case study on glioma cancer prediction. *J. Imaging* 2020, *6*, 37. [CrossRef] [PubMed]
14. Van der Velden, B.H.; Kuijf, H.J.; Gilhuijs, K.G.; Viergever, M.A. Explainable artificial intelligence (XAI) in deep learning-based medical image analysis. *Med. Image Anal.* 2022, *79*, 102470. [CrossRef] [PubMed]
15. Esmaeili, M.; Vettukattil, R.; Banitalebi, H.; Krogh, N.R.; Geitung, J.T. Explainable artificial intelligence for human-machine interaction in brain tumor localization. *J. Pers. Med.* 2021, *11*, 1213. [CrossRef]
16. Hassan, M.R.; Islam, M.F.; Uddin, M.Z.; Ghoshal, G.; Hassan, M.M.; Huda, S.; Fortino, G. Prostate cancer classification from ultrasound and MRI images using deep learning based Explainable Artificial Intelligence. *Future Gener. Comput. Syst.* 2022, *127*, 462–472. [CrossRef]
17. Kobylińska, K.; Orłowski, T.; Adamek, M.; Biecek, P. Explainable machine learning for lung cancer screening models. *Applied Sciences* 2022, *12*, 1926. [CrossRef]
18. Peng, J.; Zou, K.; Zhou, M.; Teng, Y.; Zhu, X.; Zhang, F.; Xu, J. An explainable artificial intelligence framework for the deterioration risk prediction of hepatitis patients. *J. Med. Syst.* 2021, *45*, 61. [CrossRef]
19. Watson, M.; Al Moubayed, N. Attack-agnostic adversarial detection on medical data using explainable machine learning. In Proceedings of the 2020 25th International Conference on Pattern Recognition (ICPR), Milan, Italy, 10–15 January 2021; pp. 8180–8187.
20. Idrees, M.; Sohail, A. Explainable machine learning of the breast cancer staging for designing smart biomarker sensors. *Sens. Int.* 2022, *3*, 100202. [CrossRef]
21. Xu, Y.; Yang, G.; Luo, J.; He, J. An Electronic component recognition algorithm based on deep learning with a faster SqueezeNet. *Math. Probl. Eng.* 2020, *2020*, 2940286. [CrossRef]
22. Zhang, Y.; Xu, X.; Zhang, N.; Zhang, K.; Dong, W.; Li, X. Adaptive Aquila Optimizer Combining Niche Thought with Dispersed Chaotic Swarm. *Sensors* 2023, *23*, 755. [CrossRef]
23. Bowes, B.D.; Sadler, J.M.; Morsy, M.M.; Behl, M.; Goodall, J.L. Forecasting groundwater table in a flood prone coastal city with long short-term memory and recurrent neural networks. *Water* 2019, *11*, 1098. [CrossRef]
24. Kim, A.R.; Kim, H.S.; Kang, C.H.; Kim, S.Y. The Design of the 1D CNN–GRU Network Based on the RCS for Classification of Multiclass Missiles. *Remote Sens.* 2023, *15*, 577. [CrossRef]
25. Wang, Q.; Cao, D.; Zhang, S.; Zhou, Y.; Yao, L. The Cable Fault Diagnosis for XLPE Cable Based on 1DCNNs-BiLSTM Network. *J. Control. Sci. Eng.* 2023, *2023*, 1068078. [CrossRef]
26. Zafar, M.R.; Khan, N.M. DLIME: A deterministic local interpretable model-agnostic explanations approach for computer-aided diagnosis systems. *arXiv* 2019, arXiv:1906.10263.
27. Sirinukunwattana, K.; Snead, D.R.J.; Rajpoot, N.M. A Stochastic Polygons Model for Glandular Structures in Colon Histology Images. *IEEE Trans. Med. Imaging* 2015, *34*, 2366–2378. [CrossRef]
28. Leavey, P.; Sengupta, A.; Rakheja, D.; Daescu, O.; Arunachalam, H.B.; Mishra, R. Osteosarcoma data from UT Southwestern/UT Dallas for Viable and Necrotic Tumor Assessment [Data set]. *Cancer Imaging Arch.* 2019, *14*. [CrossRef]
29. Ragab, M.; Albukhari, A. Automated Artificial Intelligence Empowered Colorectal Cancer Detection and classification Model. *Comput. Mater. Contin.* 2022, *72*, 5577–5591. [CrossRef]
30. Sarwinda, D.; Paradisa, R.H.; Bustamam, A.; Anggia, P. Deep Learning in Image Classification using Residual Network (ResNet) Variants for Detection of Colorectal Cancer. *Procedia Comput. Sci.* 2021, *179*, 423–431. [CrossRef]
31. Sirinukunwattana, K.; Raza, S.E.A.; Tsang, Y.W.; Snead, D.R.; Cree, I.A.; Rajpoot, N.M. Locality sensitive deep learning for detection and classification of nuclei in routine colon cancer histology images. *IEEE Trans. Med. Imaging* 2016, *35*, 1196–1206. [CrossRef]
32. Vaiyapuri, T.; Jothi, A.; Narayanasamy, K.; Kamatchi, K.; Kadry, S.; Kim, J. Design of a Honey Badger Optimization Algorithm with a Deep Transfer Learning-Based Osteosarcoma Classification Model. *Cancers* 2022, *14*, 6066. [CrossRef]
33. Fakieh, B.; Al-Ghamdi, A.S.A.-M.; Ragab, M. Optimal Deep Stacked Sparse Autoencoder Based Osteosarcoma Detection and Classification Model. *Healthcare* 2022, *10*, 1040. [CrossRef] [PubMed]

Disclaimer/Publisher's Note: The statements, opinions and data contained in all publications are solely those of the individual author(s) and contributor(s) and not of MDPI and/or the editor(s). MDPI and/or the editor(s) disclaim responsibility for any injury to people or property resulting from any ideas, methods, instructions or products referred to in the content.

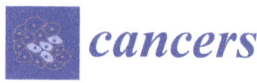

Article

Interpretable and Reliable Oral Cancer Classifier with Attention Mechanism and Expert Knowledge Embedding via Attention Map

Bofan Song [1,*], Chicheng Zhang [2], Sumsum Sunny [3], Dharma Raj KC [2], Shaobai Li [1], Keerthi Gurushanth [4], Pramila Mendonca [5], Nirza Mukhia [4], Sanjana Patrick [6], Shubha Gurudath [4], Subhashini Raghavan [4], Imchen Tsusennaro [7], Shirley T. Leivon [7], Trupti Kolur [5], Vivek Shetty [5], Vidya Bushan [5], Rohan Ramesh [7], Vijay Pillai [5], Petra Wilder-Smith [8], Amritha Suresh [3,5], Moni Abraham Kuriakose [9], Praveen Birur [4,6] and Rongguang Liang [1,*]

[1] Wyant College of Optical Sciences, The University of Arizona, Tucson, AZ 85721, USA
[2] Computer Science Department, The University of Arizona, Tucson, AZ 85721, USA
[3] Mazumdar Shaw Medical Centre, Bangalore 560099, India
[4] KLE Society Institute of Dental Sciences, Bangalore 560022, India
[5] Mazumdar Shaw Medical Foundation, Bangalore 560099, India
[6] Biocon Foundation, Bangalore 560100, India
[7] Christian Institute of Health Sciences and Research, Dimapur 797115, India
[8] Beckman Laser Institute & Medical Clinic, University of California, Irvine, CA 92617, USA
[9] Cochin Cancer Research Center, Kochi 683503, India
* Correspondence: songb@arizona.edu (B.S.); rliang@optics.arizona.edu (R.L.)

Citation: Song, B.; Zhang, C.; Sunny, S.; KC, D.R.; Li, S.; Gurushanth, K.; Mendonca, P.; Mukhia, N.; Patrick, S.; Gurudath, S.; et al. Interpretable and Reliable Oral Cancer Classifier with Attention Mechanism and Expert Knowledge Embedding via Attention Map. *Cancers* **2023**, *15*, 1421. https://doi.org/10.3390/cancers15051421

Academic Editor: Judith E. Raber-Durlacher

Received: 8 December 2022
Revised: 16 February 2023
Accepted: 18 February 2023
Published: 23 February 2023

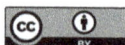

Copyright: © 2023 by the authors. Licensee MDPI, Basel, Switzerland. This article is an open access article distributed under the terms and conditions of the Creative Commons Attribution (CC BY) license (https://creativecommons.org/licenses/by/4.0/).

Simple Summary: Convolutional neural networks (CNNs) have shown promising performance in recognizing oral cancer. However, the lack of interpretability and reliability remain major challenges in the development of trustworthy computer-aided diagnosis systems. To address this issue, we proposed a neural network architecture that integrates visual explanation and attention mechanisms. It improves the recognition performance via the attention mechanism while simultaneously providing interpretability for decision-making. Furthermore, our system incorporates Human-in-the-loop (HITL) deep learning to enhance the reliability and accuracy of the system through the integration of human and machine intelligence. We embedded expert knowledge into the network by manually editing the attention map for the attention mechanism.

Abstract: Convolutional neural networks have demonstrated excellent performance in oral cancer detection and classification. However, the end-to-end learning strategy makes CNNs hard to interpret, and it can be challenging to fully understand the decision-making procedure. Additionally, reliability is also a significant challenge for CNN based approaches. In this study, we proposed a neural network called the attention branch network (ABN), which combines the visual explanation and attention mechanisms to improve the recognition performance and interpret the decision-making simultaneously. We also embedded expert knowledge into the network by having human experts manually edit the attention maps for the attention mechanism. Our experiments have shown that ABN performs better than the original baseline network. By introducing the Squeeze-and-Excitation (SE) blocks to the network, the cross-validation accuracy increased further. Furthermore, we observed that some previously misclassified cases were correctly recognized after updating by manually editing the attention maps. The cross-validation accuracy increased from 0.846 to 0.875 with the ABN (Resnet18 as baseline), 0.877 with SE-ABN, and 0.903 after embedding expert knowledge. The proposed method provides an accurate, interpretable, and reliable oral cancer computer-aided diagnosis system through visual explanation, attention mechanisms, and expert knowledge embedding.

Keywords: visual explanation; attention mechanism; human-in-the-loop deep learning; attention map; expert knowledge embedding; attention branch network

1. Introduction

Convolutional neural networks have achieved outstanding performance in many visual tasks [1–3]. However, the end-to-end learning strategy used in CNNs makes them hard to interpret. It is difficult to fully understand the CNNs' decision-making procedure that is hidden inside the network. Interpreting deep learning models has been a challenge for a long time. Many researchers have realized the significance and developed several methods for deep learning visual explanation [4]. Visual explanation generates an attention map that highlights discriminative regions used for CNN decision-making, which is a common approach for interpreting deep learning models. There are two types of visual explanations: response-based and gradient-based. Response-based approaches, such as Class Activation Mapping (CAM) [5], use the response of the convolutional layer to generate the attention map. Gradient-based approaches, such as gradient weighted-CAM (Grad-CAM) [6], use gradient and feed forward response to generate the attention map. CAM and Grad-CAM are two widely used visual explanation methods. CAM uses the K channel feature map from the convolution layer and the weight at a fully connected layer to calculate the attention map. However, this method requires modification of the CNN architectures, that is, replacing the fully connected layer of the original network with a convolutional layer and global average pooling. Grad-CAM uses the response of the convolution layer and a positive gradient in the backpropagation process to generate the attention map. Grad-CAM can be applied to interpret various models without changing network architecture or re-training.

Attention mechanism is a powerful tool that efficiently allocates the available processing resources to the most informative part of the input signal [7]. It has been applied to many fields such as computer vision and natural language processing. The attention mechanism is usually implemented in combination with a gating function such as softmax or sigmoid and sequential techniques. In image recognition tasks, previous researchers have proposed several attention-based approaches. One such approach is Squeeze-and-Excitation network (SENet) [8], which allows the network to perform feature recalibration. It can use the global information to emphasize the most informative features and suppress the less informative ones. The SE block is a lightweight gating mechanism that models channel-wise relationships in a computationally efficient manner. Another approach is Residual Attention Network [9], which employs multiple attention modules, each with a mask branch and a trunk branch. It also utilizes an attention residual learning mechanism to optimize very deep Residual Attention architecture and bottom-up top-down feedforward attention structure.

Attention branch network (ABN) [10], inspired by visual explanation and attention mechanisms, uses the attention map for both visual explanation and attention mechanism. The highlighted region in the attention map is considered an informative part and obtains more attention in image recognition. ABN has a feature extractor to extract features; the feature extractor could be various baseline models such as Resnet or VGGNet. It also consists of an attention branch and a perception branch. The attention branch extends the response-based visualization method CAM to generate an attention map. The perception branch of the ABN model utilizes the informative regions and highlighted regions in the attention map to emphasize the relevant features and suppress others to produce the final results. By integrating visual explanation and attention mechanism, the ABN model can interpret the decision-making of the deep learning network and improve the recognition performance simultaneously. Ding et al. [11] proposed a deep attention branch network by introducing two attention branches into a baseline model composed of four dense blocks, three transition layers, and a classification layer. Additionally, an entropy-guided loss weighting strategy was introduced to address the class imbalance problem. The experimental results demonstrate that the proposed method can improve the focusing ability of networks to accurately locate the discriminative lesion regions and improve the classification performance; the entropy-guided loss weighting strategy can further boost the performance.

Human-in-the-loop (HITL) deep learning [12,13] is a set of strategies that integrates human knowledge and machine intelligence to enhance the performance of deep learning models. HITL has attracted significant research interest in the machine learning community, and many studies have investigated this topic by leveraging the complementary strengths of human and machine intelligence, resulting in improved accuracy compared to machine intelligence alone. For instance, Zhu et al. [14] proposed a tool that integrates human physicians' knowledge and deep learning algorithms for efficient object detection of renal pathology. Linsley et al. [15] developed a ClickMe map that collects human feedback to train the deep learning model via the HITL framework. The method achieved better performance by introducing human knowledge to the weight of the attention mechanism. Mitsuhara et al. [16] used manually editable attention maps to embed human knowledge into deep neural networks. Human experts can intuitively understand the attention map and edit it interactively through a visual interface. The edited attention maps can improve recognition performance by reflecting human knowledge.

Oral cancer is one of the most common cancers worldwide and is the second most common cancer in India [17]. Most high-risk populations living in low- and middle-income countries do not have adequate medical resources for early diagnosis and treatment. Therefore, researchers have developed cost-effective methods for oral cancer diagnosis such as fluorescence imaging [18] and fluorescence lifetime imaging [19] to meet these pressing needs, and these methods have been successfully implemented in low-resource settings. For instance, Duran-Sierra et al. [19] developed and validated a machine-learning assisted computer aided detection system to automatically differentiate dysplastic and cancerous tissue from healthy oral tissue based on in vivo widefield autofluorescence lifetime imaging endoscopy data. This study evaluated four traditional machine learning models and did not use convolutional neural network models. Convolutional neural networks are powerful tools in medical image analysis, and multiple deep learning-based oral cancer recognition approaches have been introduced [20–23]. However, improving the accuracy, reliability, and interpretability of these models is still challenging. In this work, we use the attention branch network and Squeeze-and-Excitation blocks to apply visual explanation and attention mechanisms into the oral cancer recognition model. The attention map generated from the attention branch can interpret the model's predictions and improve the performance through the perception branch via the attention mechanism. Additionally, human experts manually edited the automatically generated attention map and fed it back to the network's perception branch. The manual editing helps to accurately highlight the oral lesion or healthy regions according to the annotation of oral oncology specialists. Our experimental results demonstrate that incorporating ABN and SE blocks improves the classification accuracy of convolutional networks. Furthermore, expert knowledge, in the form of manually edited attention maps, leads to improved reliability and performance.

2. Materials and Methods

In Section 2.1, we introduce the Attention branch network (ABN) and discuss its two main components: the attention branch and the perception branch (Sections 2.1.1 and 2.1.2). We then outline the training process for ABN in Section 2.2. In Section 2.3, we discuss how human expert knowledge can be integrated into the ABN network to improve its performance.

Additionally, in Section 2.4, we present another attention method, the Squeeze-and-Excitation, which we used to further enhance the network's performance. Finally, we describe the dataset used for this study in Section 2.5.

2.1. Attention Branch Network

Attention branch network (ABN) [10] extends the response-based visual explanation model, which is able to visualize the attention map for visual explanation while improving the CNN performance with the attention mechanism simultaneously. It consists of three components: the feature extractor that contains convolutional layers to extract feature maps from the input image; the attention branch that generates an attention map based on CAM for the attention mechanism and visual explanation; and the perception branch that outputs the probabilities of classes using the feature map from feature extractor and attention map from the attention branch. The block diagram of the attention branch network for our oral cancer classification task is shown in Figure 1.

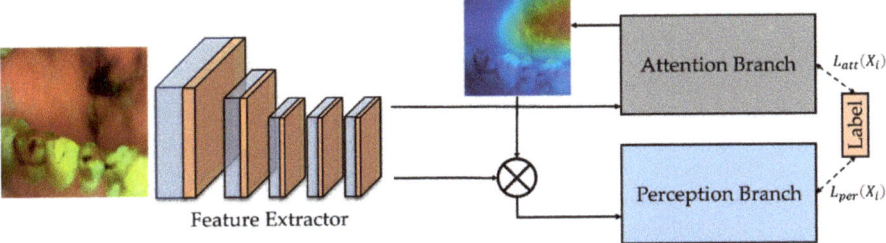

Figure 1. The block diagram of the attention branch network for our oral cancer task [10]. It has a feature extractor, an attention branch, and a perception branch. The perception branch uses the attention map generated from the attention branch to emphasize the most informative features.

2.1.1. Attention Branch

The ABN extends the CAM. CAM applies global average pooling (GAP) on the convolutional feature maps to produce the desired output. It can identify the importance of the image areas for CNN decision-making by projecting back the weights of the output layer onto the convolutional feature maps. When CAM visualizes the attention map of each class, the attention map is generated by multiplying the weighted sum of the feature map. CAM removes the fully connected layers before the final output and replaces them with convolution layers. Then, it adds a GAP and a fully connected softmax layer. This fully connected layer replacement restriction is also introduced into the attention branch. Similar to CAM, the attention branch uses convolution layer and GAP to generate an attention map. However, the attention branch replaces the fully connected layer with a Kx1x1 convolution layer (K is the number of categories) since CAM cannot generate an attention map in the training process. The Kx1x1 convolution layer imitates the last fully connected layer of CAM. The class probability output is generated using the response of GAP with the softmax function after the Kx1x1 convolution layer. The attention branch also generates an attention map for the attention mechanism. The K feature maps are convoluted by a 1x1x1 convolution layer and then normalized by the sigmoid function as the attention map.

2.1.2. Perception Branch

The perception branch outputs the classification results using the attention maps from the attention branch and feature maps from the feature extractor with an attention mechanism. In this study, the attention map $M(X_i)$ is applied to the feature map $g_c(X_i)$ by the following attention mechanism:

$$g'_c(X_i) = g_c(X_i) \cdot M(X_i)$$

2.2. Training of ABN

The loss function of ABN jointly optimizes both attention and perception branches. The combined loss function $L(X_i)$ was constructed as:

$$L(X_i) = L_{att}(X_i) + L_{per}(X_i)$$

where $L_{att}(X_i)$ is the attention branch training loss and $L_{per}(X_i)$ is the perception branch training loss. The training loss of each branch is calculated by the combination of the softmax function and cross-entropy.

2.3. Manual Editing of Attention Map

As mentioned before, in ABN, the attention map generated from the attention branch is used for the attention mechanism. The classification result could be adjusted by editing the attention map. To manually edit the attention map, one initial attention map was obtained from the attention branch of a trained ABN. Then an attention editor [16] can be used to manually edit the obtained attention maps interactively. The attention editor is created using PyQt5 [24] and PyTorch, which can add and remove an attention region easily via mouse. Since the size of the attention map generated from the attention branch is 14 × 14 pixels, the attention editor resizes it to 224 × 224 pixels and overlays it with the input oral image. After editing, the edited attention map is resized to 14 × 14 pixels, and the tool feeds it back for the attention mechanism of ABN to infer updated classification results through the perception branch. By highlighting the attention location of lesion areas and removing other regions on the attention map, the edited attention map can improve the classification results through the attention mechanism of ABN. The block diagram of the expert knowledge embedding is shown in Figure 2.

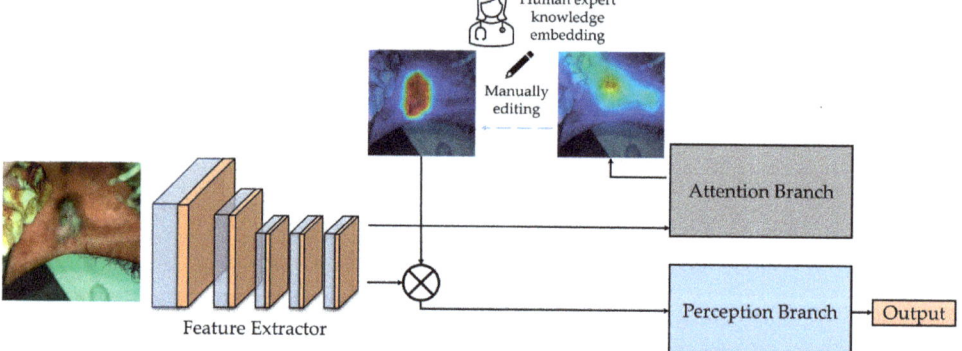

Figure 2. The block diagram shows the embedding of expert knowledge into the network [16]. The attention maps generated from the attention branch were manually edited and sent back to emphasize the most informative features.

2.4. SENet

In this study, Resnet18 was used as the baseline network to implement ABN. To further improve the performance of the Resnet18-ABN network for the oral cancer classification task, Squeeze-and-Excitation (SE) blocks were also incorporated into the network. SE block introduces a channel attention mechanism that is composed of three components: squeeze module, excitation module, and scale module.

The squeeze module uses global average pooling to generate channel-wise statistics, which reduces the feature map to a single value by taking the average of all the pixels in that feature map. If the input feature maps size is CxHxW, the output tensor will be Cx1x1 after passing through the GAP operation. Each feature map is decomposed into a singular value. The excitation module is to learn the adaptive scaling weights for the Cx1x1 tensor generated from the squeeze module. A gating mechanism with a sigmoid activation is employed. The gating mechanism is parameterized by forming a bottleneck with two fully connected layers, a dimensionality-reduction layer, a ReLU, and a dimensionality-increasing layer. The excitation module inputs the Cx1x1 tensor and outputs a weighted tensor of the same Cx1x1 size. After obtaining the Cx1x1 weighted tensor from the excitation module, it is scaled to a range of 0–1 through a sigmoid activation layer. Subsequently, the normalized weighted tensor is applied directly to the input by an element multiplication that scales each channel/feature map in the input with the corresponding learned weights.

The SE block could be applied to multiple existing network architectures and improves the network performance at a minimal additional computational cost. When adding the SE block to the residual network, it is inserted after the final convolutional layer of the residual block and before the residual is added to the skip connection.

2.5. Dataset

The dataset used in this study was captured using our customized oral cancer screening platform [25], which was obtained from patients attending the outpatient clinics of the Department of Oral Medicine and Radiology at the KLE Society Institute of Dental Sciences (KLE), the Head and Neck Oncology Department of Mazumdar Shaw Medical Center (MSMC), and the Christian Institute of Health Sciences and Research (CIHSR), India. Institutional ethics committee approval was obtained from all participating hospitals and written informed consents were collected from all subjects enrolled.

The data collection and study followed the International Conference of Harmonization recommendation on Good Clinical Practice, and all methods were carried out in accordance with relevant guidelines and regulations. The study protocol was registered in the Clinical Trial Registry of the Indian Council of Medical Research (CTRI/2019/11/022167, Registered on: 27 November 2019). The subjects were recruited at the study sub-centers, which were monitored by nodal centers in a hub-and-spoke model. Institutional Ethics Committee approvals were obtained from all nodal centers. The participants who were above 18 years of age, with a history of tobacco smoking and/or chewing, or with any oral lesion were included, and written informed consent was obtained from all the participants. The individuals currently undergoing treatment for malignancy, pregnancy, tuberculosis, or suffering from any acute illness were excluded. All the subjects included in the study were directly telediagnosed by remote specialists [26].

We used a total of 2040 oral images to validate this method for oral cancer classification. The images were separated into two categories: 'normal' (978 images), which contains normal and benign mucosal lesion images, and 'suspicious' (1062 images), which contains oral potentially malignant lesion (OPML) and malignant lesion images. The oral lesion regions for attention map editing were based on oral oncology specialists' annotations from MSMC, KLE, and CIHSR. In a previous study, we showed that oral oncology specialists' interpretation of classifying normal/benign versus OPML/malignant has high accuracy with biopsy-confirmed cases [27]. Examples of the dataset used in this study and the oncology specialists' annotations is shown in Figure 3.

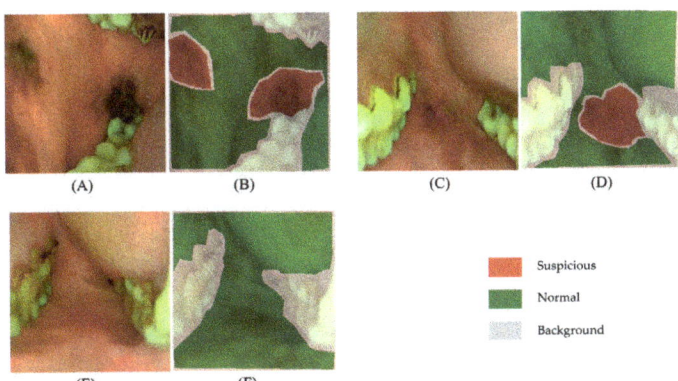

Figure 3. Examples of the dataset and oncology specialists' annotations. (**A,C,E**) are white light oral cavity images captured using our customized oral cancer screening platform. (**B,D,F**) are corresponding pixel-level annotations labeled by oral oncology specialists. The oral potentially malignant lesion and malignant lesion areas are shown in red, normal and benign areas are shown in green, and other background areas are shown in grey.

3. Results

In this study, all experiments were conducted using five-fold cross-validation. The networks were trained using the cross-entropy loss and the Adam optimization algorithm that were implemented on PyTorch. Data augmentation was applied to the training set by flipping horizontally and vertically, random rotating, and shearing while training all networks. For each training, the initial learning rate was 10^{-3}, which decayed 10 times by every 50 epochs, and the epoch number was 180 with a batch size of 32. We saved the models with the best validation accuracy.

In the first set of experiments, we trained the attention branch network and ABN with SE blocks (SE-ABN) using different baseline networks, including Resnet18, Resnet34, Resnet50, and Resnet101, to verify whether the method could improve the oral cancer classification performance. We also trained the original Resnet18, Resnet34, Resnetfive0, and Resnet101 networks with the same data and parameters for comparison purposes. Table 1 shows the five-fold cross-validation results of these experiments. Our findings show that ABN outperforms the original baseline network, and by introducing the SE blocks to ABN, the cross-validation accuracy is further increased. These results indicate that ABN can help the network pay more attention on lesion regions, leading to improved accuracy, and SE blocks can further improve the performance through its channel attention mechanism.

Table 1. The five-fold cross-validation accuracy of ABN, SE-ABN, and the original network with different baseline networks.

Five-Fold Cross-Validation Accuracy	ResNet18	ResNet34	ResNet50	ResNet101
Original Network	0.846	0.851	0.850	0.844
ABN	0.875	0.879	0.880	0.872
SE-ABN	0.877	0.880	0.881	0.876

In addition, we observed that although deeper Resnet models have more layers and require more computational time and resources, the performance difference on this oral dataset is not significant. Therefore, for the next set of attention map experiments, we will use ABN and SE-ABN with the Resnet18 baseline network.

3.1. Visualizing Attention Maps

To compare the attention maps generated by different models, we used three example cases and visualized the attention maps of the original Resnet18, ABN, and SE-ABN. The results are shown in Figure 4. While all three models highlight similar regions, the attention maps of ABN and SE-ABN are more accurate than the original Resnet18 in identifying the lesion areas. For the first and second images, the attention maps of the original Resnet18 focused more on teeth than the lesion area, while ABN and SE-ABN focused more accurately on the lesion when making decisions. The results indicate that the attention mechanism of ABN and SE block can help the network effectively focus on the lesion regions instead of background areas such as teeth. The mismatch between the classification and the attention region could degrade the reliability of the model performance, especially for medical image recognition systems. Therefore, ABN and SE-ABN networks are more reliable since they can focus more accurately on lesion areas for decision making.

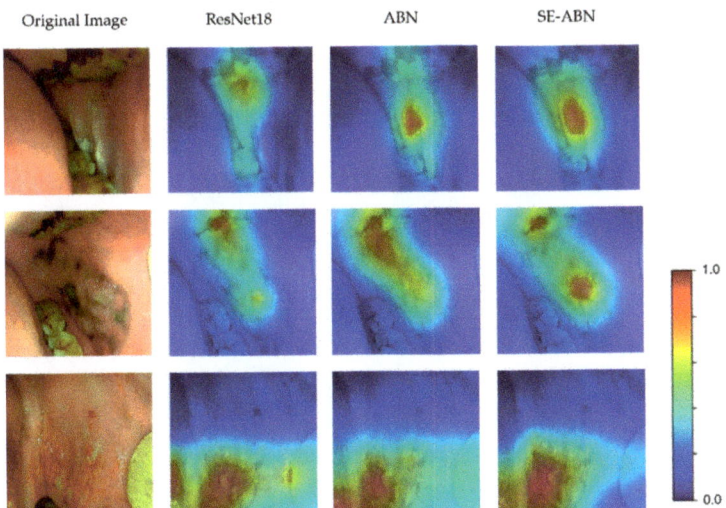

Figure 4. The attention maps of three example cases were repectively generated from the original Resnet18, ABN, and SE-ABN. The first column shows the original oral images, the second column shows the attention maps generated from the original Resnet18, the third column shows the attention maps generated from ABN (Resnet18 baseline), and the fourth column shows the attention maps generated from SE-ABN (Resnet18 baseline). Although all three models highlight similar regions, the attention maps of SE-ABN are more accurate than those of ABN in identifying the lesion areas, and both SE-ABN and ABN focused more accurately than the original Resnet18 network. For instance, in the first and second images, the attention maps of the original Resnet18 focused more on teeth than the lesion area, whereas SE-ABN clearly highlighted the lesion areas.

3.2. Incorporating Manually Edited Attention Maps

In this experiment, we employed the SE-ABN with Resnet18 backbone for attention map editing, with the aim of improving the classification performance.

To perform attention map editing, we followed the procedure outlined in Section 2.2, which involved inputting each validation image to the model and obtaining the attention map from the attention branch. The generated attention map would be overlaid with the input oral image for manual editing using the attention editor tool. Then the human experts used the editor tool to add and remove attention regions to ensure that the edited attention maps accurately and completely highlighted the corresponding regions. Finally, we sent the edited attention maps back to the attention mechanism of SE-ABN to obtain updated classification results through the perception branch.

Figure 5 presents several examples of attention map editing. In the first and third examples, the original attention maps obtained from the attention branch were incomplete and inaccurate in highlighting the lesion areas, resulting in a false classification of 'normal' for both cases. However, after manually editing the attention maps using the attention editor tool, the lesion areas were accurately and completely highlighted. The updated attention maps were then used for the attention mechanism of the model, resulting in a correct classification of 'suspicious.' Similarly, in the second example, although the model classifies the input image correctly as 'suspicious' with a probability score of 0.520, the attention map obtained from the attention branch did not completely highlight the lesion region. After manually editing the attention map, the probability score increased to 0.790. These results demonstrate that the attention map editing process can recognize more lesion features after highlighting more accurate and complete areas.

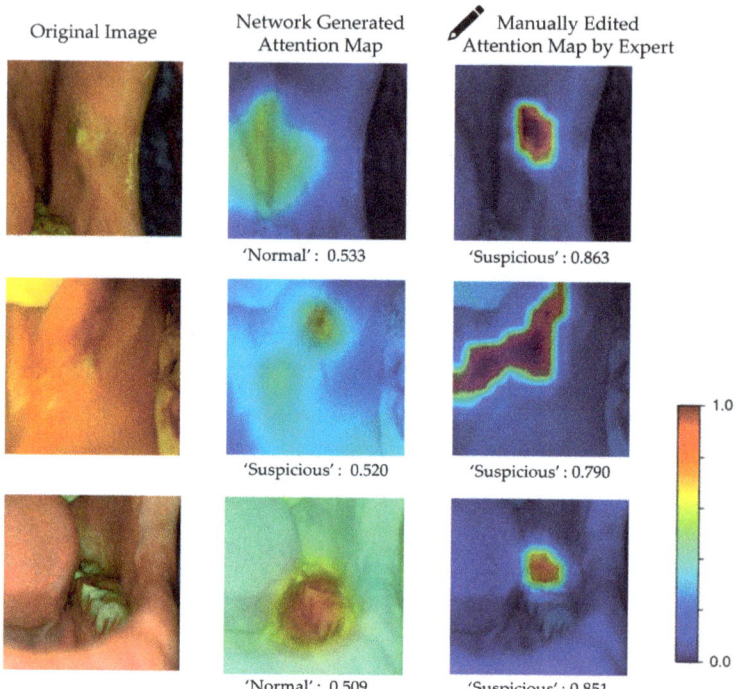

Figure 5. Three examples of manually edited attention maps, and the corresponding results before and after embedding human expert knowledge. The class label here means prediction, and the number after means the probability score. The first and third examples show that previous misclassified cases were correctly recognized after manually editing the attention maps by highlighting the lesion regions accurately and completely. The network failed to give correct predictions or focus correctly on lesion areas for the first and third cases, but after manually editing to let the network look at the accurate areas, the correct predictions were presented. Although the network gave a correct prediction for the second case, the probability score is low, while the probability score for the 'suspicious' class of the second case increased after editing.

The five-fold cross-validation accuracy of SE-ABN before and after editing the attention maps is shown in Table 2. The attention map editing process resulted in an increase in the validation accuracy from 87.7% to 90.3%. These results indicate that by editing the attention maps to highlight the accurate and complete lesion or normal areas, the network can focus on these areas via the attention branch and recognize more accurate features, resulting in improved classification accuracy.

Table 2. The performance comparison of the original network, ABN, SE-ABN, and manually edited attention maps.

	Sensitivity	0.833
	Specificity	0.857
Original ResNet18 network	Positive predictive value	0.843
	Negative predictive value	0.848
	Accuracy	0.846

Table 2. *Cont.*

ABN	Sensitivity	0.860
	Specificity	0.887
	Positive predictive value	0.876
	Negative predictive value	0.873
	Accuracy	0.875
SE-ABN	Sensitivity	0.868
	Specificity	0.886
	Positive predictive value	0.875
	Negative predictive value	0.879
	Accuracy	0.877
SE-ABN (incorporating manually edited attention maps)	Sensitivity	0.898
	Specificity	0.908
	Positive predictive value	0.899
	Negative predictive value	0.906
	Accuracy	0.903

4. Discussion

The experimental results of our proposed model have demonstrated a higher classification accuracy compared to baseline models. Additionally, the visual explanation results have shown that our proposed model can identify the lesion areas more accurately when making decisions. These results provide evidence that our proposed method improves the interpretability and reliability of the model via attention mechanism and visual explanation and successfully embeds human knowledge for the oral cancer recognition task.

The use of visual explanation and more accurate attention maps in the proposed AI model improves the model's reliability. By visualizing the areas that the model is focusing on during decision-making, we can observe whether the model is looking at correct/accurate lesion areas in addition to the classification results. The increased sensitivity and specificity makes the model more effective in cancer screening, as false positives can lead to unnecessary psychological stress, medical procedures, and increased clinical workloads. Furthermore, the manually edited attention maps generated by human experts have the potential to aid in the localization of biopsies. By highlighting the regions of interest with high accuracy and completeness, these attention maps can be used by on-site doctors to better locate biopsies.

Incorporating human expert knowledge into the decision-making process can enhance the accuracy and reliability of computer aided diagnosis system. In conjunction with our previously developed uncertainty assessment method [23], we could integrate the human expert knowledge into cases that Bayesian deep learning model is uncertain. This approach is not limited to oral cancer diagnosis, and we think any image-based cancer diagnosis approach that requires identification of the lesion areas can potentially benefit from this method.

5. Conclusions

Deep learning is a powerful tool in solving medical image analysis tasks. However, interpretability and reliability remain as challenges. In this study, we used an attention branch network for the oral cancer recognition task; it combines visual explanation and attention mechanism. The network can simultaneously interpret the decision-making and improve the recognition performance using the attention map with an attention mechanism. The attention branch of the network extends the response-based visualization method and generates an attention map, and then the perception branch uses the attention map to emphasize the most informative features extracted by the feature extractor of the network.

The attention mechanism has been widely used and has demonstrated exceptional performance in various deep learning tasks [7]. In previous attention models, the weights for the attention mechanism were obtained solely from the response value of the convolution layers during feed forward propagation in an unsupervised learning manner. However, ABN extracts the weight for an attention mechanism in image recognition by generating the attention map for visual explanation on the basis of response-based visual explanation in a supervised learning manner [10]. With ABN, the cross-validation accuracy of the oral image dataset improved to 0.875 from 0.846. After applying another attention method, the Squeeze-and-Excitation block, the accuracy further boosted to 0.877. It enables the network to perform dynamic channel-wise feature recalibration. Additionally, we incorporated the expert knowledge into the network by manually editing the attention map generated from the attention branch. The edited attention maps were then fed back into the network's perception branch and which updated the result via the attention mechanism. As a result, the cross-validation accuracy of the oral image dataset achieved 0.903.

The experiment's results have shown that the attention branch network and Squeeze-and-Excitation block can effectively improve the recognition performance as well as interpret the decision-making. Further, embedding the expert knowledge led to a further increase in accuracy. The proposed method provided an accurate, interpretable, and reliable oral cancer classifier that leverages visual explanation, attention mechanisms, and human expert knowledge embedding.

Author Contributions: Conceptualization, B.S., C.Z. and D.R.K.; methodology, B.S., C.Z. and D.R.K.; software and validation, B.S., D.R.K. and S.L.; formal analysis, B.S., C.Z., P.W.-S. and R.L.; data acquisition, annotation and curation, S.S., K.G., P.M., N.M., S.P., S.G., S.R., I.T., S.T.L., T.K., V.S., V.B., R.R., P.W.-S., A.S., M.A.K., P.B. and V.P.; writing—original draft preparation, B.S.; writing—review and editing, B.S., C.Z., P.W.-S. and R.L.; funding acquisition, B.S., P.W.-S., A.S., M.A.K., P.B. and R.L. All authors have read and agreed to the published version of the manuscript.

Funding: This research was funded by National Institute of Cancers (UH3CA239682); National Institute of Dental and Craniofacial Research (R01DE030682 and R01DE030682-02S1) of the National Institutes of Health (NIH). Tobacco-Related Disease Research Program (T31IR1825).

Institutional Review Board Statement: Institutional Ethics Committee approvals were obtained from the three nodal centers- The Karnataka Lingayat Education (KLE) Society's Institute of Dental Sciences (KLE; ECR/887/Inst/KA/2016), Bengaluru, India, Christian Institute of Health Sciences and Research (CIHSR; EC/NEW/INST/2020/782), Dimapur, Nagaland, India, and Mazumdar Shaw Medical Center (MSMC; NNH/MEC-CL-2016-394), Bengaluru, India.

Informed Consent Statement: Informed consent was obtained from all subjects involved in the study.

Data Availability Statement: Data underlying the results presented in this paper are not publicly available.

Conflicts of Interest: R.L. is the founder of Light Research Inc.

References

1. Kleppe, A.; Skrede, O.-J.; De Raedt, S.; Liestøl, K.; Kerr, D.J.; Danielsen, H.E. Designing deep learning studies in cancer diagnostics. *Nat. Rev. Cancer* **2021**, *21*, 199–211. [CrossRef]
2. Lotter, W.; Diab, A.R.; Haslam, B.; Kim, J.G.; Grisot, G.; Wu, E.; Wu, K.; Onieva, J.O.; Boyer, Y.; Boxerman, J.L.; et al. Robust breast cancer detection in mammography and digital breast tomosynthesis using an annotation-efficient deep learning approach. *Nat. Med.* **2021**, *27*, 244–249. [CrossRef]
3. Xue, P.; Wang, J.; Qin, D.; Yan, H.; Qu, Y.; Seery, S.; Jiang, Y.; Qiao, Y. Deep learning in image-based breast and cervical cancer detection: A systematic review and meta-analysis. *NPJ Digit. Med.* **2022**, *5*, 19. [CrossRef]
4. Zhang, Q.S.; Zhu, S.C. Visual interpretability for deep learning: A survey. *Front. Inf. Technol. Electron. Eng.* **2018**, *19*, 27–39. [CrossRef]

5. Zhou, B.; Khosla, A.; Lapedriza, A.; Oliva, A.; Torralba, A. Learning deep features for discriminative localization. In Proceedings of the IEEE Conference on Computer Vision and Pattern Recognition, Las Vegas, NV, USA, 27–30 June 2016; pp. 2921–2929.
6. Selvaraju, R.R.; Cogswell, M.; Das, A.; Vedantam, R.; Parikh, D.; Batra, D. Grad-CAM: Visual Explanations from Deep Networks via Gradient-Based Localization. In Proceedings of the 2017 IEEE International Conference on Computer Vision (ICCV), Venice, Italy, 22–29 October 2017; pp. 618–626.
7. Niu, Z.; Zhong, G.; Yu, H. A review on the attention mechanism of deep learning. *Neurocomputing* **2021**, *452*, 48–62. [CrossRef]
8. Hu, J.; Shen, L.; Sun, G. Squeeze-and-excitation networks. In Proceedings of the IEEE Conference on Computer Vision and Pattern Recognition, Salt Lake City, UT, USA, 18–23 June 2018; pp. 7132–7141.
9. Wang, F.; Jiang, M.; Qian, C.; Yang, S.; Li, C.; Zhang, H.; Wang, X.; Tang, X. Residual attention network for image classification. In Proceedings of the IEEE Conference on Computer Vision and Pattern Recognition, Honolulu, HI, USA, 21–26 July 2017; pp. 3156–3164.
10. Fukui, H.; Hirakawa, T.; Yamashita, T.; Fujiyoshi, H. Attention branch network: Learning of attention mechanism for visual explanation. In Proceedings of the IEEE/CVF Conference on Computer Vision and Pattern Recognition, Long Beach, CA, USA, 15–20 June 2019; pp. 10705–10714.
11. Saisai, D.; Wu, Z.; Zheng, Y.; Liu, Z.; Yang, X.; Yang, X.; Yuan, G.; Xie, J. Deep attention branch networks for skin lesion classification. *Comput. Methods Programs Biomed.* **2021**, *212*, 106447.
12. Budd, S.; Robinson, E.C.; Kainz, B. A survey on active learning and human-in-the-loop deep learning for medical image analysis. *Med. Image Anal.* **2021**, *71*, 102062. [CrossRef] [PubMed]
13. Zhao, Z.; Xu, P.; Scheidegger, C.; Ren, L. Human-in-the-loop Extraction of Interpretable Concepts in Deep Learning Models. *IEEE Trans. Vis. Comput. Graph.* **2022**, *28*, 780–790. [CrossRef] [PubMed]
14. Zhu, Z.; Lu, Y.; Deng, R.; Yang, H.; Fogo, A.B.; Huo, Y. EasierPath: An open-source tool for human-in-the-loop deep learning of renal pathology. In *Interpretable and Annotation-Efficient Learning for Medical Image Computing*; Springer: Berlin/Heidelberg, Germany, 2020; pp. 214–222.
15. Linsley, D.; Shiebler, D.; Eberhardt, S.; Serre, T. Learning what and where to attend. *arXiv* **2018**, arXiv:1805.08819.
16. Mitsuhara, M.; Fukui, H.; Sakashita, Y.; Ogata, T.; Hirakawa, T.; Yamashita, T.; Fujiyoshi, H. Embedding Human Knowledge into Deep Neural Network via Attention Map. *arXiv* **2019**, arXiv:1905.03540.
17. Sung, H.; Ferlay, J.; Siegel, R.L.; Laversanne, M.; Soerjomataram, I.; Jemal, A.; Bray, F. Global Cancer Statistics 2020: GLOBOCAN Estimates of Incidence and Mortality Worldwide for 36 Cancers in 185 Countries. *CA Cancer J. Clin.* **2021**, *71*, 209–249. [CrossRef] [PubMed]
18. Uthoff, R.D.; Song, B.; Sunny, S.; Patrick, S.; Suresh, A.; Kolur, T.; Keerthi, G.; Spires, O.; Anbarani, A.; Wilder-Smith, P.; et al. Point-of-care, smartphone-based, dual-modality, dual-view, oral cancer screening device with neural network classification for low-resource communities. *PLoS ONE* **2018**, *13*, e0207493. [CrossRef] [PubMed]
19. Duran-Sierra, E.; Cheng, S.; Cuenca, R.; Ahmed, B.; Ji, J.; Yakovlev, V.V.; Martinez, M.; Al-Khalil, M.; Al-Enazi, H.; Cheng, Y.-S.L.; et al. Machine-Learning Assisted Discrimination of Precancerous and Cancerous from Healthy Oral Tissue Based on Multispectral Autofluorescence Lifetime Imaging Endoscopy. *Cancers* **2021**, *13*, 4751. [CrossRef] [PubMed]
20. Huiping, L.; Hanshen, C.; Luxi, W.; Jiaqi, S.; Jun, L. Automatic detection of oral cancer in smartphone-based images using deep learning for early diagnosis. *J. Biomed. Opt.* **2021**, *26*, 086007.
21. Bofan, S.; Sumsum, S.; Shaobai, L.; Keerthi, G.; Pramila, M.; Nirza, M.; Sanjana, P.; Shubha, G.; Subhashini, R.; Tsusennaro, I.; et al. Mobile-based oral cancer classification for point-of-care screening. *J. Biomed. Opt.* **2021**, *26*, 065003.
22. Warin, K.; Limprasert, W.; Suebnukarn, S.; Jinapornthana, S.; Jantana, P. Automatic classification and detection of oral cancer in photographic images using deep learning algorithms. *J. Oral Pathol. Med.* **2021**, *50*, 911–918. [CrossRef] [PubMed]
23. Song, B.; Sunny, S.; Li, S.; Gurushanth, K.; Mendonca, P.; Mukhia, N.; Patrick, S.; Gurudath, S.; Raghavan, S.; Tsusennaro, I.; et al. Bayesian deep learning for reliable oral cancer image classification. *Biomed. Opt. Express* **2021**, *12*, 6422. [CrossRef] [PubMed]
24. Available online: https://pypi.org/project/PyQt5/ (accessed on 4 December 2022).
25. Ross, D.U.; Bofan, S.; Sumsum, S.; Sanjana, P.; Amritha, S.; Trupti, K.; Keerthi, G.; Kimberly, W.; Vishal, G.; Mary, E.P.; et al. Small form factor, flexible, dual-modality handheld probe for smartphone-based, point-of-care oral and oropharyngeal cancer screening. *J. Biomed. Opt.* **2019**, *24*, 106003.
26. Birur, N.P.; Song, B.; Sunny, S.P.; Mendonca, P.; Mukhia, N.; Li, S.; Patrick, S.; AR, S.; Imchen, T.; Leivon, S.T.; et al. Field validation of deep learning based Point-of-Care device for early detection of oral malignant and potentially malignant disorders. *Sci. Rep.* **2022**, *12*, 14283. [CrossRef] [PubMed]
27. Birur, N.P.; Gurushanth, K.; Patrick, S.; Sunny, S.P.; Raghavan, S.A.; Gurudath, S.; Hegde, U.; Tiwari, V.; Jain, V.; Imran, M.; et al. Role of community health worker in a mobile health program for early detection of oral cancer. *Indian J. Cancer* **2019**, *56*, 107–113. [CrossRef] [PubMed]

Disclaimer/Publisher's Note: The statements, opinions and data contained in all publications are solely those of the individual author(s) and contributor(s) and not of MDPI and/or the editor(s). MDPI and/or the editor(s) disclaim responsibility for any injury to people or property resulting from any ideas, methods, instructions or products referred to in the content.

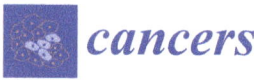

Article

Hyperparameter Optimizer with Deep Learning-Based Decision-Support Systems for Histopathological Breast Cancer Diagnosis

Marwa Obayya [1], Mashael S. Maashi [2], Nadhem Nemri [3], Heba Mohsen [4], Abdelwahed Motwakel [5,*], Azza Elneil Osman [6], Amani A. Alneil [6] and Mohamed Ibrahim Alsaid [6]

[1] Department of Biomedical Engineering, College of Engineering, Princess Nourah bint Abdulrahman University, P.O. Box 84428, Riyadh 11671, Saudi Arabia
[2] Department of Software Engineering, College of Computer and Information Science, King Saud University, Riyadh 11543, Saudi Arabia
[3] Department of Information Systems, College of Science & Art at Mahayil, King Khalid University, Abha 62529, Saudi Arabia
[4] Department of Computer Science, Faculty of Computers and Information Technology, Future University in Egypt, New Cairo 11835, Egypt
[5] Department of Information Systems, College of Business Administration in Hawtat Bani Tamim, Prince Sattam Bin Abdulaziz University, Al-Kharj 16278, Saudi Arabia
[6] Department of Computer and Self Development, Preparatory Year Deanship, Prince Sattam Bin Abdulaziz University, Al-Kharj 16278, Saudi Arabia
* Correspondence: am.ismaeil@psau.edu.sa

Simple Summary: This study develops an arithmetic optimization algorithm with deep-learning-based histopathological breast cancer classification (AOADL-HBCC) technique for healthcare decision making. The AOADL-HBCC technique employs noise removal based on median filtering (MF) and a contrast enhancement process. In addition, the presented AOADL-HBCC technique applies an AOA with a SqueezeNet model to derive feature vectors. Finally, a deep belief network (DBN) classifier with an Adamax hyperparameter optimizer is applied for the breast cancer classification process.

Abstract: Histopathological images are commonly used imaging modalities for breast cancer. As manual analysis of histopathological images is difficult, automated tools utilizing artificial intelligence (AI) and deep learning (DL) methods should be modelled. The recent advancements in DL approaches will be helpful in establishing maximal image classification performance in numerous application zones. This study develops an arithmetic optimization algorithm with deep-learning-based histopathological breast cancer classification (AOADL-HBCC) technique for healthcare decision making. The AOADL-HBCC technique employs noise removal based on median filtering (MF) and a contrast enhancement process. In addition, the presented AOADL-HBCC technique applies an AOA with a SqueezeNet model to derive feature vectors. Finally, a deep belief network (DBN) classifier with an Adamax hyperparameter optimizer is applied for the breast cancer classification process. In order to exhibit the enhanced breast cancer classification results of the AOADL-HBCC methodology, this comparative study states that the AOADL-HBCC technique displays better performance than other recent methodologies, with a maximum accuracy of 96.77%.

Keywords: decision making; healthcare; breast cancer classification; histopathological images; deep learning

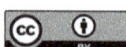

1. Introduction

Cancer is one of the most serious health concerns that threaten the health and lives of individuals [1]. The mortality rate and incidence of breast cancer seem to be increasing in recent times. Early precise diagnosis is considered to be a key to enhancing the chances of survival. The primary step in initial diagnosis is a mammogram, but it can be difficult to identify tumors in dense breast tissue, and X-ray radiation imposes a risk to the radiologist's and the patient's health [2]. The precise diagnosis of breast cancer requires skilled histopathologists, as well as large amounts of effort and time for task completion. Furthermore, the diagnosis outcomes of various histopathologists are not the same, because they mainly depend on the former knowledge of each histopathologist [3]. The average diagnosis precision is just 75%, which leads to low consistency in diagnoses. The term histopathology can be defined as the process of detailed evaluation and microscopic inspection of biopsy samples carried out by a pathologist or expert to learn about cancer growth in tissues or organs [4]. Common histopathological specimens have more structures and cells that can be dispersed and surrounded haphazardly by distinct types of tissues [5]. The physical analysis of historic pictures, along with the visual observation of such images, consumes time. This necessitates expertise and experience. In order to raise the predictive and analytical capabilities of histopathological images, the utility of computer-based image analysis represents an effective method [6]. This form of analysis is even efficient for histopathological images because it renders a dependable second opinion for consistent study, which increases output. This could aid in curtailing the time it takes to identify an issue. Thus, the burden on pathologists and the death rate can be minimized [7].

Today, machine learning (ML) is fruitfully enforced in text classification, image recognition, and object recognition. With the progression of computer-aided diagnosis (CAD) technology, ML is effectively implemented in breast cancer diagnosis [8]. Histopathological image classification related to conventional ML techniques and artificial feature extraction demands a manual model of features; however, it does not need an apparatus with more efficiency, and it has benefits in the computing period [9]. However, histopathological image classification related to deep learning (DL), particularly convolutional neural networks (CNNs), frequently needs a large number of labelled training models, whereas the labelled data are hard to gain [10]. The labeling of lesions is laborious and time-consuming work, even for professional histopathologists.

This study develops an arithmetic optimization algorithm with deep-learning-based histopathological breast cancer classification (AOADL-HBCC) technique for healthcare decision making. The presented AOADL-HBCC technique mainly aims to recognize the presence of breast cancer in HIs. At the primary level, the AOADL-HBCC technique employs noise removal based on median filtering (MF) and a contrast enhancement process. In addition, the presented AOADL-HBCC technique applies an AOA with a SqueezeNet model to derive feature vectors. Finally, a deep belief network (DBN) classifier with an Adamax hyperparameter optimizer is applied for the breast cancer classification process. In order to exhibit the enhanced breast cancer classification results of the AOADL-HBCC approach, a wide range of simulations was performed.

2. Related Works

Shankar et al. [11] established a new chaotic sparrow search algorithm including a deep TL-assisted BC classification (CSSADTL-BCC) technique on histopathological images (HPIs). The projected technique mostly concentrated on the classification and detection of BC. To realize this, the CSSADTL-BCC system initially carried out a Gaussian filter (GF) system for eradicating the presence of noise. In addition, a MixNet-oriented extracting feature system was utilized for generating a suitable group of feature vectors. Furthermore, a stacked GRU (SGRU) classifier system was utilized for allotting classes. In [12], TL and deep extracting feature approaches were employed that adjusted a pretraining CNN system to the current problem. The VGG16 and AlexNet methods were considered in the projected work for extracting features and AlexNet was employed for additional finetuning. The achieved features were then classified by SVM.

Khan et al. [13] examined a new DL infrastructure for the classification and recognition of BC from breast cytology images utilizing the model of TL. Generally, DL infrastructures demonstrated that certain problems were accomplished in isolation. In the presented structure, features in images were extracted employing pretrained CNN infrastructures such as ResNet, GoogLeNet, and VGGNet that are provided as fully connected (FC) layers to classify benign and malignant cells employing an average pooling classifier. In [14], a DL-related TL system was presented for classifying histopathological images automatically. Two famous and present pretrained CNN techniques, DenseNet161 and ResNet50, were trained as well as tested via grayscale and color images.

Singh et al. [15] examined a structure dependent upon the concept of TL for addressing this problem and concentrated their efforts on HPI and imbalanced image classifiers. The authors utilized common VGG19 as the base method and complemented it with different recent approaches for improving the entire efficiency of the technique. In [16], the conventional softmax and SVM-classifier-related TL systems were estimated for classifying histopathological cancer images in a binary BC database and a multiclass lung and colon cancer database. For achieving optimum classifier accuracy, a procedure that assigns an SVM technique to an FC layer of softmax-related TL techniques was presented. In [17], the authors' concentration on BC in HPI was attained by utilizing microscopic scans of breast tissues. The authors proposed two integrated DCNNs for extracting well-known image features utilizing TL. The pretrained Xception and Inception techniques were utilized in parallel. Afterwards, feature maps were integrated and decreased by dropout before they provided the final FC layer to classify.

3. The Proposed Model

In this work, an automated breast cancer classification method, named the AOADL-HBCC technique, was developed using HIs. The presented AOADL-HBCC technique mainly aims to recognize the presence of breast cancer in HIs. It encompasses a series of processes, namely SqueezeNet feature extraction, AOA hyperparameter tuning, DBN classification, and an Adamax optimizer. Figure 1 shows a block diagram of the AOADL-HBCC mechanism.

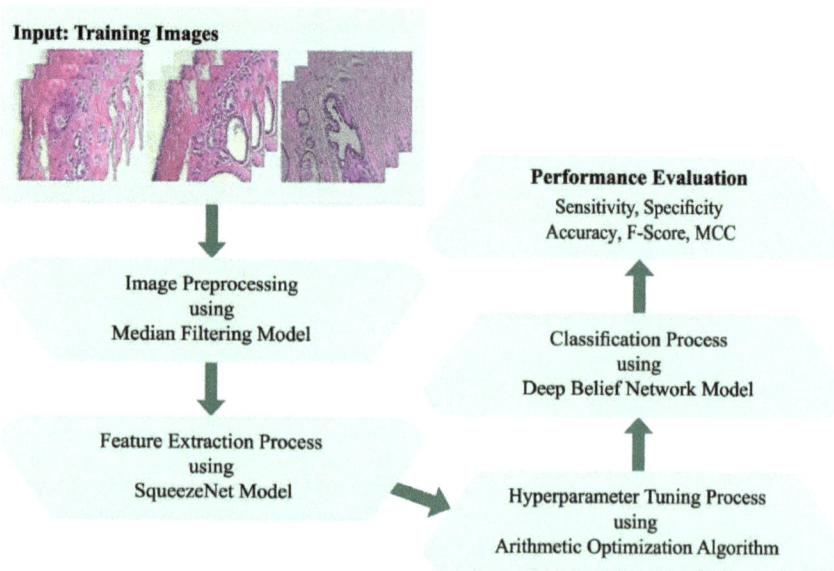

Figure 1. Block diagram of AOADL-HBCC system.

3.1. Design of AOA with SqueezeNet Model

In this study, the presented AOADL-HBCC technique utilized an AOA with a Squeeze-Net model to derive feature vectors. Presently, GoogLeNet, ResNet, VGG, AlexNet, etc., are signature techniques of DNN [18]. However, deep networks might lead to remarkable performance; this method is trained and recognition speed is reduced. Since the residual architecture does not enhance the module variable, the complexity of the trained degradation and gradient disappearance is effectively mitigated, and the convergence efficacy of the module is improved. Thus, the SqueezeNet architecture was applied as a backbone network to extract features. Figure 2 showcases the framework of the SqueezeNet method.

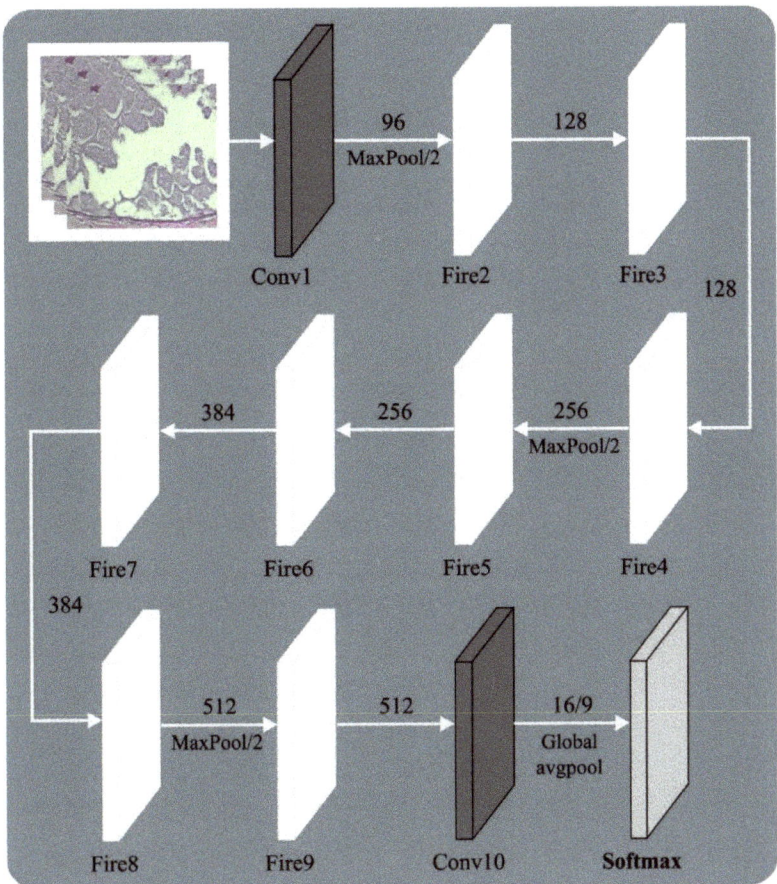

Figure 2. Architecture of SqueezeNet model.

Compared with AlexNet and VGGNet, the SqueezeNet architecture has a smaller number of parameters. The fire module was the primary approach from SqueezeNet. This approach was classified into expand and squeeze structures. The squeeze encompasses 1×1 convolutional kernels. The expand layer includes 3×3 and 1×1 convolutional kernels. The number of 3×3 convolutional kernels is $E_{3\times3}$ and the number of 1×1 convolutional kernels is $E_{1\times1}$. The model must satisfy $< (E_{1\times1} + E_{3\times3})$. Thus, 1×1 convolution is added to each inception module, the number of input networks and the convolutional kernel variable are decreased, and the computation difficulty is reduced. Lastly, a 1×1 convolutional layer is added to enhance the number of channels and feature extraction. SqueezeNet changes 3×3 convolution with a 1×1 convolutional layer to reduce the variable count to one-ninth. Image feature extraction depends on a shared convolutional layer. The lowest-level features, such as edges and angles, are detached from the basic network. The higher-level features explain that the target form is eliminated at the highest level. For demonstrating the ship target on scale, the FPN was determined to extend the backbone network; viz., it was especially efficient in the detection of smaller targets. The topmost-level feature of FPN architecture is integrated with basic features by up-sampling via each layer predicting the feature map.

To adjust the hyperparameters of the SqueezeNet method, an AOA was implemented in this work. The AOA starts with a number of arbitrary populations of objects as candidates (immersed objects) [19]. Here, the object was initialized through arbitrary location from the fluid. The initial location of each object was accomplished as follows:

$$x(i) = x_l(i) + rand \times (x_u(i) - x_l(i)) i = 1, 2, \ldots, N \quad (1)$$

In this expression, $x(i)$ describes the ith object from a population with N objects, along with $x_u(i)$ and $x_l(i)$, which indicate the upper and lower boundaries of the solution space, respectively. In addition, the following indicates the location, AOA initialized density (D), acceleration (A), and volume (V), to i^{th} object numbers:

$$V(i) = rand \quad (2)$$

$$D(i) = rand \quad (3)$$

$$A(i) = x_l(i) + rand \times (x_u(i) - x_l(i)) \quad (4)$$

Next, the cost value of the candidate is evaluated and stored as V^{best}, D^{best}, or A^{best}, based on the population. Then, the candidate is upgraded through the parameter model as follows:

$$V^{t+1}(i) = V^t(i) + rand \times \left(V^{best} - V^t(i)\right) \quad (5)$$

$$D^{t+1}(i) = D^t(i) + rand \times \left(D^{best} - D^t(i)\right) \quad (6)$$

In this case, y^{best} and D^{best} denote the density and volume, respectively, associated with the best object initiated before, and $rand$ indicates the arbitrary number that is uniformly distributed. The AOA applies a transfer operator (TF) to reach exploration–exploitation:

$$TF = \exp\left(\frac{t - t^{max}}{t^{max}}\right) \quad (7)$$

In Equation (7), TF slowly steps up from the period still accomplishing 1, and t and t^{max} indicate the iteration value and maximal iteration count, respectively. Likewise, a reduction factor of (d) density is used to offer a global–local search:

$$D^{t+1} = \exp\left(\frac{t^{max} - t}{t^{max}}\right) - \left(\frac{t}{t^{max}}\right) \quad (8)$$

In Equation (8), D^{t+1} is reduced with time that offers the ability to converge. This term renders a proper trade-off between exploitation and exploration. The exploration was stimulated on the basis of collision among objects. When $TF \leq 0.5$, a random material (mr) was preferred for upgrading acceleration of the object to $t + 1$ iteration:

$$A^{t+1} = \frac{D_{mr} + V_{mr} \times A_{mr}}{D^{t+1}(i) \times V^{t+1}(i)} \quad (9)$$

Here, $A(i)$, $V(i)$, and $D(i)$ denote the acceleration, volume, and density of the ith object. The exploitation was stimulated based on no collision among objects. When $TF > 0.5$, the object is then upgraded as follows:

$$A^{t+1}(i) = \frac{D^{best} + V^{best} \times A^{best}}{D^{t+1}(i) \times V^{t+1}(i)} \quad (10)$$

where A^{best} indicates the optimal object acceleration. The subsequent step to normalize acceleration for assessing alteration percentage is as follows:

$$A^{t+1}(\bar{i}) = u \times \frac{A^{t+1}(i) - \min(A)}{\max(A) - \min(A)} + l \qquad (11)$$

Here, $A^{t+1}(i)$ refers to the percentage of steps, and l and u correspondingly imply the normalized limit that is fixed to 0.1 and 0.9, respectively. When $TF \leq 0.5$, the location of the ith object to the succeeding round is accomplished as follows:

$$x^{t+1}(i) = x^t(i) + c_1 \times rand \times A^{t+1}(\bar{i}) \times D \times \left(x^{rand} - x^t(i)\right) \qquad (12)$$

In Equation (12), C_1 denotes the constant corresponding to 2. In addition, when $TF > 0.5$, the location of the object is upgraded:

$$x^{t+1}(i) = x^{best^t} + F \times c_2 \times rand \times A^{t+1}(\bar{i}) \times D \times \left(T \times x^{best} - x^t(i)\right) \qquad (13)$$

In this expression, c_2 denotes a constant number corresponding to 6. T enhances with time from a range $[c_3 \times 0.3, 1]$ and obtains a determined percentage in the best location. This percentage slowly enhances to diminish the variance among optimum and present locations to offer an optimal balance between exploration and exploitation. F shows the flag for changing the motion path as

$$F = \begin{cases} +1, & if\ P \leq 0.5 \\ +1, & if\ P > 0.5 \end{cases} \qquad (14)$$

while

$$P = 2 \times rand - c_4 \qquad (15)$$

Finally, the value of each object was assessed through a cost function and returned the optimal solution once the end state was satisfied.

The AOA method extracts a fitness function (FF) to receive enhanced classifier outcomes. It sets a positive value that signifies the superior outcome of the candidate's solutions. In this work, the minimized classifier error rate is indicated as the FF, as provided in Equation (16).

$$fitness(x_i) = ClassifierErrorRate(x_i) = \frac{number\ of\ misclassified\ samples}{Total\ number\ of\ samples} * 100 \qquad (16)$$

3.2. Breast Cancer Classification Using Optimal DBN Model

Finally, an Adamax optimizer with the DBN method was applied for the breast cancer classification process (Algorithm 1). A DBN is a stack of RBM, excluding the primary RBM that has an undirected connection [20]. Significantly, this network architecture creates DL possibilities and reduces training complexity. The simple and effective layer-wise trained method was developed for DBN by Hinton. It consecutively trains layers and greedily trains by tying the weight of unlearned layers, applying CD to learn the weight of a single layer and iterating until all the layers are trained. Then, the network weight was finetuned through a two-pass up-down model, and this illustrates that the network learned without pretraining, since this phase implemented as regular and assisted with the supervised optimized problem. The energy constrained from the directed approach was calculated where the maximal energy was upper-bounded and accomplished equivalence, whether the network weight was tied or not, as follows:

$$E\left(x^0, h^0\right) = -\left(\log p\left(h^0\right) + \log p\left(x^0 \big| h^0\right)\right) \qquad (17)$$

$$\log p\left(x^0\right) \geq \sum_{\forall h^0} Q(h^0|x^0)(\log p\left(h^0\right) + \log p(x^0|h^0)) - \sum_{\forall h^0} Q(h^0|x^0) \log Q(h^0|x^0) \quad (18)$$

$$\frac{\partial \log p(x^0)}{\partial \zeta_{n,m}} = \sum_{\forall h^0} Q\left(h^0|x^0\right) \log p\left(h^0\right) \quad (19)$$

Then, iteratively learning the weight of the network, the up-down approach was used to finetune the network weight. The wake-sleep approach is an unsupervised algorithm applied to train NNs from two phases: the "wake" phase was implemented on the feedforward path to compute weight and the "sleep" phase was executed on the feedback path. The up-down approach was executed to network for decreasing underfit that could usually be detected by a greedily trained network. Particularly in the primary phase, the weight on the directed connection was from named parameters or generative weight that can be adjusted by updating the weight utilizing CD, calculating the wake-phase probability, and sampling the states. Then, the prior layer was stochastically stimulated with top-down connections called inference weights or parameters. The sleep-stage probability was calculated, the state was sampled, and the result was estimated.

For optimizing the training efficacy of the DBN, the Adamax optimizer was employed for altering the hyperparameter values [21]:

$$w_t^i = w_{t-1}^i - \frac{\eta}{v_t + \epsilon} \cdot \hat{m}_t \quad (20)$$

where

$$\hat{m}_t = \frac{m_t}{1 - \beta_1^t} \quad (21)$$

$$v_t = max(\beta_2 \cdot v_{t-1}, |G_t|) \quad (22)$$

$$m_t = \beta_1 m_{t-1} + (1 - \beta_1) G \quad (23)$$

$$G = \nabla_w C(w_t) \quad (24)$$

In this expression, η denotes the learning rate, w_t represents the weight at t step, $C(.)$ indicates the cost function, and $\nabla_w C(w_t)$ specifies the gradient of the w_t weight variable. β_i is exploited to select the data needed for the old upgrade, where $\beta_i \in [0, 1]$. m_t and v_t represent the first and second moments.

Algorithm 1. Pseudocode of Adamax

η: Rate of Learning
$\beta_1, \beta_2 \in [0,1)$: Exponential decomposing value to moment candidate
$C(w)$: The cost function with variable w
w_0: Primary parameter vector
$m_0 \leftarrow 0$
$u_0 \leftarrow 0$
$i \leftarrow 0$ (Apply time step)
while w does not converge apply
$i \leftarrow i + 1$
$m_i \leftarrow \beta_1 \cdot m_{i-1} + (1 - \beta_1) \cdot \frac{\partial C}{\partial w}(w_i)$
$u_i \leftarrow max\left(\beta_2 \cdot u_{i-1}, \left|\frac{\partial C}{\partial w}(w_i)\right|\right)$
$w_{i+1} \leftarrow w_i - \left(\eta/\left(1 - \beta_1^i\right)\right) \cdot m_i/u_i$
end while
displaying w_i (end variable)

4. Experimental Validation

This section examines the breast cancer classification results of the AOADL-HBCC model on a benchmark dataset [22]. The dataset holds two sub-datasets, namely the 100× dataset and the 200× dataset, as represented in Table 1. Figure 3 illustrates some sample images.

Table 1. Dataset details.

Class	No. of Images	
	100×	200×
Benign	644	623
Malignant	1437	1390
Total No. of Images	2081	2013

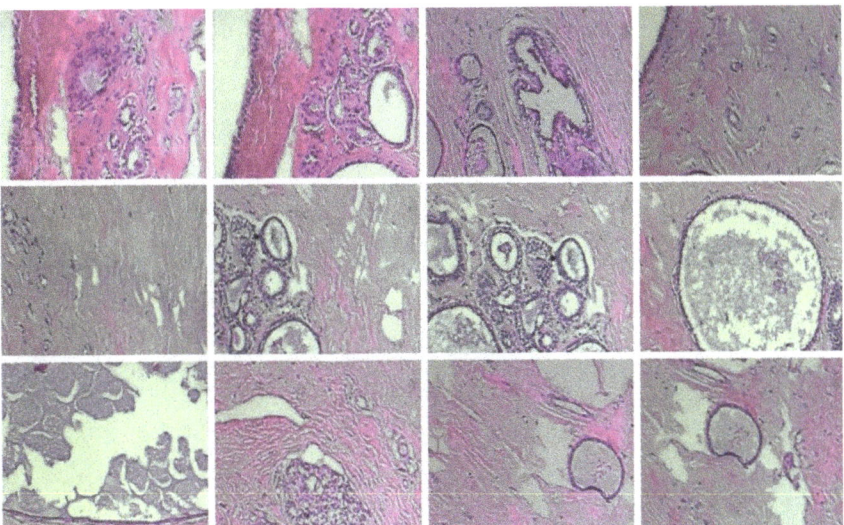

Figure 3. Sample images.

The proposed model was simulated using Python 3.6.5 tools on PC i5-8600k, GeForce 1050Ti 4 GB, 16 GB RAM, 250 GB SSD, and 1 TB HDD. The parameter settings were given as follows: learning rate: 0.01, dropout: 0.5, batch size: 5, epoch count: 50, and activation: ReLU.

The confusion matrices of the AOADL-HBCC model on the 100× dataset are reported in Figure 4. This figure implies the AOADL-HBCC method proficiently recognized and sorted the HIs into malignant and benign classes in all aspects.

Table 2 reports the overall breast cancer classification outcomes of the AOADL-HBCC method on the 100× database. The outcomes indicate that the AOADL-HBCC approach recognized both benign and malignant classes proficiently. For example, in the 80% TR database, the AOADL-HBCC method revealed an average $accu_y$ of 94.59%, $sens_y$ of 94.36%, $spec_y$ of 94.36%, F_{score} of 93.75%, and MCC of 87.55%. Simultaneously, in the 20% TS database, the AOADL-HBCC method exhibited an average $accu_y$ of 96.40%, $sens_y$ of 95.93%, $spec_y$ of 95.93%, F_{score} of 95.83%, and MCC of 91.67%. Concurrently, in the 70% TR database, the AOADL-HBCC approach displayed an average $accu_y$ of 95.60%, $sens_y$ of 93.19%, $spec_y$ of 93.19%, F_{score} of 94.62%, and MCC of 89.56%.

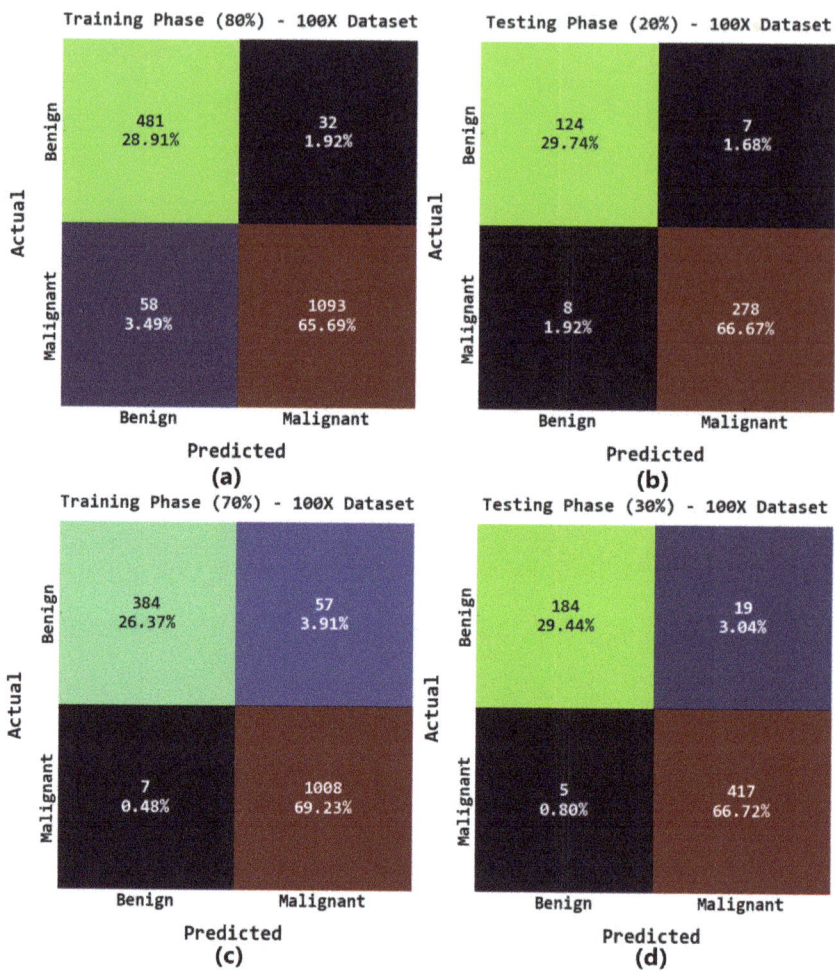

Figure 4. Confusion matrices of AOADL-HBCC system under 100× dataset: (**a,b**) TR and TS databases of 80:20, and (**c,d**) TR and TS databases of 70:30.

The TACC and VACC of the AOADL-HBCC technique under the 100× dataset are inspected on BCC performance in Figure 5. This figure indicates that the AOADL-HBCC method displayed enhanced performance with increased values of TACC and VACC. It is noted that the AOADL-HBCC algorithm gained maximum TACC outcomes.

The TLS and VLS of the AOADL-HBCC approach under the 100× dataset are tested on BCC performance in Figure 6. This figure shows that the AOADL-HBCC method exhibited better performance with minimal values of TLS and VLS. It is noted the AOADL-HBCC approach resulted in reduced VLS outcomes.

Table 2. BCC outcomes of AOADL-HBCC approach with various measures under 100× dataset.

Class	Accuracy	Sensitivity	Specificity	F-Score	MCC
Training/Testing (80:20)					
Training Phase					
Benign	94.59	93.76	94.96	91.44	87.55
Malignant	94.59	94.96	93.76	96.05	87.55
Average	94.59	94.36	94.36	93.75	87.55
Testing Phase					
Benign	96.40	94.66	97.20	94.30	91.67
Malignant	96.40	97.20	94.66	97.37	91.67
Average	96.40	95.93	95.93	95.83	91.67
Training/Testing (70:30)					
Training Phase					
Benign	95.60	87.07	99.31	92.31	89.56
Malignant	95.60	99.31	87.07	96.92	89.56
Average	95.60	93.19	93.19	94.62	89.56
Testing Phase					
Benign	96.16	90.64	98.82	93.88	91.21
Malignant	96.16	98.82	90.64	97.20	91.21
Average	96.16	94.73	94.73	95.54	91.21

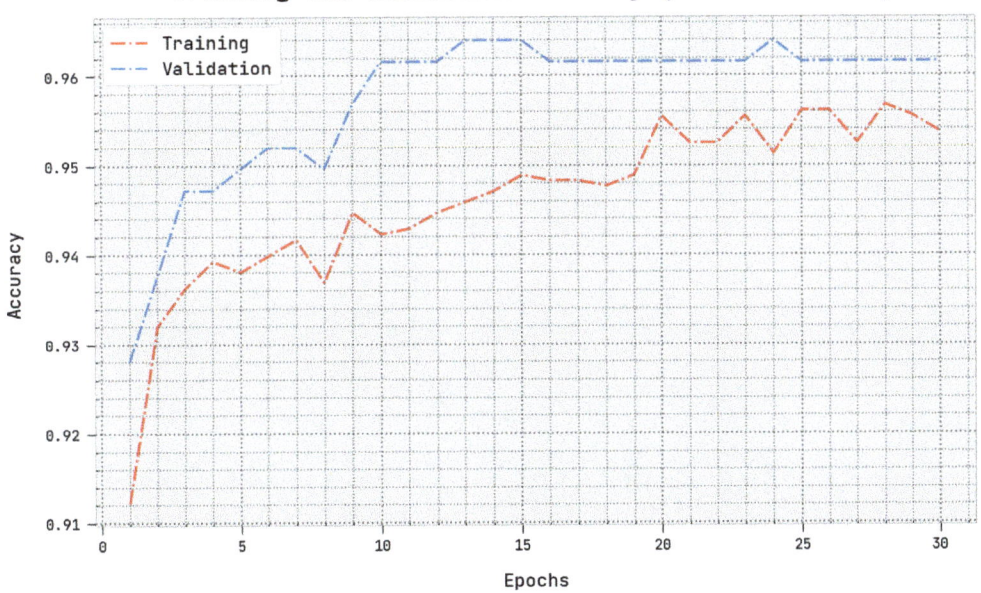

Figure 5. TACC and VACC analysis of AOADL-HBCC approach under 100× dataset.

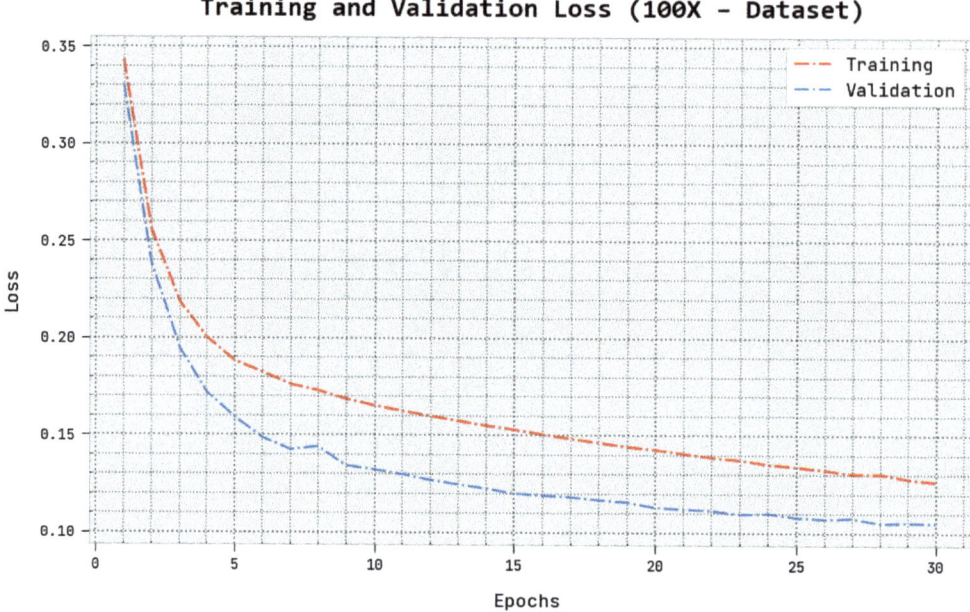

Figure 6. TLS and VLS analysis of AOADL-HBCC approach under 100× dataset.

A clear precision–recall investigation of the AOADL-HBCC methodology under the test database is given in Figure 7. This figure exhibits that the AOADL-HBCC system enhanced precision–recall values in every class label.

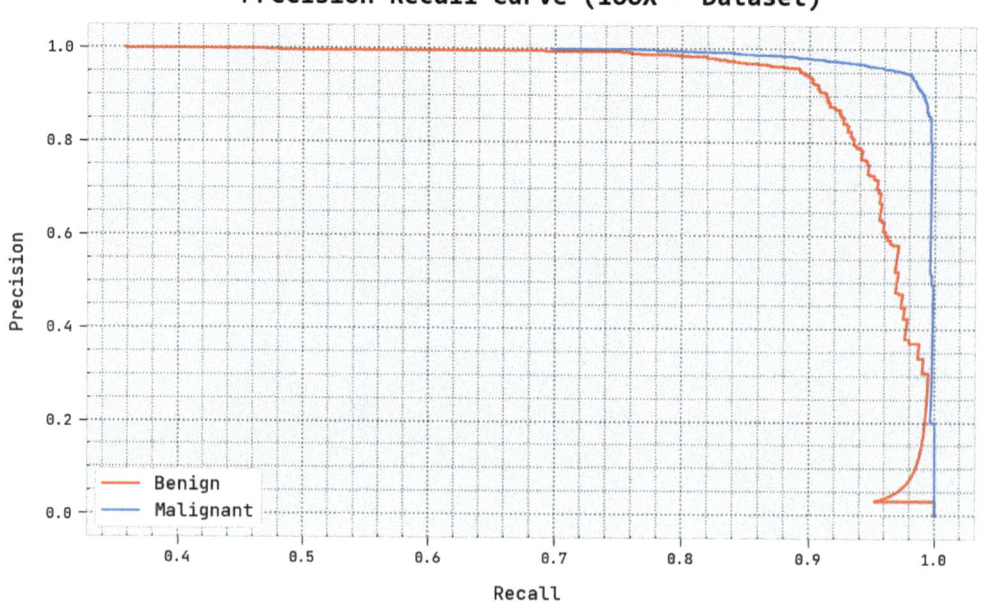

Figure 7. Precision–recall analysis of AOADL-HBCC approach under 100× dataset.

A brief ROC analysis of the AOADL-HBCC approach under the test database is shown in Figure 8. The fallouts show that the AOADL-HBCC methodology exhibited its capacity in classifying different classes in the test database.

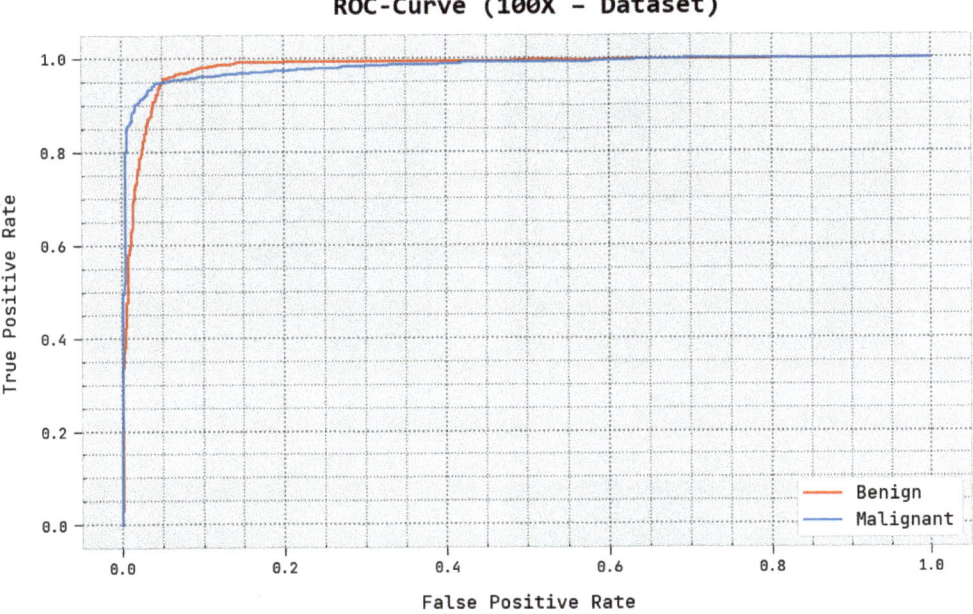

Figure 8. ROC analysis of AOADL-HBCC approach under 100× dataset.

The confusion matrices of the AOADL-HBCC approach on the 200× database are given in Figure 9. This figure indicates that the AOADL-HBCC approach proficiently recognized and sorted the HIs into malignant and benign classes in every aspect.

Table 3 shows the overall breast cancer classification results of the AOADL-HBCC approach on the 200× dataset. The results indicate that the AOADL-HBCC model recognized both benign and malignant classes proficiently. For example, in the 80% TR database, the AOADL-HBCC technique exhibited an average $accu_y$ of 96.40%, $sens_y$ of 96.18%, $spec_y$ of 96.18%, F_{score} of 95.91%, and MCC of 91.83%. Concurrently, in the 20% TS database, the AOADL-HBCC approach displayed an average $accu_y$ of 96.77%, $sens_y$ of 96.88%, $spec_y$ of 96.88%, F_{score} of 95.85%, and MCC of 91.80%. Simultaneously, in the 70% TR database, the AOADL-HBCC technique displayed an average $accu_y$ of 93.04%, $sens_y$ of 90.03%, $spec_y$ of 90.03%, F_{score} of 91.51%, and MCC of 83.45%.

The TACC and VACC of the AOADL-HBCC method under the 200× dataset are inspected on BCC performance in Figure 10. This figure shows that the AOADL-HBCC methodology displayed enhanced performance with increased values of TACC and VACC. It is noted that the AOADL-HBCC technique attained maximum TACC outcomes.

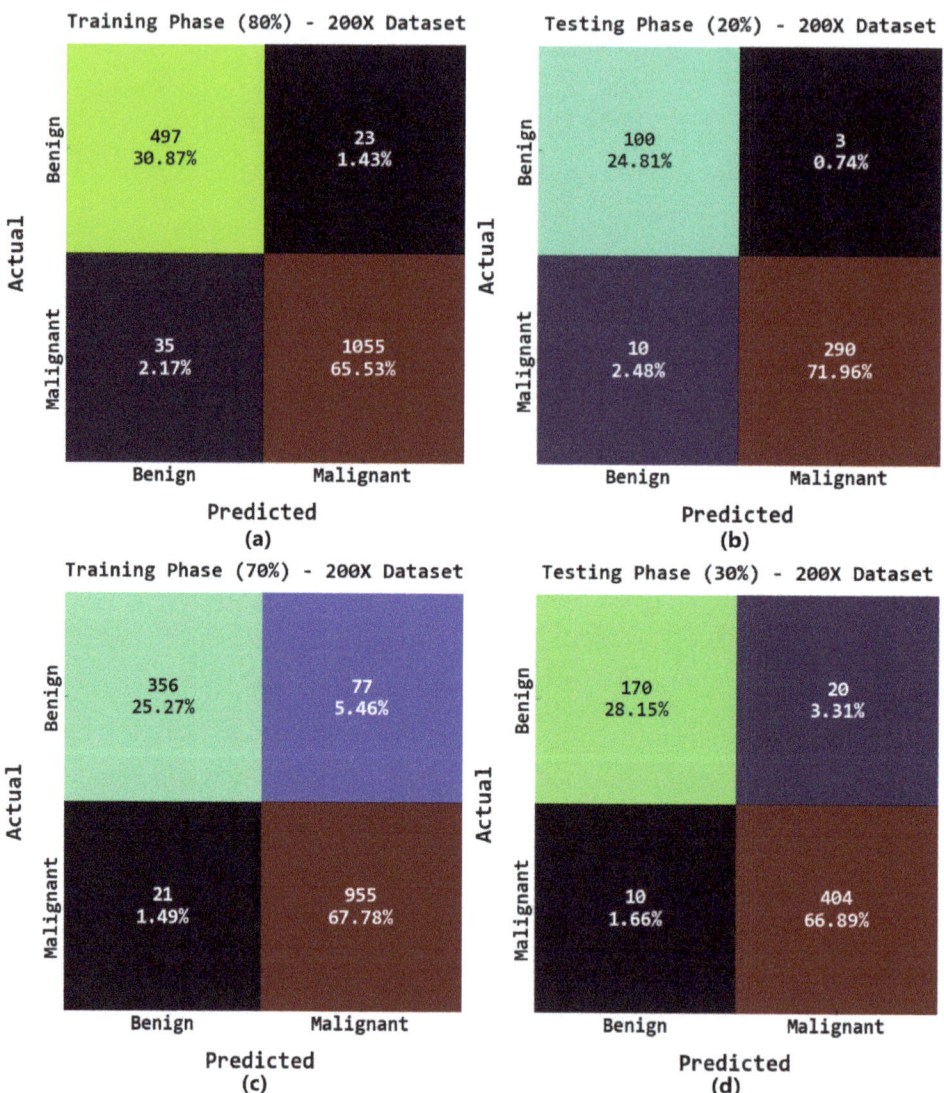

Figure 9. Confusion matrices of AOADL-HBCC system under 200× dataset: (**a**,**b**) TR and TS databases of 80:20, and (**c**,**d**) TR and TS databases of 70:30.

The TLS and VLS of the AOADL-HBCC approach under the 200× dataset are tested on BCC performance in Figure 11. This figure indicates that the AOADL-HBCC methodology revealed superior performance with minimal values of TLS and VLS. It is noted that the AOADL-HBCC method resulted in reduced VLS outcomes.

A clear precision–recall inspection of the AOADL-HBCC methodology under the test database is shown in Figure 12. This figure indicates that the AOADL-HBCC method enhanced precision–recall values in every class label.

Table 3. BCC outcomes of AOADL-HBCC approach with various measures under 200× dataset.

Class	Accuracy	Sensitivity	Specificity	F-Score	MCC
Training/Testing (80:20)					
Training Phase					
Benign	96.40	95.58	96.79	94.49	91.83
Malignant	96.40	96.79	95.58	97.32	91.83
Average	96.40	96.18	96.18	95.91	91.83
Testing Phase					
Benign	96.77	97.09	96.67	93.90	91.80
Malignant	96.77	96.67	97.09	97.81	91.80
Average	96.77	96.88	96.88	95.85	91.80
Training/Testing (70:30)					
Training Phase					
Benign	93.04	82.22	97.85	87.90	83.45
Malignant	93.04	97.85	82.22	95.12	83.45
Average	93.04	90.03	90.03	91.51	83.45
Testing Phase					
Benign	95.03	89.47	97.58	91.89	88.38
Malignant	95.03	97.58	89.47	96.42	88.38
Average	95.03	93.53	93.53	94.16	88.38

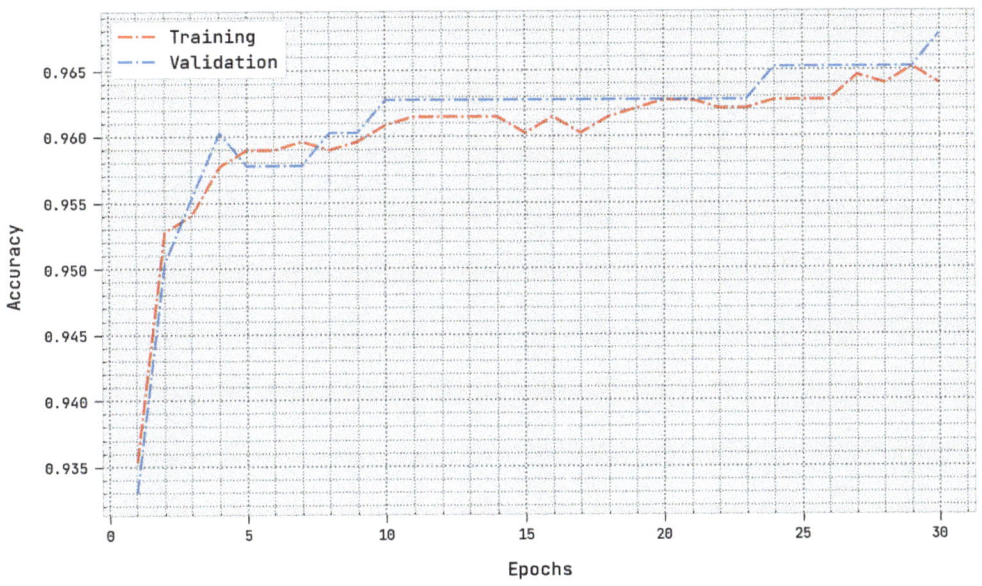

Figure 10. TACC and VACC analysis of AOADL-HBCC approach under 200× dataset.

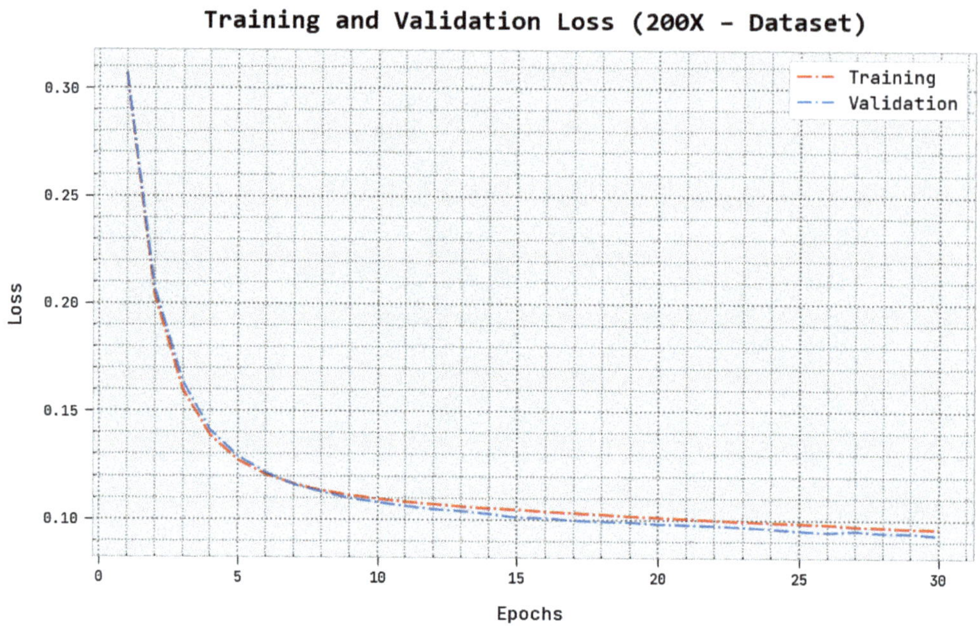

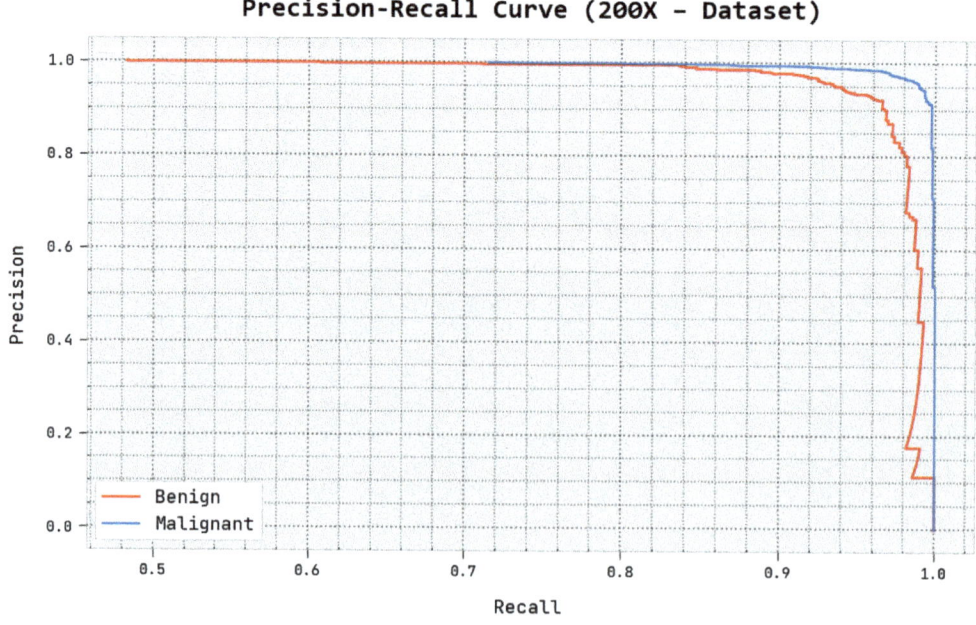

Figure 11. TLS and VLS analysis of AOADL-HBCC approach under 200× dataset.

Figure 12. Precision–recall analysis of AOADL-HBCC approach under 200× dataset.

A brief ROC study of the AOADL-HBCC system under the test database is given in Figure 13. The outcomes exhibited by the AOADL-HBCC method reveal its ability in classifying different classes in the test database.

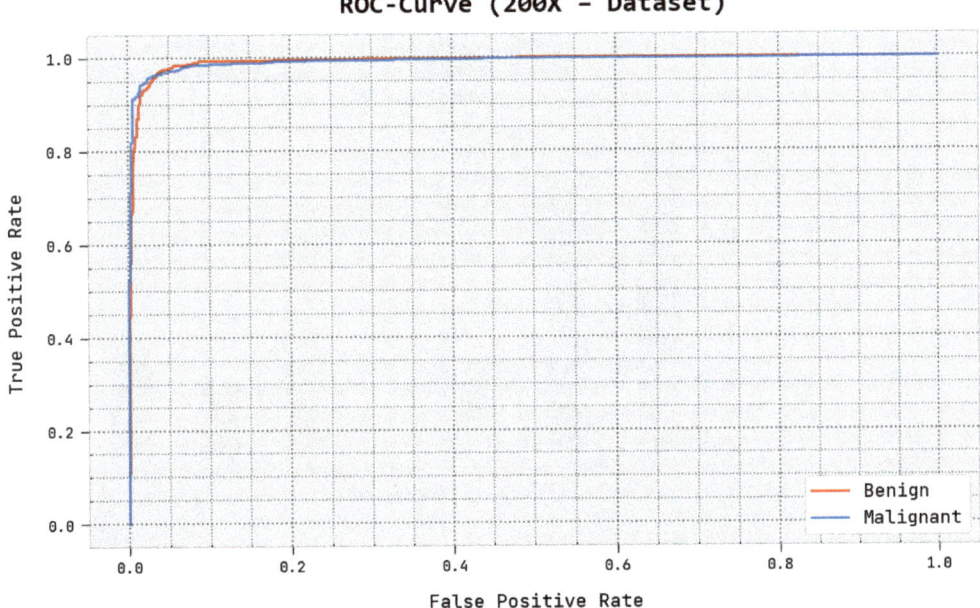

Figure 13. ROC analysis of AOADL-HBCC approach under 200× dataset.

A detailed comparative study of the AOADL-HBCC model with recent DL models is reported in Table 4 and Figure 14 [23]. The simulation values representing the Incep. V3, VGG16, and ResNet-50 models reported lower $accu_y$ of 81.67%, 80.15%, and 82.18%, respectively. Next, the Incep. V3-LSTM and Incep. V3-BiLSTM models attained reasonable $accu_y$ of 91.46% and 92.05%, respectively.

Table 4. Comparative analysis of AOADL-HBCC system with current approaches.

Methods	Accuracy
AOADL-HBCC	96.77
DTLRO-HCBC	93.52
Incep.V3	81.67
Incep.V3-LSTM	91.46
Incep.V3-BiLSTM	92.05
VGG16 Model	80.15
ResNet-50 Model	82.18

Although the DTLRO-HCBC model reached near-optimal $accu_y$ of 93.52%, the AOADL-HBCC model gained maximum $accu_y$ of 96.77%. These results ensured the enhanced outcomes of the AOADL-HBCC model over other models.

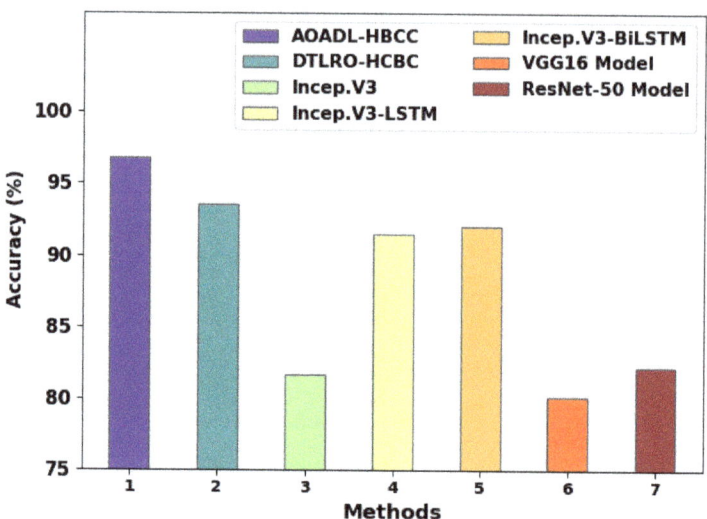

Figure 14. Comparative analysis of AOADL-HBCC system with existing approaches.

5. Conclusions

In this work, an automated breast cancer classification model, named the AOADL-HBCC technique, was developed on HIs. The presented AOADL-HBCC technique mainly aims to recognize the presence of breast cancer in HIs. At the primary level, the AOADL-HBCC technique exploited MF-based noise removal and a contrast enhancement process. In addition, the presented AOADL-HBCC technique utilized an AOA with a SqueezeNet model to derive feature vectors. Lastly, an Adamax optimizer with a DBN model was applied for the breast cancer classification process. In order to exhibit the enhanced breast cancer classification results of the AOADL-HBCC methodology, a wide range of simulations were performed. A comparative study indicated the better performance of the AOADL-HBCC technique over other recent methodologies, with a maximum accuracy of 96.77%. Therefore, the AOADL-HBCC technique can be employed for timely and accurate BC classification. In the future, ensemble-learning-based DL classifiers can be involved to boost the overall performance of the AOADL-HBCC technique. In addition, the performance of the proposed model can be tested on large-scale real-time databases.

Author Contributions: M.O.: Methodology, Project administration, Funding acquisition, Formal analysis, Writing—original draft; M.S.M.: Writing—original draft, Writing—review & editing, Validation; N.N.: Review & editing, revising critically for important intellectual content, Validation; Funding acquisition. H.M.: Formal analysis, Writing—original draft; Writing—review & editing; A.M.: Supervision, Conceptualization, data curation, Writing—original draft; A.E.O.: Software, data curation, Writing—original draft; Writing—review & editing; A.A.A.: Supervision, Writing—original draft; Writing—review & editing; M.I.A.: review & editing, revising critically for important intellectual content, Validation. All authors have read and agreed to the published version of the manuscript.

Funding: The authors extend their appreciation to the Deanship of Scientific Research at King Khalid University for funding this work through Large Groups Project under grant number (2/44). Princess Nourah bint Abdulrahman University Researchers Supporting Project number (PNURSP2023R203), Princess Nourah bint Abdulrahman University, Riyadh, Saudi Arabia. Research Supporting Project number (RSP2023R787), King Saud University, Riyadh, Saudi Arabia.

Institutional Review Board Statement: This article does not contain any studies with human participants performed by any of the authors.

Informed Consent Statement: Not applicable.

Data Availability Statement: Data sharing is not applicable to this article as no datasets were generated during the current study.

Conflicts of Interest: The authors declare that they have no conflicts of interest.

References

1. Boumaraf, S.; Liu, X.; Zheng, Z.; Ma, X.; Ferkous, C. A new transfer learning based approach to magnification dependent and independent classification of breast cancer in histopathological images. *Biomed. Signal Process. Control* **2021**, *63*, 102192. [CrossRef]
2. Bose, S.; Garg, A.; Singh, S.P. Transfer Learning for Classification of Histopathology Images of Invasive Ductal Carcinoma in Breast. In Proceedings of the 2022 3rd International Conference on Electronics and Sustainable Communication Systems (ICESC), Coimbatore, India, 17–19 August 2022; pp. 1039–1044.
3. Ahmad, N.; Asghar, S.; Gillani, S.A. Transfer learning-assisted multi-resolution breast cancer histopathological images classification. *Vis. Comput.* **2021**, *38*, 2751–2770. [CrossRef]
4. Thuy, M.B.H.; Hoang, V.T. Fusing of deep learning, transfer learning and gan for breast cancer histopathological image classification. In *International Conference on Computer Science, Applied Mathematics and Applications*; Springer: Cham, Switzerland, 2019; pp. 255–266.
5. Abbasniya, M.R.; Sheikholeslamzadeh, S.A.; Nasiri, H.; Emami, S. Classification of Breast Tumors Based on Histopathology Images Using Deep Features and Ensemble of Gradient Boosting Methods. *Comput. Electr. Eng.* **2022**, *103*, 108382. [CrossRef]
6. Chang, J.; Yu, J.; Han, T.; Chang, H.J.; Park, E. A method for classifying medical images using transfer learning: A pilot study on histopathology of breast cancer. In Proceedings of the 2017 IEEE 19th International Conference on E-Health Networking, Applications and Services (Healthcom), Dalian, China, 12–15 October 2017; pp. 1–4.
7. Ahmad, H.M.; Ghuffar, S.; Khurshid, K. Classification of breast cancer histology images using transfer learning. In Proceedings of the 2019 16th International Bhurban Conference on Applied Sciences and Technology (IBCAST), Islamabad, Pakistan, 8–12 January 2019; pp. 328–332.
8. Alzubaidi, L.; Al-Shamma, O.; Fadhel, M.A.; Farhan, L.; Zhang, J.; Duan, Y. Optimizing the performance of breast cancer classification by employing the same domain transfer learning from hybrid deep convolutional neural network model. *Electronics* **2020**, *9*, 445. [CrossRef]
9. Baghdadi, N.A.; Malki, A.; Balaha, H.M.; AbdulAzeem, Y.; Badawy, M.; Elhosseini, M. Classification of breast cancer using a manta-ray foraging optimized transfer learning framework. *PeerJ Comput. Sci.* **2022**, *8*, e1054. [CrossRef] [PubMed]
10. Sajjad, U.; Hussain, I.; Hamid, K.; Ali, H.M.; Wang, C.C.; Yan, W.M. Liquid-to-vapor phase change heat transfer evaluation and parameter sensitivity analysis of nanoporous surface coatings. *Int. J. Heat Mass Transf.* **2022**, *194*, 123088. [CrossRef]
11. Shankar, K.; Dutta, A.K.; Kumar, S.; Joshi, G.P.; Doo, I.C. Chaotic Sparrow Search Algorithm with Deep Transfer Learning Enabled Breast Cancer Classification on Histopathological Images. *Cancers* **2022**, *14*, 2770. [CrossRef] [PubMed]
12. Deniz, E.; Şengür, A.; Kadiroğlu, Z.; Guo, Y.; Bajaj, V.; Budak, Ü. Transfer learning based histopathologic image classification for breast cancer detection. *Health Inf. Sci. Syst.* **2018**, *6*, 1–7. [CrossRef] [PubMed]
13. Khan, S.; Islam, N.; Jan, Z.; Din, I.U.; Rodrigues, J.J.C. A novel deep learning based framework for the detection and classification of breast cancer using transfer learning. *Pattern Recognit. Lett.* **2019**, *125*, 1–6. [CrossRef]
14. Talo, M. Automated classification of histopathology images using transfer learning. *Artif. Intell. Med.* **2019**, *101*, 101743. [CrossRef] [PubMed]
15. Singh, R.; Ahmed, T.; Kumar, A.; Singh, A.K.; Pandey, A.K.; Singh, S.K. Imbalanced breast cancer classification using transfer learning. *IEEE/ACM Trans. Comput. Biol. Bioinform.* **2020**, *18*, 83–93. [CrossRef] [PubMed]
16. Fan, J.; Lee, J.; Lee, Y. A transfer learning architecture based on a support vector machine for histopathology image classification. *Appl. Sci.* **2021**, *11*, 6380. [CrossRef]
17. Elmannai, H.; Hamdi, M.; AlGarni, A. Deep learning models combining for breast cancer histopathology image classification. *Int. J. Comput. Intell. Syst.* **2021**, *14*, 1003. [CrossRef]
18. Escorcia-Gutierrez, J.; Gamarra, M.; Beleño, K.; Soto, C.; Mansour, R.F. Intelligent deep learning-enabled autonomous small ship detection and classification model. *Comput. Electr. Eng.* **2022**, *100*, 107871. [CrossRef]
19. Kaveh, A.; Hamedani, K.B. Improved arithmetic optimization algorithm and its application to discrete structural optimization. In *Structures*; Elsevier: Amsterdam, The Netherlands, 2022; Volume 35, pp. 748–764.
20. Zand, R.; Camsari, K.Y.; Pyle, S.D.; Ahmed, I.; Kim, C.H.; DeMara, R.F. Low-energy deep belief networks using intrinsic sigmoidal spintronic-based probabilistic neurons. In Proceedings of the 2018 on Great Lakes Symposium on VLSI, Chicago, IL, USA, 23–25 May 2018; pp. 15–20.
21. Kandel, I.; Castelli, M.; Popovič, A. Comparative study of first order optimizers for image classification using convolutional neural networks on histopathology images. *J. Imaging* **2020**, *6*, 92. [CrossRef] [PubMed]

22. Available online: https://web.inf.ufpr.br/vri/databases/breast-cancer-histopathological-database-breakhis/ (accessed on 5 July 2022).
23. Ragab, M.; Nahhas, A.F. Optimal Deep Transfer Learning Model for Histopathological Breast Cancer Classification. *CMC-Comput. Mater. Contin.* **2022**, *73*, 2849–2864. [CrossRef]

Disclaimer/Publisher's Note: The statements, opinions and data contained in all publications are solely those of the individual author(s) and contributor(s) and not of MDPI and/or the editor(s). MDPI and/or the editor(s) disclaim responsibility for any injury to people or property resulting from any ideas, methods, instructions or products referred to in the content.

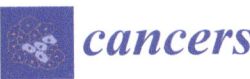

Article

A Series-Based Deep Learning Approach to Lung Nodule Image Classification

Mehmet Ali Balcı [1,*], Larissa M. Batrancea [2,*], Ömer Akgüller [1] and Anca Nichita [3]

1 Faculty of Science, Mathematics Department, Muğla Sıtkı Koçman University, 48000 Muğla, Turkey
2 Department of Business, Babeș-Bolyai University, 400174 Cluj-Napoca, Romania
3 Faculty of Economics, "1 Decembrie 1918" University of Alba Iulia, 510009 Alba Iulia, Romania
* Correspondence: mehmetalibalci@mu.edu.tr (M.A.B.); larissa.batrancea@ubbcluj.ro (L.M.B.)

Simple Summary: Medical image classification is an important task in computer-aided diagnosis, medical image acquisition, and mining. Although deep learning has been shown to outperform traditional methods based on handcrafted features, it remains difficult due to significant intra-class variation and inter-class similarity caused by the diversity of imaging modalities and clinical pathologies. This study presents an innovative method that is an intersection between 3D image analysis and series classification problems. Therefore, the self-similarity features in medical images are captured by converting the regions of interest to series with a radial scan and these series are classified with U-shape convolutional neural networks. The findings of this study are expected to be used by researchers from various disciplines working on radial scanned images, as well as researchers working on artificial intelligence in health.

Abstract: Although many studies have shown that deep learning approaches yield better results than traditional methods based on manual features, CADs methods still have several limitations. These are due to the diversity in imaging modalities and clinical pathologies. This diversity creates difficulties because of variation and similarities between classes. In this context, the new approach from our study is a hybrid method that performs classifications using both medical image analysis and radial scanning series features. Hence, the areas of interest obtained from images are subjected to a radial scan, with their centers as poles, in order to obtain series. A U-shape convolutional neural network model is then used for the 4D data classification problem. We therefore present a novel approach to the classification of 4D data obtained from lung nodule images. With radial scanning, the eigenvalue of nodule images is captured, and a powerful classification is performed. According to our results, an accuracy of 92.84% was obtained and much more efficient classification scores resulted as compared to recent classifiers.

Keywords: 4D classification; deep learning; lung nodule image; radial scanning

1. Introduction

Cancer is one of today's most serious health issues. Despite significant and promising advances in medicine, the desired level of prevention and elimination of many cancers has yet to be achieved [1–3]. Cancer is a common disease that is difficult, time-consuming, and challenging to treat. It is diverse with numerous subtypes. Some types of cancer, which are common in most people, are lethal. Cancer treatment is a difficult process, and early detection is critical. Early cancer diagnosis can be helped by a clinical follow-up of the patient in later stages. In this context, screening is the search for the presence of cancer cells in humans who have no symptoms. Screening stages are the most important steps in the fight against cancer because they are required for early diagnosis. Information obtained by imaging methods is used to determine the cancer type and its stage, which are extremely useful for disease treatment planning. As a result, the accuracy of information obtained by scanning methods can change the outcome of the disease. Patients can live a longer and more fulfilling life due to correct screening methods and treatment plans that are determined in conjunction with accurate analyses. The application of advanced technology in cancer imaging, which is required for a patient's treatment plan, as well as correct evaluation, are highly effective for determining treatment plans. Patients who have the opportunity to benefit from proper imaging techniques gain an advantage during the difficult treatment process by correctly analyzing imaging data.

Due to the high cost of equipment and personnel, as well as the difficulty of the task, it is not possible to apply known screening programs to every person. Lung nodules come in a wide range of shapes and sizes, hence identifying and characterizing abnormalities in these nodules is a difficult and delicate task. In this regard, computer-aided diagnosis (CAD) systems are critical to make clinicians' jobs easier.

Image processing and machine learning-based research on digital pathology image classification have yielded promising results. These findings suggest that digital pathology systems based on machine learning could be widely used in pathology clinics. Artificial intelligence and machine learning-based solutions will be used at a much higher rate in the coming years, particularly in pathology.

The mortality rate from lung cancer is the greatest of any kind of cancer, although this is a disease whose prognosis may be improved with early diagnosis. In order to establish which pulmonary nodules are benign and which nodules need biopsy to confirm malignancy, low-dose computed tomography has become the standard procedure for lung cancer screening. Nevertheless, lung cancer screening has a significant clinical false-positive rate because of the necessity to identify a high proportion of malignant nodules for biopsy [4,5]. Due to this, many unnecessary biopsies are conducted on people who turn out not to have cancer.

In this study, we provide a CNN architecture that combines data from volumetric radiomics series and nodule images for categorization. Qualitative and quantitative characteristics may be found in lung CT images. These characteristics illustrate the nodule's pathogenesis. Using mathematics and data characterization methods, these quantitative characteristics are retrieved from the picture. The term "radiomic" is used to describe the procedure, whereas "radiomic features" refers to the numerical characteristics that are gleaned from the data. As defined in [6], this process involves "high-throughput extraction of quantitative information from radiological pictures to build a radiomic, high-dimensional dataset followed by data mining for possibly better decision support." The radiomic characteristics of nodules primarily include their morphology, shape, and gray-level distribution. This research uses a spherical radial scan of a 3D model derived from CT scans to decode information about the nodule's volume and shape over time. The created regions in each level plane are scanned radially while the planes themselves are shifted from bottom to top. Thus, the shape shift may be considered with the gray level distributions of the CT scans collected at the various stages. Using the LIDC-IDRI dataset, we take a novel method to predict the malignancy of lung nodules by integrating hitherto unexplored image and volumetric radiomic combinations with volumetric radiomics-induced series.

CAD methods still have several limitations, despite numerous studies demonstrating that deep learning approaches outperform traditional methods based on manual features [7–10]. This is due to the fact that imaging modalities and clinical pathologies differ. Such diversity creates difficulties because of differences and similarities between classes. In this context, the new approach in our study is a hybrid method that classifies data using both medical image analysis and series features. Image-derived interest areas are subjected to a radial scan, with their centers acting as poles, in order to obtain series. A convolutional neural network (CNN) model is used to solve the series classification problem. We advance a method for classifying series obtained from lung nodule images. The eigenvalue of the nodule images is captured using radial scanning and a powerful classification is performed. According to our results, we obtained an accuracy of 92.44% and significantly higher classification scores as compared to numerous traditional classifiers.

Related Works

Many pre-diagnosis models capitalize the advantage of CNN architectures that revolutionized computer vision research by making color images usable as input data. In this context, input data are processed by a succession of cores that slide over image color channels to extract characteristics such as edges and color gradients, giving the appearance of an artificial neural network's (ANN) downstream fully linked layers. These inputs are summed and flattened before being sent on to the fully linked layer. Several different kinds of preconfigured CNN architectures are available. Radiology and digital pathology both benefit greatly from the usage of CNNs.

There has been extensive research into the development of CAD systems for lung cancer screening. Detection and segmentation of pulmonary nodules, characterization of nodules, and classification of malignancy were among the studies that stood out. Recently, very good and promising results in lung cancer screening, as well as other cancer screenings, have been obtained, with deep learning-supported studies on nodule detection, segmentation, and characterization [11–13].

Capabilities of CADs and radiomic tools to improve diagnostic accuracy and consistency across medical images help radiologists' decision-making [14,15]. CADs and radiomics rely on segmentation and quantitative feature extraction from images of identified nodules as its foundation. Moreover, machine learning algorithms use this collection of properties as a training set for classifying unseen nodule samples [16,17]. Such studies focus on the intranodular region and employ radiomic characteristics of its shape, boundary, and tissue for the most accurate identification [18–22].

Deep learning saves time for medical professionals by performing the complex classification task, which requires a significant amount of time and effort and consists of the classification of large amounts of images, while avoiding possible human-induced lines during the diagnosis phase at the same time [23–25]. Although it is well known that accurate and early diagnosis are effective in all disease types, deep learning-based methods have been successfully applied in early diagnosis, which is a crucial stage in cancer disease [26–28]. Deep network architectures have evolved and their computational power has increased as deep learning models have advanced in specific tasks. Deep neural networks have begun to be used effectively in computer vision processes such as image classification, object detection, and image segmentation as CNNs have made significant progress. Deep learning and CNN advancements have been critical in the development of medical systems for reliable scanning and image-based diagnostics. As a result, research has progressed from image segmentation and feature extraction to deep learning-based automatic classification [29,30].

Abdoulaye et al. [31] classified mammography images into three stages. First, they removed noise from the image by examining its surroundings, then they discovered the physical properties of the object and extracted patterns. In this way, they were able to create a cancer detection system based on the artificial intelligence-enabled algorithm that they trained using a pattern they obtained. Wang et al. [32] used an automatic image analysis technique to classify breast cancer histopathology images. They obtained 4 shape-based features and 138 color-space features for nodule classification. As a preprocessing step, they used bottom-up cap transformation to highlight background objects in order to locate growing cancer cells. Afterwards, they used wavelet transform to determine the location of ROIs, and as a result, they classified normal and malignant cell images with a 96.19% success rate. Jiang et al. [33] developed their own method by studying lymphatic pathologies such as chronic lymphocytic leukemia (CLL), follicular lymphoma (FL), and mantle cell lymphoma (MCL). After preprocessing the image, they extracted a feature set that included texture properties such as entropy, density mean, density standard deviation, loopy back propagation, and gray level co-occurrence matrix. They used the support vector machine (SVM) algorithm to classify pathology images based on the extracted features. As a result, their average accuracy performance value was 97.96%. Mohammed et al. [34]

trained ANNs to predict pancreatic cancer risk using clinical variables such as age, smoking status, alcohol consumption, and ethnicity.

Busnatu et al. [35] and Hunter et al. [36] present a detailed account of the recent literature studies on artificial intelligence and deep learning applications classified according to medical specialties. Readers can refer to these two studies for more comprehensive information on deep learning applications regarding cancer diagnosis based on image analysis.

Image series can be created by taking temporary images of the same scene at different ordered input. If each sequential input corresponds to the time tick, it is possible to say that the obtained series are time series. Several researchers have developed effective methods for correctly interpreting image time-series data as a result of acquiring image data [37–47]. With early diagnosis and a correct treatment, the quality of patients' lives can be substantially improved due to the analysis of biomedical time series via accurate and reliable techniques, the understanding of such data, and the rapid detection of possible abnormalities. The use of temporal correlation in time-series analysis is critical to the success of chosen methods. In this context, image time series are critical in biomedicine for monitoring disease progression.

Iakovidis et al. [37] used time series obtained from chest radiographs to track the progression of pneumonia. Contrariwise, Baur et al. [38] used canonical correlation analysis and Dynamic Bayesian Networks (DBN) to extract validated gene regulatory networks from time-series gene expression data. Likewise, Guo et al. [39] built gene regulatory networks with a feature selection algorithm based on partial least squares (PLS). In their studies, Penfold et al. [40] and Isci et al. [41] introduced Bayesian methodologies for network analysis using biological data, especially measures of time-series gene expression. Schlitt et al. [42] used Bayes and DBNs to explain gene expression variations over time in terms of regulatory network topologies. According to Ni et al. [43] and Kim et al. [44], the study of Murphy et al. [45] suggested techniques capable of expressing time-varying behavior of the underlying biological network, hence offering a more accurate representation of spatio-temporal input–output connections. In their work, Kourou et al. [46] used time-series microarray gene expression data to classify differentially expressed genes (DEGs) in cancer with great effectiveness. Imani et al. [47] expanded the analysis of radio frequency (RF) time series to enhance tissue classification at clinical frequencies by using additional time-series spectrum characteristics.

Various non-local deep learning architectures, which we also used in the comparison analysis, have been successfully used in the nodule classification task. Shen et al. [48] proposed multi-crop convolutional neural networks and Al-Shabi et al. [49] advanced gated-dilated networks for malignancy classification and obtained above 87% accuracy scores. Moreover, Ren et al. [50] built a unique manifold regularized classification deep neural network (MRC-DNN) to conduct classification directly based on the manifold representation of lung nodule images, which was motivated by the observation that genuine structure among data was typically contained on a low-dimensional manifold. Shen et al. [51] showed that the resilience of a representative DL-based lung-nodule classification model for CT images could be improved, highlighting the need of assessing and assuring model robustness while creating comparable models. To increase the depth of representation, Jiang et al. [52] first developed a contextual attention mechanism to model contextual relationships between neighboring sites. Then, authors employed a spatial attention technique to automatically find the zones that were crucial for nodule categorization. Finally, they used an ensemble of models to increase the reliability of their predictions. Al-Shabi et al. [53] suggested using residual blocks for local feature extraction and non-local blocks for global feature extraction. Furthermore, Al-Shabi et al. [54] used 3D Axial-Attention, which only needs a little amount of processing power as compared to a traditional non-local network.

2. Methodology

The 3D volumetric structure comprises the sections designated as nodules by radiologists from 2D CT scans, together with the series derived from the boundary curves of each section. The following paragraphs explain boundary curves and the process of extracting series out of them. Moreover, details on 3D models and the underlying deep learning framework are provided.

2.1. Series by Radial Scanning

A radial scan gathers image samples in a sparser distribution at the periphery of the image and in a denser distribution closer to the center of the image. This is the preferred scanning paradigm for several imaging applications, such as imaging the optic nerve head, as each B-scan acquired includes a cross-sectional image of the optic cup [55–57]. The volumetric, render, and morphometric analysis of the ensuing image may be used to see and analyze the radially obtained data samples. A straightforward radial-to-Cartesian coordinate translation may be used to resample data to a Cartesian mesh system.

Figure 1 provides a radial scan as an illustration. The region of interest of a lung nodule imaging is shown in Figure 1a. The radial scan axis is positioned at the center of the area of interest, and the boundary curve of the area of interest is depicted in Figure 1b. The boundary curve points' separation from the scanning center will vary as the scanning angle changes, resulting in a series, as illustrated in Figure 1c.

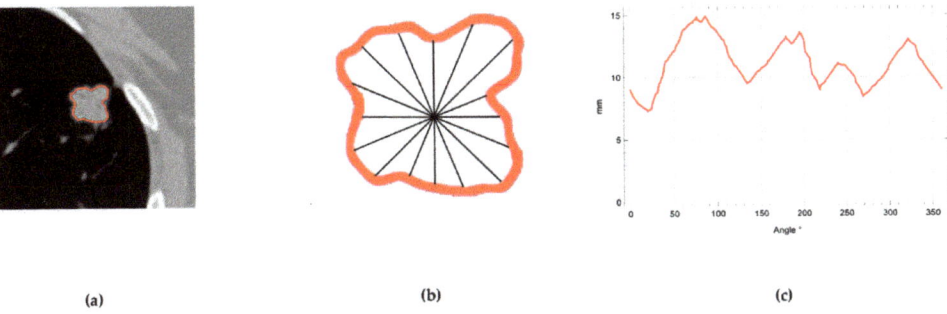

Figure 1. Method of obtaining series by radial scanning.

ROIs are portions of a designated data collection that are used for a certain objective. The term ROI is often used in a variety of application fields. For instance, in medical imaging, the borders of a tumor can be specified in an image or a volume to determine its size. For the purpose of assessing cardiac function, the endocardial boundary can be seen on an image at various points in the cardiac cycle, such as end-systole and end-diastole. The ROI establishes the perimeters of an item under inspection in computer vision and optical character recognition.

The CT images used in this study first underwent pixel-by-pixel binarization. After this morphological processing, large components in the binarized images are handled as ROIs. The center of the ROI is used to calculate the discrete center of gravity of the ROI for radial scanning. Due to the binary nature of the image, this center may be easily located without any weight.

The modified Canny edge recognition approach [58] is first applied to the ROI in each image to extract the appropriate form attributes. This extraction is made possible via the use of the improved Canny edge detector approach (one for each ROI within each image). The Canny operator employs a multi-step process to identify the edge pixels of an object. The first step is to adjust the area boundaries by using a Gaussian filter. After that, a regular 2D first derivative operator is used to compute edge strength. Pixels that are not a component of the local maximum are zeroed out when the non-maximum suppression method scans the region in the gradient direction. Lastly, a threshold is employed in order to determine the correct edge pixels. Therefore, each ROI may be represented by its own border curve.

It is essential to streamline the edges for ROI representation while extracting image features. The aim of the region boundary simplification stage is to create a smooth curve while minimizing the number of line segments used to delineate the area. This method is known as polygon approximation, and it is used to approximate a polygon curve that has a set number of vertices. The polygon curve approach looks for a subset of the initial vertices in order to minimize the objective function. The min-number problem is only one way to frame the issue. The appropriate approximation of an N-corner polygon curve is achieved by joining a certain number of straight-line M segments with another polygon curve. A common heuristic for finding a solution to the minimum number problem is the Douglas–Peucker (DP) method [59].

In this study, prior to using the Hough transform to extract features, the borders of ROIs are simplified using the Douglas–Peucker (DP) technique. The closeness of a vertex to an edge segment is a factor in the DP method. This approach operates top-down, beginning with a rough initial estimate on a simplified polygonal curve, or more specifically, on the single edge linking the first and end vertices of the polygonal curve. Then we determined the closeness of the remaining vertices to that edge. The corner that is furthest from the edge is added to the simplification if there are vertices further away from the edge than the provided tolerance ($\varepsilon > 0$). As a result, the reduced polygonal curve receives a new estimate. Recursion is used to continue this process for simplification until all vertices of the original polygonal curve fall inside the tolerance.

If the ROI border is considered a closed curve, we must figure out the optimal distribution of all neighboring vertices, including the initial one. The simplest approach is to start from the vertex with the fewest errors. Compared to the open-curve procedure, this simple method for a curve with N corners is N times more complicated to implement. There are a number of options to consider when deciding where to set off. This research makes use of a heuristic technique inspired by Sato's strategy [60]. The first step in this procedure is starting at the furthest location from the ROI's spatial center.

2.2. 3D Nodule Segmentation

In this research, computer-assisted techniques were used to identify nodules. Automatic nodule recognition and segmentation is achieved using the union of the You Only Look Once, Version 3 (YOLOv3) [61] and iW-Net [62] architectures. The short version is that the model is fine-tuned to identify lung nodules by minimizing a loss function that considers breadth, height, and center of gravity of the estimate in comparison to the baseline. In order to take 3D information into account, the algorithm is trained using 3-channel images that consist of one axial slice comprising the nodule center as well as two equally spaced neighboring slices. Candidates are joined if their bounding boxes overlap, and estimates are calculated for each axis slice. Only the first block of iW-Net, which makes a segmentation prediction, is utilized for actual segmentation. We employ an image classification method to identify nodules with a bounding box in order to facilitate the use of temporal statistical classification with the series collected from the image. This image was achieved by manually creating these marks. Each image of interest has different dimensions according to the series methodology used in this research. After the series has been normalized, this variation has no bearing on the categorization.

The LIDC-IDRI database contains thoracic CT images with highly annotated lesions for the purpose of detecting lung cancer. The series acquisition approach for the automatically segmented nodule outlined how to find the nodule border by drawing a closed curve around each nodule wherever it was present, beginning at the first pixel outside the lesion. CT scan findings are recorded in an XML file connected with each participant. Nodules in each XML file are grouped into one of three sizes based on their diameter. The locations of the nodules and their z coordinates are included in the data. With these coordinates, we were able to generate a box and mask in three dimensions that were centered on the annotated lung nodule sites and were a fixed size. Our experimental boxes are 32 pixels square and 32 slices thick. Nodule boundary curves in the sections are scanned radially in

5625-degree increments to conform to the 3D volumetric data format. By using a thickness of 32 for the slices, we may encode the nodule's border geometry as a matrix of type 32 × 32.

Figure 2 depicts a 3D segmented nodule and the aforementioned shape matrix. In order to explain the methodology, we ran 2D radial scans with an angle increase of 2 degrees and applied Laplace smoothing to the Delaunay mesh that we had derived from the boundary points shown in Figure 2. Following the smoothing of the nodule surface, 180 z-axis steps were chosen.

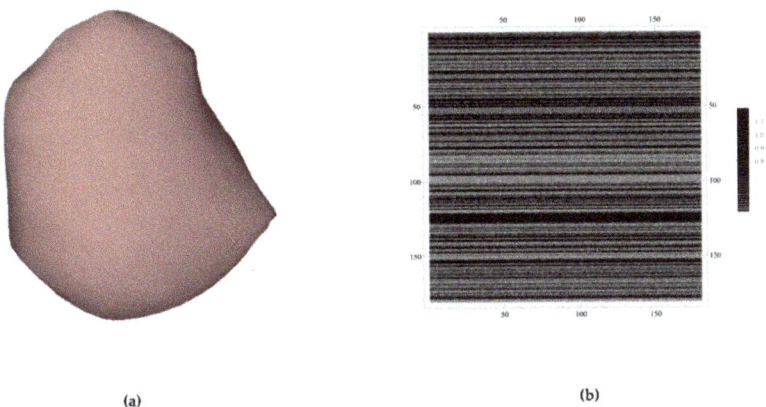

(a) (b)

Figure 2. (a) 3D segmented and smoothed nodule and (b) a 180 × 180 matrix encoding the boundary shape of each slice.

2.3. Classification with U-Net

Two-dimensional conventional CNN designs typically layer-by-layer integrate raw input data with learnable filters. It may be built using several layers, each of which is trained to recognize a particular aspect of an image. Each training image is passed through a series of filters of increasing granularity, and the resulting convolutional image serves as input for the layer below it. An image filter may begin with basic characteristics such as brightness and edges and progress to more complicated characteristics that better characterize the item being filtered. This study proposes a technique that works well inside a deep learning framework using higher-order CNNs for effective feature learning of CT image data from unprocessed information. This is accomplished by stacking many convolutional layers in order to collect a wide variety of representative characteristics. By using convolutions and trainable filters with specific filter coefficients, we can link input and output neurons.

This paper provides a solution to the 4D input issue of jointly categorizing nodule volumetric radiomic and border information. For this challenge, we use a method centered on U-Net models that generalize 2D and 3D architectures [63,64]. As shown in Figure 3, we need to calculate the shape matrix obtained from radial scanning with a tensor that takes the coordinates in mm^3 units of each volume segmented in the 3D volume and the grayscale value in these coordinates in order to train our 4D U-Net model efficiently and use it in the classification process. The model makes use of the 4D data input that it generates collectively. Lower-order models need data reduction prior to network training. In contrast, our suggested architecture makes extensive use of higher-dimensional data while performing all operations on nominally sized datasets.

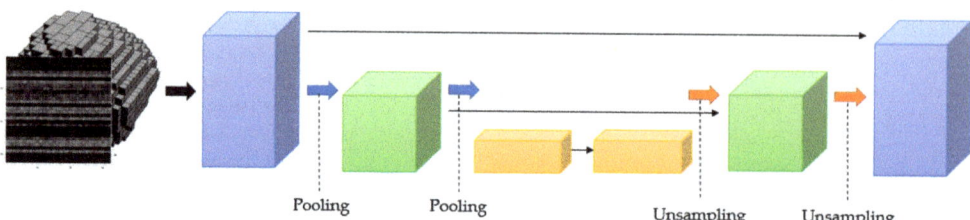

Figure 3. U-Net Architecture.

The value of a convolved output neuron at coordinates (k, l) in conventional 2D CNNs may be written as follows:

$$y_{kl} = \varphi \left(\sum_{c}^{C_{in}} \sum_{i=0}^{H-1} \sum_{j=0}^{W-1} w_{ij} x_{c(k+i)(l+j)} - b_{ij} \right), \quad (1)$$

where $\varphi(\cdot)$ is the activation function, w_{ij} is the value of the kernel connected to the current feature map at position (i, j), $x_{c(k+i)(l+j)}$ is the value of the input neuron at input channel c, b_{ij} is the bias of the computed feature map. Moreover, by following the extension method presented in [65], we can straightforwardly extend Equation (1) to 4D with

$$y_{klmn} = \varphi \left(\sum_{c}^{C_{in}} \sum_{r=0}^{R-1} \sum_{d=0}^{D-1} \sum_{i=0}^{H-1} \sum_{j=0}^{W-1} w_{ijdr} x_{c(i:i+k)(j:j+1)(d:d+m)(r:r+n)} + b_{ijdr} \right). \quad (2)$$

With our deep pixel-level categorization, each pixel can only be assigned to one of C distinct categories. Because cross-entropy may be understood as the log-likelihood function of the training samples, it was chosen as the loss function to transform the network's outputs back into probabilities. Training our models with this loss function combines the *SoftMax* activation with the cross-entropy loss to provide a probability across the C possible classes for each pixel.

3. Results

Overall, for this study, 244,559 images and 1018 CT scans from 1010 patients were provided by the Lung Image Database Consortium (LIDC) [66]. The five categories used to classify lesions in the LIDC image collection regarding pulmonary nodules are: highly likely to be benign (level 1); moderate probability of being benign (level 2); uncertain probability (level 3); moderate probability of malignancy (level 4); it is likely to be malignant (level 5). Due to the absence of a database structure, radiologists have not yet established relationships between images, examinations, and the possibility of malignancy from nodules, making the first LIDC image collection difficult to use. Thus, we choose to utilize the not only SQL (NoSQL) document-oriented Pulmonary Nodule Database (PND) [67] for our analysis.

The LIDC-IDRI study may be broken down into three major phases: image interpretation, nodule characteristic evaluation, and data recording. A radiologist was required to analyze each image of a CT examination using a computer interface and highlight lesions deemed to be nodules with in-plane dimensions between 3 and 30 mm, independent of assumed histology. As a result, these lesions may represent a primary lung cancer, a metastatic disease, a noncancerous condition, or of unknown etiology. Each nodule outline was intended to be a localizing "outside boundary" such that, according to the radiologist, the outline itself did not overlap nodule-specific pixels. According to the LIDC-IDRI literature, throughout the nodule characteristic evaluation procedure, each reader was requested to subjectively assign an integer value to nine distinct qualities. The data is stored in an eXtensible Markup Language (XML) file, and its classifications and Cartesian coordinates are based on nodule classifications. The XML file and all CT scans from a single test are kept in a folder, and all folders from all examinations were uploaded to a web server hosted on the website of the Cancer Imaging Archive (TCIA) [68]. In order to avoid unnecessary scans, PND only uses the radiologist's annotations that identify the most lesions during each exam, which amounts to 752 scans and 1944 lung nodules. To normalize the image contrast, a gray-scale lung windowing was applied by adjusting the window/level from 1600 to −600 Hounsfield units.

Nodules, which may be up to 30 mm in diameter, are a kind of lung opacity [69]. Initially, we computed the nodule size as a straightforward 2D measure of the biggest diameter in a slice, which may be done in the axial plane along the axis of the longest diameter [70]. To get these rough estimates, we measured the x and y minimum and maximum coordinates of every nodule slice. According to [71], lung nodules with a PND malignancy grade of 3 were considered too dangerous to keep. We did not include any nodules in the LIDC collection that were annotated as non-solid because of the form complexity and low density of these objects. Therefore, following this phase, 897 nodules ranging in size from 3 mm to 30 mm remained (616 benign and 281 malignant). We were restricted from selecting smaller lesions due to the LIDC requirement of a 3 mm subthreshold.

A major restriction in this study was that the dataset has an uneven distribution of classes throughout its 897 nodules. During the phase of cross-validation training, the well-known Synthetic Minority Oversampling Approach (SMOTE) [72] method was used to develop synthetic nodule samples. This approach is also known as the synthetic minority oversampling approach. The method was developed with the intention of delivering a comprehensive and well-rounded approach. At each step of the process of cross-validation, nine folds were chosen to form the training set, whereas the remaining fold was used to form the test set. Moreover, we made sure that the appropriate proportions were preserved. Training sets comprised 550 benign nodules and 252 malignant nodules. Around 298 synthetic samples are produced by the SMOTE algorithm throughout each step of the procedure. This ensures that malignant nodules are represented as precisely as possible.

To assess the performance of the developed model, we employ a number of machine learning metrics, as the problem at hand is fundamentally a pixel-level multi-class classification task. True positives (TP), false positives (FP), false negatives (FN), and true negatives (TN) are the four possible outcomes when comparing a pixel's prediction to its baseline accuracy score. True and False represent equality between the ground truth label and the predicted label, whereas Positive and Negative correspond to the class from which the metric is being calculated. In this study, common ML metrics are employed for each type of data using the above definitions. Namely, the metrics are:

$$\text{Recall} = \text{TP}/(\text{TP} + \text{FN}) \tag{3}$$

$$\text{Precision} = \text{TP}/(\text{TP} + \text{FP}) \tag{4}$$

$$\text{Accuracy} = (\text{TP} + \text{TN})/(\text{TP} + \text{FP} + \text{FN} + \text{TN}) \tag{5}$$

$$F1 = 2 \times (\text{Precision} \times \text{Recall})/(\text{Precision} + \text{Recall}) \tag{6}$$

The number of filters utilized for effective feature learning and the number of stack-layers in the proposed U-Net model are two major hyper-parameters that have a substantial impact on the model's performance. In order to determine which combination of hyper-parameters produces the best results, we conducted an ablation study.

In the experiments, the effect of increasing the number of stack levels on the performance of the U-Net is analyzed. We trained two separate 4D U-Net models, one with a depth of 3 and the other with a depth of 4. Table 1 shows that the network's generalization capacity increases when more filters are applied, suggesting that the network is becoming more robust. Naturally, the time needed to train the network grows in proportion to the number of filters, as each filter has its own set of parameters that must be learned. We also find that using only four filters in the U-Net, as opposed to eight, improves performance across the board when the depth is increased from three. Overall, the best U-Net model can be trained in around 11 h, has a depth of 3, and has a classification accuracy of 92.84%.

Table 1. Metrics for classification and training times (in minutes) for 4D U-Net models.

Depth	No. of Filters	Recall	Precision	Accuracy	Time
3	4	80.13	81.54	83.45	469.92
	8	92.41	92.63	92.84	661.8
4	4	80.04	79.63	81.22	477.74
	8	87.19	88.01	88.73	668.4

Table 2 summarizes and tabulates comparisons between our proposed method and state-of-the-art lung nodule classification methods. The results of our evaluations show that our proposed method consistently outperforms the state-of-the-art methods. Not only that, but it outperforms other non-local-based methods such as Local-Global [52], 3D Directed Partitioning Networks (DPNs) [53] and 3D Axial-Attention [54].

Table 2. The proposed method's performance compared to the state-of-the-art methods.

Method	AUC	Recall	Precision	Accuracy	F1
HSCNN [14]	85.6	70.5	N/A	84.2	N/A
Multi-Crop [48]	93.0	77.0	N/A	87.14	N/A
Local-Global [52]	95.62	88.66	87.38	88.46	88.01
Gated-Dilated [49]	95.14	92.21	91.85	92.57	92.03
3D DPN [53]	N/A	92.04	N/A	90.24	N/A
MRC-DNN [50]	N/A	81.00	N/A	90.00	N/A
Perturbated DNN [51]	91.0	90.0	N/A	83.0	N/A
3D Axial-Attention [54]	96.17	92.36	92.59	92.81	92.47
Our method	96.19	92.41	92.63	92.84	92.51

4. Discussion and Conclusions

Because lung nodules are so minuscule that they can easily blend in with the surrounding tissue and cling to complicated anatomical systems like the pleura, this work presents a deep learning strategy that additionally deals with volumetric radiomic information for classifying nodules in the lungs.

We started by obtaining 3-tensor data types representing gray levels of 3D nodule shape modeled from cross-sectional CT scans. Grayscale values between 0 and 255 are fed to this tensor at each node. Our study presents a deep learning classification solution to the age-old issue of picture classification by including the series collected from nodule segments. Our method takes into consideration the self-similarity of the boundary curves that characterize the nodule segments in order to provide a more precise categorization of nodules. By treating the series of the border curvatures of each section as rows in the matrix, we are able to solve the 4D classification issue.

For this research, we accessed a dataset hosted by LIDC. Over 95% accuracy was achieved when using the deep learning algorithms YOLOv3 and iW-Net to identify and isolate the nodules in the annotated photos. The respective photos were manually cropped and recorded in this LIDC dataset using tags. After that, we employed the image processing techniques described in the methodology section to locate the nodule's outside and innermost curves. The use of 32×32-type matrices, the scanning at 5.625 degrees and 32 section steps yielded shape matrices that were consistent with the volumetric radiomics of the nodule.

The research used a U-Net-type convolutional neural network, which proved to be successful for the 4D categorization in previous studies [73–76]. Experiments were conducted using 4 and 8-filter meshes of depths 3 and 4, respectively. When compared to other networks, the one with three depths and eight filters performed quite well (92.84% accuracy). This outcome informed the selection of the network design from our study.

In the context of volumetric radiomics, comparisons were made between the results of this research and 3D CNN networks. The provided method yields superior performance results as compared to numerous non-native solutions presently available. The method presented in our research is most comparable to the 3D Axial Attention among the non-local approaches. Due to the fact that it takes into consideration the nodule's 3D shape, the 3D Axial Attention approach is far more discriminating than earlier methods. However, the approach we present takes into account both the 3D geometry and the shape of the nodule, allowing for a 5D convolution. Although its performance is comparable to that of the 3D Axial-Attention approach, its outcomes are superior to those of prior methods. Future research may try using more radiomic variables within the framework of the 3D Axial Attention approach in order to get even more discriminating findings.

Limitations in the study design are inevitable, as is the case with every investigation. The primary barrier is the dearth of trained radiologists and experts in computer-assisted segmentation. The issue of class imbalance in the dataset may be addressed in a number of ways, all of which need careful consideration. Because the series angles derived from the radial-scanning boundary curve of the nodule follow one another in time, we may argue that the series represents a time series. An up-and-coming area of study in the field of forecasting is the use of time-series characteristics for model selection and model averaging [77–79]. However, most current methods need human intervention to choose a suitable collection of features. In modern time-series analysis, the use of machine learning techniques for automatically extracting characteristics from time series is becoming more important. Hybrid networks that can deal with radiomic features utilizing 3D geometry classification and machine learning-based time-series feature extraction may be studied in the future. Because our research demonstrates the usefulness of radial scanning, particularly in the context of medical image processing and classification, we believe it will serve as a benchmark for future studies examining other medical imaging methods.

In conclusion, we show that series from lung imaging may be used to effectively characterize lung nodules, and that a shape matrix, aided by an area of interest curve, can be used to reliably ascertain whether or not a tumor is malignant. We tested our methods using a large dataset of lung nodule pictures that was made accessible to the public, and we compared the outcomes to those produced by established methods for classifying both still photos and video over time. The requirement for our study to be repeatable prompted us to conduct these comparisons. Our research indicates that radial scanning series may be a powerful asset in the identification and categorization of lung nodules.

Author Contributions: Conceptualization, M.A.B. and Ö.A.; Methodology, M.A.B. and Ö.A.; Software, M.A.B. and Ö.A.; Validation, M.A.B. and Ö.A.; Formal analysis, M.A.B. and Ö.A.; Investigation, M.A.B., L.M.B., Ö.A. and A.N.; Resources, M.A.B., L.M.B., Ö.A. and A.N.; Data curation, M.A.B. and Ö.A.; Writing—original draft, M.A.B., L.M.B., Ö.A. and A.N.; Writing—review and editing, M.A.B., L.M.B., Ö.A. and A.N.; Visualization, M.A.B. and Ö.A.; Project administration, M.A.B. and L.M.B.; Funding acquisition, A.N. All authors have read and agreed to the published version of the manuscript.

Funding: This study was conducted with financial support from the scientific research funds of the "1 Decembrie 1918" University of Alba Iulia, Romania.

Institutional Review Board Statement: Not applicable.

Informed Consent Statement: Not applicable.

Data Availability Statement: The data presented in this study are available on request from the corresponding author.

Conflicts of Interest: The authors declare no conflict of interest.

References

1. Rowland, J.H.; Bellizzi, K.M. Cancer survivors and survivorship research: A reflection on today's successes and tomorrow's challenges. *Hematol. Oncol. Clin. N. Am.* **2008**, *22*, 181–200. [CrossRef] [PubMed]
2. Elmore, L.W.; Greer, S.F.; Daniels, E.C.; Saxe, C.C.; Melner, M.H.; Krawiec, G.M.; Phelps, W.C. Blueprint for cancer research: Critical gaps and opportunities. *CA Cancer J. Clin.* **2021**, *71*, 107–139. [CrossRef] [PubMed]
3. Benning, L.; Peintner, A.; Peintner, L. Advances in and the applicability of machine learning-based screening and early detection approaches for cancer: A primer. *Cancers* **2022**, *14*, 623. [CrossRef] [PubMed]
4. Nanavaty, P.; Alvarez, M.S.; Alberts, W.M. Lung cancer screening: Advantages, controversies, and applications. *Cancer Control* **2014**, *21*, 9–14. [CrossRef]
5. Khawaja, A.; Bartholmai, B.J.; Rajagopalan, S.; Karwoski, R.A.; Varghese, C.; Maldonado, F.; Peikert, T. Do we need to see to believe?—Radiomics for lung nodule classification and lung cancer risk stratification. *J. Thorac. Dis.* **2020**, *12*, 3303. [CrossRef]
6. Parekh, V.; Jacobs, M.A. Radiomics: A new application from established techniques. *Expert Rev. Precis. Med. Drug Dev.* **2016**, *1*, 207–226. [CrossRef]
7. Oliveira, S.P.; Neto, P.C.; Fraga, J.; Montezuma, D.; Monteiro, A.; Monteiro, J.; Cardoso, J.S. CAD systems for colorectal cancer from WSI are still not ready for clinical acceptance. *Sci. Rep.* **2021**, *11*, 14358. [CrossRef]
8. Yanase, J.; Triantaphyllou, E. A systematic survey of computer-aided diagnosis in medicine: Past and present developments. *Expert Syst. Appl.* **2019**, *138*, 112821. [CrossRef]
9. Yan, Y.; Yao, X.J.; Wang, S.H.; Zhang, Y.D. A survey of computer-aided tumor diagnosis based on convolutional neural network. *Biology* **2021**, *10*, 1084. [CrossRef]
10. Chambara, N.; Ying, M. The diagnostic efficiency of ultrasound computer-aided diagnosis in differentiating thyroid nodules: A systematic review and narrative synthesis. *Cancers* **2019**, *11*, 1759. [CrossRef]
11. Ding, J.; Li, A.; Hu, Z.; Wang, L. Accurate pulmonary nodule detection in computed tomography images using deep convolutional neural networks. In *International Conference on Medical Image Computing and Computer-Assisted Intervention*; Springer: Cham, Switzerland, 2017; pp. 559–567.
12. Wang, S.; Zhou, M.; Liu, Z.; Liu, Z.; Gu, D.; Zang, Y.; Tian, J. Central focused convolutional neural networks: Developing a data-driven model for lung nodule segmentation. *Med. Image Anal.* **2017**, *40*, 172–183. [CrossRef] [PubMed]
13. Wu, B.; Zhou, Z.; Wang, J.; Wang, Y. Joint learning for pulmonary nodule segmentation, attributes and malignancy prediction. In *2018 IEEE 15th International Symposium on Biomedical Imaging*; Curran Associates: Washington, DC, USA, 2018; pp. 1109–1113.
14. Shen, S.; Han, S.X.; Aberle, D.R.; Bui, A.A.; Hsu, W. An interpretable deep hierarchical semantic convolutional neural network for lung nodule malignancy classification. *Expert Syst. Appl.* **2019**, *128*, 84–95. [CrossRef] [PubMed]
15. Ferreira-Junior, J.R.; Koenigkam-Santos, M.; Magalhaes Tenorio, A.P.; Faleiros, M.C.; Garcia Cipriano, F.E.; Fabro, A.T.; de Azevedo-Marques, P.M. CT-based radiomics for prediction of histologic subtype and metastatic disease in primary malignant lung neoplasms. *Int. J. Comput. Assist. Radiol. Surg.* **2020**, *15*, 163–172. [CrossRef] [PubMed]
16. Firmino, M.; Angelo, G.; Morais, H.; Dantas, M.R.; Valentim, R. Computer-aided detection (CADe) and diagnosis (CADx) system for lung cancer with likelihood of malignancy. *Biomed. Eng. OnLine* **2016**, *15*, 2. [CrossRef] [PubMed]
17. Choy, G.; Khalilzadeh, O.; Michalski, M.; Do, S.; Samir, A.E.; Pianykh, O.S.; Dreyer, K.J. Current applications and future impact of machine learning in radiology. *Radiology* **2018**, *288*, 318. [CrossRef]
18. Ferreira, J.R.; Oliveira, M.C.; de Azevedo-Marques, P.M. Characterization of pulmonary nodules based on features of margin sharpness and texture. *J. Digit. Imaging* **2018**, *31*, 451–463. [CrossRef]
19. Dhara, A.K.; Mukhopadhyay, S.; Dutta, A.; Garg, M.; Khandelwal, N. A combination of shape and texture features for classification of pulmonary nodules in lung CT images. *J. Digit. Imaging* **2016**, *29*, 466–475. [CrossRef]
20. Felix, A.; Oliveira, M.; Machado, A.; Raniery, J. Using 3D texture and margin sharpness features on classification of small pulmonary nodules. In *2016 29th SIBGRAPI Conference on Graphics, Patterns and Images (SIBGRAPI)*; Curran Associates: Washington, DC, USA, 2016; pp. 394–400.
21. Beig, N.; Khorrami, M.; Alilou, M.; Prasanna, P.; Braman, N.; Orooji, M.; Madabhushi, A. Perinodular and intranodular radiomic features on lung CT images distinguish adenocarcinomas from granulomas. *Radiology* **2019**, *290*, 783. [CrossRef]
22. Uthoff, J.; Stephens, M.J.; Newell Jr, J.D.; Hoffman, E.A.; Larson, D.; Koehn, N.; Sieren, J.C. Machine learning approach for distinguishing malignant and benign lung nodules utilizing standardized perinodular parenchymal features from CT. *Med. Phys.* **2019**, *46*, 3207–3216. [CrossRef]
23. Chen, G.; Xu, Z. Usage of intelligent medical aided diagnosis system under the deep convolutional neural network in lumbar disc herniation. *Appl. Soft Comput.* **2021**, *111*, 107674. [CrossRef]
24. Bakheet, S.; Al-Hamadi, A. Computer-aided diagnosis of malignant melanoma using Gabor-based entropic features and multilevel neural networks. *Diagnostics* **2020**, *10*, 822. [CrossRef] [PubMed]
25. Maqsood, S.; Damaševičius, R.; Maskeliūnas, R. TTCNN: A breast cancer detection and classification towards computer-aided diagnosis using digital mammography in early stages. *Appl. Sci.* **2022**, *12*, 3273. [CrossRef]
26. Campanella, G.; Hanna, M.G.; Geneslaw, L.; Miraflor, A.; Werneck Krauss Silva, V.; Busam, K.J.; Fuchs, T.J. Clinical-grade computational pathology using weakly supervised deep learning on whole slide images. *Nat. Med.* **2019**, *25*, 1301–1309. [CrossRef]

27. Chlebus, G.; Schenk, A.; Moltz, J.H.; van Ginneken, B.; Hahn, H.K.; Meine, H. Automatic liver tumor segmentation in CT with fully convolutional neural networks and object-based postprocessing. *Sci. Rep.* **2018**, *8*, 15497. [CrossRef] [PubMed]
28. De Fauw, J.; Ledsam, J.R.; Romera-Paredes, B.; Nikolov, S.; Tomasev, N.; Blackwell, S.; Ronneberger, O. Clinically applicable deep learning for diagnosis and referral in retinal disease. *Nat. Med.* **2018**, *24*, 1342–1350. [CrossRef]
29. Dash, M.; Londhe, N.D.; Ghosh, S.; Semwal, A.; Sonawane, R.S. PsLSNet: Automated psoriasis skin lesion segmentation using modified U-Net-based fully convolutional network. *Biomed. Signal Process. Control* **2019**, *52*, 226–237. [CrossRef]
30. Xie, F.; Yang, J.; Liu, J.; Jiang, Z.; Zheng, Y.; Wang, Y. Skin lesion segmentation using high-resolution convolutional neural network. *Comput. Methods Programs Biomed.* **2020**, *186*, 105241. [CrossRef]
31. Abdoulaye, I.B.C.; Demir, Ö. Mamografi görüntülerinden kitle tespiti amacıyla öznitelik çıkarımı. In *Ulusal Biyomedikal Cihaz Tasarımı ve Üretmi Sempozyumu*; UBICTÜS: Istanbul, Turkey, 2017; Volume 1, pp. 33–36.
32. Wang, P.; Hu, X.; Li, Y.; Liu, Q.; Zhu, X. Automatic cell nuclei segmentation and classification of breast cancer histopathology images. *Signal Process.* **2016**, *122*, 1–13. [CrossRef]
33. Jiang, H.; Li, Z.; Li, S.; Zhou, F. An effective multi-classification method for NHL pathological images. In *2018 IEEE International Conference on Systems, Man, and Cybernetics (SMC)*; Curran Associates: Washington, DC, USA, 2018; pp. 763–768.
34. Muhammad, W.; Hart, G.R.; Nartowt, B.; Farrell, J.J.; Johung, K.; Liang, Y.; Deng, J. Pancreatic cancer prediction through an artificial neural network. *Front. Artif. Intell.* **2019**, *2*, 2. [CrossRef]
35. Busnatu, Ș.; Niculescu, A.G.; Bolocan, A.; Petrescu, G.E.; Păduraru, D.N.; Năstasă, I.; Martins, H. Clinical applications of artificial intelligence—An updated overview. *J. Clinic. Med.* **2022**, *11*, 2265. [CrossRef]
36. Hunter, B.; Hindocha, S.; Lee, R.W. The role of artificial intelligence in early cancer diagnosis. *Cancers* **2022**, *14*, 1524. [CrossRef] [PubMed]
37. Iakovidis, D.K.; Tsevas, S.; Savelonas, M.A.; Papamichalis, G. Image analysis framework for infection monitoring. *IEEE Trans. Biomed. Eng.* **2012**, *59*, 1135–1144. [CrossRef] [PubMed]
38. Baur, B.; Bozdag, S. A canonical correlation analysis-based dynamic Bayesian network prior to infer gene regulatory networks from multiple types of biological data. *J. Comput. Biol.* **2015**, *22*, 289–299. [CrossRef]
39. Guo, S.; Jiang, Q.; Chen, L.; Guo, D. Gene regulatory network inference using PLS-based methods. *BMC Bioinform.* **2016**, *17*, 545. [CrossRef]
40. Penfold, C.A.; Shifaz, A.; Brown, P.E.; Nicholson, A.; Wild, D.L. CSI: A nonparametric Bayesian approach to network inference from multiple perturbed time series gene expression data. *Stat. Appl. Genet. Mol. Biol.* **2015**, *14*, 307–310. [CrossRef] [PubMed]
41. Isci, S.; Dogan, H.; Ozturk, C.; Otu, H.H. Bayesian network prior: Network analysis of biological data using external knowledge. *Bioinformatics* **2014**, *30*, 860–867. [CrossRef]
42. Schlitt, T. Approaches to modeling gene regulatory networks: A gentle introduction. *Methods Mol. Biol.* **2013**, *1021*, 13–35.
43. Murphy, K.; Mian, S. *Modelling Gene Expression Data Using Dynamic Bayesian Networks*; Technical Report; Computer Science Division, University of California: Berkeley, CA, USA, 1999.
44. Ni, Y.; Müller, P.; Wei, L.; Ji, Y. Bayesian graphical models for computational network biology. *BMC Bioinform.* **2018**, *19*, 59–69. [CrossRef]
45. Kim, S.Y.; Imoto, S.; Miyano, S. Inferring gene networks from time series microarray data using dynamic Bayesian networks. *Brief. Bioinform.* **2003**, *4*, 228–235. [CrossRef]
46. Kourou, K.; Rigas, G.; Papaloukas, C.; Mitsis, M.; Fotiadis, D.I. Cancer classification from time series microarray data through regulatory dynamic Bayesian networks. *Comput. Biol. Med.* **2020**, *116*, 103577. [CrossRef]
47. Imani, F.; Daoud, M.; Moradi, M.; Abolmaesumi, P.; Mousavi, P. Tissue classification using depth-dependent ultrasound time series analysis: In-vitro animal study. In *Medical Imaging 2011: Ultrasonic Imaging, Tomography, and Therapy*; SPIE Medical Imaging: Lake Buena Vista, FL, USA, 2011; Volume 7968, pp. 120–126.
48. Shen, W.; Zhou, M.; Yang, F.; Yu, D.; Dong, D.; Yang, C.; Tian, J. Multi-crop convolutional neural networks for lung nodule malignancy suspiciousness classification. *Pattern Recognit.* **2017**, *61*, 663–673. [CrossRef]
49. Al-Shabi, M.; Lee, H.K.; Tan, M. Gated-dilated networks for lung nodule classification in CT scans. *IEEE Access* **2019**, *7*, 178827–178838. [CrossRef]
50. Ren, Y.; Tsai, M.Y.; Chen, L.; Wang, J.; Li, S.; Liu, Y.; Shen, C. A manifold learning regularization approach to enhance 3D CT image-based lung nodule classification. *Int. J. Comput. Assist. Radiol. Surg.* **2020**, *15*, 287–295. [CrossRef] [PubMed]
51. Shen, C.; Tsai, M.Y.; Chen, L.; Li, S.; Nguyen, D.; Wang, J.; Jia, X. On the robustness of deep learning-based lung-nodule classification for CT images with respect to image noise. *Phys. Med. Biol.* **2020**, *65*, 245037. [CrossRef] [PubMed]
52. Jiang, H.; Gao, F.; Xu, X.; Huang, F.; Zhu, S. Attentive and ensemble 3D dual path networks for pulmonary nodules classification. *Neurocomputing* **2020**, *398*, 422–430. [CrossRef]
53. Al-Shabi, M.; Lan, B.L.; Chan, W.Y.; Ng, K.H.; Tan, M. Lung nodule classification using deep local-global networks. *Int. J. Comput. Assist. Radiol. Surg.* **2019**, *14*, 1815–1819. [CrossRef]
54. Al-Shabi, M.; Shak, K.; Tan, M. 3D axial-attention for lung nodule classification. *Int. J. Comput. Assist. Radiol. Surg.* **2021**, *16*, 1319–1324. [CrossRef]
55. Bosch, C.M.; Baumann, C.; Dehghani, S.; Sommersperger, M.; Johannigmann-Malek, N.; Kirchmair, K.; Nasseri, M.A. A tool for high-resolution volumetric optical coherence tomography by compounding radial-and linear acquired B-scans using registration. *Sensors* **2022**, *22*, 1135. [CrossRef]

56. Murad, M.; Jalil, A.; Bilal, M.; Ikram, S.; Ali, A.; Khan, B.; Mehmood, K. Radial undersampling-based interpolation scheme for multislice CSMRI reconstruction techniques. *BioMed Res. Int.* **2021**, *2021*, 6638588. [CrossRef]
57. Mendoza, L.; Christopher, M.; Brye, N.; Proudfoot, J.A.; Belghith, A.; Bowd, C.; Zangwill, L.M. Deep learning predicts demographic and clinical characteristics from optic nerve head OCT circle and radial scans. *Investig. Ophthalmol. Vis. Sci.* **2021**, *62*, 2120.
58. Deng, C.X.; Wang, G.B.; Yang, X.R. Image edge detection algorithm based on improved canny operator. In *2013 International Conference on Wavelet Analysis and Pattern Recognition*; Curran Associates: Washington, DC, USA, 2013; pp. 168–172.
59. Douglas, D.H.; Peucker, T.K. Algorithms for the reduction of the number of points required to represent a digitized line or its caricature. *Cartogr. Int. J. Geograph. Inf. Geovisualization* **1973**, *10*, 112–122. [CrossRef]
60. Sato, Y. Piecewise linear approximation of plane curves by perimeter optimization. *Pattern Recognit.* **1992**, *25*, 1535–1543. [CrossRef]
61. Aresta, G.; Jacobs, C.; Araújo, T.; Cunha, A.; Ramos, I.; van Ginneken, B.; Campilho, A. iW-Net: An automatic and minimalistic interactive lung nodule segmentation deep network. *Sci. Rep.* **2019**, *9*, 11591. [CrossRef] [PubMed]
62. Aresta, G.; Araújo, T.; Jacobs, C.; Ginneken, B.V.; Cunha, A.; Ramos, I.; Campilho, A. Towards an automatic lung cancer screening system in low dose computed tomography. In *Image Analysis for Moving Organ, Breast, and Thoracic Images*; Springer: Cham, Switzerland, 2018; pp. 310–318.
63. Ronneberger, O.; Fischer, P.; Brox, T. U-net: Convolutional networks for biomedical image segmentation. In *International Conference on Medical Image Computing and Computer-Assisted Intervention*; Springer: Cham, Switzerland, 2015; pp. 234–241.
64. Çiçek, Ö.; Abdulkadir, A.; Lienkamp, S.S.; Brox, T.; Ronneberger, O. 3D U-Net: Learning dense volumetric segmentation from sparse annotation. In *International Conference on Medical Image Computing and Computer-Assisted Intervention*; Springer: Cham, Switzerland, 2016; pp. 424–432.
65. Giannopoulos, M.; Tsagkatakis, G.; Tsakalides, P. 4D U-nets for multi-temporal remote sensing data classification. *Remote Sens.* **2022**, *14*, 634. [CrossRef]
66. Armato III, S.G.; McLennan, G.; Bidaut, L.; McNitt-Gray, M.F.; Meyer, C.R.; Reeves, A.P.; Clarke, L.P. The lung image database consortium (LIDC) and image database resource initiative (IDRI): A completed reference database of lung nodules on CT scans. *Med. Phys.* **2011**, *38*, 915–931. [CrossRef]
67. Ferreira Junior, J.R.; Oliveira, M.C.; de Azevedo-Marques, P.M. Cloud-based NoSQL open database of pulmonary nodules for computer-aided lung cancer diagnosis and reproducible research. *J. Digit. Imaging* **2016**, *29*, 716–729. [CrossRef] [PubMed]
68. Clark, K.; Vendt, B.; Smith, K.; Freymann, J.; Kirby, J.; Koppel, P.; Prior, F. The Cancer Imaging Archive (TCIA): Maintaining and operating a public information repository. *J. Digit. Imaging* **2013**, *26*, 1045–1057. [CrossRef]
69. Wormanns, D.; Hamer, O.W. Glossary of terms for thoracic imaging-German version of the Fleischner Society recommendations. *RoFo* **2015**, *187*, 638–661.
70. Calheiros, J.L.L.; de Amorim, L.B.V.; de Lima, L.L.; de Lima Filho, A.F.; Ferreira Júnior, J.R.; de Oliveira, M.C. The effects of perinodular features on solid lung nodule classification. *J. Digit. Imaging* **2021**, *34*, 798–810. [CrossRef]
71. Redmon, J.; Farhadi, A. Yolov3: An incremental improvement. *arXiv* **2018**, arXiv:1804.02767.
72. Chawla, N.V.; Bowyer, K.W.; Hall, L.O.; Kegelmeyer, W.P. SMOTE: Synthetic minority over-sampling technique. *J. Artif. Intell. Res.* **2002**, *16*, 321–357. [CrossRef]
73. Huang, X.; Zhang, Y.; Chen, L.; Wang, J. U-net-based deformation vector field estimation for motion-compensated 4D-CBCT reconstruction. *Med. Phys.* **2020**, *47*, 3000–3012. [CrossRef] [PubMed]
74. Chen, G.; Zhao, Y.; Huang, Q.; Gao, H. 4D-AirNet: A temporally-resolved CBCT slice reconstruction method synergizing analytical and iterative method with deep learning. *Phys. Med. Biol.* **2020**, *65*, 175020. [CrossRef] [PubMed]
75. Choy, C.; Gwak, J.; Savarese, S. 4D spatio-temporal convnets: Minkowski convolutional neural networks. *Proc. IEEE/CVF Conf. Comput. Vis. Pattern Recognit.* **2019**, 3075–3084.
76. Liu, T.; Meng, Q.; Huang, J.J.; Vlontzos, A.; Rueckert, D.; Kainz, B. Video summarization through reinforcement learning with a 3D spatio-temporal U-net. *IEEE Trans. Image Process.* **2022**, *31*, 1573–1586. [CrossRef] [PubMed]
77. Ismail Fawaz, H.; Forestier, G.; Weber, J.; Idoumghar, L.; Muller, P.A. Deep learning for time series classification: A review. *Data Min. Knowl. Discov.* **2019**, *33*, 917–963. [CrossRef]
78. Abanda, A.; Mori, U.; Lozano, J.A. A review on distance-based time series classification. *Data Min. Knowl. Discov.* **2019**, *33*, 378–412. [CrossRef]
79. Iwana, B.K.; Uchida, S. An empirical survey of data augmentation for time series classification with neural networks. *PLoS ONE* **2021**, *16*, e0254841. [CrossRef]

Disclaimer/Publisher's Note: The statements, opinions and data contained in all publications are solely those of the individual author(s) and contributor(s) and not of MDPI and/or the editor(s). MDPI and/or the editor(s) disclaim responsibility for any injury to people or property resulting from any ideas, methods, instructions or products referred to in the content.

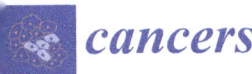

Article

APESTNet with Mask R-CNN for Liver Tumor Segmentation and Classification

Prabhu Kavin Balasubramanian [1], Wen-Cheng Lai [2,3], Gan Hong Seng [4,*], Kavitha C [5,*] and Jeeva Selvaraj [1,4]

1. Department of Data Science and Business System, Kattankulathur Campus, SRM Institute of Science and Technology, Chennai 603203, Tamil Nadu, India
2. Bachelor Program in Industrial Projects, National Yunlin University of Science and Technology, Douliu 640301, Taiwan
3. Department of Electronic Engineering, National Yunlin University of Science and Technology, Douliu 640301, Taiwan
4. Department of Data Science, UMK City Campus, University Malaysia Kelantan, Pengkalan Chepa, Kelantan 16100, Malaysia
5. Department of Computer Science and Engineering, Sathyabama Institute of Science and Technology, Chennai 600119, Tamil Nadu, India
* Correspondence: hongseng.g@umk.edu.my (G.H.S.); kavitha.cse@sathyabama.ac.in (K.C.)

Simple Summary: The classification is performed later by an interactively learning Swin Transformer block, the core unit for feature representation and long-range semantic information. In particular, the proposed strategy improved significantly and was very resilient while dealing with small liver pieces, discontinuous liver regions, and fuzzy liver boundaries. The experimental results confirm that the proposed APESTNet is more effective in classifying liver tumours than the current state-of-the-art models. Without compromising accuracy, the proposed method conserved resources. However, the proposed method is prone to slight over-segmentation or under-segmentation errors when dealing with lesions or tumours at the liver boundary. Therefore, our future work will concentrate on completely utilizing the z-axis information in 3D to reduce errors.

Abstract: Diagnosis and treatment of hepatocellular carcinoma or metastases rely heavily on accurate segmentation and classification of liver tumours. However, due to the liver tumor's hazy borders and wide range of possible shapes, sizes, and positions, accurate and automatic tumour segmentation and classification remains a difficult challenge. With the advancement of computing, new models in artificial intelligence have evolved. Following its success in Natural language processing (NLP), the transformer paradigm has been adopted by the computer vision (CV) community of the NLP. While there are already accepted approaches to classifying the liver, especially in clinical settings, there is room for advancement in terms of their precision. This paper makes an effort to apply a novel model for segmenting and classifying liver tumours built on deep learning. In order to accomplish this, the created model follows a three-stage procedure consisting of (a) pre-processing, (b) liver segmentation, and (c) classification. In the first phase, the collected Computed Tomography (CT) images undergo three stages of pre-processing, including contrast improvement via histogram equalization and noise reduction via the median filter. Next, an enhanced mask region-based convolutional neural networks (Mask R-CNN) model is used to separate the liver from the CT abdominal image. To prevent overfitting, the segmented picture is fed onto an Enhanced Swin Transformer Network with Adversarial Propagation (APESTNet). The experimental results prove the superior performance of the proposed perfect on a wide variety of CT images, as well as its efficiency and low sensitivity to noise.

Keywords: adversarial propagation; liver tumor segmentation; classification; enhanced swin transformer network; median filtering; computed tomography

Citation: Balasubramanian, P.K.; Lai, W.-C.; Seng, G.H.; C, K.; Selvaraj, J. APESTNet with Mask R-CNN for Liver Tumor Segmentation and Classification. *Cancers* 2023, *15*, 330. https://doi.org/10.3390/cancers15020330

Academic Editors: Muhammad Fazal Ijaz, Marcin Woźniak and Lorenzo Preda

Received: 29 November 2022
Revised: 21 December 2022
Accepted: 30 December 2022
Published: 4 January 2023

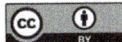

Copyright: © 2023 by the authors. Licensee MDPI, Basel, Switzerland. This article is an open access article distributed under the terms and conditions of the Creative Commons Attribution (CC BY) license (https://creativecommons.org/licenses/by/4.0/).

1. Introduction

The liver provides essential support for animals and vertebrates on this planet. Liver disease is a potentially fatal condition with no warning signs in the human body. The patient's prognosis would greatly benefit from an early diagnosis of liver illness. The incidence of liver tumours is high, making it one of the most lethal forms of cancer. Radiologists face major challenges in the early analysis and accurate staging of liver cancer. The United States reports that liver cancer ranks as the tenth foremost cause of cancer overall, the fifth foremost cause of cancer death in men, and the ninth leading motive of cancer [1,2]. When cancer is identified at an early stage, the rate of survival is significantly higher. When looking for liver tumours, CT is one of the most important and effective imaging methods [3,4]. Furthermore, CT provides entire liver pictures by contrast media injection and "multi-phase sequential scans" [5]. Due to the complexity of the CT image, manual segmentation adds significant time to the clinical workflow.

Segmentation is a crucial step in image processing and is also one of the more complex procedures involved in this field [6,7]. Automatically separating the tumour location from the liver is difficult due to factors including the liver's varying size and shape among patients. In addition, when compared to other linked organs, such as the stomach and spleen, the liver's intensity appears to be consistent throughout both high and low-contrast images [8,9]. In addition, images with low contrast and an ambiguous lesion shape make automatic segmentation of liver cancers challenging [10,11]. Issues with high susceptibility to noisy outliers and over and under-segmentation can plague several image segmentation methodologies such as active contrast segmentation, traditional segmentation technique, watershed model, and region expansion, resulting in less accurate results in less time [12,13].

Because certain lesions, such as hemangioma and metastasis, look similar to the liver, manual segmentation and organization of liver cuts from CT imageries is a lengthy task, leading to confusion and less reliable results [14]. Consequently, there is an urgent requirement for research into automated methods to aid radiotherapists in the diagnosis of liver scratches from CT scans [15]. Figure 1 demonstrates how difficult it is to detect liver regions with CT.

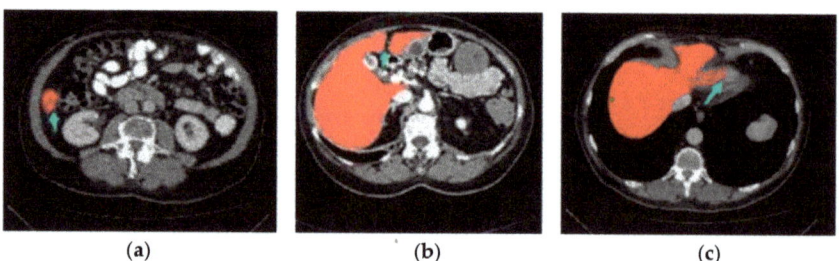

(a)   (b)   (c)

Figure 1. Three stimulating cases, including (**a**) Small liver zone, (**b**) Break liver part, (**c**) Blurred liver border.

Researchers have created a wide variety of sophisticated methods in recent decades for autonomous liver segmentation. These methods may be loosely categorized into three groups: intensity-based approaches, machine learning-based approaches, and deep learning-based approaches. As a class, intensity-based tactics are known for their speedy execution, and this is especially true of thresholding-based approaches [16,17], district growth methods, and level-set methods. Most of these methods, however, are only semi-automatic, leaving them vulnerable to noise and requiring human involvement with complex stricture situations.

They allow for substantial gains in segmentation accuracy when used with ML-based approaches [18–20]. Most machine learning (ML)-based devices, however, necessitate the manual construction of specialized features, which significantly affects precision. CNN and other deep learning-based methods have seen tremendous growth because of their sophisticated subsequent triumphs in a variety of areas, including target identification, picture segmentation, and classification [21–23]. A Fully Convolutional Network (FCN) is a popular deep learning-based technique that performs exceptionally well at classifying images down to the pixel level. The accuracy of the deep learning-based methods is significantly higher than that of existing ML-based methods [24]. There are, however, constraints on both FCN and U-Net-based approaches. Both single network training and cascade structure training employing the FCN-based method have a high failure rate when it comes to producing reliable outcomes in the liver [17,25,26]. The fundamental reason for this is that when evaluating the link among pixels, a reduction in the capacity to notice subtle visual cues occurs [27]. While the U-Net-based method is effective, it refined the feature map only after the U-Net convolution process was completed. Further, as the network's depth increases, the gradient vanishment problem becomes more easily triggered, and the picture resolution rapidly decreases due to the network's constant down-sampling operation, which would negatively affect the regions [28]. Finally, the category imbalance problem might lead to mistakes in areas and unclear liver boundaries. While a 3D network's learning effect would improve along with the z-axis information, in practice, this is difficult to achieve due to memory constraints, making the choice of the slice number tricky [29].

In most cases requiring automatic liver segmentation, the aforementioned strategies perform admirably. However, their accuracy and resilience remain insufficient when applied directly to clinical data, which severely limits their further use. The major contribution of the research work is as mentioned below:

- Three steps are only included in this study such as pre-processing, segmentation, and classification.
- Histogram Equalization and medium filtering are used for the improvement of the input images.
- Enhanced Mask R-CNN is used to segment the liver tumor from the pre-processed images. The research work introduces multistage optimization for deep learning segmentation networks. The study used a multi-optimization training system by utilizing stochastic gradient descent and adaptive moment estimation (Adam) with preprocessed CT images in enhanced Mask-RCNN.
- APESTNet is introduced in this study for classification. Overfitting issues in the Swin Transformer model are prevented by introducing Adversarial propagation in the classifier.

The following paper is constructed as follows: Section 2 discusses the related works of liver segmentation and classification. Section 3 presents a brief explanation of the proposed model. The validation analysis of proposed segmentation and classification with existing techniques are given in Section 4. Finally, the limitations and scientific contributions of the work are described in Sections 5 and 6.

2. Related Works

Rela et al. [30] use an optimization-driven segmentation and classification perfect for trying to apply a unique approach to analyzing and categorizing liver tumours. Five stages, (a) pre-processing, (b) liver segmentation, (c) tumour segmentation, (d) feature extraction, and (e) classification, are involved in the generated model's execution of the task. The acquired CT images are pre-processed in three steps, including contrast enhancement via histogram equalization and noise filtering via the median filter. In the next step after image preprocessing, CT abdominal images are segmented to isolate the liver using adaptive thresholding to train the classifier using the tumour picture segmentation. Two deep learning techniques, RNN and CNN, are utilized in the classification process. The CNN receives the segmented image of the tumour, while the RNN receives the extracted features. To further enhance the hidden neuron optimization, a hybrid classifier that has been further refined is utilized. In addition, an enhanced meta-heuristic approach.

Liver area extraction from CT scan images was proposed by Ahmad et al. [31] using a very lightweight CNN. In order to distinguish the liver from the background, the proposed CNN algorithm employs softmax across its three and two fully connected layers. Using a random Gaussian distribution to seed weights, we were able to embed these data while maintaining their semantic distances. Ga-CNN is the name of the proposed network (Gaussian-weight initialization of CNN). The MICCAI SLiver'07, 3 Dircadb01, and LiTS17 benchmark datasets are used in the experiments. Across all benchmark datasets, experimental results demonstrate the superiority of the suggested technique.

Using generative adversarial networks (GANs) and Mask R-CNN, Wei et al. [32] presented a technique for segmenting liver images. To begin, Mask R-CNN and GANs were investigated further to improve pixel-wise classification, as most output images contain noisy characteristics. To improve the segmentation performance, k-means clustering was then utilized to lock the image aspect ratio and obtain additional crucial anchors. Finally, we developed a GAN Mask R-CNN method, which outperformed state-of-the-art alternatives and the Multi-Image Classification and Analysis Improvement (MICCAI) measures. The suggested approach also outperformed ten state-of-the-art algorithms on six Boolean indications.

With its roots in the traditional U-Net, Wang et al. [33] presented a novel network design dubbed SAR-U-Net. After each convolution in the U-Net encoder, a SE block is presented to adaptively extract, hiding unimportant parts of the image and emphasizing parts that are essential to the segmentation task at hand. Second, the ASPP is used to acquire picture data at several scales and receptive fields by substituting the transition layer and the output layer. Third, the typical convolution block is swapped out for the residual structures to help with the gradient vanishment problem, and this causes the network to improve accuracy from a much higher depth. Five widely-used measures, including the Dice coefficient, VOE, RVD, ASD, and MSD, were employed in the LiTS17 database test. The proposed technique was the most accurate when compared to other similar models.

In this study, Roy et al. [34] present a novel automatic method for segmenting and classifying liver tumours. For classification purposes, the model employed a hybrid deep learning-based Convolution Neural Network (HCNN) model hybrid. The classification approach computes a multiclass categorization of the tumours discovered, while the segmentation framework seeks to distinguish between normal and malignant liver tissue. The focus of this study is on developing a method that eliminates the possibility of human mistakes in the forecasting process. On the other hand, the suggested method has recall values that are nearly as high as the best existing methods, and it delivers the highest precision for lesion identification. On average, the suggested method properly categorizes tumours in the liver as either hepatocellular carcinomas (HCC), malignant tumours other than HCC, or benign tumours or cysts. This paper's novelties lie in its implementation of MSER to segment tumour lesions and its use of a hybrid CNN-based technique to classify liver masses.

Hussain et al. [35] zeroes in on the Machine Learning (ML) techniques of multiclass liver tumour classification using Random Forest (RF). There are four types of tumours included in the dataset: hemangioma, cyst, hepatocellular carcinoma, and metastasis. The photos were gray-scaled, and the contrast was enhanced using histogram equalization. The Gabor filter was used to lessen the amount of background noise, and an image sharpening technique was used to enhance what was already there. Employing texture, binary, histogram, and rotational, scalability, and translational (RST) methods, we were able to collect 55 features for each ROI, despite their varying pixel sizes. Twenty optimal features for classification were extracted from the original set of 55 using the correlation-based feature selection (CFS) method. The outcomes demonstrated that RF and RT were more accurate (97.48% and 97.08%, respectively) than J48 and LMT. A more accurate diagnosis of liver cancers will be possible with the aid of the revolutionary framework provided.

In order to categorize multi-organ 3D CT cancer, Kaur et al. [36] used a convolutional neural network. The suggested method has been validated using a dataset consisting of 63503 CT scans of patients with liver cancer acquired from The Cancer Imaging Archive (TCIA). This strategy uses a convolutional neural network (CNN) to classify CT pictures of liver cancer. Results for the classification have been calculated. When the data-enhanced volume slices, the validation accuracy increases to 99.1% from the original volume slices' accuracy of 98.7%. When compared to other volume slices, the test accuracy of the data-augmented volume slice dataset is 93.1% higher on average. The primary benefit of this effort will be in assisting the radiation therapist in narrowing their attention to a specific region of the CT images.

Jeong et al. [37] offer an automated approach to segmenting the liver in CT scans and estimating its volume using a deep learning-based segmentation system. The framework was trained using data from 191 donors, and it showed promising results in four different segmentation tasks: for the left lobe (0.789), the right lobe (0.869), the caudate lobe (0.955), and the overall liver (0.899). Moreover, the R2 value for the volume estimate task was as high as 0.980, 0.996, 0.953, and 0.996. The outcomes proved that this strategy delivers precise and quantifiable liver segmentation outcomes, lowering the margin of error in liver volume estimation.

Militello et al. [38] generate and validate a radiomic model with radiographic features extracted from breast dynamic contrast-enhanced magnetic resonance imaging (DCE-MRI) from a 1.5 T scanner. Images were acquired using an eight-channel breast coil in the axial plane. The rationale behind this study is to demonstrate the feasibility of a radiomics-driven model that can be integrated into clinical practice using only standard-of-care DCE-MRI with the goal of reducing required image pre-processing.

The existing DL models didn't focus on overfitting issues and generally used classification techniques for classification and segmentation. This will decrease the classification accuracy, and therefore, this research work focused on addressing the overfitting issue by adding Adversarial Propagation to the Swin transformer model.

3. Materials and Methods

Radiologists currently perform a slice-by-slice examination of numerous CT scans to segment liver tumours manually. Manual methods are more difficult and time-consuming. Computer-assisted diagnosis relies on the segmented regions, and human segmentation of images may compromise diagnostic accuracy. The main challenges of automatic liver and liver tumour segmentation models are (a) low contrast between the liver tumour and healthy tissue in CT images, (b) variable size, location, and shape of liver tumours, making segmentation difficult; and (c) the liver is closely connected with the adjacent organs, and the CT value of these organs will be similar to the livers.

"(a) Image pre-processing, (b) Liver and tumor segmentation, and (c) Classification" are the three steps that make up the suggested liver tumour segmentation and classification method. The CT images are first collected, then pre-processing techniques, such as histogram equalization and median filtering are applied to them. Histogram equalization is used to increase contrast, and median filtering is used to reduce noise in the final image.

3.1. Dataset and Implementation

The experiment makes use of the labeled training sets from the LiTS17 2 and SLiver073 datasets. There is a wide range of sampling techniques included in the 131–3 D abdominal CT scan sets that make up the LiTS17-Training dataset. With an in-plane resolution of 0.55 mm × 1.0 mm and inter-slice spacing of 0.45 mm × 6.0 mm, CT images and labels have a 512 × 512 pixel size. From a total of 131 datasets, 121 were chosen at random for use in our experiment's training phase, while the remaining 10 were employed in the experiment's testing phase. Additionally, all 20 datasets from the SLiver07-Training dataset were used for evaluation. Each CT image in this dataset is 512 × 512 pixels in size.

During training, the learning rate (lr) starts at 0.001 and decreases by 0.005 per four training iterations using the Formula (1):

$$lr = initial\ lr\ (epoch/step\ scope) \qquad (1)$$

where early lr and step size are both constants. For this purpose, the tried-and-true stochastic gradient descent (SGD) algorithm was employed.

It was empirically determined that a batch size of 4 was optimal for running the suggested approach on our GPU with 11 GB of memory. Epoch is empirically chosen to 60 to guarantee efficient training, as this is the point around which the majority of the training converges. All the tests are conducted on a workstation equipped with Ubuntu (Canonical Ltd., London, UK).

3.2. Image Pre-Processing

The histogram equalization and median filtering method are used for preparing the raw CT abdominal picture.

Histogram Equalization

It's used as a preliminary processing step since it adjusts an image's brightness to boost its contrast. Let In^{im} be the input picture and define pixel value as the matrix of integer pixel intensities between 0 and 1. The number of intensity values is represented by INV, with a maximum value of 256 being the norm. Equation notation for the normalized histogram NHS of InHE with a bin to possible intensity (2). In this case, $HE = 0, 1, \ldots, (INV-1)$. The equation for the histogram-normalized image is (3) [39]:

$$NHS = \frac{Number\ of\ pixels\ with\ density\ he}{Total\ number\ of\ pixels} \quad (2)$$

$$In^{HE} = floor\left((INV-1) \sum_{he=0}^{In^{im}_{(i,Q)}} NHS\right) \quad (3)$$

The term $floor()$ in the aforementioned equation rounds down to the next integer value. Thus, a median filter is applied to further smooth out the histogram-equalized image In^{HE}. Filtering data by taking the middle value [39]: Restricting low- and high-frequency pixels, as this filter does, removes noise from an image, making it easier to see and appreciate its edges. If you want to eliminate the noise in your liver image, try using a non-linear filter, such as median filtering. This filter's primary function is to replace noisy pixels with the image's median pixel value, which is calculated by ranking each pixel according to its grayscale value. When the median filter is applied to the input image, HE, we achieved the resulting image MF, as shown in Equation (4).

$$In^{MF}(x,y) = med\left\{In^{HE}(x-u, y-v)u, v \in H\right\} \quad (4)$$

The original image and the median filtered image are represented by In^{HE} and In^{MF}, respectively, in Equation (4). As an added bonus, H represents a 2-dimensional mask. Since this is the last step in the pre-processing phase, the resulting picture, In^{MF}, is next processed using liver segmentation.

3.3. Segmentation Using Enhanced M-RCNN

The state-of-the-art in instance picture segmentation is the mask-RCNN framework, which the proposed method builds on. This framework has shown outstanding performance in a number of image segmentation studies. Figure 2 depicts the major steps that make up the proposed enhanced M-RCNN method: Backbone, Neck, DenseHead, and ROIHead (Region of Interest Head).

(1) The Backbone converts the incoming image into a raw feature map. Here, we employ a variant of ResNet-50-based on the design.
(2) The Neck joins the Spine to the Head. The original feature map is refined and rearranged. It has a vertical corridor and horizontal branches. To produce a feature

pyramid map of the same size as the raw feature map, the top-bottom route is used. Convolutional add operations between two parallel pathways' corresponding levels characterize lateral linkages.

(3) Third, the Dense Head can be used to perform dense placements of feature maps. The RPN examines each area and makes the best guess as to whether or not an object is present. The RPN's main benefit is that it doesn't need to look at the real image itself. Through the use of a fixed number of anchor boxes, the network performs a rapid scan of the feature map.

(4) ROIHead (BBoxHead, MaskHead): Using ROIAlign, extract features that affect the ROI from different feature maps while maintaining their precise spatial placements. This section takes in ROI features and then predicts task-related outcomes based on those features. At this point, you'll be doing two things at once:

   a. In the detection branch, the location of the bounding box (BBoxHead) is identified and classified for intervertebral disc (IVD) detection.
   b. In the segmentation node, the FCN created the IVD image segmentation. b. MaskHead.

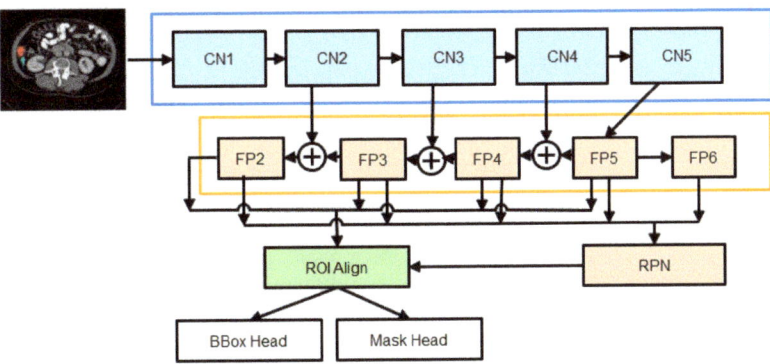

Figure 2. The diagrams of the Enhanced M-RCNN Framework.

Classification loss and mask loss are all summed together unweighted to form the loss function. SGD optimization and the Adam optimization approaches are employed by an enhanced M-RCNN. Training makes use of SGD and Adam optimization. To identify global optimums, the SGD is effective and simple to utilize. When trying to find a local optimum, SGD fails and becomes difficult to employ. When it comes to optimizing sparse gradients in noisy situations, Adam optimization combines the best features of the adaptive gradient and root mean square propagation to create an effective technique.

At its core, our feature extractor is a ResNet-50 that has been initialized using ImageNet-trained weights. Xavier initialization is used for all other weights (such as the RPN). To accomplish our tasks, a system with a single graphics processing unit is employed. The initial mask-RCNN used a batch size of 16. There are three distinct stages to the training process, the first of which involves simply training the MaskHead and not the projected ResNet-50 backbone. Parts of the backbone [beginning at layer 4 (CN4)] and the prediction heads (DenseHead and ROIHead) are fine-tuned in the second stage. The third and final stage involves joint training of the model's constituent parts (the "heads" and the "backbone"). The study employs liver image data with SGD optimization with Adam optimization during the third and final stage. Training is slowed to a crawl by setting alpha = 1.0×10^{-6} (learning rate or step size), beta1 = 0.9, beta2 = 0.999, and epsilon = 1×10^{-8}.

Starting with the smallest feature map and working our way down to larger ones via upscale operations, the study employs this top-bottom strategy to build final feature maps. A feature map is produced in layer two of the diagram, and its use of 1×1 convolutions reduces the total number of channels to 256. The up-sampled output from the previous cycle is then combined with these components. The outputs of this procedure are fed into a 33-convolution layer with stride 2 to generate the last four feature maps (FP2, FP3, FP4, and FP5). Max-pooling from FP5 yields FP6, which is considered the fifth feature map. Using these five feature maps, RPN may create candidate object bounding boxes. However, when associating with ROIs, only four feature maps (FP2, FP3, FP4, and FP5) are used.

A series of convolutional layers, followed by batch normalization and the ReLU activation function, are standard fare in the original ResNet-50 architecture's convolutional blocks and identity blocks. To better deal with training data that is jumbled together, the study employs group normalization and dropout regularization and makes many tweaks to these methods. The enhanced M-RCNN makes use of high-definition training data. Due to this, the study can only process a maximum of two photos at a time in a batch. While a small batch size can lead to an inaccurate estimation of the batch statistics, a big batch size is necessary for effective batch normalization. The model error may increase dramatically if the batch size is decreased. In this case, dropout regularization is applied after group normalization. To avoid model overfitting and boost the generalization effect, regularization is a must in deep learning. To eliminate co-adaptation issues among the hidden nodes of deep feedforward neural networks, the dropout regularization strategy has been effectively used in several deep learning models.

Loss Functions

In enhanced M-RCNN, the loss is computed as a total of losses at each stage of the model. The cost represents the weights that each stage of the model should have. For classification and bounding box regression, the ROIAlign output is fed into the BBo × Head, while for segmentation, the output is fed into the MaskHead. The output of the FCN layer is sent into a softmax layer, which performs the classification utilizing all of the characteristics. The MOM-RCNN loss function demonstrates the deviation between the predicted and observed values. As a result, the study presents a single loss function for training the bounded RCNN's box refinement regression, class prediction classification, and mask prediction generation. Mask prediction generation loss (L_{mask}) is only obtained from mask prediction generation stages, while class prediction classification loss $L_{r,class}$ and $L_{m,class}$ and bounding box refinement regression loss are obtained from both the RPN and mask prediction generation stages. It is only necessary to specify the L mask once per class, which eliminates output competition amongst masks. The resulting enhanced M-RCNN loss function is defined as (5):

$$L_{enhacned\ M-RCNN} = L_{r,class} + L_{m,class} + L_{r,box} + L_{m,box} + L_{mask} \quad (5)$$

where $L_{r,class}$: This is the monetary cost associated with an RPN's mistaken identification of anchor boxes (the presence/absence of an object). In cases where the final output model is not picking up on many objects, this value should be high so that RPN can record it. $L_{r,box}$: What this means is that the RPN is quite precise in its localization. When the object is recognized, but its bounding box needs adjusting, this is what you utilize to fine-tune the detection. $L_{m,class}$: This is the cost associated with misidentifying an item in the designated area. In the likely scenario where the object is recognized from the image but incorrectly labeled, this probability is high. $L_{m,box}$: To put it another way, this is the same as the "loss" calculated when pinpointing the precise location of the boundary of the specifically named class. It's high if the object is properly classified, but localization is off. L_{mask}: Masks were made based on the things that were detected. Therefore, this is related.

The class prediction organization error ($L_{r,class}$ and $L_{m,class}$) is calculated by (6):

$$L_{r,class} = \frac{1}{M_{class}} \sum_i -\log[pr_i^* pr_i + (1 - pr_i^*)(1 - pr_i)] \quad (6)$$

where MM class is the total number of classes and pr_i is the likelihood that the ith region of interest (ROI) contains a positive sample (liver). If the ROIs are comprised of positive samples, then =1, and else it will be 0. $L_{m,class}$ follows the same formula.

Regression loss $L_{r,class}$ and $L_{m,class}$ are calculated by plugging these two values into an Equation (7):

$$L_{r,box} = \frac{1}{M_{regress}} \sum_i pr_i^* S(trans_i, trans_i^*) \quad (7)$$

$S()$ is a smooth function where M regress is the sum of pixels in the feature map, $trans_i$ shows $L_{m,box}$ follows the same formula. The loss L mask in mask prediction generation is calculated by (8):

$$L_{mask} = -\frac{1}{n^2} \sum_{1 \leq x,y \leq n} \left[lbl_{xy}^p = (1 - lbl_{xy}) \log\left(1 - lbl_{xy}^2\right) \right] \quad (8)$$

where the label value at position (x, y) is denoted by lbl_{xy} in the n by n region, and the predicted value for the p-th class is denoted by lbl_{xy}^p.

3.4. Classification

Though the transformer was first developed for processing natural language sequences, its application to CNN for image processing is to consider the picture as a matrix for convolution operation. Unfortunately, CNN is not well-suited for direct usage in picture feature extraction. That's why patching techniques, such as patch embedding, patch merging, and masking are used.

3.4.1. Patch Embedding

Patch partition is used to divide an RGB map into individual patches that do not overlap. Here, the size of the patch is 4×4, which is multiplied by the RGB channels to yield a total size, i.e., $4 \times 4 \times 3 = 48$. To generate a feature matrix, we simply project the refined patchwork to the required dimensions.

3.4.2. Patch Merging

After partitioning the obtained feature matrix into four 22 windows and merging their respective positions, the resulting four feature matrices are concatenated.

3.4.3. Mask

When the pixels are subsequently relocated, the mask will only allow the window to focus on the continuous portion, reducing the influence of ingesting. If you shift the matrix to the right, the original window in the bottom right corner will be found. The size of the shift is proportional to window size and may be calculated using the following formula.

$$s = \left\lceil \frac{w}{2} \right\rceil \quad (9)$$

for each given shift s, the window width w must be specified.

Because the region visible in the window to the right and below does not border the section in the original matrix, it must be separated from it using the mask matrix. Both the vertical and horizontal slicing areas are [0,-window size),[-window size,-shift size),[-shift size]. The concept behind the window partition (function window partition) for the labeled mask matrix is to equally split the window size into blocks of [H/w] rows [H/w] columns and combine the dimensions for the number and the batch size. The original matrix mask will be subdivided into smaller windows so that they can be individually counted as window units.

In Figure 3, the overall design of the proposed SwinNet is seen. Encoder, bottleneck, decoder, and skip links make up SwinNet. Swin Transformer blocks are Swin-fundamental Unet's building block [40]. The medical images are divided into 4×4 non-overlapping patches for the encoder to use in transforming the inputs into sequence embeddings. After applying this partitioning strategy, the feature dimension of each patch is 4 × 4 × 3 = 48. Furthermore, the dimensions of the projected features are embedded into an arbitrary dimension using a linear embedding layer (represented as C). To create the hierarchical feature representations, the modified patch tokens are fed into multiple Swin Transformer blocks and patch merging layers. When it comes to downsampling and dimension expansion, the patch merging layer is in charge, whereas the Swin Transformer block is in charge of feature representation learning. We created a symmetric transformer-based decoder after being inspired by U-Net [24]. The decoder uses a Swin Transformer block and a patch-expanding layer. To compensate for the reduction in spatial detail brought on by down-sampling, the encoder's multiscale features are fused with the retrieved context features via skip connections. A patch expanding layer, as opposed to a patch merging layer, is purpose-built for up-sampling. Through an up-sampling ratio of 2, the patch expanding layer converts 2D feature maps into 4D feature maps. The segmentation predictions at the pixel level are generated by applying a linear projection layer to the up-sampled features, and the input resolution of the feature maps is restored via a 4 up-sampling operation carried out by the final patch expanding layer. Our breakdown of the blocks' descriptions would go as follows:

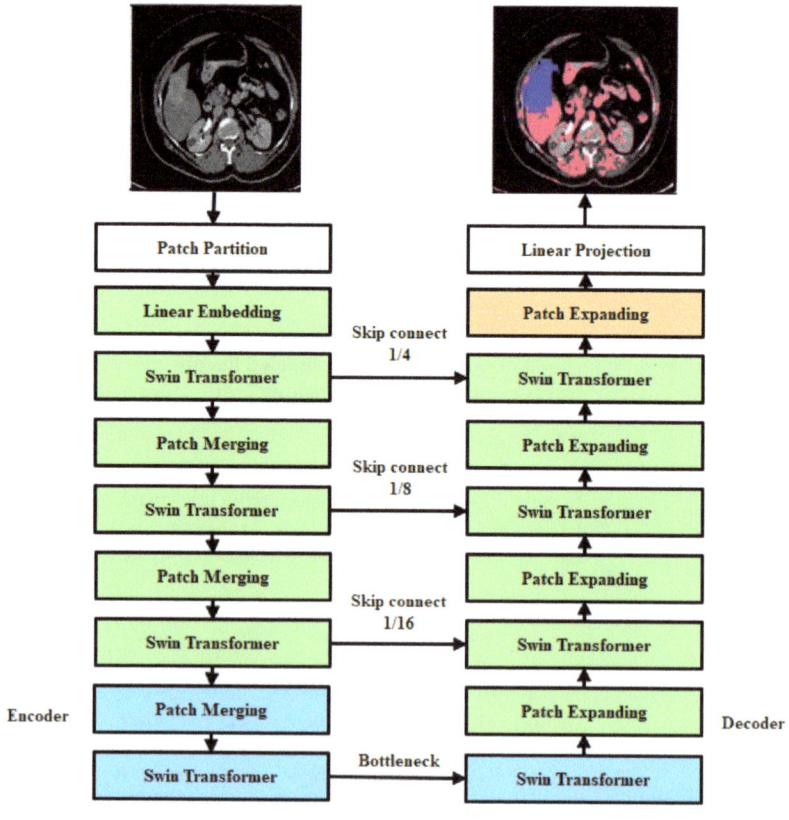

Figure 3. Encoders, bottleneck nodes, decoders, and skip links make up Swin-overall Unet's structure. The swin transformer block is the foundation of the encoder, bottleneck, and decoder.

3.4.4. Swin Transformer Block

In place of the standard multi-head self-attention (MSA) module, the swin transformer block [41] is constructed using shifted windows. Identical transformer pairs, as depicted in Figure 4. Each swin transformer block consists of LayerNorm (LN) layers, multi-head self-attention modules, residual connections, and two-layer MLPs with GELU non-linearity. A shifted window-based multi-head self-attention (SW-MSA) module is used in the first transformer block, while a window-based multi-head self-attention (W-MSA) module is used in the second. Continuous swin transformer blocks are created using this type of window partitioning (10)–(13):

$$\hat{z}^l = W - MSA\left(LN\left(z^{l-1}\right)\right) + z^{l-1} \quad (10)$$

$$z^l = MLP\left(LN\left(\hat{z}^l\right)\right) + \hat{z}^l \quad (11)$$

$$\hat{z}^{l+1} = SW - MSA\left(LN\left(z^l\right)\right) + z^l \quad (12)$$

$$z^{l+1} = MLP\left(LN\left(\hat{z}^{l+1}\right)\right) + \hat{z}^{l+1} \quad (13)$$

where $\hat{z}^l$ and z^l stand for the results produced by the lth block's SW-MSA module and the lth block's MLP module, respectively. Self-attention is calculated in the same way as in earlier publications [42,43] (14):

$$Atention(Q, K, V) = SoftMax\left(\frac{QK^T}{\sqrt{d}} + B\right)V \quad (14)$$

where Q, K, and V are the matrices in the space R(M2 d). The sum of patches in a window, $M2$, and the measurement of the query, d, are both variables. Furthermore, B is populated with numbers derived from the bias matrix $B = R((2M - 1)(2M + 1))$.

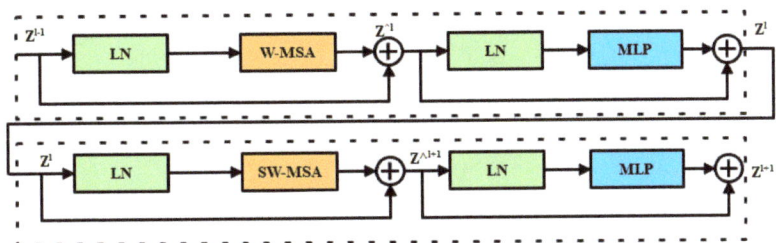

Figure 4. Swin transformer chunk.

3.4.5. Encoder

Tokenized inputs in C-dimensions at a resolution of H/4 W/4 are sent into two successive Swin Transformer blocks in the encoder for representation learning with the same feature dimension and resolution. At the same time, the patch merging layer will double the feature dimension while halving the token count. In the encoder, this process will be performed three times.

Integration layer for patches: The patch merging layer takes the input patches and combines the four subsets into one. This type of processing will result in a 2× down sampling of feature resolution. Moreover, a linear layer is applied to the concatenated features in order to reduce the feature dimension by a factor of four, making it equal to the original size of two.

3.4.6. Bottleneck

Since Transformer cannot be converged [44], the bottleneck utilized to learn the deep feature representation is made up of just two successive Swin Transformer blocks. Both the feature size and resolution are maintained in the bottleneck.

3.4.7. Decoder

The symmetric decoder is constructed using the same Swin Transformer block that was used in the encoder. Due to this, we up-sample the deep features collected by the decoder using the patch expanding layer rather than the patch merging layer. When the feature dimension is doubled.

Flare-up Expanding Layer: In order to raise the feature dimension from its initial value of (W/32 H/328 C) by 2 prior to up-sampling the features. The input characteristics are then rearrange-operated to increase their resolution by a factor of two and decrease their dimension by a factor of four (from W/32 H/3216 C to W/16 H/164 C).

3.4.8. Skip Connection

To combine the encoder's multi-scale characteristics with the up-sampled features, we use skip connections, similar to how the U-Net does. As a means of mitigating the loss of spatial information brought on by down-sampling, we join together both shallow and deep features. After an up-sampling layer, a linear layer is applied, maintaining the same dimensionality of the concatenated features as the up-sampled features. In this network, overfitting is a major issue that must be resolved to attain high classification accuracy. For this issue, adversarial propagation (AdvProp) [45] is used as an improved training scheme, which is used as a separate auxiliary batch norm for the training samples.

4. Results and Discussion

4.1. Segmentation Results

Evaluation Metrics for Segmentation

Dice coefficient (DC), Volume overlap error (VOE), Relative volume error (RVD), Average symmetric surface distance (ASD), and maximum surface distance (MSD) are the five most widely used metrics for assessing liver segmentation (MSD). The meanings of the five metrics are as follows, with A being the liver segmentation result and B representing the ground truth:

Dice coefficient (DC): the resemblance between two sets, with a range of (0,1). Greater values indicate more precise segmentation (15).

$$Dice(A, B) = \frac{2|A \cap B|}{|A| + |B|} \qquad (15)$$

Volume Overlap Error (VOE): volumetric discrepancy between segmented and raw data (16).

$$VOE = 1 - \frac{|A \cap B|}{|A \cap B|} \qquad (16)$$

RVD: Whether the result is over-segmented is measured with this metric. Values closer to 0 indicate more precise segmentation (17)–(19).

$$RVD(A, B) = \frac{|B| - |A|}{|A|} \qquad (17)$$

$$ASD(A, B) = \frac{1}{|S(A)| + |S(B)|} \left(\sum_{p \in S(A)} d(p, S(B)) + \sum_{q \in S(B)} d(q, S(A)) \right) \qquad (18)$$

$$MSD(A, B) = max \left\{ \max_{p \in S(A)} d(p, S(B)), \max_{q \in S(B)} d(p, S(A)) \right\} \qquad (19)$$

The dice measure of proposed enhanced M-RCNN achieved 0.957 on average results, where the ASD is 1.544, 0.095 of VOE, 29.144 mm of MSD, and −0.0084 of RVD on average results. A better Dice coefficient means better segmentation accuracy for an efficient proposed model. Here, the proposed model achieved better Dice, which is proved in the above Table 1. Table 2 presents the comparative analysis of the proposed segmentation model with existing techniques on the second dataset.

Table 1. The results of proposed segmentation technique on 10 LiTS17-Training datasets.

Case Num	VOE	ASD (mm)	MSD (mm)	RVD	Dice
1	0.103	1.568	28.453	−0.029	0.955
2	0.089	1.471	34.951	−0.033	0.963
3	0.100	1.382	31.259	−0.049	0.956
4	0.097	1.494	25.494	−0.048	0.968
5	0.114	1.797	28.315	−0.040	0.949
6	0.107	1.933	29.756	−0.038	0.953
7	0.094	1.229	30.657	0.034	0.960
8	0.073	0.955	39.421	0.043	0.961
9	0.086	1.673	34.598	0.036	0.954
10	0.090	1.863	28.534	0.040	0.952
Avg	0.095	1.544	29.144	−0.0084	0.957

Table 2. The results of a quantitative comparison with approaches on 20 Sliver07-Training datasets.

Methods	Dice (%)	VOE (%)	RVD (%)	ASD (mm)	MSD (mm)
Adaptive Thresholding [30]	95.60 ± 3.41	8.23 ± 5.89	−2.38 ± 2.16	2.19 ± 0.38	36.69 ± 1.45
Ga-CNN [31]	96.94 ± 1.78	5.31 ± 3.48	−0.54 ± 2.24	1.95 ± 0.34	30.66 ± 2.03
GAN Mask R-CNN [32]	96.66 ± 2.19	6.38 ± 3.93	−1.29 ± 3.58	1.80 ± 0.38	28.30 ± 2.05
Proposed Enhanced M-RCNN model	97.31 ± 1.49	5.37 ± 3.27	−1.08 ± 2.06	1.85 ± 0.30	27.45 ± 1.89

In Table 2, the experiments represent the Quantitative comparison with methods on 20 Sliver07-Training datasets. Here we have used different evaluations for the proposed method. Based on the analysis, it is clearly proven that the proposed model achieved better results than existing techniques. In the next section, the proposed classifier's validation is carried out, and the results are provided.

4.2. Classification Results

4.2.1. Performance Measure for Classification

Our ideal and comparable baseline projections are evaluated using a wide range of indicators. An exhaustive list of evaluation criteria is provided below:

- Accuracy: On test samples, accuracy is referred to as "accuracy."
- Precision: In the context of predictive value, precision refers to a positive value and is the ratio of genuine positive models to the total number of false positive samples.
- Recall: Classifier performance can be evaluated using this metric. Alternatively known as Sensitivity or True Positive Rate, which describes an organization model, Recall discards a positive prediction if it's not accurate.
- F1: Classification is an example of a machine learning task for which this measure is well-known. It is the arithmetic mean of the estimates' precision and recall.

4.2.2. Validation Analysis Using 70% of Training Data–30% of Testing Data

In the above Table 3 represents the comparative Analysis of the Proposed Model. In these evaluations, the proposed model achieves better performance than other models, such as the proposed model accuracy of 95.62%, F-1 measure of 94.53%, precision of 98.32%, and recall of 94.62%, respectively. However, the existing techniques achieved nearly 92% to 94% accuracy, 93% to 96% precision, 89% to 92% recall, and 87% to 92% F1-measure.

Table 3. Comparative Analysis of Proposed Model.

Model	Accuracy	Precision	Recall	F1
CNN-RNN [30]	80.10	87.21	80.15	80.43
Ga-CNN [31]	85.71	84.32	85.93	83.45
GAN-R-CNN [32]	92.10	92.43	92.15	91.68
SAR-U-Net [33]	92.46	93.48	92.44	91.81
HCNN [34]	89.52	90.21	89.54	89.03
RF [35]	94.53	96.61	92.52	92.24
CNN [36]	94.16	96.17	92.32	92.10
Proposed APESTNet	**95.62**	**98.32**	**94.62**	**94.53**

4.2.3. Validation Analysis Using 60% of Training Data–40% of Testing Data

In the Table 4, the results represent the Comparative Analysis of the Proposed Model. In these evaluations, the proposed model data is split into 60–40% percentages, and the performance achieves better performance than other models. For instance, the proposed model has an accuracy of 94.32% and a recall of 93.24%, respectively. Here, data plays a major role in the performance analysis, which is clearly proven in Figures 5–8.

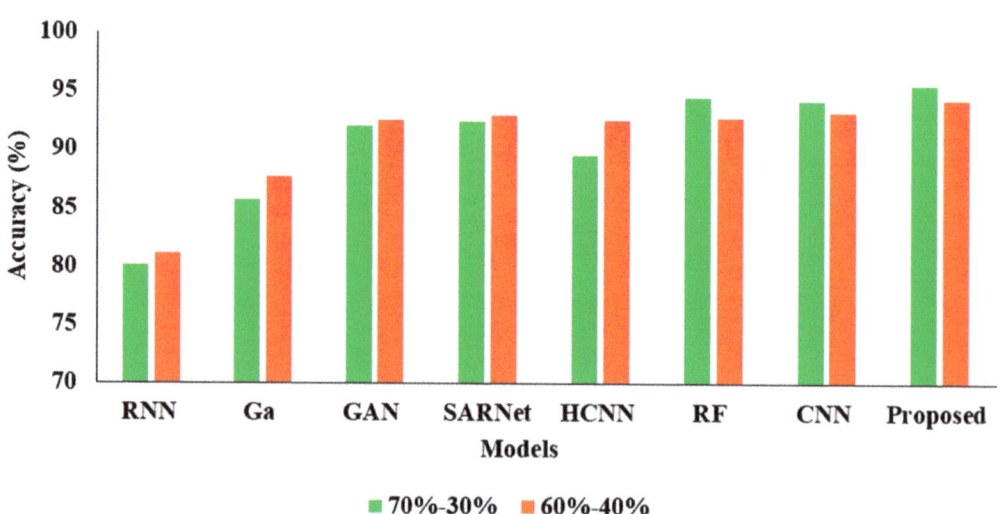

Figure 5. Accuracy Comparison for two data splits-ups.

The Table 5 represents the Comparative Analysis of the Proposed Model. From these validations, it proves that the performance of the proposed model achieves better performance than other models. For instance, the proposed model training period is 390.33, and the execution time is 0.01128 (s), respectively.

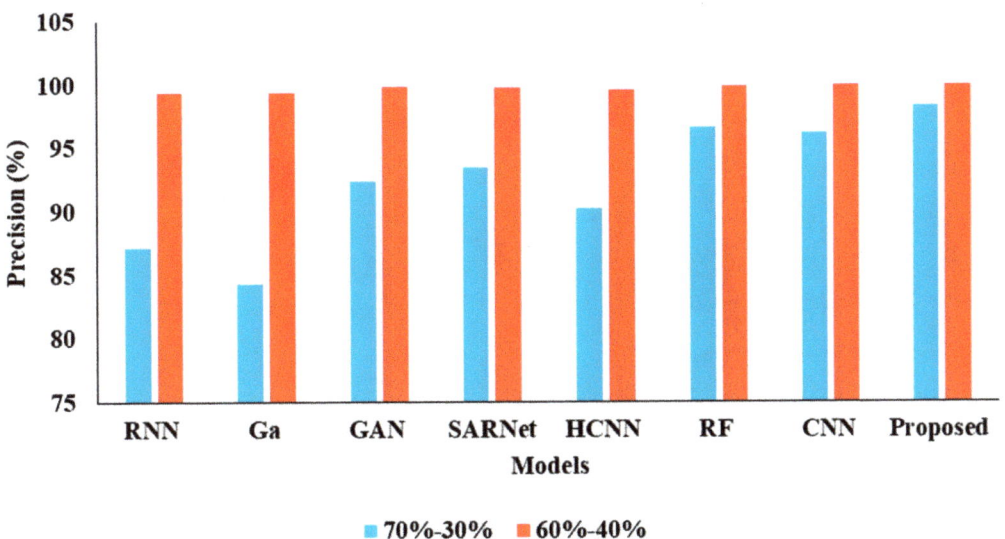

Figure 6. Precision Comparison for two data splits-ups.

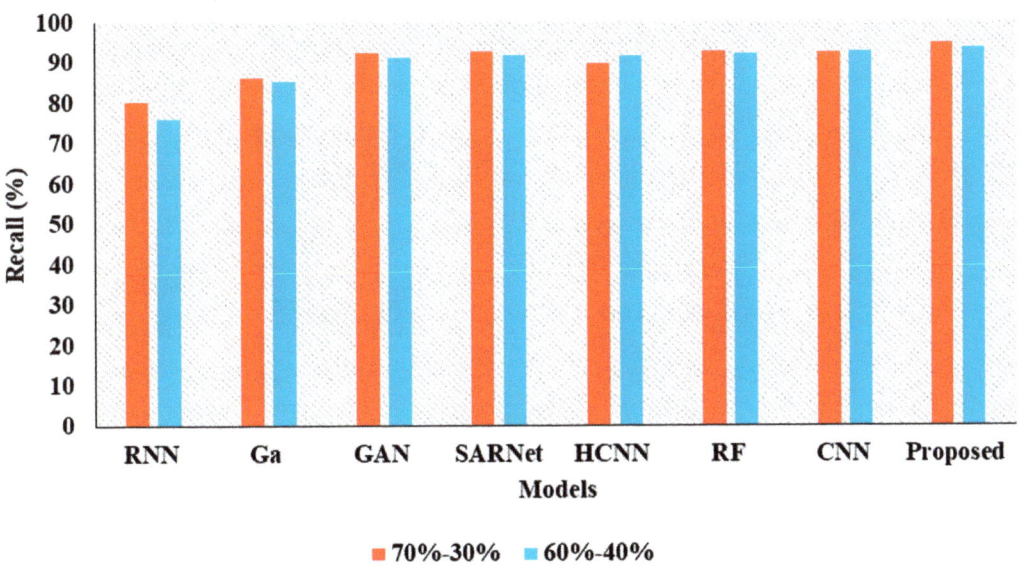

Figure 7. Recall Comparison for two data splits-ups.

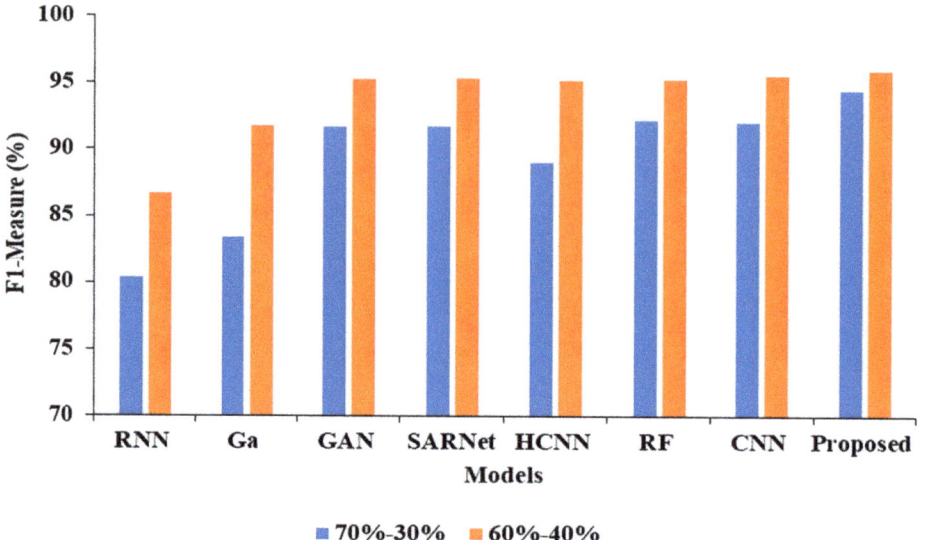

Figure 8. F1-measure Comparison for two data splits-ups.

Table 4. Comparative Analysis of Proposed Model with existing techniques.

Model	Accuracy	Precision	Recall	F1
CNN-RNN [30]	81.10	99.41	75.91	86.72
Ga-CNN [31]	87.70	99.41	85.21	91.82
GAN-R-CNN [32]	92.50	99.82	90.98	95.27
SAR-U-Net [33]	92.90	99.78	91.52	95.41
HCNN [34]	92.50	99.63	91.38	95.18
RF [35]	92.70	99.90	91.93	95.32
CNN [36]	93.27	99.91	92.47	95.63
Proposed APESTNet	**94.32**	**99.95**	**93.24**	**96.02**

Table 5. Comparison of the proposed model for different time executions.

Model	Training Time (s)	Testing Time (s)	Execution Time (s)
CNN-RNN [30]	630.01	69.17	0.01233
Ga-CNN [31]	450.53	67.38	0.01369
GAN-R-CNN [32]	543.21	65.89	0.01369
SAR-U-Net [33]	577.66	63.71	0.01657
CNN [34]	480.23	60.41	0.01309
RF [35]	583.42	59.78	0.01297
CNN [36]	423.17	59.192	0.01289
Proposed APESTNet	**390.33**	**57.621**	**0.01128**

5. Limitation

While the proposed methodology yielded some promising outcomes, there remains room for improvement. The CT pictures are 3D, but the suggested method is built on a 2D network; thus, it can easily lose crucial context information along the z-axis. In addition, the proposed technique may produce substantial mistakes around the boundary when the liver margin has lesions or tumour abnormalities.

6. Conclusions

This research introduces a novel model called APESTNet to improve the classification and categorization of liver tumours. The built-model consists of three phases: pre-processing, segmentation, and classification. The acquired CT images were subjected to histogram equalization and a median filtering technique before further analysis could be performed. After the necessary steps were taken to prepare the data, a tumour was segmented using an upgraded mask R-CNN model. The classification is then performed later by an interactively learning Swin Transformer block, the core unit for feature representation and long-range semantic information. In particular, the proposed strategy improved significantly and was very resilient while dealing with small liver pieces, discontinuous liver regions, and fuzzy liver boundaries. The experimental results confirm that the proposed APESTNet is more effective in classifying liver tumours than the current state-of-the-art models. Without compromising accuracy, the proposed method conserved resources. However, the proposed method is prone to slight over-segmentation or under-segmentation errors when dealing with lesions or tumours at the liver boundary. Therefore our future work will concentrate on completely utilizing the z-axis information in 3D to reduce errors.

Author Contributions: K.C., G.H.S.: research concept and methodology, writing—original draft preparation. J.S.: Investigation; W.-C.L.: Validation and Funding Acquisition; P.K.B.: review, revision, and editing. All authors have read and agreed to the published version of the manuscript.

Funding: This research has been funded by the National Yunlin University of Science and Technology, Douliu.

Institutional Review Board Statement: Not applicable.

Informed Consent Statement: Not applicable.

Data Availability Statement: The datasets used and/or analyzed during the current study are available from the corresponding author upon reasonable request.

Conflicts of Interest: The authors declare no conflict of interest.

References

1. Siegel, R.; Ma, J.; Zou, Z.; Jemal, A. Cancer statistics, 2014. *CA Cancer J. Clin.* **2014**, *64*, 9–29. [CrossRef]
2. Damhorst, G.L.; Murtagh, M.; Rodriguez, W.R.; Bashir, R. Microfluidics and nanotechnology for detection of global infectious diseases. *Proc. IEEE* **2015**, *103*, 150–160. [CrossRef]
3. Murakami, T.; Imai, Y.; Okada, M.; Hyodo, T.; Lee, W.-J.; Kim, M.-J.; Kim, T.; Choi, B.I. Ultrasonography, computed tomography and magnetic resonance imaging of hepatocellular carcinoma: Toward improved treatment decisions. *Oncology* **2011**, *81*, 86–99. [CrossRef]
4. Ranjbarzadeh, R.; Saadi, S.B. Automated liver and tumor segmentation based on concave and convex points using fuzzy c-means and mean shift clustering. *Measurement* **2020**, *150*, 107086. [CrossRef]
5. Hou, W.; Toh, T.B.; Abdullah, L.N.; Yvonne, T.W.Z.; Lee, K.J.; Guenther, I.; Chow, E.K.-H. Nanodiamond– manganese dual mode MRI contrast agents for enhanced liver tumor detection. *Nanomed. Nanotechnol. Biol. Med.* **2017**, *13*, 783–793. [CrossRef] [PubMed]
6. Dogantekin, A.; Ozyurt, F.; Avcı, E.; Koc, M. A novel approach for liver image classification: PH-C-ELM. *Measurement* **2019**, *137*, 332–338. [CrossRef]
7. Nasiri, N.; Foruzan, A.H.; Chen, Y.-W. Integration of a knowledge-based constraint into generative models with applications in semi-automatic segmentation of liver tumors. *Biomed Signal Process. Control* **2020**, *57*, 101725. [CrossRef]
8. Lebre, M.-A.; Vacavant, A.; Grand-Brochier, M.; Rositi, H.; Abergel, A.; Chabrot, P.; Magnin, B. Automatic segmentation methods for liver and hepatic vessels from CT and MRI volumes, applied to the Couinaud scheme. *Comput. Biol. Med.* **2019**, *110*, 42–51. [CrossRef]
9. Xu, L.; Zhu, Y.; Zhang, Y.; Yang, H. Liver segmentation based on region growing and level set active contour model with new signed pressure force function. *Optik* **2020**, *202*, 163705. [CrossRef]
10. Patil, D.D.; Deore, S.G. Medical image segmentation: A review. *Int. J. Comput. Sci. Mob. Comput.* **2013**, *2*, 22–27.
11. Cheng, D.; Guot, Y.; Zhang, Y. A novel image segmentation approach based onneutrosophic set and improved fuzzy Cmeans algorithm. *New Mat. Nat. Comput.* **2011**, *7*, 155–171. [CrossRef]

12. Budak, U.; Guo, Y.; Tanyildizi, E.; Şengür, A. Cascaded deep convolutional encoder-decoder neural networks for efficient liver tumor segmentation. *Med. Hypotheses* **2020**, *134*, 109431. [CrossRef]
13. Baazaoui, A.; Barhoumi, W.; Ahmed, A.; Zagrouba, E. Semiautomated segmentation of single and multiple Tumors in liver CT images using entropy-based fuzzy region growing. *IRBM* **2017**, *38*, 98–108. [CrossRef]
14. Tanaka, O.; Kojima, T.; Ohbora, A.; Makita, C.; Taniguchi, T.; Ono, K.; Matsuo, M.; Nagata, Y. Scores of Child-Pugh Classification Impact Overall Survival after Stereotactic Body Radiation Therapy for Primary and Metastatic Liver tumors. *J. Clin. Exp. Hepatol.* **2019**, *10*, 101–105. [CrossRef] [PubMed]
15. Perell, K.; Vincent, M.; Vainer, B.; Petersen, B.L.; Federspiel, B.; Møller, A.K.; Madsen, M.; Hansen, N.R.; Friis-Hansen, L.; Nielsen, F.C.; et al. Development and validation of a micro RNA based diagnostic assay for primary tumor site classification of liver core biopsies. *Mol. Oncol.* **2015**, *9*, 68–77. [CrossRef] [PubMed]
16. Lu, X.; Wu, J.; Ren, X. The study and application of the improved region growing algorithm for liver segmentation. *Opt. —Int. J. Light Electron Opt.* **2014**, *125*, 2142–2147. [CrossRef]
17. Li, X.; Huang, C.; Jia, F. Automatic Liver Segmentation Using Statistical Prior Models and Free-form Deformation. In *Medical Computer Vision: Algorithms for Big Data*; Springer: Cham, Switzerland, 2014; Volume 8848, pp. 181–188.
18. Shi, C.; Cheng, Y.; Wang, J.; Wang, Y.; Mori, M.; Tamura, S. Low-rank and sparse decomposition based shape model and probabilistic atlas for automatic pathological organ segmentation. *Med. Image Anal.* **2017**, *38*, 30–49. [CrossRef]
19. Wang, J.; Cheng, Y.; Guo, C.; Wang, Y.; Tamura, S. Shape–intensity prior level set combining probabilistic atlas and probability map constrains for automatic liver segmentation from abdominal CT images. *Int. J. Comput. Assist. Radiol. Surg.* **2016**, *11*, 817–826. [CrossRef]
20. Krizhevsky, A.; Sutskever, I.; Hinton, G.E. Imagenet classification with deep convolutional neural networks. In Proceedings of the 25th International Conference on Neural Information Processing Systems, Lake Tahoe, NV, USA, 3–6 December 2012; pp. 1097–1105.
21. He, K.; Zhang, X.; Ren, S.; Sun, J. Deep residual learning for image recognition. In Proceedings of the IEEE Conference on Computer Vision and Pattern Recognition, Las Vegas, NV, USA, 27–30 June 2016; pp. 770–778. Available online: https://ieeexplore.ieee.org/document/7780459 (accessed on 29 November 2022).
22. Ren, S.; He, K.; Girshick, R.; Sun, J. Faster r-cnn: Towards real-time object detection with region proposal networks. In Proceedings of the 28th International Conference on Neural Information Processing Systems, Montreal, QC, Canada, 7–12 December 2015; pp. 91–99.
23. Long, J.; Shelhamer, E.; Darrell, T. Fully convolutional networks for semantic segmentation. In Proceedings of the IEEE Conference on Computer Vision and Pattern Recognition, IEEE Computer Society, Boston, MA, USA, 7–12 June 2015; pp. 3431–3440.
24. Ronneberger, O.; Fischer, P.; Brox, T. U-Net: Convolutional Networks for Biomedical Image Segmentation. In *Medical Image Computing and Computer-Assisted Intervention—MICCAI 2015*; Springer: Cham, Switzerland, 2015; pp. 234–241.
25. Milletari, F.; Navab, N.; Ahmadi, S.-A. V-Net: Fully Convolutional Neural Networks for Volumetric Medical Image Segmentation. In Proceedings of the 2016 Fourth International Conference on 3D Vision, Stanford, CA, USA, 25–28 October 2016; pp. 565–571.
26. Rida, I.; Al-Maadeed, N.; Al-Maadeed, S.; Bakshi, S. Automatic liver and lesion segmentation in CT using cascaded fully convolutional neural networks and 3 D conditional random fields. In Proceedings of the Medical Image Computing and Computer-Assisted Intervention (MICCAI 2016), Athens, Greece, 17–21 October 2016; pp. 415–423.
27. Kaluva, K.C.; Khened, M.; Kori, A.; Krishnamurthi, G. 2d-densely connected convolution neural networks for automatic liver and tumor segmentation. *arXiv* **2018**, arXiv:1802.02182.
28. Li, X.; Chen, H.; Dou, Q.; Fu, C.W.; Heng, P.A. H-DenseU-Net: Hybrid densely connected U-Net for liver and liver tumor segmentation from CT volumes. *arXiv* **2017**, arXiv:1709.07330.
29. Han, X. Automatic liver lesion segmentation using a deep convolutional neural network method. *arXiv* **2017**, arXiv:1704.07239.
30. Rela, M.; Nagaraja Rao, S.; Ramana Reddy, P. Optimized segmentation and classification for liver tumor segmentation and classification using opposition-based spotted hyena optimization. *Int. J. Imaging Syst. Technol.* **2021**, *31*, 627–656. [CrossRef]
31. Ahmad, M.; Qadri, S.F.; Qadri, S.; Saeed, I.A.; Zareen, S.S.; Iqbal, Z.; Alabrah, A.; Alaghbari, H.M.; Rahman, M.; Md, S. A Lightweight Convolutional Neural Network Model for Liver Segmentation in Medical Diagnosis. *Comput. Intell. Neurosci.* **2022**, *2022*, 9956983. [CrossRef] [PubMed]
32. Wei, X.; Chen, X.; Lai, C.; Zhu, Y.; Yang, H.; Du, Y. Automatic Liver Segmentation in CT Images with Enhanced GAN and Mask Region-Based CNN Architectures. *BioMed Res. Int.* **2021**, *2021*, 9956983. [CrossRef] [PubMed]
33. Wang, J.; Lv, P.; Wang, H.; Shi, C. SAR-U-Net: Squeeze-and-excitation block and atrous spatial pyramid pooling based residual U-Net for automatic liver segmentation in Computed Tomography. *Comput. Methods Programs Biomed.* **2021**, *208*, 106268. [CrossRef] [PubMed]
34. Saha Roy, S.; Roy, S.; Mukherjee, P.; Halder Roy, A. An automated liver tumour segmentation and classification model by deep learning based approaches. *Comput. Methods Biomech. Biomed. Eng. Imaging Vis.* **2022**, 1–13. [CrossRef]
35. Hussain, M.; Saher, N.; Qadri, S. Computer Vision Approach for Liver Tumor Classification Using CT Dataset. *Appl. Artif. Intell.* **2022**, *36*, 2055395. [CrossRef]
36. Kaur, A.; Chauhan, A.P.S.; Aggarwal, A.K. An automated slice sorting technique for multi-slice computed tomography liver cancer images using convolutional network. *Expert Syst. Appl.* **2021**, *186*, 115686. [CrossRef]

37. Jeong, J.G.; Choi, S.; Kim, Y.J.; Lee, W.S.; Kim, K.G. Deep 3 D attention CLSTM U-Net based automated liver segmentation and volumetry for the liver transplantation in abdominal CT volumes. *Sci. Rep.* **2022**, *12*, 6370. [CrossRef]
38. Militello, C.; Rundo, L.; Dimarco, M.; Orlando, A.; Woitek, R.; D'Angelo, I.; Russo, G.; Bartolotta, T.V. 3 D DCE-MRI radiomic analysis for malignant lesion prediction in breast cancer patients. *Acad. Radiol.* **2022**, *29*, 830–840. [CrossRef]
39. Dorothy, R.; Joany, R.M.; Rathish, J.; Santhana Prabha, S.; Rajendran, S.; Joseph, S.T. Image enhancement by histogram equalization. *Int. J. Nano Corros. Sci. Eng.* **2015**, *2*, 21–30.
40. Zhu, Y.; Cheng, H. An improved median filtering algorithm for image noise reduction. *Phys Procedia.* **2012**, *25*, 609–616. [CrossRef]
41. Liu, Z.; Lin, Y.; Cao, Y.; Hu, H.; Wei, Y.; Zhang, Z.; Lin, S.; Guo, B. Swin transformer: Hierarchical vision transformer using shifted windows. In Proceedings of the IEEE/CVF International Conference on Computer Vision, Montreal, QC, Canada, 10–17 October 2021.
42. Hu, H.; Gu, J.; Zhang, Z.; Dai, J.; Wei, Y. Relation networks for object detection. In Proceedings of the 2018 IEEE/CVF Conference on Computer Vision and Pattern Recognition, Salt Lake City, UT, USA, 18–23 June 2018; pp. 3588–3597.
43. Hu, H.; Zhang, Z.; Xie, Z.; Lin, S. Local relation networks for image recognition. In Proceedings of the 2019 IEEE/CVF International Conference on Computer Vision (ICCV), Seoul, Republic of Korea, 27 October–2 November 2019; pp. 3463–3472.
44. Touvron, H.; Cord, M.; Sablayrolles, A.; Synnaeve, G.; J'egou, H. Going deeper with image transformers. *arXiv* **2021**, arXiv:2103.172392021.
45. Xie, Q.; Luong, M.-T.; Hovy, E.; Le, Q.V. Self-training with noisy student improves imagenet classication. In Proceedings of the IEEE/CVF Conference on Computer Vision and Pattern Recognition (CVPR), Seattle, WA, USA, 13–19 June 2020.

Disclaimer/Publisher's Note: The statements, opinions and data contained in all publications are solely those of the individual author(s) and contributor(s) and not of MDPI and/or the editor(s). MDPI and/or the editor(s) disclaim responsibility for any injury to people or property resulting from any ideas, methods, instructions or products referred to in the content.

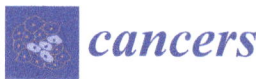

Article

An Explainable AI-Enabled Framework for Interpreting Pulmonary Diseases from Chest Radiographs

Zubaira Naz [1], Muhammad Usman Ghani Khan [1], Tanzila Saba [2], Amjad Rehman [2,*], Haitham Nobanee [3,4,5,*] and Saeed Ali Bahaj [6]

[1] Department of Computer Science, University of Engineering and Technology Lahore, Lahore 54890, Pakistan
[2] Artificial Intelligence & Data Analytics Lab, CCIS, Prince Sultan University, Riyadh 11586, Saudi Arabia
[3] College of Business, Abu Dhabi University, Abu Dhabi 59911, United Arab Emirates
[4] Oxford Center for Islamic Studies, University of Oxford, Oxford OX3 0EE, UK
[5] Faculty of Humanities & Social Sciences, University of Liverpool, Liverpool L69 7WZ, UK
[6] MIS Department, College of Business Administration, Prince Sattam bin Abdulaziz University, Alkharj 11942, Saudi Arabia
* Correspondence: arkhan@psu.edu.sa (A.R.); haitham.nobanee@liverpool.ac.uk (H.N.)

Simple Summary: Different chest diseases badly affect the human respiration system. The chest radiographs of the lungs are used to classify these diseases. Identifying diseases is essential, but the most important thing is explaining the reason behind classification results. This research provides an explanation of the classification results of different lung pulmonary diseases so that doctors can understand the reason that causes these diseases. This work achieved 97% classification accuracy. This research also evaluated the highlighted regions in the input image, during the explanation of classification results with the manifest file, where the doctor highlighted the same regions with red arrows. The automatic disease explanation and identification will help doctors to diagnose these diseases at a very early stage.

Abstract: Explainable Artificial Intelligence is a key component of artificially intelligent systems that aim to explain the classification results. The classification results explanation is essential for automatic disease diagnosis in healthcare. The human respiration system is badly affected by different chest pulmonary diseases. Automatic classification and explanation can be used to detect these lung diseases. In this paper, we introduced a CNN-based transfer learning-based approach for automatically explaining pulmonary diseases, i.e., edema, tuberculosis, nodules, and pneumonia from chest radiographs. Among these pulmonary diseases, pneumonia, which COVID-19 causes, is deadly; therefore, radiographs of COVID-19 are used for the explanation task. We used the ResNet50 neural network and trained the network on extensive training with the COVID-CT dataset and the COVIDNet dataset. The interpretable model LIME is used for the explanation of classification results. Lime highlights the input image's important features for generating the classification result. We evaluated the explanation using radiologists' highlighted images and identified that our model highlights and explains the same regions. We achieved improved classification results with our fine-tuned model with an accuracy of 93% and 97%, respectively. The analysis of our results indicates that this research not only improves the classification results but also provides an explanation of pulmonary diseases with advanced deep-learning methods. This research would assist radiologists with automatic disease detection and explanations, which are used to make clinical decisions and assist in diagnosing and treating pulmonary diseases in the early stage.

Keywords: explainable AI; class activation map; Grad-CAM; LIME; coronavirus disease; reverse transcription polymerase chain reaction; computed tomography; healthcare; health risks

---

Citation: Naz, Z.; Khan, M.U.G.; Saba, T.; Rehman, A.; Nobanee, H.; Bahaj, S.A. An Explainable AI-Enabled Framework for Interpreting Pulmonary Diseases from Chest Radiographs. *Cancers* **2023**, *15*, 314. https://doi.org/10.3390/cancers15010314

Academic Editor: Stefan Delorme

Received: 29 November 2022
Revised: 22 December 2022
Accepted: 23 December 2022
Published: 3 January 2023

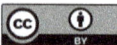

Copyright: © 2023 by the authors. Licensee MDPI, Basel, Switzerland. This article is an open access article distributed under the terms and conditions of the Creative Commons Attribution (CC BY) license (https://creativecommons.org/licenses/by/4.0/).

1. Introduction

The human respiratory system provides respiration using the lungs, which are fundamental organs of the human body. Lung pathology is observed through chest radiographs, known as chest X-rays (CXRs) [1]. Many pulmonary diseases are diagnosed by observing different pathological patterns through CXRs [2]. Computed tomography (CT) and CXR are low-cost and effective techniques for detecting pulmonary diseases such as tuberculosis, edema, nodules, and pneumonia [3]. Among all these pathologies, pneumonia is a fatal one that is clinically measured by observing lobar consolidation, interstitial opacities, and airspace opacities. Edema is identified by pulmonary vessels, patchy shadowing, increased cardiac size, and septal lines [4]. The CXRs are also used to identify tuberculosis by observing the cavities and consolidations in the upper zone of the lungs.

On the other hand, the nodules are identified as a spot in the lung zones using CXRs [5]. In the past years, there was an unexpected rise in COVID-19 patients who also had deadly lung infections such as pneumonia [6]. COVID-19 is identified by observing the airspace opacities, lobar consolidation, and patchy shadow [7,8]. This primarily affects the pulmonary system, causing a chronic inflammation that severely lowers overall lung capacity [9]. This is a severe and deadly disease due to its high transmission, absence of general population immunity, and long incubation period. CT and CXR are the primary imaging diagnostics for these pulmonary diseases [10].

This manual diagnosis process takes more time which was the main concern. Therefore, deep learning (DL)-based approaches are being employed for automated pulmonary lung disease identification [11] to deliver accurate results. DL produces highly detailed images and CT scans, the standard method for lung diagnosis and treatment [12,13]. However, it is still being determined how these DL algorithms reach the classification results and which features are more important to produce that output [14,15]. This shows deep learning algorithms' inherent black-box character and other factors, such as processing costs [16]. It originates from the inability to represent the information for a given job completed by a deep neural network, despite understanding the basic statistical principles. Easier artificial intelligence (AI) methods, such as decision trees and linear regression, are self-explanatory since the classifier boundary can be depicted in a few dimensions using the model's parameters. However, tasks such as the classification of 3D and most 2D medical images lack the complexity needed and lack the tools to check the behaviour of black-box models, thus having a negative impact on the deployment of deep learning in a variety of fields, including finance and automated vehicles and especially healthcare, where explainability and reliability of classification of disease are critical factors for end-user trust [17].

Explainable AI (XAI) has the key to opening the deep learning "black box" nature [18]. XAI is an AI model that explains goals, logic, and decision-making to laymen [19]. End users in this case could be AI system creators or those influenced by an AI model's judgment [3]. The findings show that quantitative and qualitative visual representations can help clinicians understand and make better decisions by providing more detailed data from the learned XAI algorithms' results [20]. In healthcare-related medical imaging problems, the accuracy of the prediction model is essential. Still, the visualization and localization of input medical images are more significant, which helped to identify the main regions contributing to the classification results [18]. Even though there are many reasons why XAI is substantial, research reveals that the three most critical problems are: (1) trustworthiness, (2) transparency, and (3) bias and fairness in algorithms [21]. With these features, XAI has plenty of applications in different domains for explaining deep learning algorithms' prediction. In healthcare, XAI is important for explaining deep learning algorithms' classification.

In this research, we introduced the concept of explainability for detecting the important features in medical images where the classification model gives extra attention throughout the classification task. We present the deep-learning-based framework for explaining pulmonary diseases using chest radiographs. All pulmonary diseases badly affect the lungs and respiration system of humans but have different affected zones. Due to a large number of cases of pulmonary disease COVID-19 in the past years, we took radiographs of COVID-19 for the classification results' explanation task. We achieved the goal of identifying the COVID-19 disease and provided the visualisation of input medical images contributing to the classification results. First, we provided the CXR images as input to our deep-learning-based system. The system processed the input image and provided the classification result. After that, the CXR image is passed to our XAI local interpretable model agnostic explanations (LIME) to determine which specific features helped the deep convolution neural network distinguish between COVID-19 and non-COVID-19 patients. LIME provided the highlighted regions of the input CXR images. That explains the classification results' reasons in the form of the highlighted segment of that image with different colors. In the last step, we evaluated the doctor-highlighted region with the model, and it provided the same highlighted components.

Further, this research has four main sections; Section 2 presents the in-depth state of the art; Section 3 presents the proposed methodology; Section 4 exhibits results; finally, Section 5 concludes the research.

2. Literature Survey

DL techniques enhanced the performance of medical imaging diagnostic frameworks, especially for abnormal pathologies and pulmonary diseases of lungs from CXRs [22]. Most of these systems used transfer learning approaches for identifying different lung pulmonary diseases using chest radiographs. These techniques are used to identify pulmonary disorders, i.e., edema, nodules tuberculosis, pneumonia, and COVID-19 through chest radiographs [23]. In medical imaging, disease identification is important, but explanation and interpretability also play an important role [24]. XAI provides the reason behind the specific classification and prediction results. XAI's primary goal is to investigate and develop methods for explaining the individual predictions of DL systems. We understand that a clear explanation of the reached decision is critical in medical applications depending on images. In an ideal case, the system makes a decision based on the input data and justifies which image part led to a certain classification result [25]. XAI was recently considered because of its potential to provide an understanding of the behavior and process of some complex deep-learning models. Several studies [26] showed that, using a decision tree and linear models, it is easy to explain approaches in a way that is easy to comprehend and interpret for humans. In this paper, we took the case study of COVID-19 from all pulmonary diseases. The literature survey of some of the existing XAI systems for the classification of lung diseases is presented in Table 1.

Table 1. Comparative analysis of existing explainable artificial intelligence (XAI) and classification models for lung diseases.

Methodology	Dataset	Explainability Models	Accuracy %
ResNet 101 [18]	897 CT Scans	CAM, LIME	85%
U-Net CNN [24]	1478 X-rays	Grad-CAM, LIME	83%
VGG16, ResNet [27]	3975 CXRs	GSInquire	83%
Xception [28]	2235 chest X-rays	SHAP, Grad-CAM++	87%
DenseNet, ResNet, VGGNet [29]	5959 CXRs	Grad-CAM++, LRP	90%
DenseNet169 [30]	787 CT Scans	Not Used	85%
Proposed Mode	787 CT Scans, 10,000 CXRs Scans	LIME	93%, 97%

Ye et al. [18] used ResNet 101 to identify lung pulmonary disease COVID-19 using CT scans. They also used the Class Activation Map (CAM) for global explanation and achieved a classification accuracy of 85%. They used the concept of explanation in the medical image classification and tried to explain the results using the XAI approach CAM. In another research project, Lucas O. Teixeira employed two XAI techniques to analyze the effect of human lung segmentation, predict lung diseases, and provide the explanation using LIME and Gradient-weighted Class Activation Mapping (Grad-CAM). LIME works by identifying features, such as superpixels (picture zones), that improve the likelihood of the expected class, i.e., areas that support the present model prediction. Since this model actively employs such regions to produce predictions, they might be considered important. Grad CAM examines the gradients that flow into the last convolution layers of a CNN for an input image and label. The activation mapping (AM) can then be examined visually to ensure that the model focuses on the correct area of the input image. They used UNET architecture to classify lung diseases, pneumonia, lung opacities, and COVID-19 and achieved an accuracy of 83% [24].

In another research project, Linda W et al. used the COVIDNet data set to train the VGG16 network for the classification of COVID-19 tasks. They used 3975 CXRs for training the model. GSInquire explains the classification task. They achieved an accuracy of 83% [27]. After some time, Lin Zou et al. explained pulmonary diseases, pneumonia and COVID-19 using chest X-rays. They used 2235 x-rays and explained using ensemble XAI with Grad-Cam++ and SHAP. They achieved 87% classification accuracy [28]. Similarly, Md. Rezaul Karim et al. [29] developed a system using DenseNet, ResNet, and VGGNet models named DeepCovidExplainer that provides the explanations of classification results of COVID-19. They used 5959 CXR from patients to classify the normal, COVID-19, and Pneumonia classes and achieved 90% classification accuracy. Literature studies of existing pulmonary lung disease identification using DL techniques are presented in Table 2. L. O. Hall et al. [31] examined the lung diseases pneumonia and COVID-19 from the chest X-rays using the latest techniques of DL. They used DL architectures (VGG-16 and Resnet-50) to classify the diseases into two categories. They used a small dataset containing 135 chest X-rays of COVID-19 and 320 chest X-rays of pneumonia. They achieved satisfying results of 82.2% even though the dataset used was limited. M.K. Pundit et al. used deep neural network architecture VGG16 on 1428 chest X-rays images. They focused on the identification of the lung disease COVID-19. They improved the accuracy by a little to 92% [32]. After the success of predicting COVID-19 from chest X-rays, M. Singh et al. applied a machine-learning-based algorithm (Support Vector Machine) to CT scan data to classify COVID-19. They used a transfer-learning-based support vector machine on VGG16 architecture. Their dataset consists of 718 CT Scan images; 349 of them are of COVID-19, and 376 are of non-COVID-19. Their results were promising as they achieved a ROC Score of 85.3 and an accuracy of 83.5% [33]. CoXNet, a multi-dilation CNN, was used for the automatic discovery of COVID-19 by T. Mahmud et al. They also worked on X-ray pictures but with convertible multi-accessible feature optimization. Their dataset consists of four classes, COVID-19, Normal, Viral, and Bacterial pneumonia. Each class has 305 X-ray images. They achieved 80.2% accuracies along with a ROC score of 82.0 [34].

Table 2. Comparative analysis of the existing classification models for pulmonary diseases using lung scans and X-rays.

Methodology	Dataset	Accuracy %
VGG16 [31]	455 X-rays	82.2%
VGG-16 [32]	1428 X-ray	92%
VGG16, SVM [33]	718 CT scans	83.5%
CovXNets [34]	305 X-rays	80.2%
RCNN, ResNet, ResNet101 [35]	669 CT scans	83%
SVM [36]	1380 CT scans	63%
VGG-16 [37]	1428 CT scans	82.5%

Segmentation techniques were used by M. Aleem et al. [35] to fragment the symptoms of COVID-19 in the CT SCANS of the chest. The latest techniques of DL such as RCNN were used with the backbone of Resnet. The system was trained on 669 CT scans having 313 positive COVID-19 patients and 356 healthy ones. They achieved an accuracy of 83% with ROC scores of 85. With time, researchers kept working hard and coming up with new techniques as some researchers did [36] using SVM-based analysis of X-ray images. They used support vector machines to differentiate between COVID-19 and normal subjects. The dataset that was used for training and testing their system was 1380 CT scans; however, the results were not that promising, with an accuracy of 63% and the ROC score of 72. M. Pandit et al. worked on chest radiographs to detect the lung disease COVID-19. They used techniques and achieved outstanding results. VGG-16 is used for classification purposes. The dataset used for training and testing the system contains 1428 chest radiographs with bacterial pneumonia, healthy, and COVID-19. They attained an accuracy of 82.5% [37].

Xingyi Yang et al. [30] provided a COVID CT dataset verified by the senior radiologist of Tongji Hospital, Wuhan, China. They collected the data on COVID-19 and normal CT images for the diagnosis of COVID-19; they collected data from different patients and provided the manifest file of that data as well. They also developed an automatic disease detection technique using these CT images and achieved an accuracy of 85%. We will use this COVIDNet and COVID CT dataset and improve the classification results. In the medical domain, experts are required to explain the reasons for classification results manually. We are developing a framework that visually explains the deep learning classification model results. We provide an output image highlighting the important features that participate in the classification results. We evaluate the proposed model explanation with the radiologist highlighting glass ground opacities in the CXRs.

The main contributions of this research are:

- In this research, an explainable AI framework is developed for detecting pulmonary diseases where the classification model gives extra attention throughout the classification task using chest radiographs.
- For the classification task, transfer-learning-based Resnet50 architecture is used. This developed system secures superior classification accuracies compared to the existing approaches by achieving 93% and 97% of pulmonary disease COVID-19.
- Interpretable Model-agnostic Explanations (LIME) are used to explain the classification results. This unique explanation method may explain any classifier's predictions in a comprehensible manner that provides the explanation in the form of highlighted regions in the input image in which part of the image is used in the classification result.
- For the evaluation of the explanation task, two CT images from a journal [38] are used that are diagnosed and highlighted by a verified doctor. This research paper shows that the interpretable model explains the same region that is highlighted by a doctor.

3. Proposed Methodology

The proposed methodology has a sequence of steps that include dataset understanding, in which we understand the chest radiographs of humans and the importance of various regions present in the CXRs images. The second step is feature map generation which generates the feature maps of those CXRs images. We used the concept of transfer learning in our methodology and used pre-trained Resnet50 for the classification of COVID-/NON-COVID. Our final step is to explain the pulmonary disease classification results visually using the interpretable model LIME. This developed framework takes a CXR image as input. After that, it classifies the input image as COVID and NON-COVID. Once the decision is made, we pass that image and classification prediction to the proposed explainable model LIME, and then LIME will highlight the region of the input image. That highlighted region shows which part of the CXRs images took part in the classification results. LIME highlights the important features of the image with color. We evaluate our color region with the manifest info file of the COVID-CT dataset. We check that the doctor mentioned the same region while examining the CT scan of the COVID-19 patient so our model is giving the same region. The complete workflow diagram of our methodology is shown in Figure 1.

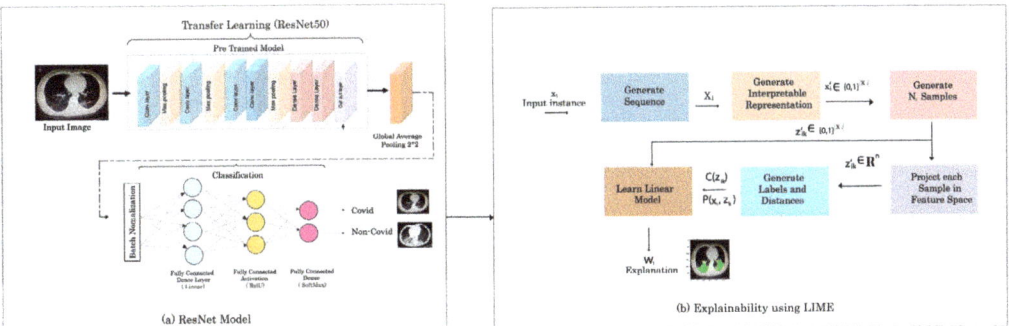

Figure 1. The architecture diagram of the proposed method.

3.1. Dataset

The datasets are the backbone of every proposed method and architecture in the computer vision and deep-learning domain. Any deep-learning system's accuracy is directly proportional to the above-mentioned parameter. Therefore, the proposed model is about a vision-related problem; a dataset is required due to deep learning. We used the COVID-CT [30] dataset and COVIDNet for COVID classification, and then we explain their classification results. The dataset's complete CXRs images and classes are given in Table 3. The COVID-CT dataset includes 349 COVID-19-positive CT scans from 216 individuals and 397 COVID-19-negative CT pictures from 397 patients. The dataset is freely available to the public in order to promote COVID-19 CT-based testing research and development. The distribution of the dataset into training, testing, and validation is shown in Table 4.

Table 3. Total sample and classes in COVID-CT and COVID-Net datasets.

Dataset	Total	Classes
COVID-CT	800	2
COVID-NET	19,000	3

Table 4. Sample data distribution in test, training, and validation of both COVID and non-COVID class.

Type	Non-COVID	COVID
Train	234	191
Test	58	60
Validate	105	98

This dataset has the manifest information of each image that helps the researcher understand the data images easily. In addition, the manifest file has information about the patients' medical history and lung scans. Figure 2 represents the distribution of the proportion of CT manifestations of COVID-19. We used these mentioned features in the explainability of chest radiographs.

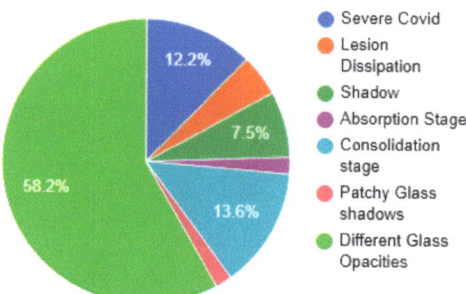

Figure 2. Chart of distribution of the proportion of CT manifestations of COVID-19.

3.2. Proposed CNN Model

Convolutional neural networks (CNNs) are a type of deep neural network that is utilized in image recognition. In order for the CNN to function, the images provided as input must be recognized by computers and translated into a processable format. As a result, CXR images are transformed to matrix format first. Then, based on CXR image differences and matrices, the system identifies which image belongs to which label. During the training phase, it learns the consequences of these changes on the label and then uses them to create predictions for fresh CXR images. We used a transfer learning technique to transfer already learned weights to pass into the current deep learning problem. The parameters of our transfer learning model are learning rates of 1×10^{-4}, 100 epochs, a batch size of 32, and two classes either "COVID" or "Non-COVID". Due to the small capacity of the dataset in the current task, deep CNN can collect general characteristics from the source dataset using the transfer learning approach. The transfer learning algorithms have a number of benefits, including avoiding overfitting whenever the number of training samples is restricted, lowering computation power, and speeding up system convergence. Figure 1a shows the complete flow of our Res-net50 model. We utilized batch normalization for each mini-batch to standardize the inputs to a layer. It normalizes the input layer and rescales it to speed up the training process and for improving stability. Equations (1)–(4) is the mathematical representation of Batch Normalization:

$$\mu = \frac{1}{n}\sum_i Z^{(i)} \qquad (1)$$

$$\sigma^2 = \frac{1}{n}\sum_i \left(Z^{(i)} - \mu\right)^2 \qquad (2)$$

$$Z^{(i)}_{norm} = \frac{Z^{(i)} - \mu}{\sqrt{\sigma^2 - \epsilon}} \qquad (3)$$

$$Z = \gamma * Z^{(i)}_{norm} + \beta \qquad (4)$$

Here, the mean is μ and the variance is σ; ϵ is a constant used for numerical stability; the activation vector is $Z^{(i)}$; γ allows for adjusting the standard deviation; β allows for adjusting the bias. Batch normalization made the training of the network faster. There are two main ways of using learning algorithms from pre-trained networks in the context of deep learning, extraction and fine-tuning of features. In our case, we used the second approach to modify and fine-tune the traditional ResNe50 architecture. That helps to outperform feature extraction and achieves better performance. The modified Resnet50 architecture generates the transfer feature map. The training of the Resnet50 model is conducted by using available CXRs data and the transfer learning pre-trained weight. For normalizing a neural network's output to a probability distribution over expected output classes, the SoftMax function was employed as the final activation function. It converts real values into probabilities by dividing the exponential of a particular class by the sum of the exponential of all classes. In class, higher probability is considered the output prediction. Totals of 349 COVID-19-positive CT scans and 397 COVID-19-negative CT were used for training the proposed model for COVID-CT data, and 19,000 CXRs were used for the COVID-NET dataset. After the training, we then saved the trained model that will be further used in the classification task. The pseudocode for modified ResNet50 is given below.

Pseudocode ResNet50

Input: Chest Radiographs
Output: classification results: Covid Or Normal
Start
    $lr \leftarrow 1 \times 10^{-4}$ ▷ lr is Initial_Learning_rate
    Batch_Size ← 32
    Number_of_Epochs ← 28
    Base_Model ← **ResNet50**(weights ← "imagenet", include_top ← False,
    input_tensor ← Input (shape ← (224, 224, 3)))   ▷ ResNet50 is the base Model

    headModel ← baseModel.output
    headModel ← AveragePooling2D(pool_size ← (7, 7))(headModel)
    headModel ← Flatten(name ← "flatten")(headModel)
    headModel ← Dense(256, activation ← "relu")(headModel)
    headModel ← Dropout(0.5)(headModel)
    headModel ← Dense(len(CLASSES), activation ← "softmax")(headModel)
    model ← Model(inputs ← baseModel.input, outputs ← headModel)
    for layer in baseModel.layers:
        layer.trainable ← True
    end for
    opt ← optimizers.Adam (lr ← INIT_LR, decay ← INIT_LR/Number_of_Epochs)
    model.compile (loss ← "binary_crossentropy", optimizer ← opt, metrics ← ["Accuracy"])
    H ← model.fit_generator (trainGen, steps_per_epoch ← totalTrain, validation_data ← valGen, validation_steps ← totalVal, epochs ← Number_of_Epochs)
End

3.3. Classification and Explanation

Instead of presenting our own architecture, available deep CNN architectures demonstrated greater performance across a wide range of classification problems. ResNet50 has a 50-layer variation of the residual neural network. Residual networks offer excellent performance and feature count balance and a high training speed. Another advantage of the residual network architecture is that it used different sizes of images for training. ResNet50′s weights are pre-trained on the ImageNet dataset. This pre-trained model can be used to classify pulmonary diseases COVID and NON-COVID. Figure 3 shows that our system took the input CXR and provided the classification. The final step of the proposed system was to explain the DL model and the reason behind the classification results.

The LIME interpretable model is used to explain and highlight the important features that contributed to the classification result of pulmonary lung diseases. The sequence of steps of the LIME Algorithm that we used to explain our classification results is given below in Algorithm 1.

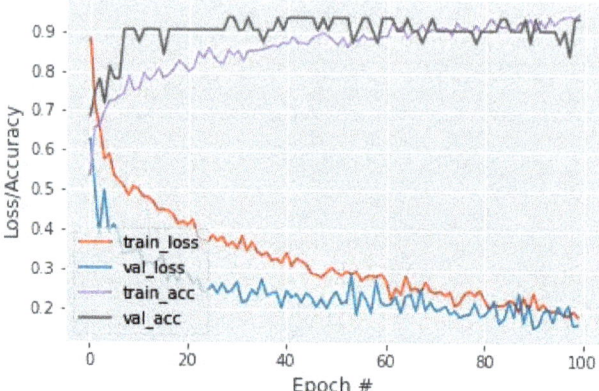

Figure 3. COVID-CT dataset training loss and accuracy.

Algorithm 1. LIME

Require: Classifier f, Number of samples N
Require: Instance x, and its interpretable version x'
Require: Similarity kernel πx, Length of explanation K
$Z \leftarrow \{\}$
for $i \in \{1, 2, 3,..., N\}$ do
 $\quad z'_i \leftarrow$ Sample around (x')
 $\quad Z \leftarrow Z \cup (z'_i, f(z^i), \pi_x (z_i))$
end for
$w \leftarrow$ K-Lasso(Z, K) $\quad\quad\quad$ ▷ with z'_i as features, f(z) as target
return w

Figure 1b shows the steps involved in the explainability using LIME. First, LIME used CXR images as input and generated the sequence present in the image. After that, it generated the interpretable representations and generated N samples. Then, it matched each sample with the featured map of the input CXR images and calculated the predicted label and distance from the predicted output. Following, these labels and distance values were passed to a linear model that provided the explanations, and a specific result was produced. LIME also highlighted the region in the CXRs image, which showed which part of the image took part of the output. The system used a CXR image as an input and classified the image as COVID and NON-COVID, and then LIME highlighted the important regions in the image, which can clearly represent and explain the reasons for classification results.

$$\xi(x) = \underset{g \epsilon G}{\operatorname{argmin}} L\left(f, g, \pi_x\right) + \Omega(g) \tag{5}$$

The Equation (5) is used for the LIME explainability calculation. In this equation, f is the model classifier, and G is a class of interpretable models. gG shows the learning of a local explainable model, and is x the proximity measure. (g) is used to measure the model complexity. The loss or distance function is denoted as L (f,g). After computing the explainability, evaluation is carried out using some images from verified doctors.

4. Results and Discussion

This section presents the complete experiment setup, performance metrics, and results of our classification deep learning models. We also discuss the results of the explainability model that we used and show the highlighted regions. Finally, we evaluate the explainability using our deep learning model highlighted region and compare it with the doctor-identified region.

4.1. Experimental Setup

In this research, we used suggested deep transfer learning models that were trained using the Python language. All experiments were run on a Google Colaboratory (COLAB) and the online cloud services with a free Central Processing Unit (CPU), NVIDIA K80 Graphics Processing Unit (GPU), and Tensor Processing Unit (TPU) hardware. By optimizing the cross-entropy value with CNN models, ResNet50 was pre-trained with some random initial weights. For overall experiments, the batch size, learning rate, and the number of epochs were set at 3, 1×10^5, and 30, respectively. All samples were randomly divided into two distinct datasets, with 80 percent used for training and 20 percent used for testing. The k-fold approach was chosen as the cross-validation method, and results were obtained using five distinct k values (k = 1–5). We first performed experiments using different CNN architectures such as DenseNet169, MobileNet, COVID LargeNet, and Resnet50. We trained these models using the COVID-CT dataset and calculated the training, testing, and validation accuracies. We found that the ResNet50 performs best of all of them. We used the transfer learning concept, fine-tuned the Resnet50, and found the best possible results. The results of different CNN models are shown in Table 5.

Table 5. Results on different CNN models.

CNN Model	Accuracy %
DenseNet169	85
MobileNet	83
COVID LargeNet	88
Our Model	93

We selected the Resnet50 model for our COVID-19 disease detection from the CXR images after performing the experiments on different CNN models as we finalized the Resnet50 model. We improved the base results; the next step was to explain the classification results. However, before moving toward the final step, we performed some more experiments and for that purpose, we trained the Resnet50 model on another dataset. The second dataset was the COVIDNet dataset which has more classes. We used that dataset for our problem and trained the Resnet50 on COVID-CT and COVIDNet datasets. We calculated the results on both datasets, shown in Table 6. For the calculation of the final results, we used some performance matrices that are discussed below.

Table 6. Classification results with ResNet50.

Measures	COVID-CT Dataset	COVID Net Dataset
	COVID or NON-COVID	COVID or NON-COVID
Precision	87-93	98-93
Recall	92-88	92-98
F1 Measure	90-90	95-95
Accuracy	93	97

4.2. Performance Matrices

In this paper, five parameters were used for measuring the performance of deep transfer learning models, having their advantages and disadvantages. We describe them one by one in the following Equations (6)–(10).

Accuracy: The correct predicted cases divided by a total number of cases gives us the accuracy [19]. High accuracy means the model is predicting accurately. It is actually a sum of true positives and negatives which is TP + TN divided by the sum of TP (True positives), TN (True Negatives), FP (False positives), and FN (False negatives).

$$\text{Accuracy} = \frac{TP + TN}{TP + TN + FP + FN} \quad (6)$$

Precision: Precision is called a number of the correct results out of the predicted results. It is calculated by dividing true positives by the sum of true positives and false positives.

$$\text{Precision} = \frac{TP}{TP + FP} \qquad (7)$$

Specificity: A number of valid negative predictions divided by a total number of negatives is known as specificity.

$$\text{Specificity} = \frac{TN}{TN + FP} \qquad (8)$$

Recall: The recall is defined as a number of the positive predicted results out of the total positive cases, also known as Sensitivity and termed as the true positivity rate. It is measured by true positives which are divided by the sum of true predictions.

$$\text{Recall} = \frac{TP}{TP + FN} \qquad (9)$$

F1. Measure: The harmonic average of precision and recall is used to get the F1 score. To refresh your memory, the harmonic mean is indeed an alternative to the more commonly used arithmetic mean. When calculating an overall average, it is very useful.

$$\text{F1 Measure} = 2 \times \text{Precision} \times \text{Recall Precision} + \text{Recall} \qquad (10)$$

By using these performance measures, the loss and accuracy of the Resnet50 model calculated and accuracy on COVID-CT testing data are shown in Figure 3. This achieved accuracy is 93% on 100 sets of epochs and for this dataset. The COVIDNet dataset has 97 accuracies on the Resnet50 model which is shown in Figure 4.

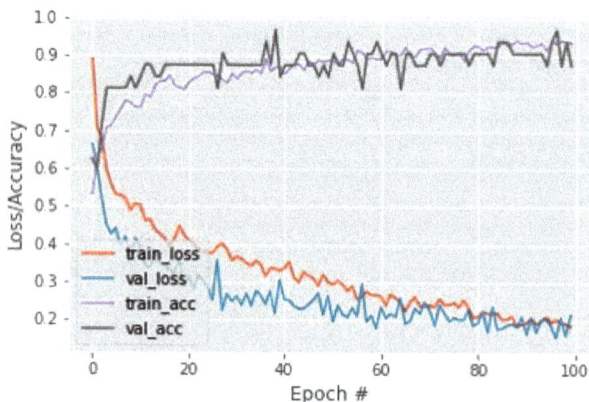

Figure 4. COVIDNet dataset training loss and accuracy.

The LIME interpretable model was used for the explainability of lung pulmonary disease COVID-19. After understanding the manifest info file of the COVID-CT dataset, we found some recurrence of the positive COVID CT images that is published in the 2020 International Journal. Figure 5 shows the region highlighted by the arrow by one of the verified doctors, and he describes the reasons that caused the COVID-19. This red arrow shows the multiple patchy ground-glass opacities in bilateral subpleural areas. These are the main features of the CT images that took part in the COVID-19 classification result.

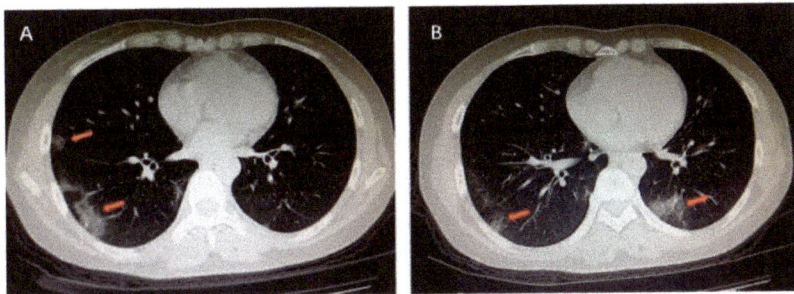

Figure 5. Multiple patchy glass ground opacities in bilateral subpleural areas (red arrow).

The main goal of this paper is to explain the same regions that are highlighted by the doctor after we classify the CT image as COVID. LIME took the same sample instance of the COVID-CT image and step-by-step process of the image as shown in Figure 6. First, it generates boundaries in the input image, finds the distance between the actual and predicted feature map, and generates the label. Then, it shows the distance using a heat map and highlights the region with color patches. These regions are the important feature that took part in the classification results.

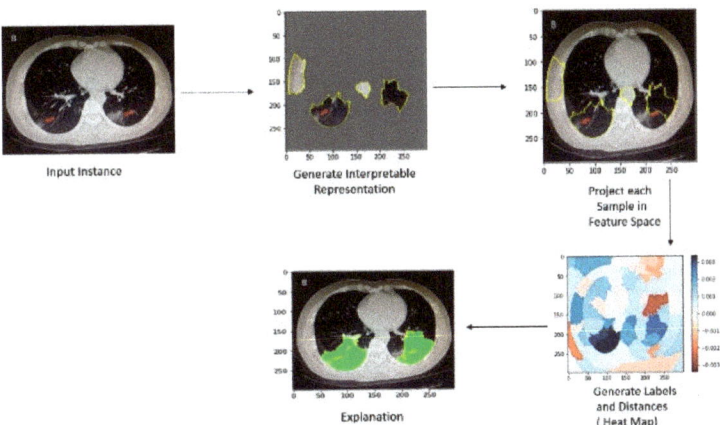

Figure 6. Explainability using LIME on CT-Image.

This research achieves the main goal using the LIME interpretable model. Further, results are evaluated using a recurrence image to verify model authenticity by cross validation of experts as shown in Figure 7.

4.3. Comparative Analysis

The qualitative and quantitative comparative analysis is conducted with the state-of-the-art methods. For quantitative analysis, we chose various state-of-the-art approaches for comparison that performed well on COVID-19 classification. Instead of analyzing each CXR image, we used the transfer learning approach to train the Resnet50 network on the entire CXR images. Meanwhile, COVID-CT and COVID-Net were used for the classification of COVID and NON-COVID. The results are shown in Table 6. We can view that our developed framework achieved the highest accuracy.

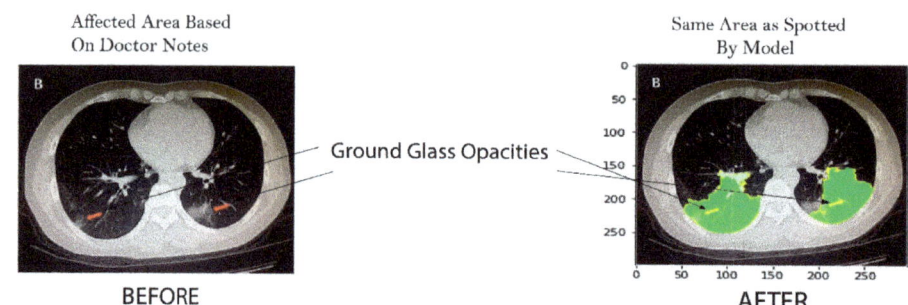

Figure 7. Before: Ground glass opacities highlighted by doctor, after: Same area highlighted by our model.

Along with its quantitative solid performance, the proposed model's explainability is also promising. To enhance the prediction to be more explainable, the activation maps are extracted by the developed method's explainable module, which we visualized in Figure 7. It can be seen that the proposed method would make a positive prediction by focusing on the most important section of the CXR image, which can be designated as the bilateral subpleural areas that show the ground glass opacities of the lungs. Furthermore, rather than focusing solely on the image's most important regions, we also consider the local regional contribution to the forecast. As previously stated, the input images were separated into many super-pixels, each of which had a similar visual pattern. This method highlighted those super-pixels in each image that greatly contributed to the prediction, and we can see that the regions with glass opacities are clearly highlighted for such a prediction. The comparative analysis of different XAI systems' clinical features is available in Table 7. This research selects more clinical features to be explained in the developed framework and provides greater explainability than the other available methods. In this research, the developed explainable AI framework provides an explanation of local and global features. As a result, it reveals that diseased areas can be easily identified using this system. The proposed method explains pulmonary disease identification that can be used as a valuable diagnostic tool for doctors.

Table 7. Clinical features analysis with XAI System.

XAI Methods	XAI Clinical Features	Agnostic or Specific	Global/Local
GSInquire [24]	Absorption Area	Specific	Local
SHAP, Grad-CAM++ [25]	Glass Opacities	Specific	Local
Grad-CAM, LIME [21]	Glass Opacities	Specific	Global
DeepCOVIDExplainer [29]	Lesion Dissipation	Agnostic	Local
Proposed XAI Model (LIME)	Lesion, Dissipation, Consolidation area, Absorption area, patchy Glass Shadow, Glass Opacities	Agnostic	Both

5. Conclusions

An explainable AI-based framework was proposed in this research to address the challenge of classification result explainability in the healthcare domain using medical images CXRs. This research presented a framework that provides the explainability of lung pulmonary diseases, i.e., edema, tuberculosis, nodules, pneumonia, and COVID-19 using chest radiographs. This research used CXRs data from the two datasets COVID-CT and COVIDNet to train the transfer-learning-based Resnet50 CNN model. This developed system achieved improved classification accuracies of 93% and 97% on both datasets. After classifying the pulmonary disease, this research further explains the classification results by using the interpretable LIME model. Our developed framework explains the classification results of the input CXRs image and highlights the region of the image that participates in the classification results. These highlighted regions are the important features that are used in the classification of diseases. After that, we evaluated our explanation results by a doctor-highlighted region image from the manifest file of the COVID-CT dataset and found that our model highlights the same ground glass opacities regions as those highlighted by the doctor. Evaluation and testing show that our approach can explain the classification results using chest radiographs. This automatic classification and explanation of lung pulmonary diseases can assist radiologists to detect and diagnose deadly lung diseases at an early stage.

Author Contributions: Z.N. and M.U.G.K. worked on this research work's conceptualization, methodology development, original draft and software. T.S. and A.R. provided their guidance in the results validation& analysis of the results, writing, review & edit. They also provided the formal analysis of the paper so that readers can learn about the algorithms used in the research. H.N. provided the data understanding, investigation, from the manifest file and helped to validate the results. S.A.B. provided the review, visualization, data curation and analysis. All authors have read and agreed to the published version of the manuscript.

Funding: This research received no external funding.

Institutional Review Board Statement: Not applicable.

Informed Consent Statement: Not applicable.

Data Availability Statement: Publicly available datasets were analyzed in this study. This data can be found here: http://arxiv.org/abs/2004.02060.

Acknowledgments: This research is technically supported by Artificial Intelligence & Data Analytics Lab (AIDA) CCIS Prince Sultan University, Riyadh, Saudi Arabia. Authors are thankful for the support.

Conflicts of Interest: The authors declare no conflict of interest.

References

1. Saba, T. Automated lung nodule detection and classification based on multiple classifiers voting. *Microsc. Res. Tech.* **2019**, *82*, 1601–1609. [CrossRef] [PubMed]
2. Centers for Disease Control and Prevention. *Pneumonia Can Be Prevented—Vaccines Can Help*; Centers for Disease Control and Prevention: Atlanta, GA, USA, 2012.
3. Saba, T.; Sameh, A.; Khan, F.; Shad, S.A.; Sharif, M. Lung nodule detection based on ensemble of hand crafted and deep features. *J. Med. Syst.* **2019**, *43*, 332. [CrossRef] [PubMed]
4. Wood, S.; Fuzaylov, G. Acute Pulmonary Edema Due to Occult Air Embolism Detected on an Automated Anesthesia Record: Illustrative Case. *J. Neurosurg. Case Lessons* **2021**, *1*, CASE2075. [CrossRef] [PubMed]
5. Kumar, V.; Abbas, A.K.; Aster, J.C. *Kumar: Robbins Basic Pathology*; Elsevier: Amsterdam, The Netherlands, 2017.
6. Haque, M.S.; Uddin, S.; Sayem, S.M.; Mohib, K.M. Coronavirus disease 2019 (COVID-19) induced waste scenario: A short overview. *J. Environ. Chem. Eng.* **2021**, *9*, 104660. [CrossRef] [PubMed]
7. Rehman, A.; Saba, T.; Tariq, U.; Ayesha, N. Deep learning-based COVID-19 detection using CT and X-ray images: Current analytics and comparisons. *IT Prof.* **2021**, *23*, 63–68. [CrossRef]
8. Javed, R.; Rahim, M.S.M.; Saba, T.; Rehman, A. A comparative study of features selection for skin lesion detection from dermoscopic images. *Netw. Model. Anal. Health Inform. Bioinform.* **2020**, *9*, 4. [CrossRef]
9. Besekar, S.M.; Sayed, S. The beneficial effect of Nintedanib in the COVID-19 Patient with the Complication of Idiopathic Pulmonary Fibrosis: A Case report. *Int. J. Case Rep. Health Sci.* **2022**, 12–18. Available online: http://ijcrhs.com/ijcrhs/article/view/3 (accessed on 10 August 2022).
10. Ksibi, A.; Zakariah, M.; Ayadi, M.; Elmannai, H.; Shukla, P.K.; Awal, H.; Hamdi, M. Improved Analysis of COVID-19 Influenced Pneumonia from the Chest X-Rays Using Fine-Tuned Residual Networks. *Comput. Intell. Neurosci.* **2022**, *2022*, 9414567. [CrossRef]
11. Abunadi, I.; Albraikan, A.A.; Alzahrani, J.S.; Eltahir, M.M.; Hilal, A.M.; Eldesouki, M.I.; Motwakel, A.; Yaseen, I. An Automated Glowworm Swarm Optimization with an Inception-Based Deep Convolutional Neural Network for COVID-19 Diagnosis and Classification. *Healthcare* **2022**, *10*, 697. [CrossRef]
12. Abunadi, I.; Senan, E.M. Multi-Method Diagnosis of Blood Microscopic Sample for Early Detection of Acute Lymphoblastic Leukemia Based on Deep Learning and Hybrid Techniques. *Sensors* **2022**, *22*, 1629. [CrossRef]
13. Pereira, R.M.; Bertolini, D.; Teixeira, L.O.; Silla, C.N.; Costa, Y.M.G. COVID-19 identification in chest X-ray images on flat and hierarchical classification scenarios. *Comput. Methods Programs Biomed.* **2020**, *194*, 105532. [CrossRef] [PubMed]

14. Lella, K.K.; Pja, A. Automatic diagnosis of COVID-19 disease using a deep convolutional neural network with multi-feature channel from respiratory sound data: Cough, voice, and breath. *Alex. Eng. J.* **2022**, *61*, 1319–1334. [CrossRef]
15. Hemdan, E.E.D.; El-Shafai, W.; Sayed, A. CR19: A framework for preliminary detection of COVID-19 in cough audio signals using machine learning algorithms for automated medical diagnosis applications. *J. Ambient. Intell. Humaniz. Comput.* **2022**, 1–13. [CrossRef] [PubMed]
16. Doornenbal, B.M.; Spisak, B.R.; van der Laken, P.A. Opening the black box: Uncovering the leader trait paradigm through machine learning. *Leadersh. Q.* **2022**, *33*, 101515. [CrossRef]
17. Khan, S.A.; Nazir, M.; Khan, M.A.; Saba, T.; Javed, K.; Rehman, A.; Akram, T.; Awais, M. Lungs nodule detection framework from computed tomography images using support vector machine. *Microsc. Res. Tech.* **2019**, *82*, 1256–1266. [CrossRef] [PubMed]
18. Ye, Q.; Xia, J.; Yang, G. Explainable AI for COVID-19 CT Classifiers: An Initial Comparison Study. In Proceedings of the 2021 IEEE 34th International Symposium on Computer-Based Medical Systems (CBMS), Aveiro, Portugal, 7–9 June 2021. Available online: https://ieeexplore.ieee.org/abstract/document/9474739/ (accessed on 2 August 2022).
19. Garg, P.K. Overview of Artificial Intelligence. In *Artificial Intelligence*; Chapman and Hall/CRC: London, UK, 2021; pp. 3–18. [CrossRef]
20. Yang, G.; Ye, Q.; Xia, J. Unbox the black-box for the medical explainable AI via multi-modal and multi-centre data fusion: A mini-review, two showcases and beyond. *Inf. Fusion* **2022**, *77*, 29–52. [CrossRef]
21. Das, A.; Rad, P. Opportunities and Challenges in Explainable Artificial Intelligence (XAI): A Survey. *arXiv* **2020**, arXiv:2006.11371. Available online: http://arxiv.org/abs/2006.11371 (accessed on 2 August 2022).
22. Rajpurkar, P.; Irvin, J.; Zhu, K.; Yang, B.; Mehta, H.; Duan, T.; Ding, D.; Bagul, A.; Langlotz, C.; Shpanskaya, K. Chexnet: Radiologist-Level Pneumonia Detection on Chest X-rays with Deep Learning. *arXiv* **2017**, arXiv:1711.05225. Available online: https://arxiv.org/abs/1711.05225 (accessed on 27 September 2022).
23. Sirshar, M.; Hassan, T.; Akram, M.U.; Khan, S.A. An incremental learning approach to automatically recognize pulmonary diseases from the multi-vendor chest radiographs. *Comput. Biol. Med.* **2021**, *134*, 104435. [CrossRef]
24. Teixeira, L.O.; Pereira, R.M.; Bertolini, D.; Oliveira, L.S.; Nanni, L.; Cavalcanti, G.D.; Costa, Y.M. Impact of Lung Segmentation on the Diagnosis and Explanation of COVID-19 in Chest X-ray Images. *Sensors* **2021**, *21*, 7116. [CrossRef]
25. Ribeiro, M.T.; Singh, S.; Guestrin, C. 'Why Should I Trust You?' Explaining the Predictions of Any Classifier. In Proceedings of the 22nd ACM SIGKDD International Conference on Knowledge Discovery and Data Mining, San Francisco, CA, USA, 13–17 August 2016. [CrossRef]
26. Ahsan, M.M.; Gupta, K.D.; Islam, M.M.; Sen, S.; Rahman, M.L.; Hossain, M.S. COVID-19 Symptoms Detection Based on NasNetMobile with Explainable AI Using Various Imaging Modalities. *Mach. Learn. Knowl. Extr.* **2020**, *2*, 490–504. [CrossRef]
27. Wang, L.; Lin, Z.Q.; Wong, A. COVID-Net: A tailored deep convolutional neural network design for detection of COVID-19 cases from chest X-ray images. *Sci. Rep.* **2020**, *10*, 19549. [CrossRef] [PubMed]
28. Zou, L.; Goh, H.L.; Liew, C.J.Y.; Quah, J.L.; Gu, G.T.; Chew, J.J.; Kumar, M.P.; Ang, C.G.L.; Ta, A. Ensemble image explainable AI (XAI) algorithm for severe community-acquired pneumonia and COVID-19 respiratory infections. *IEEE Trans. Artif. Intell.* **2022**, 1. [CrossRef]
29. Karim, M.R.; Dohmen, T.; Cochez, M.; Beyan, O.; Rebholz-Schuhmann, D.; Decker, S. DeepCOVIDExplainer: Explainable COVID-19 Diagnosis from Chest X-ray Images. In Proceedings of the 2020 IEEE International Conference on Bioinformatics and Biomedicine, BIBM 2020, Seoul, Republic of Korea, 16–19 December 2022; pp. 1034–1037. [CrossRef]
30. Yang, X.; He, X.; Zhao, J.; Zhang, Y.; Zhang, S.; Xie, P. COVID-CT-Dataset: A CT Scan Dataset about COVID-19. *arXiv* **2020**, arXiv:2003.13865. Available online: http://arxiv.org/abs/2003.13865 (accessed on 26 July 2022).
31. Hall, L.O.; Paul, R.; Goldgof, D.B.; Goldgof, G.M. Finding Covid-19 from Chest X-rays using Deep Learning on a Small Dataset. *arXiv* **2020**, arXiv:2004.02060. Available online: http://arxiv.org/abs/2004.02060 (accessed on 10 January 2022).
32. Pandit, M.K.; Banday, S.A. SARS n-CoV2-19 detection from chest x-ray images using deep neural networks. *Int. J. Pervasive Comput. Commun.* **2020**, *16*, 419–427. [CrossRef]
33. Singh, M.; Bansal, S.; Ahuja, S.; Dubey, R.K.; Panigrahi, B.K.; Dey, N. Transfer learning based ensemble support vector machine model for automated COVID-19 detection using lung computerized tomography scan data. *Med. Biol. Eng. Comput.* **2021**, *5*, 825–839. [CrossRef]
34. Mahmud, T.; Rahman, M.A.; Fattah, S.A. CovXNet: A multi-dilation convolutional neural network for automatic COVID-19 and other pneumonia detection from chest X-ray images with transferable multi-receptive feature optimization. *Comput. Biol. Med.* **2020**, *122*, 103869. [CrossRef]
35. Aleem, M.; Raj, R.; Khan, A. Comparative performance analysis of the ResNet backbones of Mask RCNN to segment the signs of COVID-19 in chest CT scans. *arXiv* **2020**, arXiv:2008.09713. Available online: http://arxiv.org/abs/2008.09713 (accessed on 10 January 2021).
36. Soin, K.S. Detection and Diagnosis of COVID-19 via SVM-Based Analyses of X-ray Images and Their Embeddings. 2020. Available online: www.ijisrt.com644 (accessed on 10 January 2021).

37. Pandit, M.; Banday, S.; Naaz, R.; Chishti, M. Automatic detection of COVID-19 from chest radiographs using deep learning. *Radiography* **2021**, *27*, 483–489. Available online: https://www.sciencedirect.com/science/article/pii/S1078817420302285 (accessed on 9 January 2021). [CrossRef]
38. Chen, D.; Xu, W.; Lei, Z.; Huang, Z.; Liu, J.; Gao, Z.; Peng, L. Recurrence of positive SARS-CoV-2 RNA in COVID-19: A case report. *Int. J. Infect. Dis.* **2020**, *93*, 297–299. [CrossRef] [PubMed]

Disclaimer/Publisher's Note: The statements, opinions and data contained in all publications are solely those of the individual author(s) and contributor(s) and not of MDPI and/or the editor(s). MDPI and/or the editor(s) disclaim responsibility for any injury to people or property resulting from any ideas, methods, instructions or products referred to in the content.

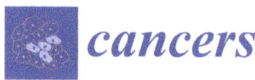

Article

Attention Cost-Sensitive Deep Learning-Based Approach for Skin Cancer Detection and Classification

Vinayakumar Ravi

Center for Artificial Intelligence, Prince Mohammad Bin Fahd University, Khobar 34754, Saudi Arabia; vravi@pmu.edu.sa

Simple Summary: According to skin disease reports by healthcare organizations, the number of cases of skin disease is growing gradually over the years globally. In skin disease diagnosis, dermatologists examine skin cells by using a dermatoscope. Due to the global shortage of expert dermatologists, mainly in developing countries, an accurate early skin disease diagnosis is not possible. To automate the examination of skin disease images, computer-aided diagnosis-based tools are used in healthcare and medical environments. Computer-aided diagnosis employs machine learning including deep learning models on skin disease images to detect and classify skin diseases. The present work proposes a deep learning-based model to accurately detect skin diseases and classify them into a family of skin diseases using skin disease images. The proposed system demonstrated a performance improvement of 4% accuracy for skin disease detection and 9% accuracy for skin disease classification compared to the existing deep learning-based models. The proposed computer-aided tool can be used as an early skin diagnosis tool to assist dermatologists in healthcare and medical environments.

Abstract: Deep learning-based models have been employed for the detection and classification of skin diseases through medical imaging. However, deep learning-based models are not effective for rare skin disease detection and classification. This is mainly due to the reason that rare skin disease has very a smaller number of data samples. Thus, the dataset will be highly imbalanced, and due to the bias in learning, most of the models give better performances. The deep learning models are not effective in detecting the affected tiny portions of skin disease in the overall regions of the image. This paper presents an attention-cost-sensitive deep learning-based feature fusion ensemble meta-classifier approach for skin cancer detection and classification. Cost weights are included in the deep learning models to handle the data imbalance during training. To effectively learn the optimal features from the affected tiny portions of skin image samples, attention is integrated into the deep learning models. The features from the finetuned models are extracted and the dimensionality of the features was further reduced by using a kernel-based principal component (KPCA) analysis. The reduced features of the deep learning-based finetuned models are fused and passed into ensemble meta-classifiers for skin disease detection and classification. The ensemble meta-classifier is a two-stage model. The first stage performs the prediction of skin disease and the second stage performs the classification by considering the prediction of the first stage as features. Detailed analysis of the proposed approach is demonstrated for both skin disease detection and skin disease classification. The proposed approach demonstrated an accuracy of 99% on skin disease detection and 99% on skin disease classification. In all the experimental settings, the proposed approach outperformed the existing methods and demonstrated a performance improvement of 4% accuracy for skin disease detection and 9% accuracy for skin disease classification. The proposed approach can be used as a computer-aided diagnosis (CAD) tool for the early diagnosis of skin cancer detection and classification in healthcare and medical environments. The tool can accurately detect skin diseases and classify the skin disease into their skin disease family.

Keywords: skin disease; deep learning; transfer learning; attention; cost-sensitive; meta-classifier

Citation: Ravi, V. Attention Cost-Sensitive Deep Learning-Based Approach for Skin Cancer Detection and Classification. *Cancers* **2022**, *14*, 5872. https://doi.org/10.3390/cancers14235872

Academic Editors: Muhammad Fazal Ijaz and Marcin Woźniak

Received: 10 November 2022
Accepted: 23 November 2022
Published: 29 November 2022

Publisher's Note: MDPI stays neutral with regard to jurisdictional claims in published maps and institutional affiliations.

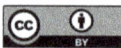

Copyright: © 2020 by the authors. Licensee MDPI, Basel, Switzerland. This article is an open access article distributed under the terms and conditions of the Creative Commons Attribution (CC BY) license (https://creativecommons.org/licenses/by/4.0/).

1. Introduction

In the present era, skin diseases are one of the leading infectious diseases among people globally. Skin diseases are common in fair-skinned populations. Skin diseases can be permanent or temporary and these are painless or painful. The number of cases of skin cancer has been high in the recent year in the United States and Australia [1]. In addition, the total cost involved in the treatment of skin diagnosis has been high compared to other cancers and this was reported by the government of Australia and the United States. A report by the Skin Cancer Foundation shows that the number of skin disease cases continues to increase worldwide in the future [2,3]. Dermoscopy is a non-invasive imaging technology that can examine skin lesions with a dermatoscope. This technology removes the surface reflection of the skin and obtains more informative visual information by going into deeper levels of the skin. This type of technology has enhanced the diagnosis of skin cancer detection and classification. In developing countries and in the world, the number of dermatologists is not sufficient, as skin diseases become high every year. Moreover, dermatologists need to be experts with good experience in achieving good accuracy otherwise the performance of dermatologists in accurately detecting skin disease will not be high [2]. There may be a possibility that the appearance of multiple skin diseases is similar and expert dermatologists' accuracy on similar multiple skin disease diagnoses will not be high.

To automate the diagnosis of skin lesion data samples, CAD tools were introduced [4]. CAD tools can be used for an early skin disease diagnosis. In the development of CAD-based tools, to automate the process of skin disease detection and classification, researchers employed various data mining and machine learning algorithms on the images of skin diseases [5]. Various feature engineering and feature selection approaches were investigated to accurately detect skin cancers by passing the features into various machine learning and data mining algorithms. The survey of skin disease detection and classification shows that there are various studies based on supervised, semi-supervised, and unsupervised approaches [3]. The performance of supervised-based methods is high compared to the semi-supervised and unsupervised approaches [6]. Thus, the current study considered the supervised-based approach to accurately detect skin diseases and classify them into their skin disease family. The major issue that exists in data mining and machine learning-based skin disease detection and classification is that the model's performance relies on optimal features [7]. These features are extracted manually and require a domain-level knowledge of image processing and skin diseases. This type of feature engineering and feature selection process is not easy. This may require more cost, and time complexity will be high. Most importantly, the attacker can compromise the CAD-based system if the features are known using the concepts available in the domain of adversarial machine learning. So, the machine learning-based CAD approach for skin disease detection and classification may not be completely considered robust in an adversarial environment, since the current healthcare system is connected to the internet and the healthcare networks and their connected devices are open to attacks. In addition to the performance of the model, the security of the model for skin disease detection and classification is important in the healthcare environment. In addition to the robustness of the model, the generalization of the model is important, i.e., there may be a possibility that the machine learning-based model may not work well for new skin diseases or the variants of the existing skin disease detection and classification.

A recent literature survey demonstrates that deep learning-based approaches were employed for skin disease detection and classification [8]. The deep learning-based approaches outperformed machine learning and data mining-based approaches in skin disease detection and classification, using samples of skin images. Various studies reported that the performance of deep learning is higher compared to the data mining and machine learning-based studies on benchmark data sets, i.e., the International Skin Imaging Collaboration (ISIC) archive. The studies have finetuned ImageNet-based pretrained models for skin disease detection and classification and reported that the finetuned model performances are higher compared to the non-finetuned models. In addition to that, the pretrained models require less time compared to the non-pretrained models. This is mainly due to the reason that the ImageNet-based pretrained models were trained with very big databases of natural images with several different classes. Though the medical images are different compared to natural images, the weights learned on natural images are finetuned with the medical images. This type of finetuned model shows better performances in various medical image classification tasks including skin disease detection and classification. The existing studies for skin disease classification using deep learning-based pretrained models used SoftMax at the last layer with a fully connected network for classification [3]. However, instead of using SoftMax, the features of the finetuned models can be further passed into other classical machine learning classifiers and this type of approach can be called a large-scale machine learning classifier. This type of classifier has the capability to show better performances compared to the SoftMax with a fully connected network. In addition to using one pretrained model for skin disease detection and classification, an ensemble of pretrained models can be employed. Since each pretrained model has the capability to extract its own features, there may be a possibility that ensemble-based models can enhance the performance of individual models. The survey shows that this type of ensemble approach demonstrates a better performance compared to the individual classifiers [5]. The classes in the benchmark datasets of skin diseases are highly imbalanced and most of the existing models for skin disease classification are not effective in handling rare skin diseases. In order to handle the data imbalance, authors have used data augmentation and Generative Adversarial Network (GAN)-based approaches. However, these are not effective in handling the data imbalance of skin diseases and though the studies reported good performances, there may be a possibility that the models may not perform well on the datasets that are from different modalities or patients from different regions. The proposed work's major contributions are given below

- The current work proposed an attention-cost-sensitive deep learning-based feature fusion ensemble meta-classifier approach for skin cancer detection and classification.
- Detailed investigation and analysis of convolutional neural network (CNN)-based pretrained model for skin disease detection and classification.
- Fusion of features from CNN-based pretrained models is proposed to enhance the performance for skin disease detection and skin disease classification.
- Attention is integrated into the CNN-based pretrained model to extract the optimal features to accurately detect skin diseases.
- Cost-weights are introduced during the training of a model to handle data imbalance in the skin disease dataset.
- To improve the performance of the SoftMax-based fully connected network classifiers, a two-stage classification model is proposed.
- Comparison of the proposed model with other CNN-based pretrained models and other existing studies.

The remaining parts of the paper are organized as follows. The literature survey of skin disease detection and classification is included in Section 2. Detailed information on the proposed method is discussed in Section 3. The description of datasets is included in Section 4 and statistical metrics are included in Section 5. Results and discussion of the proposed approach for skin disease detection and classification are included in Section 6. Finally, the conclusion and feature works are included in Section 7.

2. Literature Survey

Skin disease detection and its classification is a long-standing problem in the field of artificial intelligence. Prior to deep learning, various feature engineering methods were employed on the skin disease image database and further various classical machine learning algorithms were employed for skin disease detection and its skin disease family classification. However, with the recent surge of deep learning methods in performance improvement in various applications in medical imaging, the literature survey shows that methods of deep learning have been employed for skin disease identification and skin disease classification. The detailed literature survey summary of the existing methods for skin disease detection, skin disease classification, and available datasets for skin disease is discussed in detail by authors [2,3,5,8]. The literature survey shows that deep learning and artificial intelligence-based approaches outperform dermatologists' performance in accurately detecting skin diseases and classifying them into their skin disease family. However, there are various scenarios in which the best-performed model in the existing survey may not perform well. One such case study is rare skin diseases or skin diseases that have a smaller number of data samples. In addition to this, the performance of the models can be enhanced by adding clinical features. In this literature survey section, the existing works summary and its main limitations are discussed by comparing it with the proposed work.

The GoogleNet Inception v3 CNN architecture was employed for skin disease classification and its performances were evaluated against dermatologists against different test cases [9]. However, the model performances were not evaluated in detail and the models are not robust and generalizable. The ResNet50-based model was proposed for skin disease classification [10]. The model performances were assessed in different test cases with the involvement of healthcare and dermatologists. Though the proposed model achieved better performances compared to the existing methods, the models cannot be employed in a real-time environment, and in addition, this study cannot be considered for benchmarking the machine learning and deep learning models. The reason is the dataset was collected from different publically available sources and there may be overlapping of samples in training, validation, and testing datasets. This is one of the reasons the study reported good performances in all the test cases. Multichannel CNN with Gabor wavelet-based approach is proposed for skin disease classification [11]. The authors reported the performance of the proposed model by using ISIC 2017 datasets. Since the dataset is highly imbalanced, the proposed method's detailed study of handling rare skin diseases is required. Without this, the proposed method may not be considered robust for skin disease classification. In addition to that, the authors have considered only a smaller number of classes from the dataset, mainly the performance of the study demonstrated for melanoma skin disease. A hybrid of classical image processing feature engineering, clinical features, and automated feature engineering using ResNet-50 models is proposed for skin disease classification [12]. The performances of the proposed study were demonstrated on the datasets NIH SBIR dermoscopy studies and ISIC 2018. Though the model reported better performances on both datasets, the authors did not show the performance of the proposed model in handling rare skin diseases.

To develop a generalized skin disease classification model, the authors adopted the domain adaptation deep learning approach using CycleGAN and its performance shown on the HAM10000 dataset [13]. The proposed model is generalized, and its experiments and results reported by the authors show that the model was able to classify the skin disease samples by handling different cohorts with different shifts. The patch-based attention approach is proposed for skin disease classification [14]. To handle the data imbalance after patching the skin disease samples, the proposed approach uses various cost-sensitive approaches. The authors report that the proposed approach performs better than the existing methods and handles data imbalances during training. The performance of the methods was shown on more than one skin disease dataset, including the HAM10000 dataset. CNN-based approach with a novel optimizer-based approach is proposed for skin disease classification using the ISIC skin disease dataset [15]. However, the authors did not demonstrate a detailed analysis of the proposed model to identify the robustness and generalization to accurately detect skin diseases. In [16], the authors used the support of binary classification and enhanced the performance of the GoogLeNet and Inception-v3 model by 7% in skin disease classification with seven classes. The proposed model is not effective in an imbalanced skin disease database, and in addition, the model is not effective in extracting the tiny portions of the infected region from the overall skin image. To increase the number of data samples for rare skin diseases, StyleGANs approach is employed. Later, the authors developed a method for skin disease classification by fusing the CNN-based pretrained models. Though the proposed method alleviates the data samples for rare skin diseases, the proposed StyleGANs may not generate samples that are similar to the samples collected from the patients in real time. This type of GAN-based approach may not be considered accurate to handle rare skin diseases.

A fusion of handcrafted features and automated features from a CNN-based deep learning model was used in accurately detecting skin diseases [17]. Since the proposed model depends on hand-crafted feature engineering, the model time complexity is high and this type of approach may not be appropriate in a real-time skin-disease classification system in the healthcare environment. This is because deep learning itself can identify the optimal features and in addition to this, segmentation using deep learning can be incorporated. A two-stage approach was proposed for skin disease classification [18]. The first stage does the segmentation and classification of the segmented data classified in the classification stage. The authors employed fully resolution CNN in the first stage for segmentation and Inception-v3, ResNet-50, Inception-ResNet-v2, and DenseNet-201 for classification. The authors have conducted a detailed study using ISIC 2016, 2017, and 2018 datasets. The rare disease in ISIC datasets is handled using augmentation. However, the data augmentation approach may not be the right approach to handle the data imbalance and the literature survey on data augmentation shows that it cannot improve the performance of rare skin diseases. To handle various image sizes of skin disease, the authors have proposed a multiscale model with an ensemble of more than one CNN-based pretrained model for skin disease classification [19]. The proposed approach performances are demonstrated on the ISIC 2017 and 2018 datasets. Since the proposed approach is cost-insensitive, the model performance may not be considered good in the rare skin disease classification. With the aim to handle rare skin diseases in the ISIC 2018 dataset, the authors proposed a GAN-based approach for data augmentation and CNN for classification [20]. The authors reported that the GAN-based data augmentation approach with CNN performed better than the CNN. Data augmentation is not the right approach to handle the imbalance in the skin disease data sets. It may be possible that the GAN-based generated images are not entirely new samples and there will be a bias in learning.

The authors reported 7% improvement in accuracy by using clinical information along with a skin disease image database [21]. This database is a privately collected dataset using a phone camera. The dataset is balanced and moreover, there may be bias in training and testing datasets. Since the authors have not demonstrated the datasets of training and testing collected in different healthcare environments with different patients, the proposed approach may not be considered robust for skin disease classification. An ensemble of various pretrained model performances was shown for skin disease classification using the ISIC 2018 dataset [22]. The proposed model may not be effective in achieving good performance in classifying the rare disease as the proposed method is not giving any kind of importance to the minor classes of skin disease during the training of an ensemble model. To detect skin disease accurately, segmentation was employed before the classification [23]. The authors compared the proposed segmentation approach performance with U-Net, and in all the test cases, the proposed approach demonstrated better performances. The performance of CNN and other classical machine learning models' performances were demonstrated for classification. With several test cases, authors have demonstrated that the proposed model shows better performances compared to the existing approaches using the ISIC 2018 skin disease dataset. Though the proposed model is robust in accurately detecting skin diseases, the authors did not show the proposed method's performance in handling rare skin diseases. A fusion of CNN-based pretrained models was proposed for skin disease classification [24]. The performance of the proposed models was evaluated on the ISIC 2016 dataset. The authors report that the fused model demonstrates better performances in detecting skin disease compared to the non-fused and existing studies. However, the detailed performance of the proposed study is not evaluated on ISIC 2016. Since the dataset is highly imbalanced, it may be possible that the bias existed during learning a skin disease model in training. The ResNeXt101-based model is evaluated for multi-class skin disease classification using the HAM10000 dataset [25]. The authors reported that the proposed model performed better than the non-pretrained and pretrained models. However, the detailed performance of the proposed model is not shown for handling rare skin diseases.

A 34-layer residual network-based approach is proposed for skin disease classification using the HAM10000 dataset [26]. The performance of the proposed approach is evaluated in various clinical settings and the authors reported that the proposed approach performs better than the existing methods, and in some test cases outperforms the dermatologists. However, the robustness and generalizability of the proposed approach are not shown in detail for skin disease classification. A decision fusion of GoogleNet, ResNet-101, and NasNet-Large is proposed and its performances are shown on the skin disease classification using the ISIC 2019 dataset [27]. The proposed method demonstrated better performances compared to the related existing methods. However, the detailed evaluation and analysis of the proposed method are not evaluated on rare skin disease classification. The inception-v4-based model was proposed for skin disease classification [28]. The model uses a hybrid of clinical features and images of skin disease and classifies the patient skin samples into 27 classes. The model performance on rare skin diseases is required to understand the robustness of the proposed method in handling the imbalanced data set of skin diseases. ResNet152 and InceptionResNet-V2 with a triplet loss-based approach were proposed for identifying the skin disease and their performance was shown on a publically available dataset [29]. The authors demonstrate that the method performed well compared to the other methods, however, the detailed performance of the method is not demonstrated for rare skin diseases or the minority classes of skin diseases. CNN-based model is proposed for skin disease classification. The proposed model supports the multi-class skin disease classification [30]. The performance of the proposed model is shown on the datasets of ISIC-17, ISIC-18, and ISIC-19. These three datasets are well-known datasets and are used for benchmarking the models of machine learning and deep learning in detecting skin disease and classifying the detected skin disease to its skin disease family. All of these three datasets are highly imbalanced, such as, some skin disease are rare, and contain a smaller number of data samples. This may be one of the reasons that the proposed method reports good performances even by using a non-pretrained CNN model. To handle rare skin diseases, an attention-based GAN deep learning approach is proposed [31]. The authors demonstrate that the proposed method generates skin disease samples that are from different distributions and it is considered to be more effective than data augmentation. However, even though the attention-based GAN has the capability to generate skin disease samples from different distributions, the generated sample may not be the same as the data samples collected from patients in real time.

The authors propose a three-stage approach for skin disease classification [32]. The first stage employs MaskRCNN for segmentation and feature extraction using DenseNet in the second stage and classification using a support vector machine (SVM). The proposed model performances are demonstrated on the datasets of ISBI2016, ISBI2017, and HAM10000. The experiments reported in the paper demonstrate that the proposed model achieves better performances compared to the existing models. The proposed model is computationally expensive and in addition, the proposed model performances are not shown in detail for rare skin diseases. DenseNet201 network-based approach is proposed for skin disease classification using HAM10000 dataset [33]. The proposed method demonstrated better performances compared to the existing non-pretrained models. The authors did not show detailed experiments on the generalization and robustness of the proposed method in skin disease classification. A hybrid of MobileNet V2 and the long short-term memory (LSTM)-based approach is proposed for skin disease classification [34]. This method has outperformed the existing methods by showing more than 85% accuracy on the HAM10000 dataset. The robustness and generalizability of the proposed method for skin disease classification are not discussed in detail. The authors have demonstrated that the CNN-based model performance is similar to the performance obtained from clinical experts [35]. However, the authors did not show a detailed analysis of the proposed approach in different experimental settings. Thus, the proposed method cannot be considered robust and accurate. The summary of the existing works on skin disease detection and skin disease classification is summarized in Table 1.

Table 1. Summary of existing methods for skin disease classification.

Reference	Methodology	Dataset	Pretrained Model	Effective for Class Imbalance	Accuracy	Attention	Large-Scale Learning	Feature Fusion
[9]	GoogleNet Inception v3	ISIC Archive	Yes	No	93.3%	No	No	No
[10]	ResNet50	ISIC Archive	Yes	No	82%	No	No	No
[11]	CNN	ISIC 2017	Yes	No	83%	No	No	No
[12]	ResNet-50	ISIC 2018	Yes	No	94%	No	No	Yes
[13]	ResNet-152	HAM10000	Yes	No	92%	No	No	No
[14]	SE-Resnext50	HAM10000	Yes	Yes	-	Yes	No	Yes
[15]	CNN	ISIC Archive	No	No	97.49	No	No	No
[16]	GoogLeNet Inception-v3	ISIC 2018	Yes	No	67–73%	No	No	No
[36]	VGG, ResNet, AlexNet	ISIC 2019	Yes	No	95%	No	No	No
[17]	VGG, ResNET-50, Inception, MobileNet, DenseNet, Xception	ISIC 2018	Yes	No	92.4	No	Yes	Yes
[18]	Inception, ResNet	ISIC 2016, 2017, and 2018	Yes	No	81.79	No	No	No
[19]	EfficientNet	ISIC 2016, ISIC 2017	Yes	No	86.2%	No	No	Yes
[20]	ResNet	ISIC 2018	Yes	No	95.2	Yes	No	No
[21]	ResNet	Private dataset	Yes	No	79%	No	No	No
[22]	EfficientNet, ResNet	ISIC 2019	Yes	No	-	No	No	No
[23]	CNN and Naïve Bayes	ISIC Archive	No	No	93.6%	No	Yes	No
[24]	VGG ResNet DenseNet	ISIC 2018	Yes	Yes	87.06%	No	Yes	Yes
[25]	ResNeXt101	HAM 10000	Yes	No	92.83%	No	No	No
[26]	ResNet	HAM 10000	Yes	No	80–90%	No	No	No
[27]	GoogleNet, ResNet-101, & NasNet-Large	ISIC 2019	Yes	No	89%	No	No	Yes
[28]	Inception	Private dataset	Yes	No	70–75%	No	No	No
[35]	CNN	Private dataset	No	No	-	No	No	No
[29]	ResNet152 and InceptionResNet-V2	Private dataset	Yes	No	87.42	No	No	No
[30]	CNN	ISIC 2017 ISIC 2018 ISIC 2019	No	No	85–90%	No	No	No
[31]	ResNet	ISIC 2018	Yes	Yes	70.1%	Yes	No	No
[32]	DenseNet	ISBI 2016 ISBI 2017 HAM10000	Yes	No	93.6%	No	Yes	No
[33]	DenseNet	HAM10000	Yes	No	96.18	No	No	No
[34]	MobileNet	HAM10000	Yes	No	85%	No	Yes	No
Proposed	EfficientNetV2B0, EfficientNetV2B1, & EfficientNetV2B2	HAM10000, ISIC Archive	Yes	Yes	99%	Yes	Yes	Yes

The detailed literature survey of the aforementioned works shows that ImageNet-based pretrained models are employed for skin disease detection and its family classification with the aim to enhance the performance of non-pretrained models. However, the existing studies on skin disease databases demonstrate that the available standard database in the literature is highly imbalanced, and also, some skin diseases are rare. As a result, rare skin diseases contain very a much smaller number of data samples. Thus, the existing models are not accurate in predicting this rare skin disease and the existing models are highly dominant to the skin disease that are common and have a very high number of data samples. In a skin image database, the disease is a tiny portion of the overall skin image and it may be possible that the existing study might miss this type of important tiny region in accurately identifying the skin disease. Even though the CNN-based models have the capability to extract the important regions from the skin disease image, extraction of important and optimal features from the infected region in the overall image is limited by the CNN-based pretrained models. In addition, each CNN-based pretrained models have the capability to extract its own features to accurately identify the skin disease and classify the skin disease to its family. The features are unique and disjoint from each other. In the proposed work, cost-sensitive learning is introduced to the CNN-based pretrained model to avoid bias in learning during training, and equal importance is given to all the classes of skin disease. The various EfficientNetV2-based pretrained models were extracted and further, the dimension of the feature was reduced using the dimensionality reduction approach, i.e., PCA. Further, the features are combined and passed into the meta-classifier for skin disease detection and skin disease classification. The stacked classifier is a two-level approach; the first level includes the random forest (RFTree) and SVM for the prediction of skin disease, and later these predictions were classified accurately using the logistic regression in the second level.

3. Proposed Methodology for Skin Cancer Detection and Classification

The proposed methodology for skin disease detection and skin disease classification is shown in Figure 1. The details of the proposed architecture are given below.

The skin images of patients are preprocessed in the input layer. The preprocessing includes transforming the dimension of the image into input dimensions of the CNN-based pretrained model. After reading the image data, the data are transformed into the [0–1] range by applying normalization.

The existing literature survey shows that the CNN-based pretrained models have been employed for skin disease detection and classification. The pretrained models of the ImageNet database are finetuned on the skin image database. This type of finetuned model has demonstrated better performances compared to the non-finetuned models. This work employs various CNN-based pretrained models for skin disease detection and classification. The pretrained models considered in this work are Xception, VGG16, MobileNet, ResNet50, InceptionV3, DenseNet121, EfficientNetB0, EfficientNetV2B0, EfficientNetV2B1, and EfficientNetV2B2. All these models have an input layer, more than one hidden layer, and a classification layer. In the hidden layer, the pretrained models contain more than one convolution layer, pooling layer, and fully connected layers. Between the convolution and fully connected layers, the model contains batch normalization and dropout layers.

The current work employs EfficientNetV2 model for skin disease detection and classification. EfficientNetV2 model is a pretrained model on the ImageNet database. This database contains 1000 classes of natural images and the models have learned a rich feature representation by training a model using a very big image database. In this work, the EfficientNetV2 pretrained model is finetuned on skin disease detection with two classes by replacing the last layer of the EfficientNetV2 pretrained model and skin disease classification with seven classes by replacing the last layer of the EfficientNetV2 pretrained model.

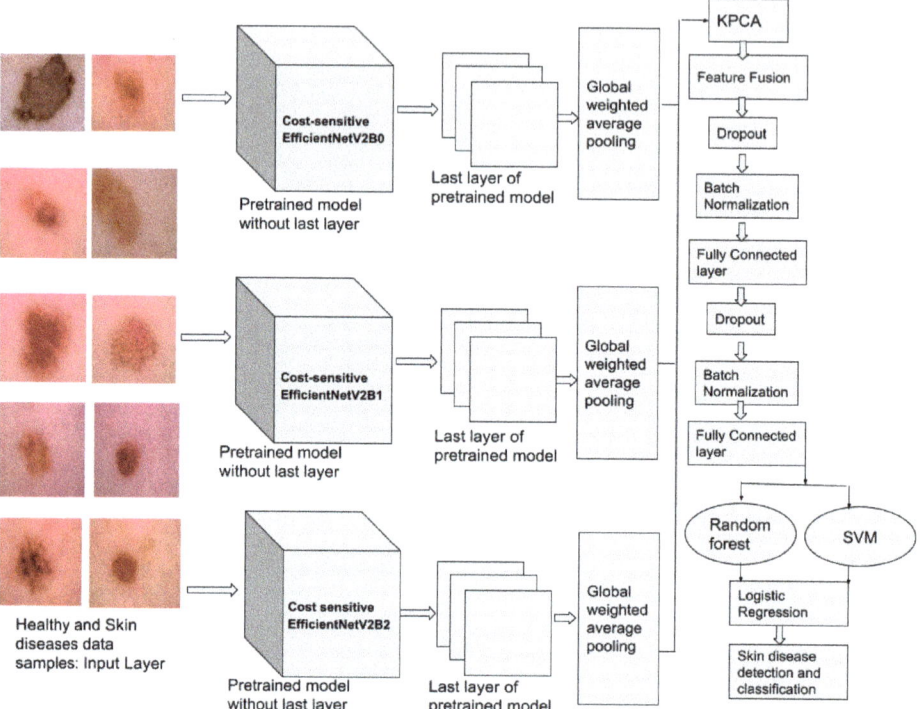

Figure 1. Proposed methodology for skin disease detection and skin disease classification.

Recent years' work demonstrates that many experiments carried out by researchers find out the efficient CNN architecture in deep learning. The architecture maintains a balance among accuracy, speed, FLOPs, etc. For example, to improve the performance of the model with better accuracy, DenseNet and EfficientNet model were introduced. The same authors of EfficienNet architecture studied the limitations of the EfficientNet architecture and developed a new architecture called EfficientNetV2. EfficientNetV2 is a family of models such as EfficientNetV2B0, EfficientNetV2B1, EfficientNetV2B2, EfficientNetV2B3, EfficientNetV2S, EfficientNetV2M, and EfficientNetV2L. In EfficientNetV2 architecture, the authors developed techniques to improve the model performances with a smaller number of parameters and improve the model inference time. The authors included the following techniques in EfficientNetV2:

- Neural architecture search (NAS): To find optimal parameters and model design, the authors employ random search and reinforcement learning techniques.
- Scaling: Authors have employed the compound scaling rule of the EfficientNet model. However, the modification was conducted to the compound scaling scheme to avoid memory issues due to the increase in the size of the image.
- Training: Authors employ new regularization methods, and training model guidelines to improve the efficiency during training of an EfficeienNetV2 model.
- Progressive learning: The training of the model is accelerated by progressively increasing the size of the image.
- Convolutions and their building blocks: The EfficientNetV2 models use various types of convolutions, mainly Fused-MB Conv instead of MB Conv. The detailed architecture information of Fused-MB Conv and MB Conv is shown in Figure 2.

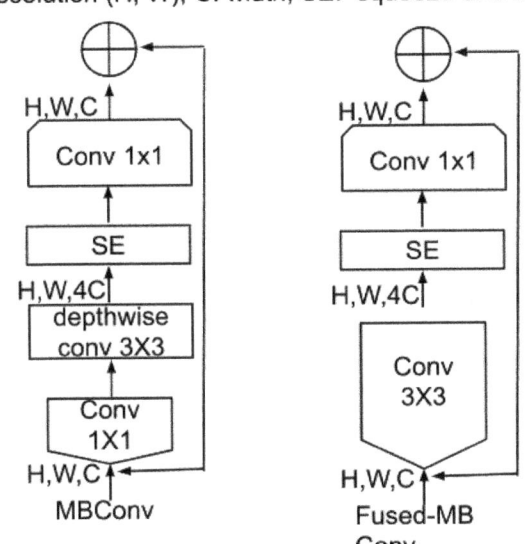

Figure 2. Architecture of MBConv and Fused-MBConv.

The above-modified methods make the EfficientNetV2 model achieve better performance by increasing the speed during training a model compared to EfficientNet models ranging from B0 to B7.

Since the CNN-based pretrained models are ineffective in handling the imbalanced datasets, the current work integrates a cost-sensitive learning approach for CNN-based pretrained models. During backpropogation, the current work follows an algorithmic approach to include the misclassification costs to handle the bias in the training of a model. The skin disease sample of patient S is connected with a cost item $[C[class(S), t]$, where $class(S)$ and t are the actual and predicted class, respectively. The current work assigns less cost to the classes that contain more data samples and high cost to the classes that contain a lesser number of skin disease data samples. Since the values of the cost matrix are empty at the beginning, the current work follows the Gaussian distribution to assign the values for the cost matrix. These values in the cost matrix are finetuned across epochs. The loss function for cost-insensitive CNN-based pretrained models is defined as

$$J = - \sum_{s \in samples} \sum_{n} t^n \log pred^n \qquad (1)$$

The loss function for the cost-sensitive model is given below:

$$J = - \sum_{s \in samples} \sum_{n} t^n \log pred^n C[class(s), n] \qquad (2)$$

where S is a loss function, $pred^n$ denotes the predicted output of the nth output neuron, t^n is the target value, $C[class(s), n]$ denotes the cost with $class(s)$ and is the exact value of sample s, and n is the predicted class of sample s.

The EfficientNetV2 models such as EfficientNetV2B0, EfficientNetV2B1, and EfficientNetV2B2 networks contain more than one convolutional layer and pooling layers followed by a series of fully connected layers. There may be a possibility that passing the high-dimensional feature representation learned from the series of a convolutional and pooling layer to a fully connected layer results in overfitting and hinders the model's generalization ability. Since more than one fully connected layer is involved at the end of the networks before classification, dropout and regularization layers are required. There may be a possibility that the dropout and regularization layers result in the loss of important features. To overcome the series of fully connected layers with dropout and regularization layers, in this work, instead of passing the extracted features from finetuned model to global average pooling, the current work sends the extracted features to an attention layer. Global average pooling is a simple approach that estimates the average output of each feature map in the previous layer. Since some of the features are more important than others in each feature map of the previous layer, an attention mechanism is introduced that turns pixels in the GAP on or off. Next, rescale results on the number of pixels. The attention approach employed in this work is similar to global weighted average pooling. Since the dimensionality of the features of the finetuned model is high, KPCA is used. This helps to reduce the dimension of the features. KPCA is an improved version of PCA. It employs a kernel that allows projecting the data onto a higher dimensional space where the data points become linearly separable. Though there are many types of kernels available, this work employs the Radial basis function (rbf). This is mainly due to the reason that the data samples of skin disease are highly non-linearly separable. This is mainly due to the reason that the skin disease is very similar to each other. There may be a possibility that other kernels might perform better than the rbf kernel. Thus, a detailed analysis of the importance of kernel and other hyperparameters of KPCA will be considered as future work. The reduced feature representation of EfficientNetV0, EfficientNetV1, and EfficientNetV2 are fused. Since there are many advanced feature fusion methods available in the literature, employing them in the current work to learn better feature representation to accurately detect skin disease and classify them into their skin disease family will be considered as one of the significant directions toward future work. Further, the reduced features were passed into the ensemble meta-classifier.

The meta-classifier is a two-stage classifier, the first stage contains SVM and RFTree for prediction and the second stage contains the logistic regression for classification. SVM is a kernel-based machine learning algorithm used for solving problems related to classification and regression. SVM considers each data point in skin disease data samples in an n-dimensional plane and partitions them into two classes. The hyperplane line is selected based on the maximum margin among the two classes' data points to distinguish the two classes. The selection of the kernel plays an important role in achieving good performance. The most commonly used kernels are rbf, linear, and poly. RFTree randomly constructs multiple decision trees and applies the input datasets. The output classification of each decision tree is considered to perform the ensemble learning to determine the final output. One of the well-known ensemble methods used in classification is the maximum number of RFTree trees voted for any particular class, considered as the outcome of the given input. Logistic regression is the probability modeling of the outcome given an input variable. Logical regression can be used for solving binary or multi-class problems. The logistic function will be a Sigmoid function taking any input value and classifying it as 0 or 1 for the binary classification of skin diseases. These machine learning classifiers are used in our framework to perform the ensemble meta-classifier-based feature fusion skin disease detection and classification. The SVM, RFTree, and logistic regression classifiers have parameters. The optimal performance depends on the parameters. This work has run several trials of experiments to identify the best parameters for SVM, RFTree, and logistic regression. The best parameters for SVM are tolerance = 0.0001, max iter = 5000, kernel = linear, and regularization parameter C = 1.0. The important parameters and the values of RFTree are n_estimators = 100 and max depth = 200. For both SVM and RFTree, random_state is set to 50. In logistic regression, tolerance, max_iter, and c is set to 0.0001, 100, and 1.0, respectively.

The steps involved in skin disease detection and skin disease classification using the proposed model are shown in Algorithm 1. Skin disease and Healthy samples are inputs to the proposed model and after that, the images are passed through several hidden layers to extract the features to recognize skin diseases. Finally, the proposed model outputs the label for the skin samples as either Healthy or Malignant in skin disease detection, and in the case of skin disease classification, the skin samples are classified into corresponding skin disease families.

Algorithm 1: Skin disease detection and classification.

Input: A set of Healthy and skin disease color images $img_1, img_2,..., img_n$.
Output: Labels $y_1, y_2,..., y_n$.
for *each color image img_i* **do**

    // EfficientNetV2B0 architecture
    feature maps $Fm0$ = ConvolutionalLayers(img_i);
    gwap features $G0$ = GlobalWeightedAveragePooling($Fm0$);

    // EfficientNetV2B1 architecture
    feature maps $Fm1$ = ConvolutionalLayers(img_i);
    gwap features $G1$ = GlobalWeightedAveragePooling($Fm1$);

    // EfficientNetV2B2 architecture
    feature maps $Fm2$ = ConvolutionalLayers(img_i);
    gwap features $G2$ = GlobalWeightedAveragePooling($Fm2$);

    // Dimensionality reduction
    reduced features $RFB0$ = KPCA($G0$);
    reduced features $RFB1$ = KPCA($G1$);
    reduced features $RFB2$ = KPCA($G2$);

    // Feature Fusion
    fused features $FF = RFB0 + RFB1 + RFB2$;

    // Ensemble meta-level classifier
    // Stage 1: Base-level classifiers
    prediction P_1 = SVM(FF);
    prediction P_2 = RandomForestClassifier(FF);

    // Stage 2: Meta-level classifier
    Compute y_i = LogisticRegression(P_1, P_2);
    // Skin disease detection
    y_i: 0 (Healthy) and y_i: 1 (Skin disease);
    // Skin disease classification
    y_i: 0 (Melanocytic nevi), y_i: 1 (Melanoma), y_i: 2 (Benign keratosis-like lesions), y_i: 3 (Basal cell carcinoma), y_i: 4 (Actinic keratoses), y_i: 5 (Vascular lesions), y_i: 6 (Dermatofibroma);

end

The proposed model takes skin disease image samples as input and outputs a value as either skin disease or healthy. Further, the model classifies the detected skin disease into its skin disease family.

4. Description of Datasets

The detailed statistics of skin diseases databases used in skin disease detection and skin disease classification are provided in Tables 2 and 3, respectively. The data statistics show that the datasets are highly imbalanced. Without the proper handling of this type of dataset during training a model, there may be a possibility that due to bias, the models demonstrate better accuracy. The models might not learn better feature representation of the minority classes of skin diseases. To avoid this, the current work assigns the higher cost weights for the minority classes and lower-cost weights for the majority classes of skin disease during training a model. This type of assignment of cost-weights during training a model helps to avoid bias and gives importance to all skin diseases.

Skin disease samples of Healthy and Malignant are shown in Figure 3. These images are randomly chosen from the skin disease detection dataset. The images for skin disease detection are taken from the publicly available data repository, the ISIC archive. The images shown in Figure 3 demonstrate that the skin samples, both healthy and malignant, have higher intra-class and inter-class similarity. Since most of the samples of healthy and malignant look similar, there may be a chance that misclassification can be performed by the dermatologists. The chances of misclassification rate are very high. To avoid this, this work proposed a CAD-based tool by using an advanced deep learning approach with meta-classifier learning that extract the optimal features to accurately discriminate between the healthy and malignant.

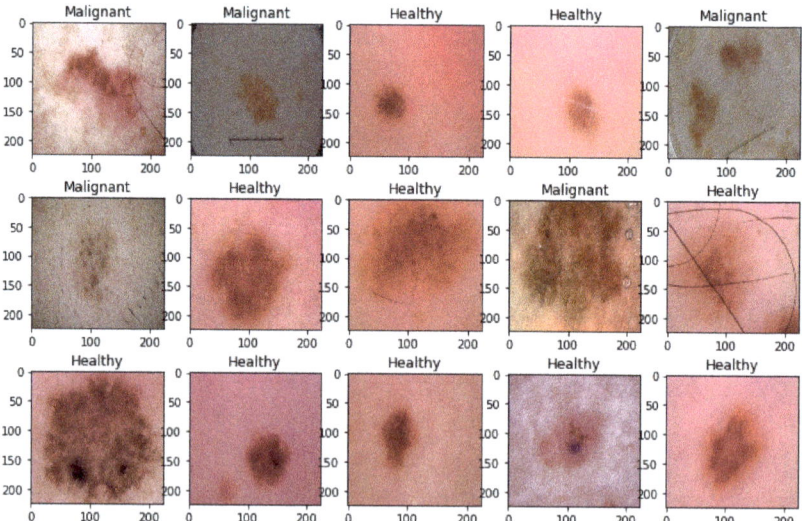

Figure 3. Skin image samples of healthy and malignant from skin disease dataset.

A benchmark dataset for the development of CAD-based tools provided by the ISIC. The HAM10000 ("Human Against Machine with 10000 training images") skin disease dataset is publicly available in the ISIC archive. The HAM10000 dataset is considered to be one of the well-known datasets and it is used in many studies to benchmark the machine learning and deep learning models for skin disease detection and skin disease classification. This dataset was collected from different populations with different modalities. Patients are from both male and female groups and most patients' ages are in the range of 30 to 44. The data of skin disease classification shows that the skin disease increases with the increase in the age. Skin diseases are less for children aged less than 10. Skin diseases are most prominent if males are compared to females according to the skin disease classification dataset i.e., HAM10000. The most found skin disease among people is melanocytic nevi and the least found is dermatofibroma. Skin diseases are taken from the different regions of the body. The regions are the back, lower extremity, trunk, upper extremity, abdomen, face, chest, foot, neck, scalp, hand, ear, genital, and sacral. Most patients are affected by skin disease in the back region and it is most prominent in men. Benign keratosis-like lesions are affected in the region face and Melanocytic nevi are affected in body parts of the patients except for the face. Melanocytic nevi diseases are the most prominent skin disease in the age group between 0–75. People aged 80–90 are affected more by Benign keratosis lesions. Skin disease in HAM10000 datasets is discovered by using histopathology (53.3%), follow-up examination (37.0%), expert consensus (9.0%), and confirmation by in-vivo confocal microscopy (0.7%). The samples were taken from different places in the patient's body. This dataset is composed of 10,015 dermatoscopic images. The ground truth of the images is conducted by expert pathologists and medical experts. The images in the HAM10000 dataset were collected from the Department of Dermatology at the Medical University of Vienna, Austria, and Cliff Rosendahl in Queensland, Australia for a time period of around 20 years. Thus, the database is good and contains skin patient samples for various skin diseases. The images in HAM10000 are from seven different skin diseases. The detailed information on skin diseases and the technology involved in the database creation is discussed in detail by the authors [37].

Table 2. Statistics of skin disease detection dataset.

Class	Training	Testing	Total
Healthy	1440	360	1800
Malignant or Skin Cancer	1197	360	1557
Total	2637	720	3357

Table 3. Statistics of skin disease classification dataset.

Class	Training	Testing	Total
Melanocytic nevi (nv)	6034	671	6705
Melanoma (mel)	1005	108	1113
Benign keratosis-like lesions (bkl)	989	110	1099
Basal cell carcinoma (bcc)	463	51	514
Actinic keratoses (akiec)	290	37	327
Vascular lesions (vasc)	130	12	142
Dermatofibroma (df)	102	13	115
Total	9013	1002	10,015

The samples of healthy and skin disease samples are shown in Figure 3. Skin disease samples of seven classes are shown in Figure 4. As shown in Figures 3 and 4, the samples belonging to various classes in both datasets of skin disease detection, skin disease classification are similar and they have high intra-class and inter-class variance. In addition to that, the tiny affected region is important in accurately detecting and classifying the skin disease to its family of skin diseases. There may be a possibility that the CNN-based models might not give importance to these tiny regions. To avoid this, the current work integrates attention to the CNN architecture that can focus on the infected regions in the skin disease image.

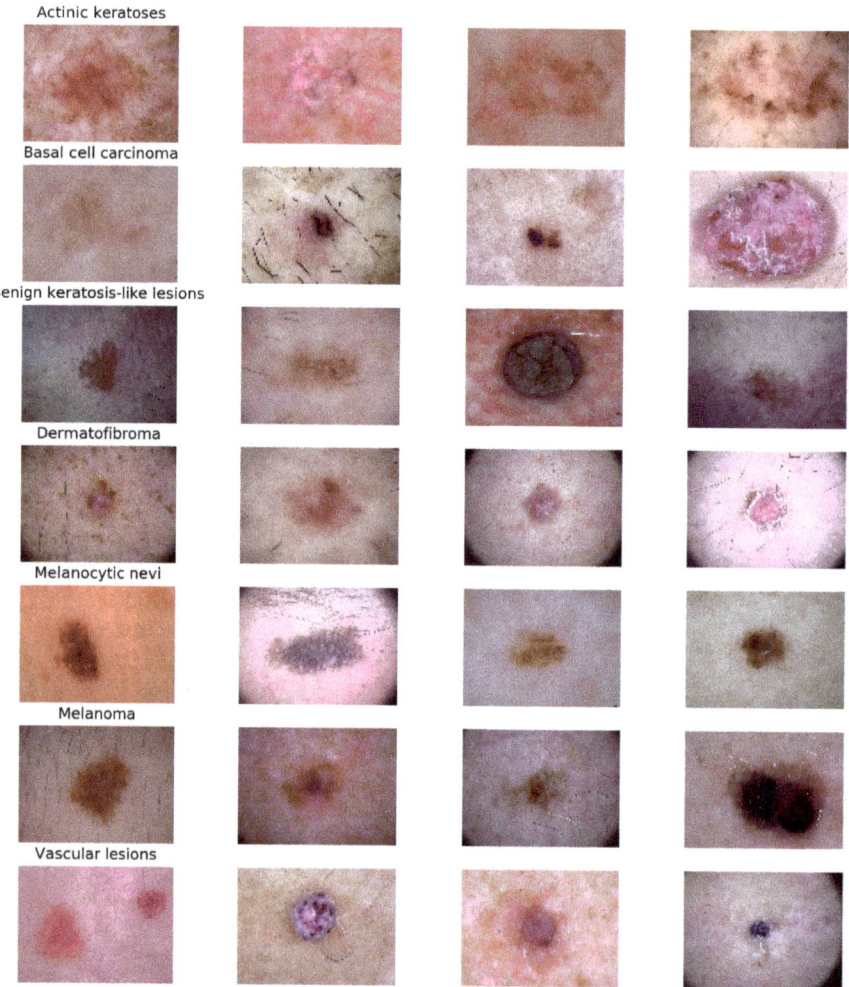

Figure 4. Skin disease samples of 7 classes in skin disease classification.

5. Statistical Metrics

The proposed model for skin disease detection and skin disease classification is evaluated using the following statistical measures

Accuracy: The accuracy measure is estimated by dividing the total of correctly classified skin data samples by the total number of skin disease data samples. The accuracy metric gives equal importance to all the classes in the skin disease dataset. This may not be considered to be a good metric to evaluate the proposed model because the dataset used in skin disease classification is highly imbalanced.

$$Accuracy = \frac{TP + TN}{TP + TN + FP + FN} \qquad (3)$$

Precision: It is also called positive predictive value. It is the correct classification of the skin disease samples to the sum of the correct classification of the skin disease and incorrect classification of the skin disease in the given model. False positives should be less to get high precision.

$$Precision = \frac{TP}{TP+FP} \quad (4)$$

Recall: It is also called sensitivity. It is the correct classification of the skin disease to the sum of the correct classification of the skin disease and the missed classification of the skin disease in the given model. False negative should be less to obtain high recall.

$$Recall = \frac{TP}{TP+FN} \quad (5)$$

F1-score: It is the harmonic mean of precision and recall

$$F1\ score = 2 \times \frac{Precision \times Recall}{Precision + Recall} \quad (6)$$

For a good skin disease detection and classification model, the precision, recall, and f1-score is close to 1.

TP, TN, FP, and FN denote true positive, true negative, false positive, and false negative, respectively, in accuracy, precision, recall, and f1-score. These are defined in the skin disease dataset, as given below

- TP: The number of skin disease data samples correctly predicted as skin disease.
- FN: The number of skin disease data samples wrongly predicted as normal.
- TN: The number of healthy patient data samples predicted as healthy.
- FP: The number of healthy patient data samples predicted as skin disease.

Using a confusion matrix, the TP, TN, FP, and FN are obtained. The confusion matrix counts the distribution of predictions across the actual labels of the skin disease dataset. The dimension of the confusion matrix is nXn, and n denotes the number of classes in the skin disease dataset. To estimate the performances of the proposed model at the class level in both skin disease detection and skin disease classification, precision, recall, and f1-score statistical metrics were considered in this work. The performances are reported for both the macro and weighted metrics of precision, recall, and f1-score. Macro measures are considered to be better for imbalanced datasets because the classes in the skin disease datasets are considered equally while computing the arithmetic mean of precision, recall, and f1-score of all the skin diseases. In the weighted metric, a support score is assigned while computing the arithmetic mean of precision, recall, and f1-score of all the skin diseases. The models are considered to be good if it shows high precision and high recall for rare skin diseases.

6. Results and Discussions

The experiments were conducted on the Kaggle GPU platform with hardware configurations: GPU P100 with 16 GB GPU memory, 13 GB CPU RAM, and 73.1 GB hard disk and libraries such as Keras, TensorFlow, scikit-learn with Python 3.5 for machine learning and deep learning model development.

CNN-based pretrained models were trained on skin disease detection and skin disease classification. The CNN-based pretrained models considered in this work are Xception, VGG16, MobileNet, ResNet50, InceptionV3, DenseNet121, EfficientNetB0, EfficientNetV2B0, EfficientNetV2B1, and EfficientNetV2B2. These models contain several network parameters and network structures. The optimal performance depends on these network parameters and network structures. To find the best parameters for the network, various trials of experiments were run for the parameters' optimizer, learning rate, epochs, and batch size. During training, the data samples in training and validation sets are shuffled to avoid bias in the training of a model. The optimal parameters for learning rate, epochs, batch size, and optimizer were 0.001, 50, 64, and adam, respectively. Various trials of experiments were run for optimizers such as adam, sgd, Adagrad, Adamax, and Nadam. The experiments with adam demonstrated successive improvement in training accuracy and validation accuracy and successive decrement in training loss and validation loss across epochs. Based on this, the optimizer parameter value is set to adam for the rest of the experiments. Next, to identify the optimal learning rate, the experiments were run for the learning rate in the range of 0.0001–0.5. The experiment with 0.001 demonstrated better training accuracy, validation accuracy, training loss, and validation loss during training. Thus, the learning rate is set to 0.001. To find the optimal parameters for batch size, the experiments were run for batches 32, 64, and 128. Due to limited access to memory, the batch size was not increased after 128. The experiments with 64 and 128 were almost similar in training accuracy and validation accuracy across epochs. Thus, the batch size is set to 64. Though batch size 128 slightly shows better performances for training accuracy and training loss, the batch size is set to 64. Because some of the CNN-based pretrained models result in memory issues, to find out the best parameter for epochs, the experiments were run for 70 epochs. However, all the models have not demonstrated any successive improvement in training accuracy and successive decrease in training loss after 50 epochs. Thus, we decided to set 50 epochs as optimal for the training of a model to detect skin diseases and classify them into the skin disease family. The training accuracy and training loss for the CNN-based pretrained models across 50 epochs for skin disease detection is shown in Figure 5. Figure 6 shows the training accuracy and training loss for the CNN-based pretrained models for skin disease classification. The models belonging to the EfficientNetV2 family demonstrated better accuracy by showing successive improvement in training accuracy and successive decrement in training loss compared to other CNN-based pretrained models in both skin disease detection and skin disease classification. Though the other models attained closer performance of training accuracy and training loss as EfficientNetV2, most of the models other than EfficientNetV2 did not show the same performance during testing. This is mainly due to the reason that most of the models other than EfficientNetV2 have reached the phase of overfitting and the models were not able to discriminate well among classes during testing for the new variants of skin disease images. VGG16 and MobileNet models demonstrated less performance in training accuracy and training loss compared to other CNN-based pretrained models in both skin disease detection and skin disease classification. Xception, DensNet121, ResNet50, and InceptionV3 models' performance in terms of training accuracy and training loss were almost similar across epochs 50 but less compared to the models of a family of EfficientNet in both skin disease detection and skin disease classification. For skin disease detection, most of the models have demonstrated above 96% training accuracy and less than 0.1 training loss. EfficientNet models have reached above 99% training accuracy and less than 0.001 training loss for skin disease detection at the end of epochs 50. Most of the models have reached an accuracy of 95% and loss of less than 1 by epochs in the range of 15–20 for skin disease detection. The experiments were run to 50 epochs because the models have demonstrated successive improvement in training accuracy and training loss after 20 epochs. Similar performances were demonstrated by the CNN-based pretrained models for skin disease classification. In particular, the family of EfficientNet models has achieved 99% training accuracy with less than 0.01 training loss for skin disease classification. Most of the CNN-based models have demonstrated above 95% training accuracy and less than 0.1 training loss at epochs in the range 20–25. The experiments were continued until epoch 50 because the model has demonstrated a little successive improvement after epoch 25.

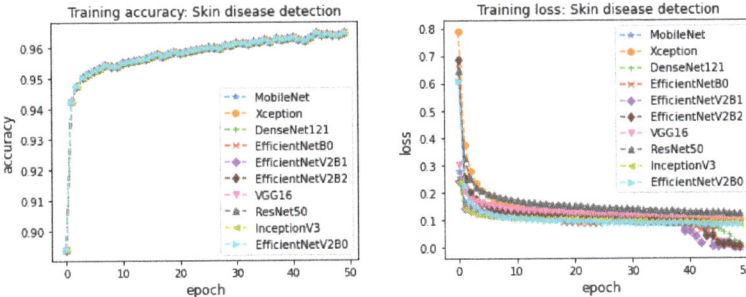

Figure 5. Training accuracy and training loss of CNN-based finetuned models for skin disease detection (left to right).

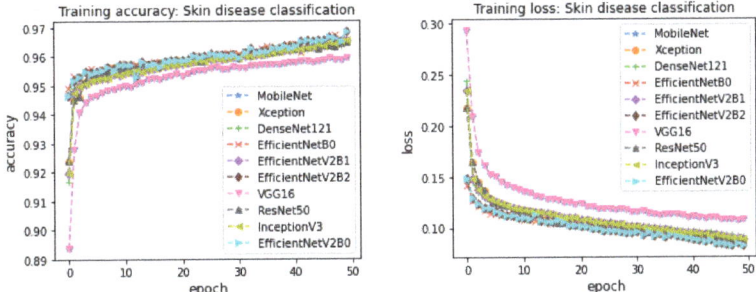

Figure 6. Training accuracy and training loss of CNN-based finetuned models for skin disease classification (left to right).

The total parameters for Xception, VGG16, MobileNet, ResNet50, InceptionV3, DenseNet121, EfficientNetB0, EfficientNetV2B0, EfficientNetV2B1, EfficientNetV2B2 are 23025711, 15306055, 4344519, 25751943, 23967015, 8153159, 5427363, 5427363, 7953031, and 9277433, respectively. The train parameters for Xception, VGG16, MobileNet, ResNet50, InceptionV3, DenseNet121, EfficientNetB0, EfficientNetV2B0, EfficientNetV2B1, fficientNetV2B2 are 22971183, 15306055, 4322631, 25698823, 23932583, 8069511, 5385347, 5385347, 7890983, and 9209865, respectively. The non-train parameters for Xception, VGG16, MobileNet, ResNet50, InceptionV3, DenseNet121, EfficientNetB0, EfficientNetV2B0, EfficientNetV2B1, fficientNetV2B2 are 54528, 0, 21888, 53120, 34432, 84648, 42016, 42016, 62048, and 67568, respectively. The trained models' performances of CNN finetuned models for skin disease detection are reported in Table 4. Table 4 shows that the proposed model outperformed all the CNN-based pretrained models for skin disease detection with an accuracy of 99%. Results of the CNN-based models are reported in terms of Accuracy, weighted and macro precision, weighted and macro recall, and weighted and macro f1-score. The proposed model has improved the accuracy by 2% of the family of EfficientNetV2 models and 3% of the family of EfficientNet models. This shows that each CNN-based pretrained models learn its own feature representation and these features are unique. The proposed model takes advantage of the fusion of features of the family EfficientNetV2 models to accurately detect skin disease. Models such as ResNet50, InceptionV3, DenseNet121, and Xception demonstrated an accuracy of 92%, 93%, 93%, and 93%, respectively. These models performed lesser than the proposed model by accuracy in the range of 6–7%. In addition, the performances shown by ResNet50, InceptionV3, DenseNet121, and Xception on the test dataset for skin disease classification are lesser compared to the family of models of EfficientNet. Both the MobileNet and VGG16 demonstrated performances in terms of accuracy in the range of 88–89% for skin disease detection which is lesser than 10% accuracy compared to the proposed model. Overall, both MobileNet and VGG16 performed lesser than the proposed model, a family of EfficientNet models, and models such as ResNet50, InceptionV3, DenseNet121, and Xception. Along with accuracy, the performances for skin disease detection are reported in terms of macro and weighted precision, recall, and f1-score. The proposed model macro precision, macro recall, and macro f1-score is 99%, 99%, and 99%, respectively. Similar to the macro score, the proposed model showed 99% for weighted precision, weighted recall, and weighted f1-score. This indicates that the proposed model is effective in handling the imbalanced dataset. Macro and weighted performances of the proposed model are 2–3% higher compared to the family of EfficientNet models, 6–7% higher compared to the models such as ResNet50, InceptionV3, DenseNet121, and Xception, and 10–12% higher compared to the models such as VGG16 and MobileNet. Overall, the proposed method outperformed the existing CNN-based models and a family of EfficientNet models with better accuracy, precision, recall, and f1-score metrics for skin disease detection. The less performance in terms of accuracy, precision, recall, and f1-score are shown by the models such as MobileNet and VGG16.

Table 4. Detailed results for skin disease detection.

Model	Accuracy	Type	Precision	Recall	F1-Score	Confusion Matrix
Xception	0.93	Macro	0.93	0.93	0.93	[342 18]
		Weighted	0.93	0.93	0.93	[34 326]
VGG16	0.89	Macro	0.89	0.89	0.89	[333 27]
		Weighted	0.89	0.89	0.89	[50 310]
MobileNet	0.88	Macro	0.89	0.88	0.88	[330 30]
		Weighted	0.89	0.88	0.88	[53 307]
ResNet50	0.92	Macro	0.92	0.92	0.92	[336 24]
		Weighted	0.92	0.92	0.92	[36 324]
InceptionV3	0.93	Macro	0.93	0.93	0.93	[338 22]
		Weighted	0.93	0.93	0.93	[31 329]
DenseNet121	0.93	Macro	0.93	0.93	0.93	[340 20]
		Weighted	0.93	0.93	0.93	[32 328]
EfficientNetB0	0.96	Macro	0.96	0.96	0.96	[350 10]
		Weighted	0.96	0.96	0.96	[19 341]
EfficientNetV2B0	0.97	Macro	0.97	0.97	0.97	[352 8]
		Weighted	0.97	0.97	0.97	[16 344]
EfficientNetV2B1	0.97	Macro	0.97	0.97	0.97	[355 5]
		Weighted	0.97	0.97	0.97	[16 344]
EfficientNetV2B2	0.97	Macro	0.97	0.97	0.97	[355 5]
		Weighted	0.97	0.97	0.97	[16 344]
Proposed	0.99	Macro	0.99	0.99	0.99	[357 3]
		Weighted	0.99	0.99	0.99	[5 355]

For skin disease classification, the current work employed CNN-based pretrained models, and its results are reported in Table 5. The proposed approach outperformed all the other methods for skin disease classification in all the settings of test experiments. The table contains the results of the CNN-based pretrained models in terms of Accuracy, weighted and macro precision, weighted and macro recall, and weighted and macro F1-score. Since the dataset of skin disease classification is highly imbalanced, the work considers macro precision, macro recall, and macro f1-score. To demonstrate the differences between macro and weighted, this work reports the performances of all the models in both macro and weighted. As can be observed from the Table 5, the models show high precision, high recall, and high f1-score even though the misclassification rate is high in some rare skin diseases such as Dermatofibroma and Vascular lesions. The proposed model showed macro precision, macro recall, and macro f1-score of 97%, 100%, and 99%, respectively, and weighted precision, weighted recall, and weighted f1-score of 99%, 99%, and 99%, respectively. Though there is misclassification in the skin disease classes, the weighted measure shows 99% for precision, recall, and F1-score. However, macro precision, macro recall, and macro f1-score are considered to be best compared to weighted metrics because these metrics facilitate showing the individual class's score with support instead of taking the average of all the classes. The family of EfficientNetV2 models showed better macro precision, macro recall, and macro f1-score over EfficientNetB0. The EfficientNetV2 models improved the macro precision, macro recall, and macro weighted metric of EfficientNetB0 model by 18%, 8%, and 13%, respectively. In a family of EfficientNetV2 models, EfficientNetV2B2 models outperformed the models EfficientNetV2B0 and EfficientNetV2B1 in all the settings of the experiments during testing a model for skin disease classification. The experiments are stopped at EfficientNetV2B2 models because there was no performance improvement by using other EfficientNetV2 models. Macro and weighted metrics of ResNet50, InceptionV3, and DenseNet121 models are in the range of 50–65%, 50–65% and 80–90%, respectively. These models' performances are 30% lesser than the proposed model and a family of EfficientNet model compared to macro metrics and 20% lesser compared to weighted metrics of the proposed model and a family of EfficientNet models. Xception, VGG16, and MobileNet models showed macro precision, macro recall, and macro f1-score in the range of 40–60% and weighted precision, weighted recall, and weighted f1-score in the range of 80–90%. These model performances are almost 30% less compared to the macro metric of the proposed model and 10% less compared to the weighted metric of the proposed model. The proposed models showed an accuracy of 99% for skin disease classification by improving the accuracy in the range of 8–9% for the family of EfficientNet models. Models such as DenseNet121, InceptionV3, and ResNet50 showed an accuracy of 93%, 93%, and 92%, respectively, and their performances are lesser compared to the proposed model and the family of EfficientNet models. Similar to skin disease classification, models such as Xception, VGG16, and MobileNet showed an accuracy of 83%, 79%, and 76%, respectively. The model performances of Xception, VGG16, and MobileNet are lesser compared to the proposed model and other CNN-based pretrained models such as a family of EfficientNet models, DenseNet121, InceptionV3, and ResNet50. Overall, the proposed model showed better performances in accuracy and both macro and weighted metrics compared to the other CNN-based pretrained models. Since the proposed model has shown better performances in macro metrics compared to the existing CNN-based models on skin disease classification, the proposed model is considered to be effective in handling imbalanced skin disease datasets. Moreover, the proposed model is able to detect and classify rare skin diseases such as Vascular lesions and Dermatofibroma more accurately compared to other existing CNN-based pretrained models.

Table 5. Detailed results for skin disease classification.

Model	Accuracy	Type	Precision	Recall	F1-Score
Xception	0.83	Macro	0.57	0.59	0.58
		Weighted	0.84	0.83	0.84
VGG16	0.79	Macro	0.50	0.51	0.50
		Weighted	0.80	0.79	0.80
MobileNet	0.76	Macro	0.46	0.44	0.44
		Weighted	0.78	0.76	0.77
ResNet50	0.85	Macro	0.56	0.55	0.54
		Weighted	0.86	0.85	0.85
InceptionV3	0.89	Macro	0.59	0.60	0.59
		Weighted	0.88	0.89	0.88
DenseNet121	0.90	Macro	0.61	0.63	0.61
		Weighted	0.89	0.90	0.89
EfficientNetB0	0.91	Macro	0.78	0.76	0.75
		Weighted	0.91	0.91	0.91
EfficientNetV2B0	0.93	Macro	0.82	0.83	0.82
		Weighted	0.93	0.93	0.93
EfficientNetV2B1	0.94	Macro	0.91	0.84	0.86
		Weighted	0.95	0.94	0.94
EfficientNetV2B2	0.96	Macro	0.96	0.84	0.88
		Weighted	0.96	0.96	0.96
Proposed	0.99	Macro	0.97	1.00	0.99
		Weighted	0.99	0.99	0.99

The detailed results of each class in skin disease detection and skin disease classification is reported in Tables 6 and 7, respectively. In skin disease detection, the proposed approach demonstrated 99% accuracy, 99% precision, 99% recall, and 99% f1-score for both Healthy and Malignant classes. For skin disease classification, the proposed model showed 100% precision, 100% recall, and 100% f1-score for the skin diseases Actinic keratoses, Dermatofibroma, and Vascular lesions. For Melanoma and Melanocytic nevi, the proposed model demonstrated 96% precision, 100% recall, 98% f1-score, and 100% precision, 98% recall, and 99% f1-score, respectively. The proposed model for skin diseases such as Basal cell carcinoma and Benign keratosis-like showed 89% precision, 100% recall, 94% f1-score and 97% precision, 100% recall, and 99% f1-score, respectively. Overall, the proposed approach demonstrated better performance in all the classes in both skin disease detection and skin disease classification compared to other existing CNN-based pretrained models.

Table 6. Detailed results of Healthy and Malignant classes in skin disease detection.

Class	Precision	Recall	F1-Score
Healthy	0.99	0.99	0.99
Malignant	0.99	0.99	0.99
accuracy	0.99		
macro avg	0.99	0.99	0.99
weighted avg	0.99	0.99	0.99

Table 7. Detailed results of each classes in skin disease classification.

Class	Precision	Recall	F1-Score
Actinic keratoses (akiec)	1.00	1.00	1.00
Basal cell carcinoma (bcc)	0.89	1.00	0.94
Benign keratosis-like lesions (bkl)	0.97	1.00	0.99
Dermatofibroma (df)	1.00	1.00	1.00
Melanoma (mel)	0.96	1.00	0.98
Melanocytic nevi (nv)	1.00	0.98	0.99
Vascular lesions (vasc)	1.00	1.00	1.00
accuracy	0.99		
macro avg	0.97	1.00	0.99
weighted avg	0.99	0.99	0.99

The confusion matrix for the CNN-based pretrained models for skin disease detection is included in Table 2. The proposed approach misclassification rate is 0.0111, which is lesser compared to all the other CNN-based pretrained models. The model misclassifies the three samples of Healthy as Malignant and five samples of Malignant as Healthy. The misclassification rate of EfficientNetB0, EfficientNetV2B0, EfficientNetV2B1, and EfficientNetV2B2 are 0.0401, 0.0333, 0.0292, and 0.0292, respectively. Models such as ResNet50, InceptionV3, Xception, and DenseNet121 showed misclassification rates of 0.0811, 0.0736, 0.0722, and 0.0722, respectively. The high misclassification rate is shown by models such as VGG16 and MobileNet. The misclassification rate of VGG16 and MobileNet are 0.1021 and 0.1153, respectively. All the models including the proposed approach demonstrated a high misclassification rate for the Malignant. This indicates that the model's enhancement is required to avoid these misclassifications. There may be a possibility to avoid misclassification in the Malignant class by providing more data samples from different patients across different ages from different modalities. In addition to that, a detailed investigation and analysis of the proposed method needs to be analyzed to understand the misclassification. The optimal features that are used to accurately detect the Malignant data samples need to be analyzed in detail to understand the misclassification. This type of study of the proposed model can be considered as one of the significant directions toward future work.

The confusion matrix for the CNN-based pretrained model for skin disease classification is shown in Figure 7. The proposed model showed a 0.0138 misclassification rate, which is less compared to all the CNN-based pretrained models. The misclassification rate of EfficientNetB0, EfficientNetV2B0, EfficientNetV2B1, and EfficientNetV2B2 are 0.09, 0.07, 0.06, and 0.04, respectively. Models such as ResNet50, InceptionV3, and DenseNet121 showed a high misclassification rate compared to the models of a family of EfficientNet. The high misclassification shown by the models Xception, VGG16, and

MobileNet is compared to all the other CNN-based pretrained models in skin disease classification. The proposed approach classified all the samples of Actinic keratoses, Basal cell carcinoma, Benign keratosis-like lesions, Dermatofibroma, Melanoma, and Vascular lesions. For Melanocytic nevi, the proposed model misclassified six samples as Basal cell carcinoma, three samples as Benign keratosis-like lesions, and five samples as Melanoma. Most importantly, except the proposed models, the other existing models have shown a high misclassification rate for rare skin diseases such as Vascular lesions and Dermatofibroma. The models such as ResNet50, InceptionV3, VGG16, MobileNet, Xception, and DenseNet121 have failed to classify a single sample correctly for Vascular lesions and Dermatofibroma. This indicates that these models are not effective in highly imbalanced skin disease datasets. Though these models are effective in other classes and demonstrated accuracy above 85%, the existing models are not effective for rare skin diseases in both skin disease detection and skin disease classification. In addition to rare skin diseases, the models other than the proposed approach and a family of EfficientNet showed a high misclassification rate. Since the proposed approach is a fused model of a family of EfficientNetV2, it outperformed a single-finetuned EfficientNetV2 model and EfficientNet model in both skin disease detection and skin disease classification. Overall, the proposed model has demonstrated less misclassification rate for all the classes in skin disease classification compared to other CNN-based pretrained models.

The proposed model has outperformed the CNN-based pretrained models in all the test settings in both skin disease detection and skin disease classification. Most importantly, the proposed model integrates the cost weight to the deep learning model, which helped to demonstrate a better classification rate compared to the existing approaches. In addition to that, the proposal of a meta-classifier in the final classification helped to achieve generalization and to make the model to be more robust in detecting the skin disease and classifying the skin disease to its family. Since the proposed model is an ensemble of various EfficientNetV2 models, the model has learned better feature representation to accurately detect and classify skin diseases. The result of the ensemble feature representation of pretrained model has performed better than the single CNN-based pretrained model. In the proposed work, the CNN-based pretrained model and the classification model are not integrated together during training in skin disease detection and the skin disease classification model. Thus, proposing a loss function to integrate the CNN-based pretrained model and classification model will be considered one of the significant directions toward future work. The proposed model employs a KPCA-based dimensionality reduction to reduce the features of CNN-based pretrained models. There may be a possibility that the loss of features can happen in this stage. Detailed analysis and experiments can be demonstrated using the different dimensions of features for skin disease detection and classification. This type of experimental work can be considered future work. The proposed model is a hybrid of CNN-based pretrained models and meta-classifiers. The detailed model parameters of the CNN-based pretrained models for skin disease detection and classification are reported. However, discussion of algorithm complexity analysis to the experimental part in skin disease detection and classification is important and this will be another direction towards future works.

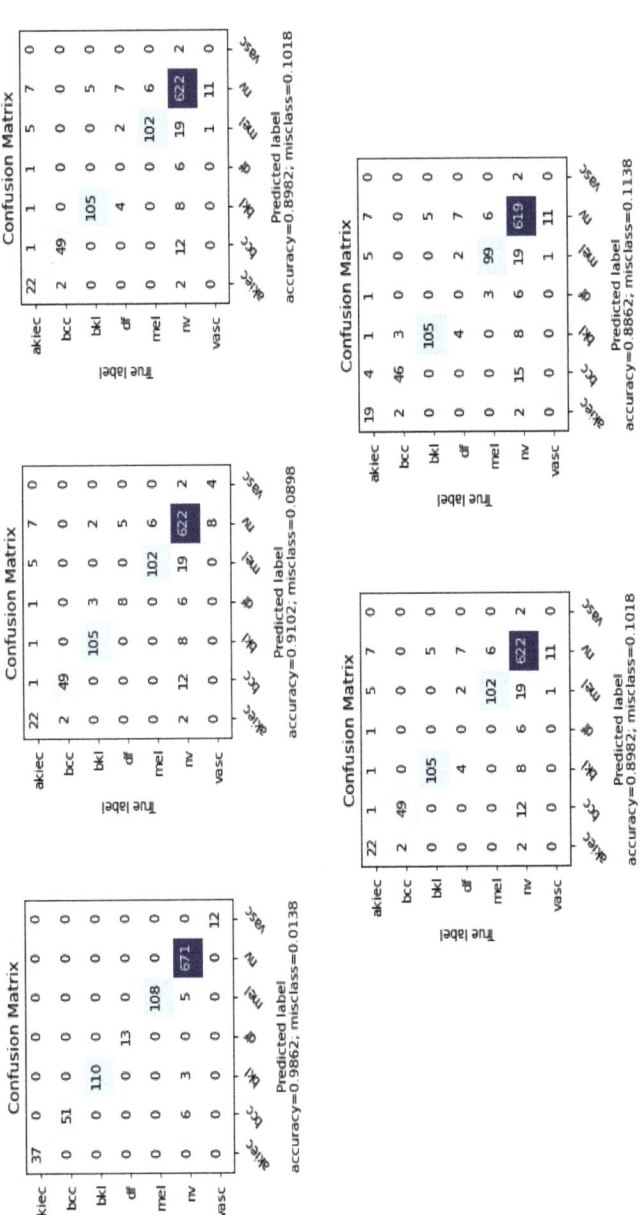

Figure 7. Skin disease classification confusion matrix using Proposed Model, EfficientNetB0, ResNet50, InceptionV3, and DenseNet121 (left to right).

7. Conclusions and Future Works

This paper proposed an attention-cost-sensitive deep learning-based feature fusion ensemble meta-classifier approach for skin cancer detection and classification. The proposed model integrates attention to the deep learning model to detect the infected tiny regions of the overall skin image. To give importance to the minority classes during the training, cost-weights were introduced. The proposed work assigns higher class weights to the classes that have fewer skin disease data samples and lower-class weights to the classes that have a high number of skin disease data samples. The proposed model fuses the features of EfficientNetV2 pretrained models, and the dimensionality reduction of the features is conducted using KPCA. Further, the reduced features are passed into ensemble meta-classifiers. In the first stage of the ensemble meta-classifiers, the prediction of the skin disease is conducted using RFTree and SVM, and the logistic regression performs the classification by considering the probability of the first-stage classifiers as features. In all the experimental settings of the proposed model, the proposed model outperformed the existing methods for both skin cancer detection and skin cancer classification. The proposed model improves the accuracy by 4% compared to the existing approaches for skin disease detection and 9% for skin disease classification. Since clinical features play an important role in enhancing the detection rate of skin diseases, the clinical features of skin diseases can be included along with skin images. This type of fused features of clinical and non-clinical can improve the performance of the model in accurately detecting the skin disease and classifying them into their disease family. The deep learning models are not robust in an adversarial environment and there may be a possibility that the deep learning models can be bypassed by following the techniques available in the field of adversarial machine learning. Thus, the detailed evaluation of the proposed model to detect and classify skin diseases in an adversarial environment will be considered as future work.

Funding: This research received no external funding.

Institutional Review Board Statement: Not applicable.

Informed Consent Statement: Not applicable.

Data Availability Statement: Data available on request from the author.

Conflicts of Interest: The author declares no conflict of interest.

References

1. Chang, W.Y.; Huang, A.; Yang, C.Y.; Lee, C.H.; Chen, Y.C.; Wu, T.Y.; Chen, G.S. Computer-aided diagnosis of skin lesions using conventional digital photography: A reliability and feasibility study. *PloS ONE* **2013**, *8*, e76212.
2. Goyal, M.; Knackstedt, T.; Yan, S.; Hassanpour, S. Artificial intelligence-based image classification methods for diagnosis of skin cancer: Challenges and opportunities. *Comput. Biol. Med.* **2020**, *127*, 104065.
3. Li, H.; Pan, Y.; Zhao, J.; Zhang, L. Skin disease diagnosis with deep learning: A review. *Neurocomputing* **2021**, *464*, 364–393.
4. Houssein, E.H.; Hassaballah, M.; Ibrahim, I.E.; AbdElminaam, D.S.; Wazery, Y.M. An automatic arrhythmia classification model based on improved marine predators algorithm and convolutions neural networks. *Expert Syst. Appl.* **2022**, *187*, 115936.
5. Li, L.F.; Wang, X.; Hu, W.J.; Xiong, N.N.; Du, Y.X.; Li, B.S. Deep learning in skin disease image recognition: A review. *IEEE Access* **2020**, *8*, 208264–208280.
6. Abdel Hameed, M.; Hassaballah, M.; Hosney, M.E.; Alqahtani, A. An AI-Enabled Internet of Things Based Autism Care System for Improving Cognitive Ability of Children with Autism Spectrum Disorders. *Comput. Intell. Neurosci.* **2022**, *2022*, 2247675.
7. Villa-Pulgarin, J.P.; Ruales-Torres, A.A.; Arias-Garzon, D.; Bravo-Ortiz, M.A.; Arteaga-Arteaga, H.B.; Mora-Rubio, A.; Alzate-Grisales, J.A.; Mercado-Ruiz, E.; Hassaballah, M.; Orozco-Arias, S.; et al. Optimized convolutional neural network models for skin lesion classification. *Comput. Mater. Contin.* **2022**, *70*, 2131–2148.
8. Jones, O.; Matin, R.; van der Schaar, M.; Bhayankaram, K.P.; Ranmuthu, C.; Islam, M.; Behiyat, D.; Boscott, R.; Calanzani, N.; Emery, J.; et al. Artificial intelligence and machine learning algorithms for early detection of skin cancer in community and primary care settings: A systematic review. *Lancet Digit. Health* **2022**, *4*, e466–e476.
9. Esteva, A.; Kuprel, B.; Novoa, R.A.; Ko, J.; Swetter, S.M.; Blau, H.M.; Thrun, S. Dermatologist-level classification of skin cancer with deep neural networks. *Nature* **2017**, *542*, 115–118.

10. Maron, R.C.; Weichenthal, M.; Utikal, J.S.; Hekler, A.; Berking, C.; Hauschild, A.; Enk, A.H.; Haferkamp, S.; Klode, J.; Schadendorf, D.; et al. Systematic outperformance of 112 dermatologists in multiclass skin cancer image classification by convolutional neural networks. *Eur. J. Cancer* **2019**, *119*, 57–65.
11. Serte, S.; Demirel, H. Gabor wavelet-based deep learning for skin lesion classification. *Comput. Biol. Med.* **2019**, *113*, 103423.
12. Hagerty, J.R.; Stanley, R.J.; Almubarak, H.A.; Lama, N.; Kasmi, R.; Guo, P.; Drugge, R.J.; Rabinovitz, H.S.; Oliviero, M.; Stoecker, W.V. Deep learning and handcrafted method fusion: Higher diagnostic accuracy for melanoma dermoscopy images. *IEEE J. Biomed. Health Inform.* **2019**, *23*, 1385–1391.
13. Gu, Y.; Ge, Z.; Bonnington, C.P.; Zhou, J. Progressive transfer learning and adversarial domain adaptation for cross-domain skin disease classification. *IEEE J. Biomed. Health Inform.* **2019**, *24*, 1379–1393.
14. Gessert, N.; Sentker, T.; Madesta, F.; Schmitz, R.; Kniep, H.; Baltruschat, I.; Werner, R.; Schlaefer, A. Skin lesion classification using CNNs with patch-based attention and diagnosis-guided loss weighting. *IEEE Trans. Biomed. Eng.* **2019**, *67*, 495–503.
15. Albahar, M.A. Skin lesion classification using convolutional neural network with novel regularizer. *IEEE Access* **2019**, *7*, 38306–38313.
16. Harangi, B.; Baran, A.; Hajdu, A. Assisted deep learning framework for multi-class skin lesion classification considering a binary classification support. *Biomed. Signal Process. Control* **2020**, *62*, 102041.
17. Almaraz-Damian, J.A.; Ponomaryov, V.; Sadovnychiy, S.; Castillejos-Fernandez, H. Melanoma and nevus skin lesion classification using handcraft and deep learning feature fusion via mutual information measures. *Entropy* **2020**, *22*, 484.
18. Al-Masni, M.A.; Kim, D.H.; Kim, T.S. Multiple skin lesions diagnostics via integrated deep convolutional networks for segmentation and classification. *Comput. Methods Programs Biomed.* **2020**, *190*, 105351.
19. Mahbod, A.; Schaefer, G.; Wang, C.; Dorffner, G.; Ecker, R.; Ellinger, I. Transfer learning using a multi-scale and multi-network ensemble for skin lesion classification. *Comput. Methods Programs Biomed.* **2020**, *193*, 105475.
20. Qin, Z.; Liu, Z.; Zhu, P.; Xue, Y. A GAN-based image synthesis method for skin lesion classification. *Comput. Methods Programs Biomed.* **2020**, *195*, 105568.
21. Pacheco, A.G.; Krohling, R.A. The impact of patient clinical information on automated skin cancer detection. *Comput. Biol. Med.* **2020**, *116*, 103545.
22. Gessert, N.; Nielsen, M.; Shaikh, M.; Werner, R.; Schlaefer, A. Skin lesion classification using ensembles of multi-resolution EfficientNets with meta data. *MethodsX* **2020**, *7*, 100864.
23. Ali, A.R.; Li, J.; Yang, G.; O'Shea, S.J. A machine learning approach to automatic detection of irregularity in skin lesion border using dermoscopic images. *PeerJ Comput. Sci.* **2020**, *6*, e268.
24. Bakkouri, I.; Afdel, K. Computer-aided diagnosis (CAD) system based on multi-layer feature fusion network for skin lesion recognition in dermoscopy images. *Multimed. Tools Appl.* **2020**, *79*, 20483–20518.
25. Chaturvedi, S.S.; Tembhurne, J.V.; Diwan, T. A multi-class skin Cancer classification using deep convolutional neural networks. *Multimed. Tools Appl.* **2020**, *79*, 28477–28498.
26. Tschandl, P.; Rinner, C.; Apalla, Z.; Argenziano, G.; Codella, N.; Halpern, A.; Janda, M.; Lallas, A.; Longo, C.; Malvehy, J.; et al. Human–computer collaboration for skin cancer recognition. *Nat. Med.* **2020**, *26*, 1229–1234.
27. El-Khatib, H.; Popescu, D.; Ichim, L. Deep learning–based methods for automatic diagnosis of skin lesions. *Sensors* **2020**, *20*, 1753.
28. Liu, Y.; Jain, A.; Eng, C.; Way, D.H.; Lee, K.; Bui, P.; Kanada, K.; de Oliveira Marinho, G.; Gallegos, J.; Gabriele, S.; et al. A deep learning system for differential diagnosis of skin diseases. *Nat. Med.* **2020**, *26*, 900–908.
29. Ahmad, B.; Usama, M.; Huang, C.M.; Hwang, K.; Hossain, M.S.; Muhammad, G. Discriminative feature learning for skin disease classification using deep convolutional neural network. *IEEE Access* **2020**, *8*, 39025–39033.
30. Iqbal, I.; Younus, M.; Walayat, K.; Kakar, M.U.; Ma, J. Automated multi-class classification of skin lesions through deep convolutional neural network with dermoscopic images. *Comput. Med. Imaging Graph.* **2021**, *88*, 101843.
31. Abdelhalim, I.S.A.; Mohamed, M.F.; Mahdy, Y.B. Data augmentation for skin lesion using self-attention based progressive generative adversarial network. *Expert Syst. Appl.* **2021**, *165*, 113922.
32. Khan, M.A.; Akram, T.; Zhang, Y.D.; Sharif, M. Attributes based skin lesion detection and recognition: A mask RCNN and transfer learning-based deep learning framework. *Pattern Recognit. Lett.* **2021**, *143*, 58–66.
33. Thurnhofer-Hemsi, K.; Domínguez, E. A convolutional neural network framework for accurate skin cancer detection. *Neural Process. Lett.* **2021**, *53*, 3073–3093.
34. Srinivasu, P.N.; SivaSai, J.G.; Ijaz, M.F.; Bhoi, A.K.; Kim, W.; Kang, J.J. Classification of skin disease using deep learning neural networks with MobileNet V2 and LSTM. *Sensors* **2021**, *21*, 2852.
35. Weber, P.; Tschandl, P.; Sinz, C.; Kittler, H. Dermatoscopy of neoplastic skin lesions: Recent advances, updates, and revisions. *Curr. Treat. Options Oncol.* **2018**, *19*, 1–17.
36. Gong, A.; Yao, X.; Lin, W. Dermoscopy image classification based on StyleGANs and decision fusion. *IEEE Access* **2020**, *8*, 70640–70650.
37. Tschandl, P.; Rosendahl, C.; Kittler, H. The HAM10000 dataset, a large collection of multi-source dermatoscopic images of common pigmented skin lesions. *Sci. Data* **2018**, *5*, 1–9.

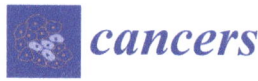

Article

Integrated Design of Optimized Weighted Deep Feature Fusion Strategies for Skin Lesion Image Classification

Niharika Mohanty [1], Manaswini Pradhan [1], Annapareddy V. N. Reddy [2], Sachin Kumar [3,*] and Ahmed Alkhayyat [4]

[1] Department of Information and Communication Technology, Fakir Mohan University, Balasore 756089, India
[2] Department of Information Technology, Lakireddy Bali Reddy College of Engineering, Mylavaram 521230, India
[3] Big Data and Machine Learning Lab, South Ural State University, Chelyabinsk 454080, Russia
[4] College of Technical Engineering, The Islamic University, Najaf 54001, Iraq
* Correspondence: kumars@susu.ru

Simple Summary: The reported global incidences of skin cancer led to the development of automated clinical aids for making proper clinical decision models. Correctly classifying the skin lesions during the early stage may increase the chances of being cured before cancer. However, the skin lesion dataset images pose many critical challenges related to available features to develop classification models with cross-domain adaptability and robustness. This paper made an attempt to select important features from skin lesion datasets for proper skin cancer classification by proposing some feature fusion strategies. Three pre-trained models were utilized to select the important features and then an adaptive weighted mechanism of choosing important features was explored to propose model-based and feature-based optimized feature fusion strategies by optimally and adaptively choosing the weights using a meta-heuristic artificial jellyfish algorithm. The empirical evidence shows that choosing the weights of the pre-trained networks adaptively in an optimized way gives a good starting point for initialization to mitigate the chances of exploding or vanishing gradients.

Abstract: This study mainly focuses on pre-processing the HAM10000 and BCN20000 skin lesion datasets to select important features that will drive for proper skin cancer classification. In this work, three feature fusion strategies have been proposed by utilizing three pre-trained Convolutional Neural Network (CNN) models, namely VGG16, EfficientNet B0, and ResNet50 to select the important features based on the weights of the features and are coined as Adaptive Weighted Feature Set (AWFS). Then, two other strategies, Model-based Optimized Weighted Feature Set (MOWFS) and Feature-based Optimized Weighted Feature Set (FOWFS), are proposed by optimally and adaptively choosing the weights using a meta-heuristic artificial jellyfish (AJS) algorithm. The MOWFS-AJS is a model-specific approach whereas the FOWFS-AJS is a feature-specific approach for optimizing the weights chosen for obtaining optimal feature sets. The performances of those three proposed feature selection strategies are evaluated using Decision Tree (DT), Naïve Bayesian (NB), Multi-Layer Perceptron (MLP), and Support Vector Machine (SVM) classifiers and the performance are measured through accuracy, precision, sensitivity, and F1-score. Additionally, the area under the receiver operating characteristics curves (AUC-ROC) is plotted and it is observed that FOWFS-AJS shows the best accuracy performance based on the SVM with 94.05% and 94.90%, respectively, for HAM 10000 and BCN 20000 datasets. Finally, the experimental results are also analyzed using a non-parametric Friedman statistical test and the computational times are recorded; the results show that, out of those three proposed feature selection strategies, the FOWFS-AJS performs very well because its quick converging nature is inculcated with the help of AJS.

Keywords: skin lesion classification; feature selection; VGG16; EfficientNet B0; ResNet50; HAM 10000 dataset; BCN 20000 dataset

Citation: Mohanty, N.; Pradhan, M.; Reddy, A.V.N.; Kumar, S.; Alkhayyat, A. Integrated Design of Optimized Weighted Deep Feature Fusion Strategies for Skin Lesion Image Classification. *Cancers* **2022**, *14*, 5716. https://doi.org/10.3390/cancers14225716

Academic Editors: Muhammad Fazal Ijaz and Marcin Woźniak

Received: 14 October 2022
Accepted: 11 November 2022
Published: 21 November 2022

Publisher's Note: MDPI stays neutral with regard to jurisdictional claims in published maps and institutional affiliations.

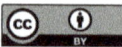

Copyright: © 2022 by the authors. Licensee MDPI, Basel, Switzerland. This article is an open access article distributed under the terms and conditions of the Creative Commons Attribution (CC BY) license (https://creativecommons.org/licenses/by/4.0/).

1. Introduction

Skin lesion mainly refers to a skin area with distinctive characteristics, such as color, shape, size, and texture, from the other surrounding areas of skin. The leading cause of this may be sunburn or contact dermatitis, which causes localized damage to the skin [1–3]. The American Society for Dermatologic Surgery describes a skin lesion as an abnormal lump, bump, ulcer, sore, or colored skin area. Other causes of skin lesions or skin patches include any underlying disorder, infections, diabetes, or genetic disorders. It has been seen that this type of skin type may be benign non-harmless or malignant, or premalignant, leading to skin cancer. Freckles or small patches of light brown skin color can be the reason for exposure to the sun. Flat moles are the best examples of skin lesions, and a growing mole with color variation, itching, and bleeding may lead to melanoma lesions, as shown in Figure 1 for regular lesions (Figure 1a) and melanoma lesions (Figure 1b) [4].

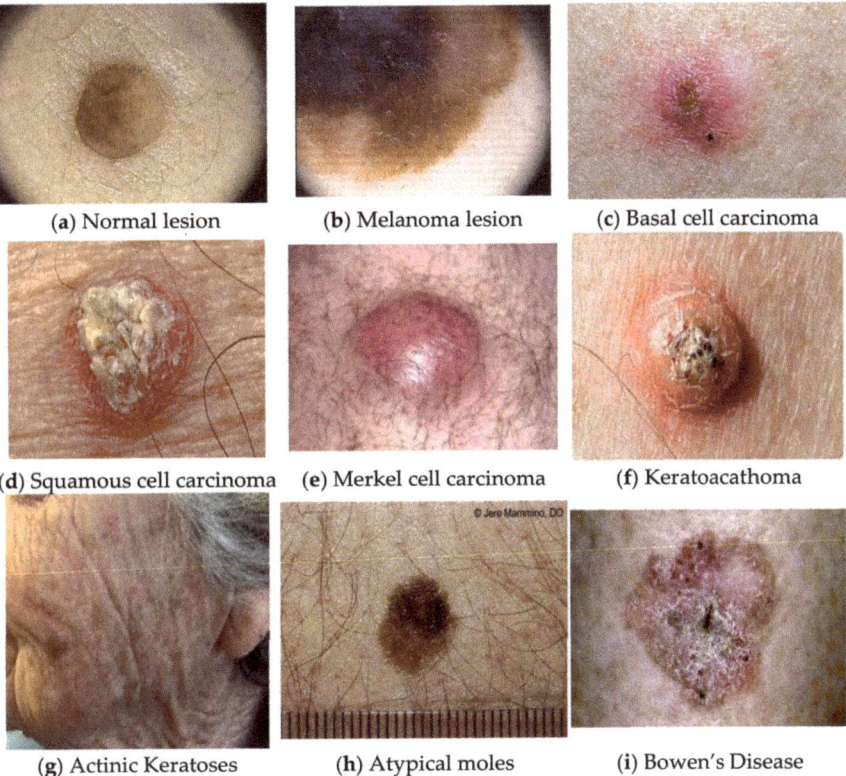

Figure 1. Examples of normal lesions and melanoma in skin lesion images [4]. (**a**) Normal lesion, (**b**) Melanoma lesion, (**c**) Basal cell carcinoma, (**d**) Squamous cell carcinoma, (**e**) Merkel cell carcinoma, (**f**) Keratoacathoma, (**g**) Actinic Keratoses, (**h**) Atypical moles, (**i**) Bowen's Disease.

The study reveals that this skin cancer is the 17th most common cancer worldwide and is a warning phase for researchers and academicians to develop an early detection system for this skin cancer in the form of a computer-based system for effective treatment and better outcomes treatment. The computer-assisted dermoscopic image classification has attracted significant research for its potential to timely and accurately diagnose skin lesions [4–7]. Scientists, clinicians, analyzers, and experimenters are trying to delve into this area of research to develop models and strategies by exploring artificial intelligence (AI)-, machine learning (ML)-, and deep learning (DL)-based approaches [8–11].

It is evident that DL strategies are being widely used for structure detection by researchers for localization and interpolation of anatomical structures in medical images and to accomplish this task of distinguishing the image features [10,11]. Additionally, the DL methods are highly effective in handling large samples during the training stage, and this network learns valuable representations of the features directly. For example, the convolutional neural network's (CNN's) pre-trained architectures can effectively identify and remove the artifacts from the images such as noise. In medial image processing, especially in skin lesion recognition, it is essential to pre-process the image concerning feature selection and feature extraction leading to feature engineering to design an effective and correctly working algorithm [12–15]. The evolution of transfer learning and its advantages of saving resources with improved efficiency concerning cost and time-consuming issues have widely used CNN's pre-trained networks in the image analysis research domain [2,11]. In other words, this transfer learning is an ML-based approach where a pre-trained model is reused and customized to develop a new model for a new dataset. For image recognition tasks, the pre-trained models are great because they are easier to use and typically perform better with less training time. It also enables the models to train fast and accurately by extracting the relatively useful features or features of importance at the beginning of training learned from the large datasets [16,17]. The feature level fusion in the classification task has shown improved recognition performance by combining the results of multiple feature selection strategies, thereby identifying a compact set of salient features without losing any data that can improve the recognition accuracy compared to the single base models. Feature fusion, or in other words, the combination of features from different networks, is an omnipresent part of the model learning mechanisms, which is achieved in many ways. The simplest form is the concatenation of outputs of participating networks or using some means or methods of optimizing the weights of the opinions of the participating networks to obtain a good fusion of features having relative discriminative power to design a classification model [18–20]. The importance of using optimization in feature fusion is not only to just rank the ranking of features to obtain an optimized version of features, but also the optimized weights help to decide the impact of each feature even if a feature of first rank will have some weighted importance. Being motivated by the advantages of DL-based recognition systems, the use of transfer learning mechanism through CNN's pre-trained networks, and the feature fusion approach, in this study, we attempted to design a few feature fusion methodologies which call for active fusion approaches resulting to an effective and robust skin lesion classification model. Our prime contributions in this research are: the transfer learning strategy was exploited with the help of CNN's pre-trained networks for feature selection and feature fusion [2,16–18]; the advantages of visual geometry group network (VGG16), EfficientNet B0, and residual neural network (ResNet50) such as low number of parameters and small size filters, multi objective neural architecture optimizing the accuracy and floating point operations with a balanced depth, width, and resolution producing a scalable, accurate and easily deployable model; and the ability to solve the problem of vanishing gradients of those three pre-trained networks have been explored deeply while designing this deep feature fusion model [12–15]. The key advantages of the ensemble learning mechanism to design a robust feature selection model by proposing combined feature fusion strategies [19–21], such as combined feature set (CFS), adaptive weighted feature set (AWFS), model-based optimized weighted feature set (MOWFS), and feature-based optimized weighted feature set (FOWFS), are experimented and validated. In order to reduce the losses and selection of optimized weights of those three pre-trained networks, the advantages of a new meta-heuristic optimizer artificial jellyfish optimizer (AJS) [22–29] was used and finally, the performance of the proposed feature fusion strategies are likened to other combinations of the models with genetic algorithm (GA) [30] and particle swarm optimization (PSO) [31] such as MOWFA-GA, MOWFS-PSO, FOWFS-GA, and FOWPS-PSO, and it was observed that the proposed combination of FOWFS-AJS outperforms the other models used for classification of skin lesion diagnosis.

The rest of the article is organized as follows: the literature on CNN's pre-trained networks and feature fusion approaches are discussed in Section 2. The pre-trained CNN feature extraction models are discussed in Section 3, the experimentations, results, and discussions are detailed in Section 4. Finally, the conclusion and future scope are given in Section 5.

2. Literature Survey

The key challenge associated with the available skin lesion datasets includes the selection of features of importance giving rise to feature selection and/or feature extraction as one the pre-processing task to improve the classification accuracy of the classifiers. This section mainly reviews some related feature selection and feature extraction approaches for image datasets including feature fusion or ensemble techniques. In early studies, the researchers usually used few traditional feature selection methods such as correlation-based feature selection, consistency-based filter, information gain, ReliefF etc., then they shifted their attention to using CNN to extract features. For instance, dense convolutional network (DenseNet), VGG16, Inceptionv3 (GoogLeNet), ResNet, EfficientNet, etc. are the most commonly used pre-trained models for fine-tuning the datasets to improve classification accuracy [2,12–15].

Lingzhi Kong and Jinyong Cheng [32] proposed classification of COVID-19 X-ray images using DenseNet and VGG models and fine-tuned feature fusion model. First, they applied pre-processing of images and then segmented those images for classification. In addition to this, authors also attempted to resolve the data imbalance problem by introducing fine-tuned global attention block and category attention block to obtain more detailed information of small lesions. Manjary P et al. [33] proposed a classification model to distinguish between natural and computer-generated images by designing a multi-color-space fused EfficientNet using transfer learning methodology which operates in three different color spaces. Ying Guo et al. [34] proposed an EfficientNet based multi view feature fusion model for cervical cancer screening. This proposed model takes the colposcopy images as inputs and tries to extract the features which lead to cervical intraepithelial neoplasia lesions by avoiding the negative effects caused by individual differences and non-cervical intraepithelial neoplasia lesions. An interesting study was carried out by David McNeely-White et al. [35] for comparing the utility of inception and ResNet for as a feature extractor. Authors observed that the features extracted by Inception are very similar to features extracted using ResNet, i.e., the feature set can be very well approximated by an affine transformation of the other. In other words, this literature suggests that for the CNNs, the selection of training set is more important than the selection of pre-trained models.

Yan Wang et al. [36] focused on accurate skin lesion classification by adversarial multimodal fusion with attention mechanism for classification, but before this process, they adopted a discriminator based on adversarial learning to extract the correlated features. This proposed multimodal feature extraction strategy tries to extract the features of the lesion area to enhance the feature vector to obtain more discriminative features. Moreover, the main focus was to consider both correlated and complementary information to design a multimodal fusion strategy. Lina Liu et al. [37] created an automated skin lesion classification model by extracting the region of interest from skin lesson images using ResNet and DenseNet. The authors tried to obtain the mid-level features by studying the relationships among different images based on distance metric learning and gave as an input to the classifiers instead of using the extracted features directly. A study on understanding the efficiency of 17 commonly pre-trained CNN models used for feature extraction was carried out by Samia Benyahia et al. [38]. It has been observed that DenseNet201 along with k-nearest neighbor and support sector machine (SVM) outperformed with respect to classification accuracy for the ISIC 2019 dataset. Di Zhuang et al. [39] proposed a cost-sensitive multi-classifier fusion approach for skin lesion image classification by taking the advantage of subjective weights assigned to datasets. That study utilized a concept of cost-sensitive feature by adapting to the different customized cost matrices and twelve different CNN architectures to evaluate the fusion approaches performance.

As per the study, it was seen that the ensemble learning or fusion approach made better predictions and achieved better performance than the single contributing feature or model. The higher predictive accuracy compared to individual models of this ensemble strategy gained wide use in the case of classification. Considering this advantage, many researchers are trying to use this either in the feature level or classifier level. In this section, some works done on this approach are described. Amirreza Mahbod et al. [40] proposed an automatic skin lesion ensemble-based classification model for ISIC 2017 skin lesion classification challenge dataset by combining intra and inter architecture network fusion with multiple sets of CNNs and in that model, the CNNs are pre-trained architectures. Those pre-trained CNNs are able to identify fine-tuned dermoscopic lesion images for the different settings of those models. Similarly, Nils Gessert et al. [41] also proposed an ensemble-based classification model for ISIC 2017 skin lesion classification challenge using EfficientNets, SENet, and ResNeXt WSL. Mohamed A. Elashiri et al. [19] proposed an ensemble-based classification model with the weighted deep concatenated features with long short-term memory. These ensembles of weighted features are basically concatenated features from three CNNs pre-trained models, namely DeepLabv3, ResNet50, and VGG16 integrating the optimal weights of each feature using their proposed hybrid squirrel butterfly search algorithm. Amira S. Ashour et al. [42] also proposed an ensemble-based bag of features strategy for classification of COVID-19 X-ray images.

Redha Ali et al. [43,44] proposed DL-based skin lesion analysis models in 2019 and 2022. In [43], the authors proposed a CNN-based ensemble method by utilizing VGG19-UNet, DeeplabV3+, and a few other pre-processing methodologies using the ISIC 2018 challenge dataset. Similarly, a DL-based incremental modular network named IMNets was proposed in [44] for medical imaging by using small network modules called as SubNets capable of generating salient features for a particular problem, then larger and more powerful networks were designed by combining these SubNets in different configurations. At each stage, only one new SubNet module underwent learning updates, thereby reducing the computational resource requirements for training in network optimization. Xinzi He et al. [45] proposed a segmentation and classification model by improving the CNNs through a fully transformer network to learn long-range contextual information for skin lesion analysis.

3. Methodologies

The preliminary details of VGG16, EfficientNet B0, and ResNet 50 along with their architectures are discussed in this section along with the theory and working process of AJS optimization algorithm. The broad scope of this study along with the proposed deep feature fusion strategies are also detailed along with their workflow diagrams.

3.1. CNNs' Pre-Trained Models for Feature Selection

CNNs' pre-trained models are saved networks that were previously trained on a large dataset for large-scale image classification and can be used as is or may be customized as per the requirements. This type of architecture of applying the gained knowledge from one source to a different but similar task is widely known as transfer learning. There are many pre-trained models of CNN available and they are being widely used in the field of image processing, such as LeNet, AlexNet, ResNet, GoogleNet or InceptionNet, VGG, DenseNet, EfficientNet, PolyNet, and many more. CNN is basically originated from neural network with convolution layers, pooling layers, activation layers, etc., and those mentioned pre-trained networks are specific CNNs designed for various applications, such as classification and localization [2,12–17,31–34,37].

In this work of designing feature fusion strategy for feature selection, three pre-trained CNNs, namely VGG16, EfficientNet B0, and ResNet50 were utilized. The VGG stands for Visual Geometry Group, consisting of blocks composed of 2D convolution and max pooling layers. This has two variants, VGG16 and VGG19, representing 16 and 19 layers in each of them and it has been seen that the performance of VGG16 is equivalent to VGG19; therefore, VGG16 is widely used rather than VGG19. VGG16 was proposed in [46] at the Visual Geometry Lab in Oxford University, United Kingdom in 2014; it is denser with small 3 × 3 filters which provides the effect of a big size filters such as 5 × 5 and 7 × 7, as shown in Figure 2a. The lowering of number of parameters and use of small size filters in the VGG16 network shows the benefit of low computational complexity which gave a new research trend to work with low filters.

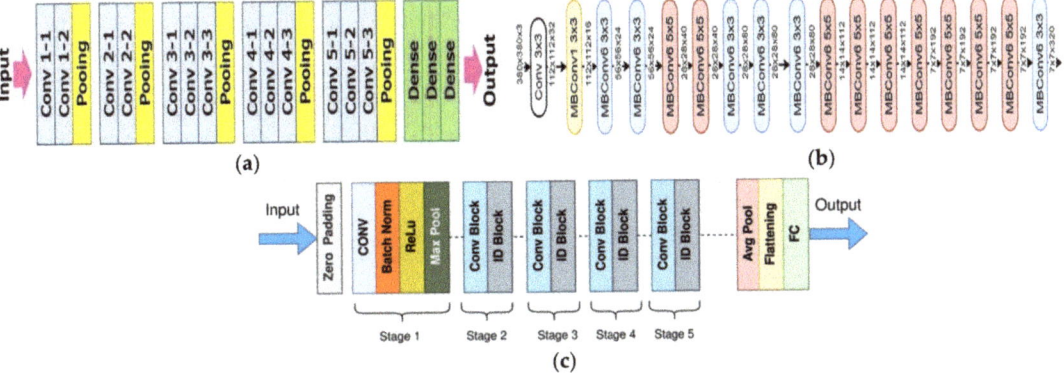

Figure 2. VGG16, EfficientNet B0, and ResNet 50 pre-trained networks architecture. (a) VGG16 network architecture [46], (b) EfficientNet B0 network architecture [47], (c) ResNet50 network architecture [48].

EfficientNet uses the neural architecture search to design a new network and it has been scaled up to obtain a family of deep learning models. The EfficientNet B0 was developed using a multi-objective neural architecture optimizing the accuracy and floating point operations. It has been found that this network achieves better accuracy and efficiency in comparison to standard CNN models and taking this EfficientNet B0 as a baseline model, a full family of EfficientNets from EfficientNet B1 to EfficientNet B7 are being developed, and they have shown their accuracy and efficiency on ImageNet. The total number of layers in EfficientNet Bo is 237 and 11 M trainable parameters and the detailed architecture in shown in Figure 2b [47]. This model exacts features throughout the layers by using multiple convolution layers using 3 × 3 receptive field and mobile inverted bottleneck convolution layer. This network employs a balanced depth, width, and resolution which produce a scalable, accurate, and easily deployable model. This EfficientNet was proposed by Mingxing Tan and Quoc V. Le of Google Research in 2019.

Residual network or ResNet is a classic neural network used for many computer vision and image processing tasks and allowed to train more than 150 layers, being the extremely deep neural networks, leading to solving the problem of vanishing gradients introduced by Kaiming He, Xiangyu Zhang, Shaoqing Ren, and Jian Sun in 2015. ResNet50 is a deep network with 5 stages that contains 3 convolutional layers and 1 identity block, which is trained over 23 million parameters and can work very well with 50 neural network layers as shown in Figure 2c [48]. A skip connection is used in the ResNet50 to fetch the earlier parameters to the layers close to the output. It overcomes the vanishing gradient problem.

The concept of wider, deeper, and higher resolution properties of those pre-trained networks giving the network with more filters, more convolution layers and the ability to process the images with larger depth has gained popularity in the field of image processing. Considering those general advantages as well as a few other advantages, such as VGG16 is good at image classification, the effectiveness of model scaling, the proper use of baseline network in EfficientNet B0, and the principle of ResNet50 to build deeper networks and efficiency to obtain number of optimized layers to overcome the vanishing gradient problem, has been the motivation behind this work to design a deep feature fusion strategy for feature selection leading to an effective skin lesion image classification [2,8–15,17–20].

3.2. Artificial Jellyfish Search Algorithm (AJS)

This AJS is one of the newly proposed meta-heuristic swarm-based optimization algorithms derived by simulating the locomotion and dietary patterns [22–29] of jellyfish. Jellyfish are the most efficient swimmers of all aquatic animals widely seen in the oceans having umbrella-shaped bells and trailing tentacles. Their bodies are made up of 98% water which helps them to survive by blending themselves with the direction of current of ocean. The jellyfish swims in the water in such a way that creates two vortex rings, which in turn allows the jellyfish to travel 30% farther on each swimming cycle. From a study, it was observed that jellyfish are excellent swimmers and they utilizes less energy and less oxygen to travel within the water. They have a very simple nervous system which acts as a good receptor to detect light, vibration, and chemicals in the water. They also have a great ability to sense the gravity which allows the jellyfish to traverse in the ocean. The gelatinous skin of this jellyfish helps them to absorb oxygen and their thin hairs help them to bite the food. Jellyfish have stinging cells called nematocysts with tiny needle-like stingers known as tentacles to paralyze the prey before eating. The rising sea temperatures and the dead zones created for other fish or aquatic animals have given a better opportunity to the jellyfish to bloom.

The jellyfish bloom or flock is being affected by the ecosystem significantly, i.e., the amount of food varies from place to place the jellyfish moves or visits to determine the best place which contains more food. Considering this movement of jellyfish to search for more food in an ocean motivated the design of an AJS based on three idealistic rules:

(a) The movement of the jellyfish is either drawn by the current of the ocean or looking at the swarm and controlling the switching between the mentioned two movements by a time controlled approach;

(b) Being efficient swimmers, jellyfish swim to search for food and try to obtain the locations where a large amount of food is available.

The location simply depends on the quantity of food found and the corresponding objective function of it (i.e., location of jellyfish);

The AJS algorithm basically depends on four ingredients considering the above three rules, namely ocean current; bloom of jellyfish; the time controlled mechanism; and boundary conditions in search spaces and are mathematically formulated and detailed as follows.

(a) Ocean current: The jellyfish is attracted to the large amount of food based on the direction ($\rightarrow$) of the current of the ocean and the new location of the jellyfish can be formulated using Equations (1) and (2), respectively.

$$\overrightarrow{Ocean}_{Current} = JF^{\#} - \varphi \times rand(0,1) \times MeanLocation_{JF} \quad (1)$$

$$JF_i(t+1) = JF_i(t) + rand(0,1) \times \overrightarrow{Ocean}_{Current} \quad (2)$$

where, $JF^{\#}$ represents the jellyfish currently at the best location in a swarm or bloom; φ is the distribution coefficient and is >0 related to the direction of $\overrightarrow{Ocean}_{Current}$, JF_i represents the *jellyfish i*, and $MeanLocation_{JF}$ represents the new location of each jellyfish.

(b) Jellyfish bloom or swarm: The mobility of the jellyfish is of two types, i.e., passive and active motion, and most jellyfish initially show passive motion during the formation of bloom and they progressively show active motion. Basically, the passive motion of the jellyfish is around their own locations and the corresponding updated location of each jellyfish can be obtained using Equation (3). The $Upper_{bound}$ and $Lower_{bound}$ are the upper and lower bounds of the search space and ω is the length of the movement around the jellyfish's locations and is called as motion coefficient.

$$JF_i(t+1) = JF_i(t) + \omega \times rand(0,1) \times (Upper_{bound} - Lower_{bound}) \tag{3}$$

The active motion can be simulated as

(a) either JF_i moves towards JF_j or moves away;
(b) JF_j other than a JF_i is randomly chosen and a vector from JF_i to the chosen JF_j is used to determine the direction of the movement of jellyfish or motion;
(c) when the food quantity exceeds at the chosen location of JF_j that the location of JF_i, a JF_i moves towards a JF_j;
(d) and if the quantity of the food available to the chosen JF_j is lower than that available to a JF_i, it moves away from it;

This leads every jellyfish to move in a better direction to find food in a bloom and the direction of motion is simulated and the location of the jellyfish is updated using Equations (4) and (5), respectively, where f is an objective function of location of jellyfish.

$$Motion\ \vec{Direction} = \begin{cases} JF_j(t) - JF_i(t) & if\ f(JF_i) \geq f(JF_j) \\ JF_i(t) - JF_j(t) & if\ f(JF_i) < f(JF_j) \end{cases} \tag{4}$$

$$JF_i(t+1) = JF_i(t) + rand(0,1) \times Motion\ \vec{Direction} \tag{5}$$

(c) Time Controlled Mechanism: The passive or active motions of jellyfish in a bloom over a time need to be determined to control the motions of jellyfish towards the ocean current. This time controlled mechanism can be formulated using a time control function $f(T_C)$ which is a random value that changes between $(0, 1)$ over time and a constant c as shown in Equation (6), where maximum number of iterations is given as $Iterations_{max}$ and t is the time specified with respect to the iteration number.

$$f(T_C) = \left| \left(1 - \frac{t}{Iterations_{max}}\right) \times (2 \times rand(0,1) - 1) \right| \tag{6}$$

Equation (6) computes the $f(T_C)$ and when this function increases the value of constant c, it signifies that, the jellyfish follow the $\vec{Ocean}_{Current}$ and when $f(T_C) < c$, the jellyfish move inside the bloom. In this case, $f(T_C) = c$ is not known as the time control changes.

(d) Boundary Conditions: The boundary conditions represent the maximum search space defined for the jellyfish. With respect to these boundary conditions (as represented in Equation (7)), when a jellyfish progresses outside the bounds of search area, it will return to the opposite bound. In this equation, $JF_{i,d}$, $JF'_{i,d}$, $Upper_{bound,d}$, and $Lower_{bound,d}$ represent the location of the ith jellyfish in d^{th} dimension, upper, and lower bounds of the search spaces, respectively.

$$\begin{cases} JF'_{i,d} = (JF_{i,d} - Upper_{bound,d}) + Lower_{bound}(d) & if\ JF_{i,d} > Upper_{bound,d} \\ JF'_{i,d} = (JF_{i,d} - Lower_{bound,d}) + Upper_{bound}(d) & if\ JF_{i,d} > Lower_{bound,d} \end{cases} \tag{7}$$

3.3. Proposed Deep Feature Fusion Approach for Feature Selection

The broad scope of the proposed deep feature fusion strategy for feature selection of skin lesion classification is outlined in Figure 3. The original feature sets are given as input to the three variants of pre-trained CNN models as an initial phase of experimentation. Considering the contributing factors of ensemble techniques such as (a) the final prediction obtained by combining the results from several base models have achieved better performance and (b) the spread or dispersion of the predictions and model performance are more robust, this study mainly focused on design of ensemble-based feature fusion strategy exploring the deep learning architecture. In this work, four ensemble feature fusion strategies, namely CFS, AWFS, MOWFS, and FOWFS, are proposed, experimented, and validated.

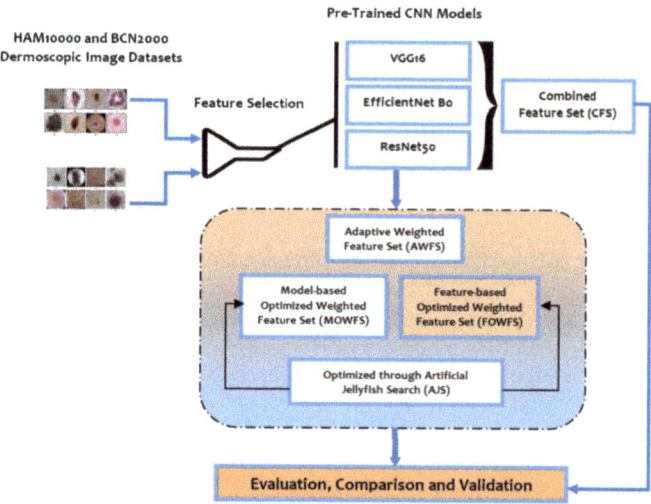

Figure 3. Layout of proposed feature fusion approach for skin lesion data classification.

The predicted features by VGG16, EfficientNet B0, and ResNet50 are 512, 1024, and 1024, respectively, while the input to those three models are images from HAM 10000 [49] and BCN 20000 [50] datasets represented as $\{I_1 \cdots I_m \cdots I_k\}$. The CFS is one of simplest form of ensemble techniques which simply concatenates the outputs of the three pre-trained models to form a batch of feature set as illustrated in Figure 4a. In the AWFS approach, the weights of those three pre-trained models are initialized to (0, 1) and then the combined feature set is formed by adaptively selecting weights concatenated by the extracted features from the respective pre-trained models, namely $[w_1 \times F_{VGG16}]$, $\left[w_2 \times F_{EfficientNet\ B0}\right]$, and $[w_3 \times F_{ResNet50}]$ as shown in Figure 4b.

The workflow of the proposed MOWFS is illustrated in Figure 4c, in which initially, the combined feature set is formed same as the AWFS strategy and then, the technique of identifying optimum point considering two special cases (active and passive) motion of AJS optimization algorithm helps to find best cost. In this model-based approach, any one of the classifiers (in our experimentation DT, NB, MLP and SVM) is considered as *cost function*, where the measured MSE of the opted classification model is taken as the cost and the weights (w_1, w_2 and w_3) are taken as *decision variables*. This total process is continued for 50 iterations to obtain optimized weights from all three pre-trained models. Then the final ensemble of features is formed for test set as $([w_1]_{1 \times 1} \times F_{VGG16})$, $\left([w_2]_{1 \times 1} \times F_{EfficientNet\ B0}\right)$, $([w_3]_{1 \times 1} \times F_{ResNet50})$. The process of FOWFS strategy focuses on feature-based optimization of adaptively chosen weights for formation of combined weighted feature set, such as $[w_1]_{1 \times 512} \times F_{VGG16}$, $[w_2]_{1 \times 1024} \times F_{EfficientNet\ B0}$, and $[w_3]_{1 \times 1024} \times F_{ResNet50}$ with total weights (512+1024+1024). Then, the process of obtaining optimized weights is performed the same as the MOWFS strategy and finally it returns 512 + 1024 + 1024 number of optimized weights based on each feature and the combined feature set is formed as $[w_1]_{1 \times 512} \times F_{VGG16}$, $[w_2]_{1 \times 1024} \times F_{EfficientNet\ B0}$, $[w_3]_{1 \times 1024} \times F_{ResNet50}$. The total process of this strategy is detailed in Figure 4d. Then, features having weights more than 0.5 are considered as best performing features and are considered for final classification. Finally, the performance of the proposed deep feature fusion strategies such as CFS, AWFS, MOWFS, and FOWFS are evaluated based on each classification model and the proposed optimized strategies are compared with GA and PSO two widely used meta-heuristic optimization techniques though accuracy, precision, sensitivity, and F1-score.

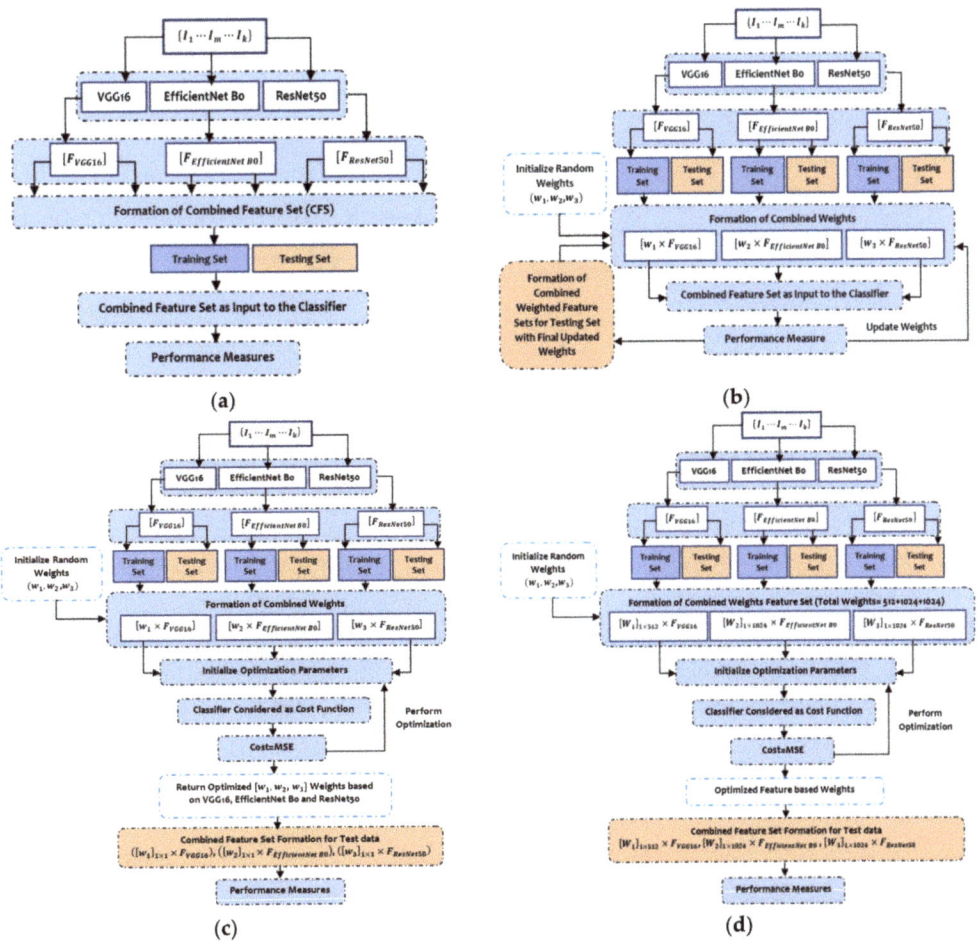

Figure 4. The steps of (**a**) Combined Feature Set (CFS) generation process; (**b**) Adaptive Weighted Feature Set (AWFS) generation process; (**c**) Model-based Optimized Weighted Feature Set (MOWFS) generation process; and (**d**) Feature-based Optimized Weighted Feature Set (FOWFS) generation process.

4. Experiments, Results, and Discussion

This segment focuses on the experimental stages in order to effectively illustrate the study's findings. Broadly, the section discusses the datasets and parameter descriptions, the algorithm of the proposed FOWFS feature fusion approach. The experimentation was performed using Intel(R) Core(TM) i5-7200U CPU @ 2.50G Hz with 2.71 GHz processor, 4.00 GB (3.88 GB usable) RAM, 64-bit operating system, x64-based processor operating system, and executed on the platform Google Colab.

4.1. Datasets Description

This study of feature selection and classification was performed on two skin lesion datasets, HAM 10000 and BCN 20000, collected from [49,50]. The HAM 10000 dataset is the abbreviated form of Human Against Machine and it has 10,000 training images for detection of pigmented skin lesions with seven classes. The BCN 20000 dataset is composed of 19,424 demoscopic images of skin lesion collected from a hospital clinic in Barcelona during the period 2010 to 2016 and this dataset has eight classes as detailed in Table 1 and Figure 5a,b.

Table 1. Datasets and description of skin lesion classes.

Dataset	Classes
HAM 10000	Actinic keratoses and intraepithelial carcinoma/Bowen's disease (AKIEC), basal cell carcinoma (BCC), benign keratosis-like lesions (BKL), dermatofibroma (DF), melanoma (MEL), melanocytic nevi (NV) and vascular lesions (VASC).
BCN 20000	Nevus, melanoma (MEL), basal cell carcinoma (BCC), seborrheic keratosis (SK), actinic keratosis (AK), squamos cell carcinoma (SCC), dermatofibroma (DF), and vascular lesions (VASC).

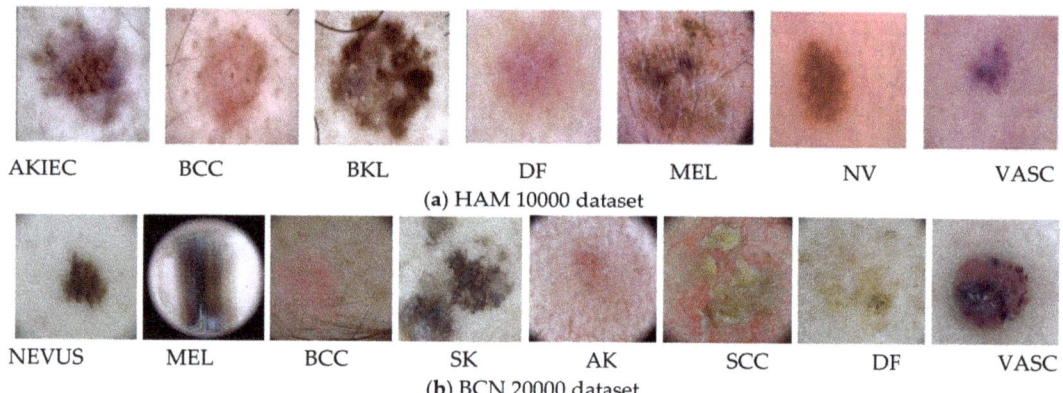

Figure 5. The skin lesions of (**a**) HAM 10000 and (**b**) BCN 20000 datasets.

4.2. Parameters Discussion

The various parameters of the network models and optimization techniques used for experimentation of this study and their chosen values are discussed in Table 2.

Table 2. Parameters and their chosen values.

Network Models and Optimization Techniques	Parameters and Their Associated Values
VGG16	16 weight layers
EfficientNet B0	237 weight layers
ResNet50	50 weight layers
AWFS	Total weights:3; w_1 dimension = 1×1; w_2 dimension = 1×1; w_2 dimension = 1×1
MOWFS	Total weights:3; w_1 dimension = 1×1; w_2 dimension = 1×1; w_2 dimension = 1×1
FOWFS	Total weights:3; w_1 dimension = 1×504; w_2 dimension = 1×1024; w_2 dimension = 1×1024
GA	Number of decision variables = 3; Maximum number of iterations = 50; Population size = 10; Selection method-Roulette wheel
PSO	Number of decision variables = 3; Maximum number of iterations = 50; Number of particles = 10; Inertia weight = 1; Inertia weight damping ratio = 0.99; Personal learning coefficient = 1.5; Global learning coefficient = 2.0
AJS	Number of decision variables = 3; Maximum number of iterations = 50; Population size = 10

4.3. Algorithm of Proposed FOWFS Feature Fusion Strategy

The working principle of the four feature fusion strategies, CFS, AWFS, MOWFS, and FOWFS, are depicted in Figure 4a–d. The MOWFS and FOWFS strategies are based on optimizing the chosen weights using AJS algorithm. The optimization steps of both are the same, the only difference lies in the formation of combined feature weights as detailed in Section 3.3. The hybridization of AJS for formation of combined feature sets exploring the model-based optimization and each feature-based optimization is depicted in an algorithmic form as given in Algorithm 1.

Algorithm 1 MOWFS and FOWFS: Optimized deep feature fusion strategies

---

For 100 population $(Total_{pop})$ initialize $(w_1, w_2$ and $w_3)$;
    For $i = 1 : Total_{pop}$
        Calculate MSE using extracted features and *cost function* of SVM/DT/NB/MLP classifier;
    For $i = 1 : Total_{pop}$;
        Calculate *time control function* $f(T_C)$ for t;
        If $f(T_C)(t) \geq 0.5$
            Update w_1, w_2 and w_3 using Equation (2);
        Else
            If $rand(0,1) > (1 - f(T_C)(t)$
            Update w_1, w_2 and w_3 using Equation (3);
            Else
                Update w_1, w_2 and w_3 using Equation (5);
            End if
        End for
    End for
Check the boundary conditions such as $Upper_{bound}$ and $Lower_{bound}$, whether w_1, w_2 and w_3 range between 0~1;
Choose w_1, w_2 and w_3 with minimum MSE;
End for: Iterate over 50 iterations;

4.4. Result Analysis and Validation

This section discusses the experimental results of all the proposed deep feature fusion approach for skin lesion classification of HAM 10000 and BCN 20000 datasets along with the evaluation and validation of the feature selection strategies. In the first phase of experimentation, the benefit of transfer learning mechanism was achieved for obtaining the better performance with less computational effort. Here, three CNNs' pre-trained learning models, VGG16, EfficientNet B0, and ResNet50, were used to extract the meaningful features from the new images.

Table 3 shows the experimental results of those three pre-trained models for both the skin lesion image datasets, which demonstrates the feature acquisition time (in minutes) with respect to the original features. A straightforward comparison was carried out for the accuracy validation with respect to fused feature sets and the highest ranked feature sets (features whose $weight > 0.5$) obtained from three pre-trained models using Decision Tree (DT), Naïve Bayesian (NB), Multi-Layer Perceptron (MLP), and Support Vector Machine (SVM) classifiers as discussed in Table 4, Table 5, Table 6, Table 7, respectively. From those three tables, it can be seen that for both the datasets, initially, the number of features selected from three pre-trained models is 2560 features, which form a fused feature set and the CFS selects 2560 features and as all the features are selected for the classification process, the ranking of features has not been done, therefore there is no improvement in validation accuracy.

Table 3. Feature acquiring time.

CNN Pre-Trained Models	Datasets	Original No. of Features	Feature Acquisition Time
VGG16	HAM 10000	512	10.11
EfficientNet B0		1024	8.24
ResNet50		1024	5.42
VGG16	BCN 20000	512	17.21
EfficientNet B0		1024	15.11
ResNet50		1024	10.29

Table 4. Validation accuracy of fused feature sets vs. ranked feature sets based on DT.

Fused Feature Configurations	Datasets	Dimensionality (Fused Feature Set)	Validation Accuracy (Fused Feature Set)	Dimensionality (Highest Ranked Feature Set)	Validation Accuracy (Highest Ranked Feature Set)
CFS	HAM 10000	2560	0.9110	2560	0.9110
AWFS		2560	0.9124	512+1024	0.9410
MOWFS-GA		2560	0.9116	512	0.9411
MOWFS-PSO		2560	0.9215	512	0.9412
MOWFS-AJS		2560	0.9219	1024	0.9401
FOWFS-GA		2560	0.9310	1015	0.9312
FOWFS-PSO		2560	0.9322	954	0.9412
FOWFS-AJS		2560	0.9322	914	0.9422
CFS	BCN 20000	2560	0.8847	2560	0.8847
AWFS		2560	0.8925	512	0.9610
MOWFS-GA		2560	0.8948	512 + 1024	0.9611
MOWFS-PSO		2560	0.9012	512 + 1024 + 1024	0.9612
MOWFS-AJS		2560	0.8999	1121	0.9602
FOWFS-GA		2560	0.9015	998	0.9512
FOWFS-PSO		2560	0.9128	1019	0.9611
FOWFS-AJS		2560	0.9198	925	0.9622

Table 5. Validation accuracy of fused feature sets vs. ranked feature sets based on NB.

Fused Feature Configurations	Datasets	Dimensionality (Fused Feature Set)	Validation Accuracy (Fused Feature Set)	Dimensionality (Highest Ranked Feature Set)	Validation Accuracy (Highest Ranked Feature Set)
CFS	HAM 10000	2560	0.9118	2560	0.9118
AWFS		2560	0.9211	512	0.9411
MOWFS-GA		2560	0.9124	512	0.9421
MOWFS-PSO		2560	0.9158	1024	0.9422
MOWFS-AJS		2560	0.9199	1024 + 1024	0.9428
FOWFS-GA		2560	0.9210	995	0.9391
FOWFS-PSO		2560	0.9214	961	0.9438
FOWFS-AJS		2560	0.9218	1015	0.9448
CFS	BCN 20000	2560	0.9001	2560	0.9001
AWFS		2560	0.9191	512 + 1024	0.9611
MOWFS-GA		2560	0.9125	1024	0.9621
MOWFS-PSO		2560	0.9215	512 + 1024	0.9622
MOWFS-AJS		2560	0.9244	512 + 1024 + 1024	0.9628
FOWFS-GA		2560	0.9248	1115	0.9594
FOWFS-PSO		2560	0.9314	1245	0.9632
FOWFS-AJS		2560	0.9325	998	0.9648

Table 6. Validation accuracy of fused feature sets vs. ranked feature sets based on MLP.

Fused Feature Configurations	Datasets	Dimensionality (Fused Feature Set)	Validation Accuracy (Fused Feature Set)	Dimensionality (Highest Ranked Feature Set)	Validation Accuracy (Highest Ranked Feature Set)
CFS	HAM 10000	2560	0.9211	2560	0.9211
AWFS		2560	0.9214	1024	0.9550
MOWFS-GA		2560	0.9244	512 + 1024	0.9552
MOWFS-PSO		2560	0.9214	512 + 1024	0.9558
MOWFS-AJS		2560	0.9254	512	0.9561
FOWFS-GA		2560	0.9311	915	0.9342
FOWFS-PSO		2560	0.9324	898	0.9537
FOWFS-AJS		2560	0.9345	975	0.9562
CFS	BCN 20000	2560	0.9112	2560	0.9112
AWFS		2560	0.9119	512+1024	0.9650
MOWFS-GA		2560	0.9132	1024+1024	0.9652
MOWFS-PSO		2560	0.9124	512	0.9658
MOWFS-AJS		2560	0.9312	512+1024	0.9661
FOWFS-GA		2560	0.9365	1124	0.9549
FOWFS-PSO		2560	0.9378	954	0.9649
FOWFS-AJS		2560	0.9411	929	0.9669

Table 7. Validation accuracy of fused feature sets vs. ranked feature sets based on SVM.

Fused Feature Configurations	Datasets	Dimensionality (Fused Feature Set)	Validation Accuracy (Fused Feature Set)	Dimensionality (Highest Ranked Feature Set)	Validation Accuracy (Highest Ranked Feature Set)
CFS	HAM 10000	2560	0.9225	2560	0.9225
AWFS		2560	0.9315	1024 + 1024	0.9599
MOWFS-GA		2560	0.9311	512	0.9611
MOWFS-PSO		2560	0.9347	512 + 1024	0.9712
MOWFS-AJS		2560	0.9348	512 + 1024	0.9612
FOWFS-GA		2560	0.9378	1125	0.9479
FOWFS-PSO		2560	0.9399	897	0.9679
FOWFS-AJS		2560	0.9425	867	0.9779
CFS	BCN 20000	2560	0.9147	2560	0.9147
AWFS		2560	0.9110	1024	0.9599
MOWFS-GA		2560	0.9118	1024 + 512	0.9611
MOWFS-PSO		2560	0.9210	1024 + 1024	0.9712
MOWFS-AJS		2560	0.9211	512	0.9612
FOWFS-GA		2560	0.9212	1005	0.9579
FOWFS-PSO		2560	0.9245	905	0.9688
FOWFS-AJS		2560	0.9311	899	0.9779

From Table 4, it can be seen that, for the HAM 10000 dataset, the AWFS selects highest ranked feature set with weights of VGG16 (with 512 features) and any one of the other two pre-trained models (with 1024 features) based on DT classifier with an improved accuracy of 94.10%. It can also be inferred that the MOWFS-AJS and FOWFS-AJS have validation accuracy of 94.24% and 94.22%, respectively, with the highest ranked feature set of 1024 and 914 number of features. Considering the improvement in accuracy with respect to CFS, MOWFS-AJS, and FOWFS-AJS, it is clearly evident that with a lower number of feature sets, MOWFS-AJS and FOWFS-AJS achieve 3.14% and 3.12% improved accuracy for HAM 10000 dataset based on DT classifier. Similarly, for the BCN 20000 dataset, the improvement of MOWFS-AJS and FOWFS-AJS over CFS was found to be 7.77% and 7.75%, respectively, with a lower number of features selected as ranked fused feature set based on DT classifier.

The performance based on NB classifier from Table 5 can be detailed as follows. The observed improvements for HAM 10000 dataset of MOWFS-AJS and FOWFS-AJS over CFS were found to be 3.1% and 3.3%, respectively with 1024 + 1024 and 1015 ranked feature sets. Similarly, for the BCN 20000 dataset, the recorded improvements of MOWFS-AJS and FOWFS-AJS over CFS were 6.27% and 6.47%. Additionally, it was seen that the number of features selected for classification by FOWFS-AJS is only 998 features, which is much less in comparison to both strategies.

Table 6 depicts the performance of all proposed feature fusion strategies based on the MLP classifier. From this table, it can be seen that the FOWFS-AJS is outperformed over the rest of the compared methods for both the datasets. The observed improvements for HAM 10000 dataset of MOWFS-AJS and FOWFS-AJS over CFS were found to be 3.3% and 3.58%, respectively, with 512 and 975 features in ranked feature set. Similarly, for the BCN 20000 dataset, the recorded improvements of MOWFS-AJS and FOWFS-AJS over CFS are 5.49% and 5.57% with 512 + 1024 and 929 selected features from the ranked feature set.

Similarly, the performance based on the SVM classifier for both the datasets are recorded in Table 7. From this table, we can see that the improvements for the HAM 10000 dataset of MOWFS-AJS and FOWFS-AJS over CFS was found to be 3.87% and 5.54%, respectively with 512+1024 and 876 features in the ranked feature set. For the BCN 20000 dataset, the recorded improvements of MOWFS-AJS and FOWFS-AJS over CFS were 4.65% and 6.32% with 512 and 899 selected features from the ranked feature set. From Table 5 to Table 7, the FOWFS-AJS outperformed rest of the proposed feature fusion strategies with respect to validation accuracy measured using NB, MLP, and SVM for both the skin lesion datasets except the performance recorded using DT shows MOWFS-AJS better results in comparison to other strategies (Table 4), but when compared with FOWFS-AJS, it has only 0.02% improved result for both the datasets.

The recognition performance of the three CNNs' pre-trained models and the proposed strategies, namely CFS, AWFS, MOWFS-GA, MOWFS-PSO, MOWFS-AJS, FOWFS-GA, FOWFS-PSO, and FOWFS-AJS, are recorded in Tables 8 and 9 for HAM 10000 and BCN 20000 datasets, respectively, by measuring the accuracy, precision, sensitivity, and F1-score based on all four classification algorithms. From both tables, it is observed that the SVM shows better recognition performance and FOWFS-AJS is showing improved recognition rate with respect to all the models considered for comparison.

Table 8. Recognition performance with respect to CNNs' pre-trained models, CFS, and feature fusion configurations for HAM 10000 dataset.

Classifiers	Performance Measures	CNN Pre-Trained Models			CFS	AWFS	Feature Fusion Configurations					
		VGG16	EfficientNet B0	ResNet50			MOWFS-GA	MOWFS-PSO	MOWFS-AJS	FOWFS-GA	FOWFS-PSO	FOWFS-AJS
DT	Accuracy	0.9302	0.9321	0.9315	0.9412	0.9410	0.9411	0.9412	0.9424	0.9312	0.9412	0.9422
	Precision	0.9100	0.9112	0.9187	0.9189	0.9128	0.9254	0.9288	0.9321	0.9124	0.9311	0.9318
	Sensitivity	0.9125	0.9144	0.9128	0.9214	0.9311	0.9301	0.9299	0.9298	0.9388	0.9258	0.9301
	F1-Score	0.9115	0.9132	0.9120	0.9199	0.9205	0.9289	0.9289	0.9298	0.9298	0.9299	0.9304
NB	Accuracy	0.9308	0.9302	0.9311	0.9332	0.9411	0.9421	0.9422	0.9428	0.9398	0.9438	0.9448
	Precision	0.9104	0.9106	0.9111	0.9154	0.9128	0.9118	0.9187	0.9144	0.9218	0.9217	0.9288
	Sensitivity	0.9114	0.9114	0.9125	0.9128	0.9177	0.9178	0.9188	0.9198	0.9189	0.9200	0.9202
	F1-Score	0.9108	0.9110	0.9121	0.142	0.9135	0.9158	0.9187	0.9158	0.9199	0.9211	0.9245
MLP	Accuracy	0.9302	0.93	0.9342	0.9369	0.9550	0.9552	0.9558	0.9561	0.9349	0.9549	0.9569
	Precision	0.9114	0.9115	0.9105	0.9200	0.9189	0.9344	0.9341	0.9358	0.9219	0.9347	0.9382
	Sensitivity	0.9148	0.9198	0.9200	0.9258	0.9301	0.9289	0.9299	0.9351	0.9374	0.9387	0.9403
	F1-Score	0.9151	0.9144	0.9184	0.9235	0.9215	0.9288	0.9306	0.9352	0.9254	0.9355	0.9389
SVM	Accuracy	0.9412	0.9341	0.9416	0.9477	0.9599	0.9611	0.9712	0.9612	0.9479	0.9679	0.9779
	Precision	0.9204	0.9205	0.9345	0.9200	0.9301	0.9301	0.9289	0.9447	0.9321	0.9498	0.9524
	Sensitivity	0.9200	0.9236	0.9124	0.9258	0.9256	0.9306	0.9401	0.9400	0.9389	0.9498	0.9499
	F1-Score	0.9200	0.216	0.9205	0.9250	0.9289	0.9302	0.325	0.9411	0.9322	0.9497	0.9510

Table 9. Recognition performance with respect to CNN's pre-trained models, CFS, and feature fusion configurations for BCN 20000 dataset.

Classifiers	Performance Measures	CNN Pre-Trained Models			CFS	AWFS	Feature Fusion Configurations					
		VGG16	EfficientNet B0	ResNet50			MOWFS-GA	MOWFS-PSO	MOWFS-AJS	FOWFS-GA	FOWFS-PSO	FOWFS-AJS
DT	Accuracy	0.9402	0.9461	0.9415	0.9512	0.9610	0.9611	0.9612	0.9624	0.9512	0.9612	0.9622
	Precision	0.9348	0.9311	0.9321	0.9348	0.9410	0.9422	0.9148	0.9522	0.9432	0.9498	0.9509
	Sensitivity	0.9218	0.9302	0.9109	0.9358	0.9389	0.9401	0.9487	0.9451	0.9422	0.9502	0.9511
	F1-Score	0.9225	0.9310	0.9215	0.9250	0.9399	0.9410	0.9255	0.9458	0.9425	0.9500	0.9510
NB	Accuracy	0.9421	0.9402	0.9451	0.9532	0.9611	0.9621	0.9622	0.9628	0.9598	0.9638	0.9648
	Precision	0.9215	0.9244	0.9348	0.9324	0.9422	0.9502	0.9248	0.9100	0.9458	0.9519	0.9588
	Sensitivity	0.9257	0.9301	0.9108	0.9458	0.9109	0.9002	0.9315	0.9487	0.9518	0.9505	0.9522
	F1-Score	0.9222	0.9241	0.9210	0.9344	0.324	0.9542	0.9268	0.9214	0.9461	0.9510	0.9544
MLP	Accuracy	0.9502	0.9538	0.9542	0.9569	0.9650	0.9652	0.9658	0.9661	0.9549	0.9649	0.9669
	Precision	0.9325	0.9328	0.9212	0.9318	0.9458	0.9428	0.9478	0.9488	0.9498	0.9500	0.9582
	Sensitivity	0.9388	0.9399	0.9458	0.9222	0.9331	0.9411	0.9501	0.9499	0.9502	0.9312	0.9401
	F1-Score	0.9341	0.9349	0.9332	0.9288	0.9339	0.9412	0.9481	0.9492	0.9499	0.9514	0.9554
SVM	Accuracy	0.9522	0.9541	0.9546	0.9572	0.9599	0.9611	0.9712	0.9612	0.9579	0.9679	0.9779
	Precision	0.9401	0.9388	0.9406	0.9399	0.9401	0.9402	0.9500	0.9502	0.9501	0.9515	0.9624
	Sensitivity	0.9358	0.9412	0.9402	0.9388	0.9385	0.9366	0.9488	0.9412	0.9499	0.9489	0.9539
	F1-Score	0.9366	0.9391	0.9404	0.9389	0.9390	0.9389	0.9489	0.9488	0.9488	0.9490	0.9568

Further, a straightforward comparison was made considering the observed validation accuracy of all the proposed feature fusion strategies for the combined or fused feature sets and the feature sets obtained after ranking based on all four classifiers for both of the datasets as given in Figure 6, Figure 7, Figure 8, Figure 9. The differences in validation accuracy based on DT classifier for HAM 10000 and BCN 20000 datasets are represented in Figure 6a,b respectively and from this figure, we can see the significant improvement of MOWFS-AJS and FOWFS-AJS over the remaining six strategies and the MOWFS-AJS performed better in this case of classification with 1.09% (fused feature set) and 2.91% (ranked feature set) for HAM 10000 and 3.51% and 7.75% for BCN 20000 datasets. The FOWFS-AJS showed better validation accuracy with respect to the rest of the proposed strategies based on NB, MLP, and SVM classifiers. From Figure 7a,b, it can be seen that FOWFS-AJS over CFS showed improvement of 1% (fused feature set) and 2% (ranked feature set) and 3.24% (fused feature set) and 6.47% (ranked feature set) for HAM 10000 and BCN 20000 datasets, respectively. Similarly, the accuracy recorded based on MLP and SVM classifiers can be summarized as 1.34% (fused feature set),3.51% (ranked feature set), 2% (fused feature set), 5.54% (ranked feature set) for HAM 10000 dataset (Figures 8a and 9a) and 2.99% (fused feature set), 5.57% (ranked feature set) and 1.64% (fused feature set) and 6.35% (ranked feature set) for BNC dataset respectively (Figures 8b and 9b).

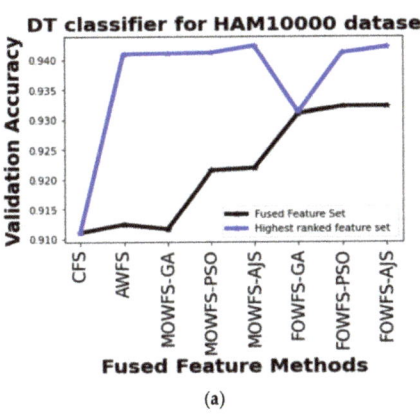
(a)

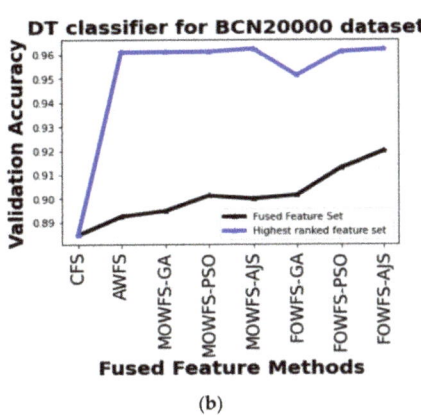
(b)

Figure 6. Comparison of validation accuracy for fused feature set and highest ranked feature set using DT classifier for (a) HAM 10000 dataset and (b) BCN 20000 dataset.

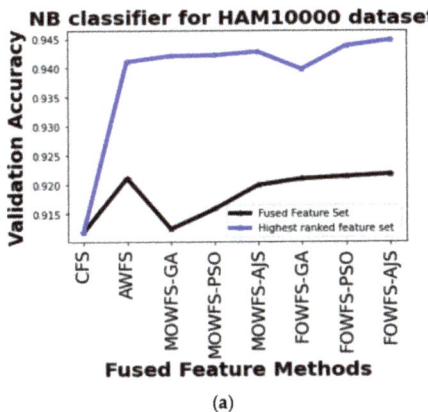
(a)

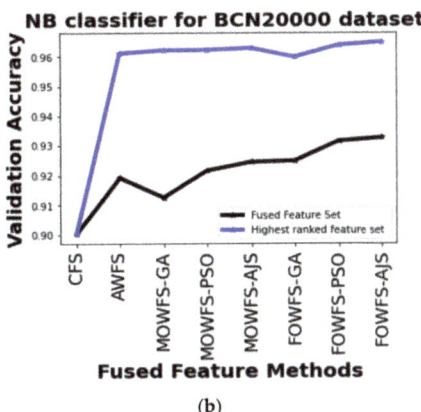
(b)

Figure 7. Comparison of validation accuracy for fused feature set and highest ranked feature set using NB classifier for (a) HAM 10000 dataset and (b) BCN 20000 dataset.

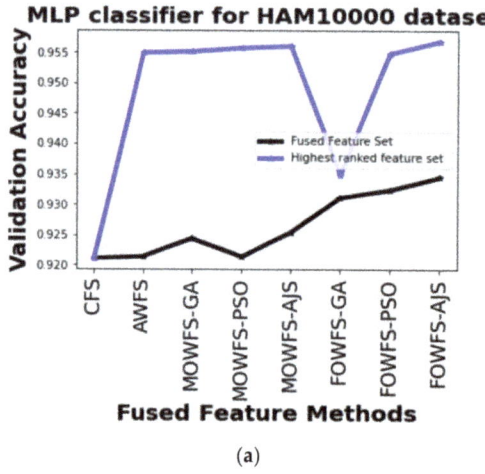
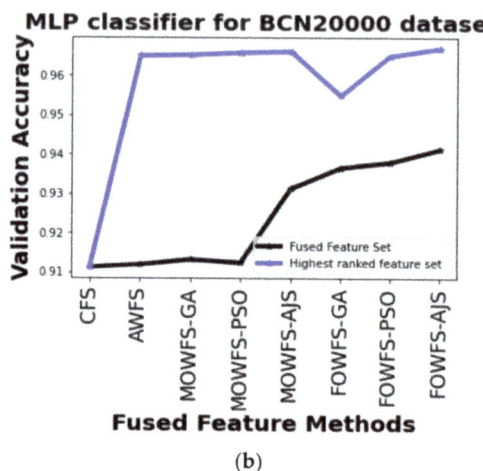

Figure 8. Comparison of validation accuracy for fused feature set and highest ranked feature set using MLP classifier for (**a**) HAM 10000 dataset and (**b**) BCN 20000 dataset.

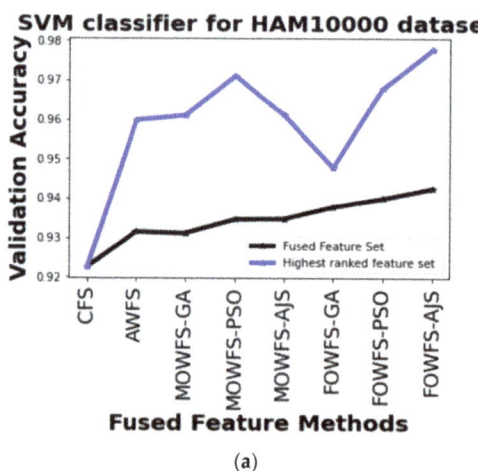
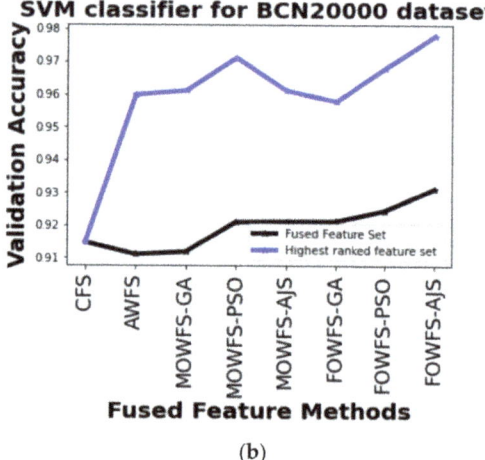

Figure 9. Comparison of validation accuracy for fused feature set and highest ranked feature set using SVM classifier for (**a**) HAM 10000 dataset and (**b**) BCN 20000 dataset.

Additionally, the area under the receiver operating characteristics curves (AUC-ROC) were plotted to measure the performance and degree of separability amongst the proposed three strategies AWFS, MOWFS-AJS, and FOWFS-AJS to describe how well the models are capable of distinguishing between the classes which are represented in Figure 10, Figure 11, Figure 12, Figure 13 for both datasets based on DT, NB, MLP, and SVM classifiers. From Figure 10a,b, it is observed that FOWFS-AJS showed best accuracy performance with 90.9% and 91.06% for HAM 10000 and BCN 20000 datasets, respectively. Similarly, the recorded performance of the three remaining classifiers can be summarized as: based on NB classifier, the best recorded performance of FOWFS-AJS was 92.84% and 93.21% for HAM 10000 and BCN 20000 datasets, respectively (Figure 11a,b); based on MLP, FOWFS-AJS showed 93.24% and 93.81% for HAM 10000 and BCN 20000 datasets, respectively (Figure 12a,b);

and similarly, the SVM recorded a performance of FOWFS-AJS as 94.05% and 94.90%, respectively, for HAM 10000 and BCN 20000 datasets (Figure 13a,b).

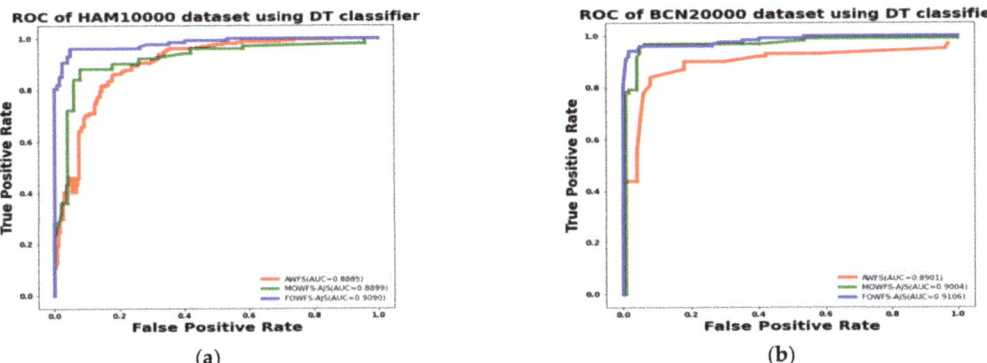

Figure 10. ROC using DT classifier for (**a**) HAM 10000 dataset and (**b**) BCN 20000 dataset.

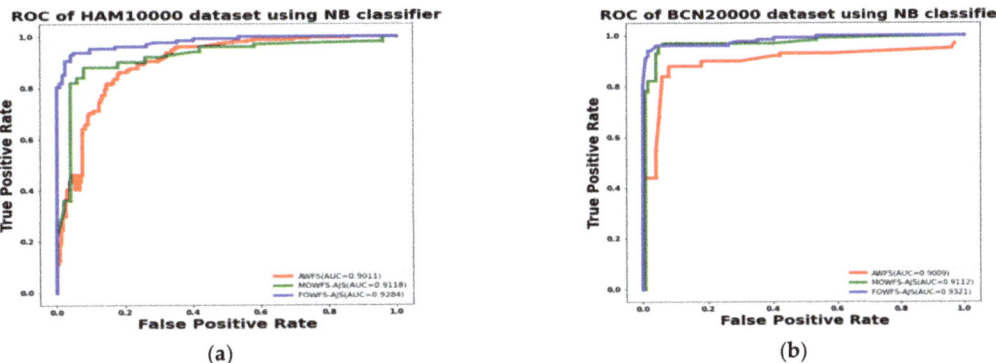

Figure 11. ROC using NB classifier for (**a**) HAM 10000 dataset and (**b**) BCN 20000 dataset.

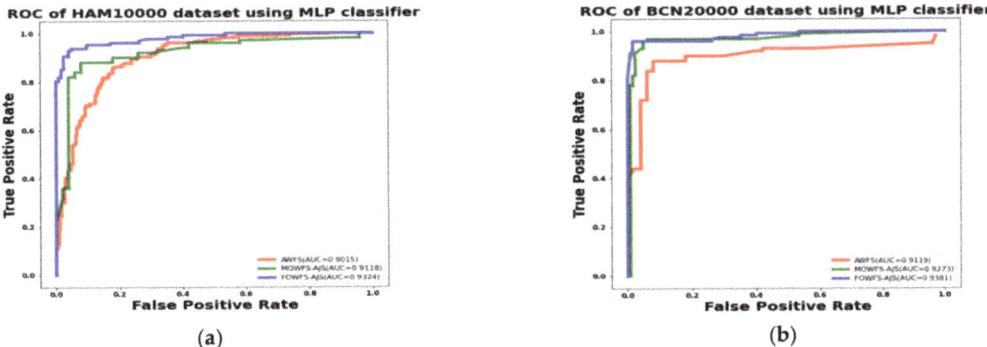

Figure 12. ROC using MLP classifier for (**a**) HAM 10000 dataset and (**b**) BCN 20000 dataset.

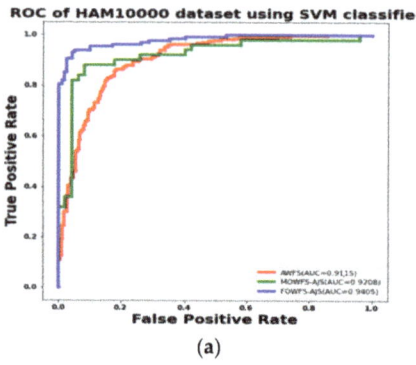
(a)

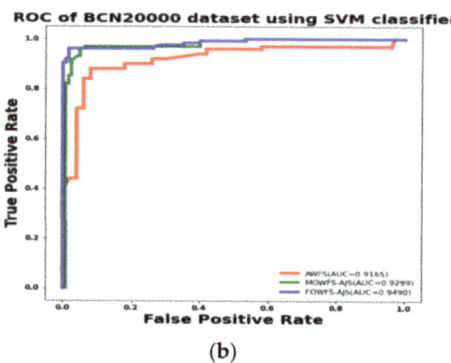
(b)

Figure 13. ROC using SVM classifier for (**a**) HAM 10000 dataset and (**b**) BCN 20000 dataset.

Finally, a computational comparison (in minutes) was made between the feature acquisition time by the proposed deep feature fusion strategies and the mean of time taken for classification algorithms to classify the skin lesson datasets with the updated feature sets and is shown in Figure 14a,b for HAM 10000 and BCN 20000 datasets, respectively. From those two figures, it is also evident that the proposed FOWFS-AJS comparatively showed better performance with respect to both feature acquisition and classification time for both the datasets.

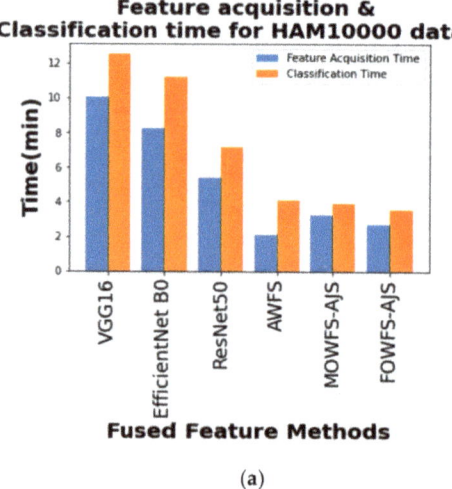
(a)

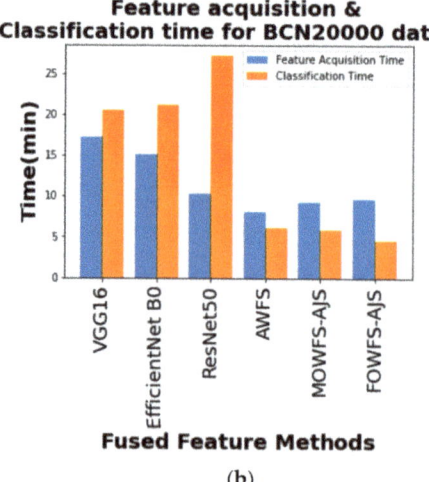
(b)

Figure 14. Comparison of mean feature acquisition time vs. classification time of DT, NB, MLP, and SVM classifiers for (**a**) HAM 10000 dataset and (**b**) BCN 20000 dataset.

4.5. Validation through Statistical Test

The experimental results were further analyzed using a non-parametric Friedman statistical test [51,52] to determine whether or not there is a statistical difference observed between the models or strategies experimented and compared. Here, this statistical test was utilized to deal with the issue of comparison between all three pre-trained CNNs' models and the proposed fusion strategies on both HAM 10000 and BCN 20000 datasets. To analyze the performance of VGG16, EfficientNet B0, ResNet50, CFS, AWFS, MOWFS-GA, MOWFS-PSO, MOWFS-AJS, FOWFS-GA, FOWFS-PSO, and FOWFS-AJS, the test was performed from the perspective of average ranking. This Friedman test, which is under the null hypothesis, was computed as follows using Equation (8):

$$\begin{aligned}
FM_{Stat} &= \left[\frac{12}{(N \times k \times (k+1))}\right] \times \sum R^2 - [3 \times N \times (k+1)] \\
FM_{Stat} &= \left[\frac{12}{(N \times k \times (3+1))}\right] \times \sum 32^2 + 27^2 + 13^2 - [3 \times 12 \times (3+1)] \\
FM_{Stat} &= \left[\frac{12}{144}\right] \times \sum \times [1024 + 729 + 169] - 144 \\
FM_{Stat} &= [0.083 \times 1922] - 144 = 15.526
\end{aligned} \quad (8)$$

where FM_{Stat}, N, k, and R represent the statistical value, number of datasets, the number of strategies used, and average ranking respectively. The statistical value FM_{Stat} is distributed in line with the Fisherman distribution with $(k-1)$ and $((k-1)()(T-1))$ degrees of freedom. The result of this test is $R = [21\ 21\ 18\ 16\ 12\ 10\ 4\ 8\ 14\ 6\ 2]$ and the calculated $FM_{Stat} = 19.7988$. The critical value is 2.9782 under the significance level $\alpha = 0.05$ for $N = 2$ and $k = 11$; it is evident that the critical value is smaller than the observed values of all FM_{Stat} on all evaluation metrics. This means that the null hypothesis on all evaluations metrics is rejected under this test and the proposed FOWFS-AJS deep feature fusion strategy achieves satisfactory performance on two datasets and eleven compared models.

4.6. Discussions on Key Findings

The key findings of this research are as follows. The performance of the transfer learning at the feature level based on the CNNs' three pre-trained networks achieved optimal performance faster than any other traditional feature selection models and the ensemble learning of features used to design the feature fusion models (for example, CFS) from the output of those three pre-trained networks showed their good performance to design a robust classifier for skin lesion datasets. From the experimentation, it was seen that only designing a CFS model based on basic fusion strategy does not achieve better leverage, therefore the weighted approach of selecting features and forming features sets through AWFS was experimented and shown to have better performance over CFS. Rather than only using feature fusion, it was seen that the strategy for decision on feature fusion approach by utilizing the AJS optimizer to identify the optimum point considering two special cases (active and passive) motions of this algorithm helped to find the best cost. In this study, two decision-based feature fusion models, namely model-based and feature based strategies formed by adaptively choosing the optimal weights such as MOWFS-AJS and FOWFS-AJS have showed their relatively good performance. The MSE of both model-based and feature-based strategies are measured as *cost function*, where the measured MSE of the opted classification model is taken as the cost and the weights $(w_1, w_2\ and\ w_3)$ are taken as *decision variables*. This total process was continued for 50 iterations to obtain optimized weights from all three pre-trained models. Thus, the final ensemble of features was formed for test set as $([w_1]_{1\times 1} \times F_{VGG16})$, $([w_2]_{1\times 1} \times F_{EfficientNet\ B0})$, $([w_3]_{1\times 1} \times F_{ResNet50})$ for model-based strategy. The feature-based strategy focused on feature-based optimization of adaptively chosen weights for formation of combined weighted feature set such as $[w_1]_{1\times 512} \times F_{VGG16}$, $[w_2]_{1\times 1024} \times F_{EfficientNet\ B0}$ and $[w_3]_{1\times 1024} \times F_{ResNet50}$ with total weights (512 + 1024 + 1024). Then, the process of obtaining optimized weights is performed and finally it returns 512 + 1024 + 1024 optimized weights based on each feature and the combined feature set is formed as $[w_1]_{1\times 512} \times F_{VGG16}$, $[w_2]_{1\times 1024} \times F_{EfficientNet\ B0}$, $[w_3]_{1\times 1024} \times F_{ResNet50}$. Then, features having *weights* > 0.5 were considered as best performing features and were considered for final classification. The performance of the proposed deep feature fusion strategies was evaluated based on each classification model and the proposed optimized strategies were compared with GA and PSO, two widely used meta-heuristic optimization techniques, through accuracy, precision, sensitivity, and F1-score. Finally, the Friedman statistical test was performed to statistically validate the proposed strategies.

The empirical evidence showed that choosing the weights of the pre-trained networks adaptively in an optimized way gave a good starting point for initialization to mitigating the chances of exploding or vanishing gradients, thus the performance of FOWFS-AJS with SVM learning leveraged the existing network for both the skin lesion datasets and the advantage of properly selecting rich and informative beneficial feature through this feature-based optimized approach received better attention during the experimentation and validation processes.

5. Conclusions

Visual inspection and manual examination of skin lesion images has been a burden to the physicians and clinicians to detect melanoma. With the advancements of technology and computational resources, academicians and researchers are trying to develop computational models and AI, ML, and DL have given a new direction to this area of research. In this work, we tried to propose feature level fusion strategies by exploring the DL approaches which in turn help for proper classification. An empirical study was attempted for design of combined, weighted, and optimized strategies of feature selection by exploring the feature fusion approach for classification of skin lesion image classification. The key advantages of transfer learning through the CNNs' pre-trained networks, fusion approach, selection of features sets by adaptively choosing the weights (model based and feature based) with a new meta-heuristic optimizer AJS was experimented for two skin lesion datasets and then validated through four state-of-the art classifiers, namely DT, NB, MLP, and SVM. The validations of the proposed strategies were performed based on classification accuracies, precision, sensitivity, and F1-score, the difference between the validation accuracies and the AUC-ROC curves were plotted. Extensive comparative studies and the computational time taken for acquisition of features to form features along with statistical validations were performed and the outcome of this empirical research led to conclude that in this experimental setting, the feature sets generated through the proposed FOWFS-AJS leveraged the SVM classifier to classify the HAM 10000 and BCN 20000 skin lesion datasets. This work only explored three pre-trained networks and can be further experimented for few more pre-trained networks to establish the capability of transfer learning. Further, this research can be implemented for other domains of research and specifically, the decision fusion approach can be further explored by utilizing many other upcoming meta-heuristic optimization techniques and a few other skin lesion datasets can also be experimented.

Author Contributions: Conceptualization, N.M., A.V.N.R., and S.K.; methodology, N.M. and M.P.; software, A.A.; validation, N.M. and M.P.; formal analysis, N.M.; investigation, N.M.; writing—original draft preparation, N.M. and M.P.; writing—review and editing, N.M. and M.P.; supervision, S.K. and M.P.; funding acquisition, A.A. All authors have read and agreed to the published version of the manuscript.

Funding: This research received no external funding.

Institutional Review Board Statement: Not applicable.

Informed Consent Statement: Not applicable.

Data Availability Statement: Data will be made available on request to the first author.

Acknowledgments: This work was supported by the Ministry of Science and Higher Education of the Russian Federation (Government Order FENU-2020-0022).

Conflicts of Interest: The authors declare no conflict of interest.

References

1. Talavera-Martínez, L.; Bibiloni, P.; Giacaman, A.; Taberner, R.; Hernando, L.J.D.P.; González-Hidalgo, M. A novel approach for skin lesion symmetry classification with a deep learning model. *Comput. Biol. Med.* **2022**, *145*, 105450. [CrossRef] [PubMed]
2. Hasan, K.; Elahi, T.E.; Alam, A.; Jawad, T.; Martí, R. DermoExpert: Skin lesion classification using a hybrid convolutional neural network through segmentation, transfer learning, and augmentation. *Informatics Med. Unlocked* **2022**, *28*, 100819. [CrossRef]

3. Batista, L.G.; Bugatti, P.H.; Saito, P.T. Classification of Skin Lesion through Active Learning Strategies. *Comput. Methods Programs Biomed.* **2022**, *226*, 107122. [CrossRef] [PubMed]
4. Lucieri, A.; Bajwa, M.N.; Braun, S.A.; Malik, M.I.; Dengel, A.; Ahmed, S. ExAID: A multimodal explanation framework for computer-aided diagnosis of skin lesions. *Comput. Methods Programs Biomed.* **2022**, *215*, 106620. [CrossRef] [PubMed]
5. Calderón, C.; Sanchez, K.; Castillo, S.; Arguello, H. BILSK: A bilinear convolutional neural network approach for skin lesion classification. *Comput. Methods Programs Biomed. Updat.* **2021**, *1*, 100036. [CrossRef]
6. Hameed, N.; Shabut, A.; Hameed, F.; Cirstea, S.; Hossain, A. Chapter 7—Achievements of neural network in skin lesions classification. In *State of the Art in Neural Networks and their Applications*; El-Baz, A.S., Suri, J.S., Eds.; Academic Press: Cambridge, MA, USA, 2021; pp. 133–151.
7. Khan, M.A.; Zhang, Y.-D.; Sharif, M.; Akram, T. Pixels to Classes: Intelligent Learning Framework for Multiclass Skin Lesion Localization and Classification. *Comput. Electr. Eng.* **2021**, *90*, 106956. [CrossRef]
8. Goyal, M.; Knackstedt, T.; Yan, S.; Hassanpour, S. Artificial intelligence-based image classification methods for diagnosis of skin cancer: Challenges and opportunities. *Comput. Biol. Med.* **2020**, *127*, 104065. [CrossRef]
9. Tschandl, P.; Codella, N.; Akay, B.N.; Argenziano, G.; Braun, R.P.; Cabo, H.; Gutman, D.; Halpern, A.; Helba, B.; Hofmann-Wellenhof, R.; et al. Comparison of the accuracy of human readers versus machine-learning algorithms for pigmented skin lesion classification: An open, web-based, international, diagnostic study. *Lancet Oncol.* **2019**, *20*, 938–947. [CrossRef]
10. Hameed, N.; Shabut, A.M.; Ghosh, M.K.; Hossain, M. Multi-class multi-level classification algorithm for skin lesions classification using machine learning techniques. *Expert Syst. Appl.* **2020**, *141*, 112961. [CrossRef]
11. Shankar, K.; Dutta, A.K.; Kumar, S.; Joshi, G.P.; Doo, I.C. Chaotic Sparrow Search Algorithm with Deep Transfer Learning Enabled Breast Cancer Classification on Histopathological Images. *Cancers* **2022**, *14*, 2770. [CrossRef]
12. Iqbal, I.; Younus, M.; Walayat, K.; Kakar, M.U.; Ma, J. Automated multi-class classification of skin lesions through deep convolutional neural network with dermoscopic images. *Comput. Med Imaging Graph.* **2021**, *88*, 101843. [CrossRef] [PubMed]
13. Spyridonos, P.; Gaitanis, G.; Likas, A.; Bassukas, I.D. A convolutional neural network based system for detection of actinic keratosis in clinical images of cutaneous field cancerization. *Biomed. Signal Process. Control* **2023**, *79*, 104059. [CrossRef]
14. Ali, K.; Shaikh, Z.A.; Khan, A.A.; Laghari, A.A. Multiclass skin cancer classification using EfficientNets—A first step towards preventing skin cancer. *Neurosci. Inform.* **2022**, *2*, 100034. [CrossRef]
15. Tan, M.; Le, Q.V. EfficientNet: Rethinking Model Scaling for Convolutional Neural Networks. In Proceedings of the 36th International Conference on Machine Learning, PMLR 97, Long Beach, CA, USA, 9–15 June 2019.
16. Guo, S.; Yang, Z. Multi-Channel-ResNet: An integration framework towards skin lesion analysis. *Inform. Med. Unlocked* **2018**, *12*, 67–74.
17. Rodrigues, D.D.A.; Ivo, R.F.; Satapathy, S.C.; Wang, S.; Hemanth, J.; Filho, P.P.R. A new approach for classification skin lesion based on transfer learning, deep learning, and IoT system. *Pattern Recognit. Lett.* **2020**, *136*, 8–15. [CrossRef]
18. Ali, S.; Miah, S.; Haque, J.; Rahman, M.; Islam, K. An enhanced technique of skin cancer classification using deep convolutional neural network with transfer learning models. *Mach. Learn. Appl.* **2021**, *5*, 100036. [CrossRef]
19. Elashiri, M.A.; Rajesh, A.; Pandey, S.N.; Shukla, S.K.; Urooj, S.; Lay-Ekuakille, A. Ensemble of weighted deep concatenated features for the skin disease classification model using modified long short term memory. *Biomed. Signal Process. Control* **2022**, *76*, 103729. [CrossRef]
20. Talukder, A.; Islam, M.; Uddin, A.; Akhter, A.; Hasan, K.F.; Moni, M.A. Machine learning-based lung and colon cancer detection using deep feature extraction and ensemble learning. *Expert Syst. Appl.* **2022**, *205*, 117695. [CrossRef]
21. Oliveira, R.B.; Pereira, A.S.; Tavares, J.M.R. Skin lesion computational diagnosis of dermoscopic images: Ensemble models based on input feature manipulation. *Comput. Methods Programs Biomed.* **2017**, *149*, 43–53. [CrossRef]
22. Shafiullah, M.; Abido, M.A.; Al-Mohammed, A.H. Chapter 2—Metaheuristic optimization techniques. In *Power System Fault Diagnosis*; Shafiullah, M., Abido, M.A., Al-Mohammed, A.H., Eds.; Elsevier: Amsterdam, The Netherlands, 2022; pp. 27–68.
23. Khare, A.; Kakandikar, G.M.; Kulkarni, O.K. An Insight Review on Jellyfish Optimization Algorithm and Its Application in Engineering. *Rev. Comput. Eng. Stud.* **2021**, *9*, 31–40. [CrossRef]
24. Chou, J.-S.; Truong, D.-N. Multiobjective optimization inspired by behavior of jellyfish for solving structural design problems. *Chaos Solitons Fractals* **2020**, *135*, 109738. [CrossRef]
25. Chou, J.-S.; Truong, D.-N. A novel metaheuristic optimizer inspired by behavior of jellyfish in ocean. *Appl. Math. Comput.* **2021**, *389*, 125535. [CrossRef]
26. Desuky, A.S.; Elbarawy, Y.M.; Kausar, S.; Omar, A.H.; Hussain, S. Single-Point Crossover and Jellyfish Optimization for Handling Imbalanced Data Classification Problem. *IEEE Access* **2022**, *10*, 11730–11749. [CrossRef]
27. Al-Qarafi, A.; Alsolai, H.; Alzahrani, J.S.; Negm, N.; Alharbi, L.A.; Al Duhayyim, M.; Mohsen, H.; Al-Shabi, M.; Al-Wesabi, F.N. Artificial Jellyfish Optimization with Deep-Learning-Driven Decision Support System for Energy Management in Smart Cities. *Appl. Sci.* **2022**, *12*, 7457. [CrossRef]
28. Abdel-Basset, M.; Mohamed, R.; Chakrabortty, R.; Ryan, M.; El-Fergany, A. An Improved Artificial Jellyfish Search Optimizer for Parameter Identification of Photovoltaic Models. *Energies* **2021**, *14*, 1867. [CrossRef]
29. Farhat, M.; Kamel, S.; Atallah, A.M.; Khan, B. Optimal Power Flow Solution Based on Jellyfish Search Optimization Considering Uncertainty of Renewable Energy Sources. *IEEE Access* **2021**, *9*, 100911–100933. [CrossRef]

30. Handels, H.; Roß, T.; Kreusch, J.; Wolff, H.; Pöppl, S. Feature selection for optimized skin tumor recognition using genetic algorithms. *Artif. Intell. Med.* **1999**, *16*, 283–297. [CrossRef]
31. Tan, T.Y.; Zhang, L.; Neoh, S.C.; Lim, C.P. Intelligent skin cancer detection using enhanced particle swarm optimization. *Knowl.-Based Syst.* **2018**, *158*, 118–135. [CrossRef]
32. Kong, L.; Cheng, J. Classification and detection of COVID-19 X-ray images based on DenseNet and VGG16 feature fusion. *Biomed. Signal Process. Control* **2022**, *77*, 103772. [CrossRef] [PubMed]
33. Gangan, M.P.; Anoop, K.; Lajish, V.L. Distinguishing natural and computer generated images using Multi-Colorspace fused EfficientNet. *J. Inf. Secur. Appl.* **2022**, *68*, 103261. [CrossRef]
34. Guo, Y.; Wang, Y.; Yang, H.; Zhang, J.; Sun, Q. Dual-attention EfficientNet based on multi-view feature fusion for cervical squamous intraepithelial lesions diagnosis. *Biocybern. Biomed. Eng.* **2022**, *42*, 529–542. [CrossRef]
35. McNeely-White, D.; Beveridge, J.R.; Draper, B.A. Inception and ResNet features are (almost) equivalent. *Cogn. Syst. Res.* **2020**, *59*, 312–318. [CrossRef]
36. Wang, Y.; Feng, Y.; Zhang, L.; Zhou, J.T.; Liu, Y.; Goh, R.S.M.; Zhen, L. Adversarial multimodal fusion with attention mechanism for skin lesion classification using clinical and dermoscopic images. *Med Image Anal.* **2022**, *81*, 102535. [CrossRef]
37. Liu, L.; Mou, L.; Zhu, X.X.; Mandal, M. Automatic skin lesion classification based on mid-level feature learning. *Comput. Med Imaging Graph.* **2020**, *84*, 101765. [CrossRef]
38. Benyahia, S.; Meftah, B.; Lézoray, O. Multi-features extraction based on deep learning for skin lesion classification. *Tissue Cell* **2022**, *74*, 101701. [CrossRef]
39. Zhuang, D.; Chen, K.; Chang, J.M. Morris Chang, CS-AF: A cost-sensitive multi-classifier active fusion framework for skin lesion classification. *Neurocomputing* **2022**, *491*, 206–216. [CrossRef]
40. Mahbod, A.; Schaefer, G.; Ellinger, I.; Ecker, R.; Pitiot, A.; Wang, C. Fusing fine-tuned deep features for skin lesion classification. *Comput. Med. Imaging Graph.* **2019**, *71*, 19–29. [CrossRef] [PubMed]
41. Gessert, N.; Nielsen, M.; Shaikh, M.; Werner, R.; Schlaefer, A. Skin lesion classification using ensembles of multi-resolution EfficientNets with meta data. *MethodsX* **2020**, *7*, 100864. [CrossRef] [PubMed]
42. Ashour, A.S.; Eissa, M.M.; Wahba, M.A.; Elsawy, R.A.; Elgnainy, H.F.; Tolba, M.S.; Mohamed, W.S. Ensemble-based bag of features for automated classification of normal and COVID-19 CXR images. *Biomed. Signal Process. Control* **2021**, *68*, 102656. [CrossRef] [PubMed]
43. Ali, R.; Hardie, R.C.; Narayanan, B.N.; Kebede, T.M. IMNets: Deep Learning Using an Incremental Modular Network Synthesis Approach for Medical Imaging Applications. *Appl. Sci.* **2022**, *12*, 5500. [CrossRef]
44. Ali, R.; Hardie, R.C.; Narayanan Narayanan, B.; De Silva, S. Deep learning ensemble methods for skin lesion analysis towards melanoma detection. In Proceedings of the IEEE National Aerospace and Electronics Conference (NAECON), Dayton, OH, USA, 15–19 July 2019; pp. 311–316.
45. He, X.; Tan, E.L.; Bi, H.; Zhang, X.; Zhao, S.; Lei, B. Fully transformer network for skin lesion analysis. *Med. Image Anal.* **2022**, *77*, 102357. [CrossRef] [PubMed]
46. Available online: https://www.geeksforgeeks.org/vgg-16-cnn-model/ (accessed on 10 January 2022).
47. Putra, T.A.; Rufaida, S.I.; Leu, J.-S. Enhanced Skin Condition Prediction Through Machine Learning Using Dynamic Training and Testing Augmentation. *IEEE Access* **2020**, *8*, 40536–40546. [CrossRef]
48. Available online: https://commons.wikimedia.org/wiki/File:ResNet50.png (accessed on 15 January 2022).
49. Available online: https://www.kaggle.com/datasets/kmader/skin-cancer-mnist-ham10000 (accessed on 12 January 2022).
50. Available online: https://paperswithcode.com/dataset/bcn-20000 (accessed on 14 January 2022).
51. Available online: https://www.statisticshowto.com/friedmans-test/ (accessed on 17 March 2022).
52. Available online: https://www.york.ac.uk/depts/maths/tables/friedman.pdf (accessed on 20 March 2022).

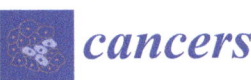

Article

A Deep Learning-Aided Automated Method for Calculating Metabolic Tumor Volume in Diffuse Large B-Cell Lymphoma

Russ A. Kuker [1], David Lehmkuhl [1], Deukwoo Kwon [2], Weizhao Zhao [3], Izidore S. Lossos [4], Craig H. Moskowitz [4], Juan Pablo Alderuccio [4,*,†] and Fei Yang [5,*,†]

1. Department of Radiology, Division of Nuclear Medicine, University of Miami Miller School of Medicine, Miami, FL 33136, USA
2. Department of Public Health Sciences, University of Miami Miller School of Medicine, Miami, FL 33136, USA
3. Department of Biomedical Engineering, University of Miami, Coral Gables, FL 33146, USA
4. Sylvester Comprehensive Cancer Center, Department of Medicine, Division of Hematology, University of Miami Miller School of Medicine, Miami, FL 33136, USA
5. Sylvester Comprehensive Cancer Center, Department of Radiation Oncology, University of Miami Miller School of Medicine, Miami, FL 33136, USA
* Correspondence: jalderuccio@med.miami.edu (J.P.A.); fei@miami.edu (F.Y.)
† These authors contributed equally to this work.

Simple Summary: In recent years metabolic tumor volume (MTV) has been shown to predict outcomes in lymphoma. However, the current methods used to measure MTV are time-consuming and require manual input from the nuclear medicine reader. Therefore, we aimed to develop a deep-learning-aided automated method to calculate MTV. We tested this approach in 100 patients with diffuse large B-cell lymphoma enrolled in a clinical trial cohort. We observed a high correlation between nuclear medicine readers and the automated method, underscoring the potential of this approach to integrate PET-based biomarkers in clinical research.

Abstract: Metabolic tumor volume (MTV) is a robust prognostic biomarker in diffuse large B-cell lymphoma (DLBCL). The available semiautomatic software for calculating MTV requires manual input limiting its routine application in clinical research. Our objective was to develop a fully automated method (AM) for calculating MTV and to validate the method by comparing its results with those from two nuclear medicine (NM) readers. The automated method designed for this study employed a deep convolutional neural network to segment normal physiologic structures from the computed tomography (CT) scans that demonstrate intense avidity on positron emission tomography (PET) scans. The study cohort consisted of 100 patients with newly diagnosed DLBCL who were randomly selected from the Alliance/CALGB 50,303 (NCT00118209) trial. We observed high concordance in MTV calculations between the AM and readers with Pearson's correlation coefficients and interclass correlations comparing reader 1 to AM of 0.9814 ($p < 0.0001$) and 0.98 ($p < 0.001$; 95%CI = 0.96 to 0.99), respectively; and comparing reader 2 to AM of 0.9818 ($p < 0.0001$) and 0.98 ($p < 0.0001$; 95%CI = 0.96 to 0.99), respectively. The Bland–Altman plots showed only relatively small systematic errors between the proposed method and readers for both MTV and maximum standardized uptake value (SUVmax). This approach may possess the potential to integrate PET-based biomarkers in clinical trials.

Keywords: artificial intelligence; deep learning; U-Net; PET/CT; diffuse large B-cell lymphoma; metabolic tumor volume

1. Introduction

Diffuse large B-cell lymphoma (DLBCL) is the most common histologic subtype of non-Hodgkin lymphomas, with an estimated incidence of 150,000 new cases annually worldwide [1–3]. DLBCL is a curable disease in nearly 60% of patients treated with

Citation: Kuker, R.A.; Lehmkuhl, D.; Kwon, D.; Zhao, W.; Lossos, I.S.; Moskowitz, C.H.; Alderuccio, J.P.; Yang, F. A Deep Learning-Aided Automated Method for Calculating Metabolic Tumor Volume in Diffuse Large B-Cell Lymphoma. *Cancers* 2022, 14, 5221. https://doi.org/10.3390/cancers14215221

Academic Editors: Marcin Woźniak and Muhammad Fazal Ijaz

Received: 23 August 2022
Accepted: 20 October 2022
Published: 25 October 2022

Publisher's Note: MDPI stays neutral with regard to jurisdictional claims in published maps and institutional affiliations.

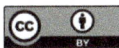

Copyright: © 2022 by the authors. Licensee MDPI, Basel, Switzerland. This article is an open access article distributed under the terms and conditions of the Creative Commons Attribution (CC BY) license (https://creativecommons.org/licenses/by/4.0/).

anthracycline-containing immunochemotherapy such as rituximab, cyclophosphamide, doxorubicin, vincristine, and prednisone (R-CHOP) and dose-adjusted etoposide, prednisone, vincristine, cyclophosphamide, doxorubicin, and rituximab (EPOCH-R) [4,5]. Patients with refractory DLBCL, however, demonstrate poor outcomes, with a median overall survival of only 6.3 months [6]. Therefore, the early identification of patients at risk for treatment failure remains a critical need in an effort to consider alternative treatment strategies in this population.

Prognosis in patients with DLBCL is commonly determined by the International Prognosis Index (IPI) score comprised of clinical and laboratory variables [7]. The IPI score was developed in the early 1990s, undergoing subsequent validations and revisions associated with better risk assessment [8,9]. However, significant advances in the understanding of disease biology that occurred over the last two decades uncovered substantial molecular heterogeneity and associated divergent survival, which was not fully captured in the IPI score [10,11]. Furthermore, this index is not included in the treatment selection of frontline or subsequent lines of therapy, underscoring the need to develop biomarker-driven therapies in patients with DLBCL.

^{18}F-fluorodeoxyglucose (FDG) positron-emission tomography with computed tomography (PET/CT) is routinely incorporated in clinical practice for the staging and assessment of treatment response in DLBCL [1,12–14]. The Lugano classification criteria is the most commonly used staging system for the evaluation of treatment efficacy for established and experimental therapies [15]. Metabolic tumor volume (MTV) calculated from FDG-PET/CT has been shown to be a robust prognostic biomarker across different lymphomas [16–18]. In patients with DLBCL, MTV demonstrated prognostication in the frontline and relapsed settings [19–21]. Investigators from the SAKK38/07 trial developed a prognostic model, including mutation profiling and baseline FDG-PET/CT metrics, in patients enrolled in the study. Patients with high MTV and metabolic heterogeneity demonstrated the highest risk of relapse [22]. Furthermore, Mikhaeel et al. recently developed the International Metabolic Prognostic index integrating MTV with individual components of the IPI score, such as age and stage, enabling individualized estimates of patient outcome [23]. Therefore, the implementation of MTV in clinical practice is expected to be imminent.

Despite encouraging prognostication defined by MTV, several challenges remain for its broad implementation. Calculating MTV can be tedious and time-consuming when using currently available semiautomatic software [24]. There can also be inherent variability in calculating MTV that requires manual input from the readers [25–29]. The goal of the present study was to develop a fully automated method for calculating MTV. We first explored the feasibility of a fully automated method (AM) to calculate MTV in a clinical trial dataset and, subsequently, we compared the results obtained by the AM with the results obtained by two blinded readers. The contributions of our study include:

- Developing a novel fully automated machine learning approach for MTV calculation in DLBCL.
- Validating the developed approach against experienced nuclear medicine readers in determining MTV and maximum standardized uptake value (SUVmax).
- Enabling the integration of a machine learning approach in DLBCL clinical research.

2. Materials and Methods
2.1. Study Cohort

The clinical trial cohort consisted of 491 eligible patients with newly diagnosed DLBCL who were enrolled in the Alliance/CALGB 50,303 (NCT00118209) trial, an intergroup, randomized phase III study aimed to compare six cycles of dose-adjusted EPOCH-R with standard R-CHOP as a frontline therapy for DLBCL [30]. Eligible patients included untreated DLBCL confirmed by central pathology review. Before enrollment, limited field radiation or fewer than 10 days of glucocorticoid treatment for urgent disease complications were allowed. Additional eligibility included age ≥ 18 years, stage II to IV DLBCL (stage I primary mediastinal B-cell lymphoma was allowed), Eastern Cooperative Oncology Group performance status 0 to 2, and acceptable cardiac, renal, hematological, and liver function. The presence of central nervous system involvement and human immunodeficiency virus infection represented exclusion criteria. In the Alliance/CALGB 50,303 study dose-adjusted EPOCH-R was more toxic and did not improve progression-free survival or overall survival compared with standard R-CHOP [30,31]. Among those 491 patients, 155 whole-body FDG-PET/CT scans at study enrollment were publicly available at The Cancer Imaging Archive (TCIA) [32]. We randomly selected 100 patients to analyze for the present study.

2.2. Imaging Data

Imaging examinations of the selected patients were acquired from three different types of PET/CT scanners including Siemens Biograph (Siemens Medical System, Erlangen, Germany), Philips GEMINI (Philips Healthcare, Best, The Netherlands), and GE Discovery (General Electric Co., Milwaukee, WI, USA). As per the trial protocol, after confirming plasma glucose level <200 mg/dL and at least a 4-h fasting period, patients were intravenously injected with 8–20 mCi of FDG and PET/CT scans were obtained approximately 60 to 80 min afterward. Concomitant low-dose CTs, extending mainly from the skull base to thighs for anatomic localization and attenuation correction, were performed at 110–140 kVp with a reference dose of 200 mAs and iteratively reconstructed with a slice thickness ranging from 2 mm to 4 mm. PET scans were reconstructed using algorithms ranging from ordered-subset expectation maximization (OSEM) to blob-based iterative time-of-flight (BLOB-OS-TF) to point spread function (PSF) modeling with and without time-of-flight (PSF-TF). PET scan slice thickness ranged from 2 mm to 4.25 mm, with the most typical being 3.25 mm or 4.25 mm (83%). In addition, 50 whole-body CT scans from the TCIA collection of the whole-body FDG-PET/CT dataset [33] were used to fine-tune the employed deep-learning-based segmentation model. Imaging parameters of these CT scans were as follows: tube voltage of 120 kV, reference dose of 200 mAs, and slice thickness of 2–3 mm. Contours of the brain, heart, kidneys, and bladder were provided by a consensus exercise of two expert radiologists. The local institutional review board (IRB) waived the study from review as only publicly available aggregated patient datasets were utilized.

2.3. Segmentation of Anatomic Structures with Physiologic FDG Avidity

Anatomic structures with avid physiologic FDG uptake, such as the brain, heart, kidneys, and bladder, complicate the interpretation of PET imaging data for MTV determination. To alleviate this, a deep convolutional neural network model was deployed to segment these structures on the CTs. The segmentation model was built off the pre-trained 2D dilated residual U-net architecture by Manteia Medical Technologies (Milwaukee, WI, USA) [34]. Residual U-net was adopted due to its ability to alleviate the vanishing gradient problem as the depth of the network increases. Figure 1 illustrates the network architecture of the deployed model. Both the encoder and decoder were composed of five cascades of residual blocks. In addition, a shortcut connection was implemented between the corresponding feature maps between the encoder and decoder. Each residual block was composed of two convolution layers, and the size of the convolution kernel was 3×3. Each residual block was cascaded with the down-sampling layer or the upper-sampling layer. The down-sampling method used was maximum pooling and the upper-sampling method was the bilinear interpolation. Furthermore, batch normalization was also applied to reduce the internal covariate shift [35].

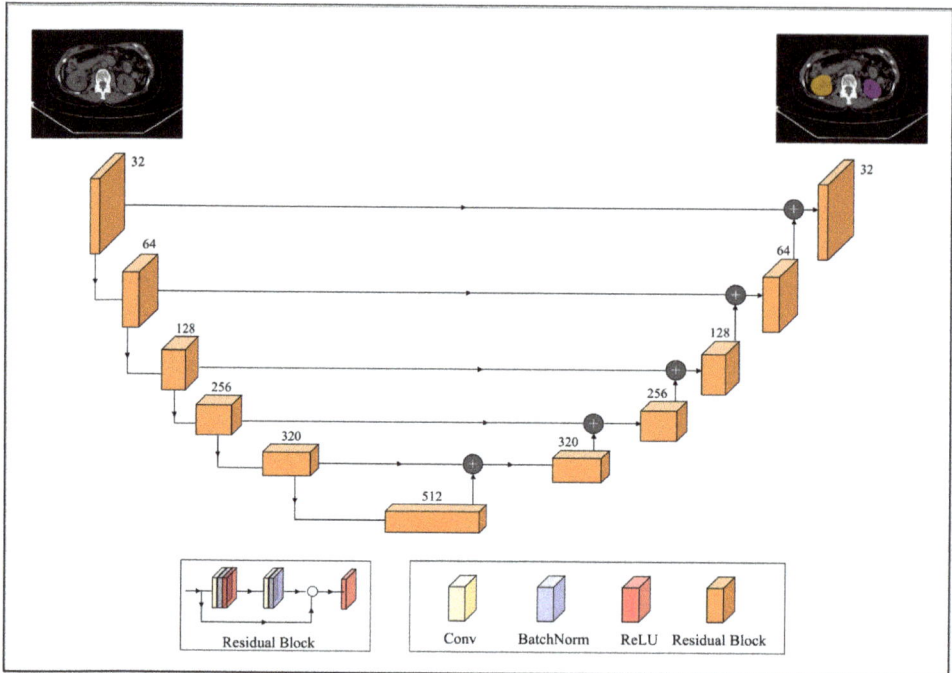

Figure 1. A schematic overview of the employed 2D dilated residual U-net-based segmentation model. The encoder and decoder were composed of 5 cascades of residual blocks. Each residual block was composed of two convolution layers and was cascaded with the downsampling layer (maximum pooling; down arrow) or the upper sampling layer (bilinear interpolation; upper arrow). A shortcut connection (horizontal arrow) was implemented between the corresponding feature maps between the encoder and decoder.

To fine-tune the pre-trained model towards the purpose of this work, the weights of the final output layer of the original model were reset to random values, resulting in a total of 165 trainable parameters. The dataset used for fine-tuning the pretrained model comprised the aforementioned 50 whole-body CTs annotated for the brain, heart, kidneys, and bladder, which were divided at the ratio of 5:1:4 for training, validation, and testing sets, respectively. Data preprocessing included clipping image intensity to 1–99% of the maximum and Z-Score standardization. The modified model was trained with a maximum number of training epochs of 100. The learning rate was initialized as 3×10^{-4} and decreased to 3×10^{-6} after about 60 epochs. Regarding data augmentation for training, techniques based on affine transforms such as rotation, translation, scaling, and flipping were employed. The objective function was a combination of cross-entropy and Dice loss, and adaptive moment estimation (ADAM) was utilized to update the parameters with a weight decay of 1×10^{-4}. Training loss went from 1.3317 to 0.0190, from 1.4233 to 0.0551, from 1.2526 to 0.0774, and from 1.6453 to 0.0576 for the brain, heart, kidneys, and bladder, respectively. Training accuracy by the Dice coefficient for the brain, heart, kidneys, and bladder were 0.9885, 0.9441, 0.9145, and 0.9045, respectively. Testing accuracy by the Dice coefficient for the four target organs was 0.9524, 0.9023, 0.9107, and 0.8809, respectively. Regarding the implementation environment for the described fine-tuning process, PyTorch (v1.10) [36] was employed.

Upon being obtained on the CTs, contours of the above-mentioned FDG avid structures were transferred to the PET scans with automatic adjustment for their respective PET presentations by the aid of an array of ad hoc image-processing algorithms including region-growing, active contours, and fast matching [37–39] (Figure 2).

Step 1. PET/CT scan
Deploy a deep-learning based volumetric segmentation algorithm to identify physiologic avid structures such as the brain, heart, kidneys, and bladder on the CT

Step 2. Segmented regions of interest (ROIs)
We then transfer the contours obtained for these structures to the PET with adaptation being carried out automatically based on their respective presentations on the PET

Step 3. Identified lesions on Maximum Intensity Projection (MIP)
Metabolic tumor volumes are derived by thresholding with respect to SUV and volume

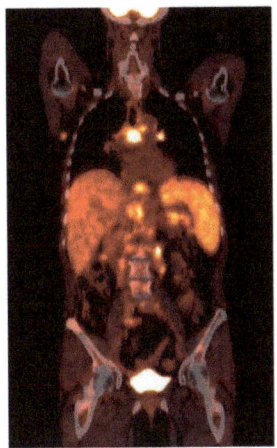
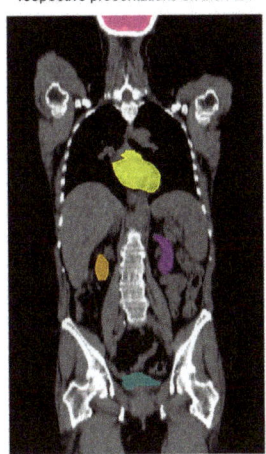
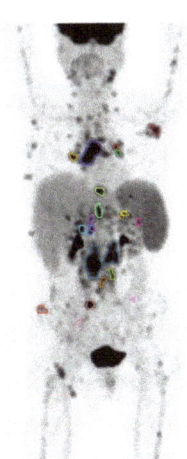

Figure 2. Step-by-step demonstration of deep-learning-aided metabolic tumor volume calculations.

2.4. Automated Determination of MTV on FDG-PET

Prior to MTV calculation, a narrow trapezoid-shaped zone was established based on PET-adapted kidney and bladder contours. The zone extended in the cranial–caudal direction from the superior poles of the kidneys to the central cross-sectional plane of the bladder, in the anterior–posterior direction from the anterior to the posterior surfaces of the kidneys on the top base while on the bottom base from the anterior to the posterior borders of the bladder, as shown in the central cross-sectional plane, and in the left-right direction between the midlines of the two kidneys on the top base while, on the bottom base, between the lateral borders of the bladder, a central cross-sectional plane is shown. The rationale for creating such a zone was to aid in the identification of focal uptake by the ureters, which, incidentally, posed a challenge to the employed deep learning-based segmentation model given both the paucity of accurate training data and the wide anatomical variation of the ureters. In addition, establishing such a zone was also of help in the detection of isolated and scattered areas of focal uptake resulting from the kidneys and bladder.

The MTV determination was conducted within the volume defined by the PET-imaged whole-body volume excluding the aforementioned anatomical structures being transferred and adapted to PET scans, including the brain, heart, kidneys, and bladder. This volume was determined by a threshold with respect to 41% of the SUVmax, [40] followed by clustering of the contiguous supra-threshold voxels into isolated regions under an additional constraint of retaining only the ones with size greater than 1 cm^3. This resulted in the formation of a set of candidate lesion regions of interest (ROI), which was then further screened for exclusion of the ones with size less than 2 cm^3 as well as those falling in the defined trapezoid-shaped zone. In scenarios where the candidate lesion ROI with the SUVmax was screened out, its volume was removed from the defined MTV analyzing space, and the process was repeated, until all the criteria laid out above were met. Of note, the whole described process was automatic, without requiring any manual intervention.

2.5. Semiautomatic Method for MTV Measurement

All FDG-PET/CT images were independently reviewed using the Hermes Affinity Viewer by two experienced nuclear medicine readers. ROIs selected by the software were manually adjusted in three planes to exclude adjacent physiologic FDG avid structures. SUVmax was defined as the maximum voxel intensity within the volumetric region of interest. Bone marrow involvement was only included in volume measurement if there was focal uptake. The spleen was considered as involved if there was focal uptake or diffuse uptake higher than 150% of the liver background. MTV was obtained by summing the metabolic volumes of all individual lesions using the previously reported 41% of SUVmax threshold and volume ≥ 1 cm^3. Nuclear medicine readers were blinded for the automated results and vice versa.

2.6. Statistical Analysis

MTV and SUVmax were compared to the fully automated results from the developed algorithm. To examine agreement, we estimated Pearson's correlation coefficients and inter-class correlation coefficients (ICCs), along with corresponding 95% confidence intervals and p-values. For visualization, we displayed scatter plots along with regression lines and Bland–Altman plots between readers and the automated method. All tests were two-sided and statistical significance was considered when $p < 0.05$. Statistical software R was used for all statistical analyses.

3. Results

We sought to investigate the performance of a three-dimensional deep learning-aided AM for MTV calculation in 100 patients with DLBCL enrolled in the Alliance/CALGB 50,303 clinical trial. There were 17 centers participating in this trial and the PET/CT systems employed included: Siemens ($n = 53$), GE ($n = 30$), and Philips ($n = 17$). Among the randomly selected patients, the mean MTV calculated by reader 1 was 226.470 mL (standard deviation (SD) 260.066 and coefficient of variation (CV) 114.834), for reader 2 was 226.799 mL (SD 261.965 and CV 115.505) and for AM was 205.704 mL (SD 245.825 and CV 119.504).

Comparing reader 1 to reader 2, the Pearson's correlation coefficients and ICCs were 0.9997, $p < 0.0001$ and 1, $p < 0.0001$ (95%CI = 1 to 1) for MTV and 1, $p < 0.0001$ and 1, $p < 0.0001$ (95%CI = 1 to 1) for SUVmax, respectively (Figure 3A,B). Comparing reader 1 to AM, the Pearson's correlation coefficients and ICCs were 0.9814, $p < 0.0001$ and 0.98, $p < 0.0001$ (95%CI = 0.96 to 0.99) for MTV and 0.9868, $p < 0.0001$ and 1, $p < 0.0001$ (95%CI = 0.99 to 1) for SUVmax, respectively (Figure 3C,D). Comparing reader 2 to AM, the Pearson's correlation coefficients and ICCs were 0.9818, $p < 0.0001$ and 0.98, $p < 0.0001$ (95%CI = 0.96 to 0.99) for MTV and 0.9868, $p < 0.0001$ and 1, $p < 0.0001$ (95%CI = 0.99 to 1) for SUVmax, respectively (Figure 3E,F).

When we assessed the data sorted by the type of PET/CT system, we observed small differences in SUVmax between the readers and AM only on images obtained by Philips scanners (readers and AM: ICC 0.81, $p < 0.0001$ (95%CI = 0.57 to 0.93)) (Supplemental Table S1). We did not observe differences by the type of scanner in MTV volumes. (Supplemental Table S2).

The Bland–Altman plots showed only relatively small systematic errors between the proposed method and the manual readings across the entire data range being examined for both MTV (Figure 4) and SUVmax (Figure 5).

Subsequently, we calculated the Root-Mean-Squared Error (RMSE) between readers (average) and the proposed AM as a measure of accuracy and positive difference and negative difference between the two measurements as a bias. For MTV calculations, the RMSE was 54.7, with a positive bias of 28.4 and a negative bias of 0.27 (Supplemental Figure S1A). The mean difference between readers was 20.92 (95% limits of agreement of −49.77 and 91.63). AM demonstrated smaller MTV values compared to those of the nuclear medicine readers. For SUVmax calculations, we found an RMSE of 1.93 with a positive bias of 15.4 and a negative bias of 1.26 (Supplemental Figure S1B). The mean difference between readers was −0.03 (95% limits of agreement of −3.34 and 3.26). Again, AM demonstrated smaller values of SUVmax compared to the nuclear medicine readers.

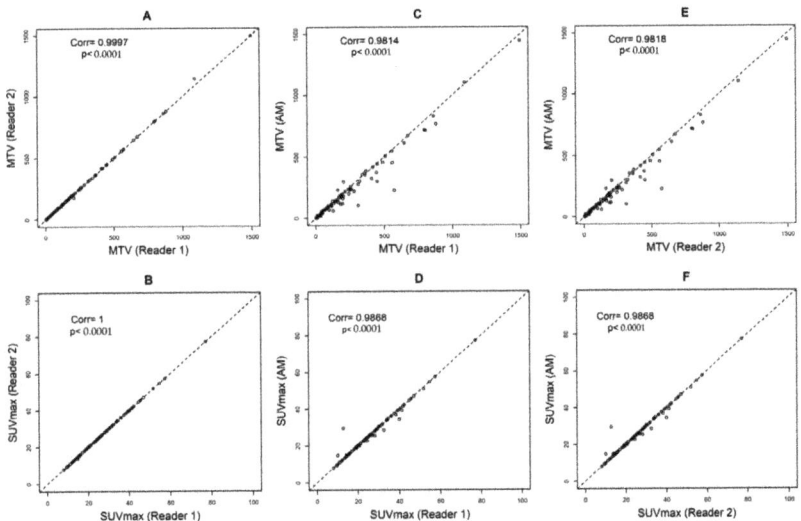

Figure 3. Pearson's correlation coefficients calculating metabolic tumor volumes (MTV) with a threshold of 41% and SUVmax between Reader 1 and Reader 2 (**A**,**B**), Automated Method (AM) approach and Reader 1 (**C**,**D**), and AM and Reader 2 (**E**,**F**).

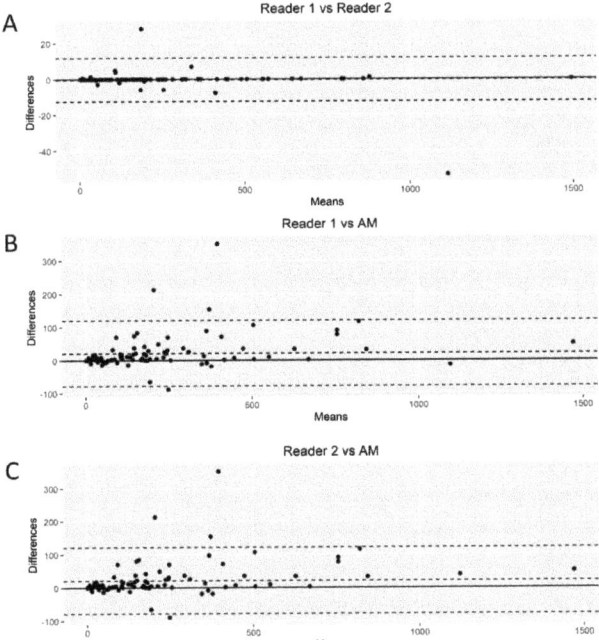

Figure 4. Bland–Altman plot. Graphical display for bias between two readers and automated method (AM) in metabolic tumor volume calculation (**A**–**C**).

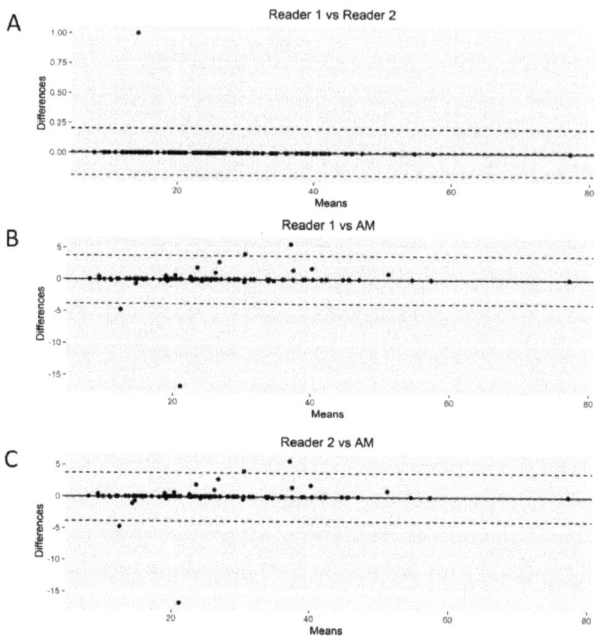

Figure 5. Bland–Altman plot. Graphical display for bias between two readers and automated method (AM) in SUVmax calculation (**A–C**).

4. Discussion

In this study, we showed that a deep-learning-aided method can accurately segment lymphoma lesions, allowing for a fully automated assessment of MTV in a homogeneously treated patient population. SUVmax and tumor volumes measured by our proposed method were highly correlated with those determined by independent readers using a semiautomatic software, validating these results. No subjects were excluded due to failure of the automated method. Furthermore, the algorithm was highly accurate in classifying FDG-avidity in patients from a multicenter clinical trial involving 17 centers that obtained images on different scanner models with variable reconstruction settings.

Deep learning is a subtype of representation learning aimed to describe complex data representations using simpler hierarchized structures defined from a set of specific features [41]. Convolutional neural networks represent the core of deep learning methods for imaging and are multilayered artificial neural networks with weighted connections between neurons that are iteratively adjusted through repeated exposure to training data. These networks may be used for the automation of various time-consuming tasks including image detection, segmentation, and classification [42]. This method possesses the potential to decrease reading time and increase the reproducibility of measurements and has been associated with similar accuracy to semiautomatic methods that require reader input [43–45].

The availability of predictive factors of response to standard and experimental regimens remains an unmet need in DLBCL. More recently, several automated segmentation methods have been proposed in DLBCL [45–49]. Capobianco et al. examined a machine learning approach to generate MTV in DLBCL [47]. The authors tested an investigational software prototype (PET-Assisted Reporting System (PARS); Siemens Medical Solutions USA, Inc., Malvern, PA, USA) to estimate MTV in 301 patients enrolled in the REMARC clinical trial [47,50]. The automated whole-body high-uptake segmentation algorithm identified all three-dimensional regions of interest with increased tracer uptake. The resulting

ROIs were processed using a convolutional neural network trained on an independent cohort. They observed a similar correlation between PARS-based MTV with reference MTV calculated by two experienced readers ($\rho = 0.76$; $p < 0.001$). Subsequently, Jiang et al. trained a 3-D U-Net architecture on patches randomly sampled within PET images in 414 patients with DLBCL [48]. Authors found a strong positive correlation (linear regression analysis; R^2 linear = 0.882, $p < 0.001$) between ground-truth MTV and predictive MTV in training and validation (R^2 linear = 0.939, $p < 0.001$) cohorts. Most recently, Revailler et al. completed a training dataset of 407 patients in 93 h underscoring the speed of current deep-learning models to compute MTV [45].

The automated method proposed here brings a new solution to the problem of MTV calculation in DLBCL and has several advantages compared to the previous methods. First, when compared to the previous methods, which are more or less "black box" models that are difficult to interpret and often provide little insight into how decisions are made, the proposed method is more explicit and more direct in emulating how nuclear medicine physicians reason through DLBCL PET/CT imaging data. Moreover, the inherent human bias induced by inter- and intra-observer perception errors in reading PET/CT scans for MTV calculation is eliminated by the proposed method since it does not need the massive quantities of annotated training data on which others rely. In addition, the proposed method with the use of segmentation of physiologic FDG avid structures on CTs may be advantageous for patient cases featuring a low tumor burden, for which the previous methods are particularly problematic.

Limitations of the present study include the applicability of our results to other lymphoma subtypes and cancer groups and the need to further validate and refine our automated method. Although our sample size is relatively small, patients were randomly selected from a homogeneous dataset, and we observed similar results across our cohort. Furthermore, the presented performance of the developed method should be interpreted with caution, given that the method was validated against readings collected from only one, although generally accepted and widely used, dedicated semiautomatic MTV calculation software. In addition, the manual readings for this study were performed by readers from the same institution, which may lend itself to potential reader bias. We did not seek to develop a predictive or prognostic model due to the incomplete availability of PET/CT scans from TCIA. Our goal was limited to validating our automated method approach. Finally, the performance of the proposed automated MTV calculation method may deteriorate in some rare but complicated clinical scenarios, such as tumor activity being located in close proximity to normal physiologic structures such as the bladder or kidneys, or when normal anatomy is distorted either due to the disease process or image artifacts, including misregistration or patient motion amongst others.

Nonetheless, the proposed automated method is strengthened by its ability to calculate MTV with a high correlation to analysis by expert readers in the company of automation and high throughput (median process time: 5 min for the proposed method vs. 20 min for expert analysis). Developing a fully automated method, such as ours, for calculating MTV that is accurate and reproducible may facilitate the application of MTV in clinical research, providing real-time risk stratification. Future studies should prospectively explore treatment decisions based on MTV data.

5. Conclusions

We demonstrated that a deep-learning-aided, fully automated method is capable of calculating MTV in patients with DLBCL. The resulting MTV values were highly concordant with the results obtained by two blinded nuclear medicine readers. Employing deep learning for the calculation of MTV offers many advantages over semiautomated methods, including time efficiency and the reproducibility of results across different PET/CT systems. The proposed automated method is unique in that it emulates how nuclear medicine readers analyze PET/CT images and does not require massive quantities of annotated training data.

We believe that an accurate and highly reproducible automated method for calculating MTV has great potential for incorporation into clinical research.

Supplementary Materials: The following supporting information can be downloaded at: https://www.mdpi.com/article/10.3390/cancers14215221/s1, Figure S1: (A) Bland-Altman plot. Graphical display for bias and Root-Mean-Squared Error (RMSE) between average of reader 1 and reader 2 versus automated method in metabolic tumor volume calculations, (B) Bland-Altman plot. Graphical display for bias and Root-Mean-Squared Error (RMSE) between average of reader 1 and reader 2 versus automated method in SUVmax calculations; Table S1: Concordance between readers in SUVmax values by scanner type; Table S2: Concordance between readers in MTV values by scanner type.

Author Contributions: R.A.K., J.P.A. and F.Y. conceptualized and designed the study, analyzed the data, and wrote the manuscript; F.Y. performed deep learning analysis of this study; D.L., D.K., W.Z., I.S.L. and C.H.M. collected and analyzed the data and wrote the manuscript. All authors have read and agreed to the published version of the manuscript.

Funding: This research was supported by the Sylvester Comprehensive Cancer Center National Cancer Institute (NCI) core grant P30CA240139.

Institutional Review Board Statement: The local institutional review board (IRB) waived this study from review on account of only publicly available aggregated patient data being utilized.

Informed Consent Statement: Patient consent was waived due to the publicly available database.

Data Availability Statement: The Cancer Imaging Archive is a service which de-identifies and hosts a large archive of medical images of cancer accessible for public download. https://www.cancerimagingarchive.net/ (accessed on 1 October 2021).

Acknowledgments: I.S.L. is supported by grant 1R01CA233945 and U01 CA195568 from the National Cancer Institute, the Intramural Funding Program from the University of Miami SCCC, by the Dwoskin and Anthony Rizzo Families Foundations and Jaime Erin Follicular Lymphoma Research Consortium. J.P.A. is supported by Peykoff Initiative from the Lymphoma Research Foundation and the Dwoskin Family Foundation. We acknowledge the services and expertise provided by the Biostatistics and Bioinformatics Shared Resource of Sylvester Comprehensive Cancer Center.

Conflicts of Interest: I.S.L. has served on the advisory boards Adaptive Biotechnologies. J.P.A. consultant for and research funding for ADC Therapeutics. An immediate family member has served on the advisory boards of Puma Biotechnology, Inovio Pharmaceuticals, Agios Pharmaceuticals, Forma Therapeutics, and Foundation Medicine.

References

1. Sehn, L.H.; Salles, G. Diffuse Large B-Cell Lymphoma. *N. Engl. J. Med.* **2021**, *384*, 842–858. [CrossRef] [PubMed]
2. Campo, E.; Jaffe, E.S.; Cook, J.R.; Quintanilla-Martinez, L.; Swerdlow, S.H.; Anderson, K.C.; Brousset, P.; Cerroni, L.; de Leval, L.; Dirnhofer, S.; et al. The International Consensus Classification of Mature Lymphoid Neoplasms: A Report from the Clinical Advisory Committee. *Blood* **2022**, *140*, 1229–1253. [CrossRef]
3. Swerdlow, S.H.; Campo, E.; Lee Harris, N.; Jaffe, E.S.; Pileri, S.A.; Stein, H.; Thiele, J.; Arber, D.A.; Hasserjian, R.P.; Le Beau, M.M.; et al. *WHO Classification of Tumours of Haematopoietic and Lymphoid Tissues*, 4th ed.; IARC Press: Lyon, France, 2017.
4. Coiffier, B.; Lepage, E.; Brière, J.; Herbrecht, R.; Tilly, H.; Bouabdallah, R.; Morel, P.; Van Den Neste, E.; Salles, G.; Gaulard, P.; et al. CHOP Chemotherapy plus Rituximab Compared with CHOP Alone in Elderly Patients with Diffuse Large-B-Cell Lymphoma. *N. Engl. J. Med.* **2002**, *346*, 235–242. [CrossRef] [PubMed]
5. Wilson, W.H.; Grossbard, M.L.; Pittaluga, S.; Cole, D.; Pearson, D.; Drbohlav, N.; Steinberg, S.M.; Little, R.F.; Janik, J.; Gutierrez, M.; et al. Dose-adjusted EPOCH chemotherapy for untreated large B-cell lymphomas: A pharmacodynamic approach with high efficacy. *Blood* **2002**, *99*, 2685–2693. [CrossRef] [PubMed]
6. Crump, M.; Neelapu, S.S.; Farooq, U.; Van Den Neste, E.; Kuruvilla, J.; Westin, J.; Link, B.K.; Hay, A.; Cerhan, J.R.; Zhu, L.; et al. Outcomes in refractory diffuse large B-cell lymphoma: Results from the international SCHOLAR-1 study. *Blood* **2017**, *130*, 1800–1808. [CrossRef] [PubMed]
7. International Non-Hodgkin's Lymphoma Prognostic Factors Project. A Predictive Model for Aggressive Non-Hodgkin's Lymphoma. *N. Engl. J. Med.* **1993**, *329*, 987–994. [CrossRef] [PubMed]
8. Ruppert, A.S.; Dixon, J.G.; Salles, G.; Wall, A.; Cunningham, D.; Poeschel, V.; Haioun, C.; Tilly, H.; Ghesquieres, H.; Ziepert, M.; et al. International prognostic indices in diffuse large B-cell lymphoma: A comparison of IPI, R-IPI, and NCCN-IPI. *Blood* **2020**, *135*, 2041–2048. [CrossRef]

9. Sehn, L.H.; Berry, B.; Chhanabhai, M.; Fitzgerald, C.; Gill, K.; Hoskins, P.; Klasa, R.; Savage, K.J.; Shenkier, T.; Sutherland, J.; et al. The revised International Prognostic Index (R-IPI) is a better predictor of outcome than the standard IPI for patients with diffuse large B-cell lymphoma treated with R-CHOP. *Blood* **2007**, *109*, 1857–1861. [CrossRef]
10. Chapuy, B.; Stewart, C.; Dunford, A.J.; Kim, J.; Kamburov, A.; Redd, R.A.; Lawrence, M.S.; Roemer, M.G.M.; Li, A.J.; Ziepert, M.; et al. Molecular subtypes of diffuse large B cell lymphoma are associated with distinct pathogenic mechanisms and outcomes. *Nat. Med.* **2018**, *24*, 679–690. [CrossRef]
11. Schmitz, R.; Wright, G.W.; Huang, D.W.; Johnson, C.A.; Phelan, J.D.; Wang, J.Q.; Roulland, S.; Kasbekar, M.; Young, R.M.; Shaffer, A.L.; et al. Genetics and Pathogenesis of Diffuse Large B-Cell Lymphoma. *N. Engl. J. Med.* **2018**, *378*, 1396–1407. [CrossRef]
12. NCCN. Clinical Practice Guidelines in Oncology. B-Cell Lymphomas, Version 3.2022. Available online: https://www.nccn.org/login?ReturnURL=https://www.nccn.org/professionals/physician_gls/pdf/b-cell.pdf (accessed on 1 August 2022).
13. Tilly, H.; da Silva, G.; Vitolo, U.; Jack, A.; Meignan, M.; Lopez-Guillermo, A.; Walewski, J.; Andre, M.; Johnson, P.W.; Pfeundschuh, M.E.; et al. Diffuse large B-cell lymphoma (DLBCL): ESMO Clinical Practice Guidelines for diagnosis, treatment and follow-up. *Ann Oncol.* **2015**, *26* (Suppl. 5), 116–125. [CrossRef] [PubMed]
14. Barrington, S.F.; Trotman, J. The role of PET in the first-line treatment of the most common subtypes of non-Hodgkin lymphoma. *Lancet. Haematol.* **2021**, *8*, e80–e93. [CrossRef]
15. Cheson, B.D.; Fisher, R.I.; Barrington, S.F.; Cavalli, F.; Schwartz, L.H.; Zucca, E.; Lister, T.A. Recommendations for initial evaluation, staging, and response assessment of Hodgkin and non-Hodgkin lymphoma: The Lugano classification. *J. Clin. Oncol.* **2014**, *32*, 3059–3068. [CrossRef]
16. Moskowitz, A.J.; Schöder, H.; Gavane, S.; Thoren, K.L.; Fleisher, M.; Yahalom, J.; McCall, S.J.; Cadzin, B.R.; Fox, S.Y.; Gerecitano, J.; et al. Prognostic significance of baseline metabolic tumor volume in relapsed and refractory Hodgkin lymphoma. *Blood* **2017**, *130*, 2196–2203. [CrossRef] [PubMed]
17. Delfau-Larue, M.-H.; van der Gucht, A.; Dupuis, J.; Jais, J.-P.; Nel, I.; Beldi-Ferchiou, A.; Hamdane, S.; Benmaad, I.; Laboure, G.; Verret, B.; et al. Total metabolic tumor volume, circulating tumor cells, cell-free DNA: Distinct prognostic value in follicular lymphoma. *Blood Adv.* **2018**, *2*, 807–816. [CrossRef] [PubMed]
18. Vercellino, L.; Di Blasi, R.; Kanoun, S.; Tessoulin, B.; Rossi, C.; D'Aveni-Piney, M.; Obéric, L.; Bodet-Milin, C.; Bories, P.; Olivier, P.; et al. Predictive factors of early progression after CAR T-cell therapy in relapsed/refractory diffuse large B-cell lymphoma. *Blood Adv.* **2020**, *4*, 5607–5615. [CrossRef]
19. Vercellino, L.; Cottereau, A.S.; Casasnovas, O.; Tilly, H.; Feugier, P.; Chartier, L.; Fruchart, C.; Roulin, L.; Oberic, L.; Pica, G.M.; et al. High total metabolic tumor volume at baseline predicts survival independent of response to therapy. *Blood* **2020**, *135*, 1396–1405. [CrossRef]
20. Alderuccio, J.P.; Kuker, R.A.; Barreto-Coelho, P.; Martinez, B.M.; Miao, F.; Kwon, D.; Beitinjaneh, A.; Wang, T.P.; Reis, I.M.; Lossos, I.S.; et al. Prognostic value of presalvage metabolic tumor volume in patients with relapsed/refractory diffuse large B-cell lymphoma. *Leuk. Lymphoma* **2022**, *63*, 43–53. [CrossRef]
21. Dean, E.A.; Mhaskar, R.S.; Lu, H.; Mousa, M.S.; Krivenko, G.S.; Lazaryan, A.; Bachmeier, C.A.; Chavez, J.C.; Nishihori, T.; Davila, M.L.; et al. High metabolic tumor volume is associated with decreased efficacy of axicabtagene ciloleucel in large B-cell lymphoma. *Blood Adv.* **2020**, *4*, 3268–3276. [CrossRef]
22. Genta, S.; Ghilardi, G.; Cascione, L.; Juskevicius, D.; Tzankov, A.; Schär, S.; Milan, L.; Pirosa, M.C.; Esposito, F.; Ruberto, T.; et al. Integration of Baseline Metabolic Parameters and Mutational Profiles Predicts Long-Term Response to First-Line Therapy in DLBCL Patients: A Post Hoc Analysis of the SAKK38/07 Study. *Cancers* **2022**, *14*, 1018. [CrossRef]
23. Mikhaeel, N.G.; Heymans, M.W.; Eertink, J.J.; Vet, H.C.W.d.; Boellaard, R.; Dührsen, U.; Ceriani, L.; Schmitz, C.; Wiegers, S.E.; Hüttmann, A.; et al. Proposed New Dynamic Prognostic Index for Diffuse Large B-Cell Lymphoma: International Metabolic Prognostic Index. *J. Clin. Oncol.* **2022**, *40*, 2352–2360. [CrossRef] [PubMed]
24. Camacho, M.R.; Etchebehere, E.; Tardelli, N.; Delamain, M.T.; Vercosa, A.F.A.; Takahashi, M.E.S.; Brunetto, S.Q.; Metze, I.; Souza, C.A.; Cerci, J.J.; et al. Validation of a Multifocal Segmentation Method for Measuring Metabolic Tumor Volume in Hodgkin Lymphoma. *J. Nucl. Med. Technol.* **2020**, *48*, 30–35. [CrossRef]
25. Yang, F.; Young, L.; Yang, Y. Quantitative imaging: Erring patterns in manual delineation of PET-imaged lung lesions. *Radiother. Oncol.* **2019**, *141*, 78–85. [CrossRef] [PubMed]
26. Johnson, P.B.; Young, L.A.; Lamichhane, N.; Patel, V.; Chinea, F.M.; Yang, F. Quantitative imaging: Correlating image features with the segmentation accuracy of PET based tumor contours in the lung. *Radiother. Oncol.* **2017**, *123*, 257–262. [CrossRef] [PubMed]
27. Yang, F.; Young, L.; Yang, Y. Data for erring patterns in manual delineation of PET-imaged lung lesions. *Data Brief* **2020**, *28*, 104846. [CrossRef] [PubMed]
28. Yang, F.; Simpson, G.; Young, L.; Ford, J.; Dogan, N.; Wang, L. Impact of contouring variability on oncological PET radiomics features in the lung. *Sci. Rep.* **2020**, *10*, 369. [CrossRef]
29. Yang, F.; Grigsby, P.W. Delineation of FDG-PET tumors from heterogeneous background using spectral clustering. *Eur. J. Radiol.* **2012**, *81*, 3535–3541. [CrossRef]
30. Bartlett, N.L.; Wilson, W.H.; Jung, S.H.; Hsi, E.D.; Maurer, M.J.; Pederson, L.D.; Polley, M.C.; Pitcher, B.N.; Cheson, B.D.; Kahl, B.S.; et al. Dose-Adjusted EPOCH-R Compared With R-CHOP as Frontline Therapy for Diffuse Large B-Cell Lymphoma: Clinical Outcomes of the Phase III Intergroup Trial Alliance/CALGB 50303. *J. Clin. Oncol.* **2019**, *37*, 1790–1799. [CrossRef]

31. Schöder, H.; Polley, M.-Y.C.; Knopp, M.V.; Hall, N.; Kostakoglu, L.; Zhang, J.; Higley, H.R.; Kelloff, G.; Liu, H.; Zelenetz, A.D.; et al. Prognostic value of interim FDG-PET in diffuse large cell lymphoma: Results from the CALGB 50303 Clinical Trial. *Blood* **2020**, *135*, 2224–2234. [CrossRef]
32. Clark, K.; Vendt, B.; Smith, K.; Freymann, J.; Kirby, J.; Koppel, P.; Moore, S.; Phillips, S.; Maffitt, D.; Pringle, M. The Cancer Imaging Archive (TCIA): Maintaining and operating a public information repository. *J. Digit. Imaging* **2013**, *26*, 1045–1057. [CrossRef]
33. Gatidis, S.; Kuestner, T. A whole-body FDG-PET/CT dataset with manually annotated tumor lesions (FDG-PET-CT-Lesions) [Dataset]. *Cancer Imaging Arch.* **2022**, *9*, 601. [CrossRef]
34. U.S. Food and Drug Administration; Picture Archiving and Communications System. AccuContour K191928 Approval Letter. 2020. Available online: https://www.accessdata.fda.gov/scripts/cdrh/cfdocs/cfpmn/pmn.cfm?ID=K191928 (accessed on 1 October 2021).
35. Ioffe, S.; Szegedy, C. Batch normalization: Accelerating deep network training by reducing internal covariate shift. *Proc. Int. Conf. Mach. Learn.* **2015**, *37*, 448–456.
36. Paszke, A.; Gross, S.; Massa, F.; Lerer, A.; Bradbury, J.; Chanan, G.; Killeen, T.; Lin, Z.; Gimelshein, N.; Antiga, L. Pytorch: An imperative style, high-performance deep learning library. *Adv. Neural Inf. Process Syst.* **2019**, *32*.
37. Chan, T.F.; Vese, L.A. Active contours without edges. *IEEE Trans. Image Process.* **2001**, *10*, 266–277. [CrossRef] [PubMed]
38. Sethian, J.A. *Level Set Methods and Fast Marching Methods: Evolving Interfaces in Computational Geometry, Fluid Mechanics, Computer Vision, and Materials Science*; Cambridge University Press: Cambridge, UK, 1999; Volume 3.
39. Yang, F.; Grigsby, P.W. A segmentation framework towards automatic generation of boost subvolumes for FDG-PET tumors: A digital phantom study. *Eur. J. Radiol.* **2012**, *81*, 4123–4130. [CrossRef]
40. Meignan, M.; Sasanelli, M.; Casasnovas, R.O.; Luminari, S.; Fioroni, F.; Coriani, C.; Masset, H.; Itti, E.; Gobbi, P.G.; Merli, F.; et al. Metabolic tumour volumes measured at staging in lymphoma: Methodological evaluation on phantom experiments and patients. *Eur. J. Nucl. Med. Mol. Imaging* **2014**, *41*, 1113–1122. [CrossRef]
41. Montagnon, E.; Cerny, M.; Cadrin-Chênevert, A.; Hamilton, V.; Derennes, T.; Ilinca, A.; Vandenbroucke-Menu, F.; Turcotte, S.; Kadoury, S.; Tang, A. Deep learning workflow in radiology: A primer. *Insights Into Imaging* **2020**, *11*, 22. [CrossRef]
42. Cheng, P.M.; Montagnon, E.; Yamashita, R.; Pan, I.; Cadrin-Chênevert, A.; Romero, F.P.; Chartrand, G.; Kadoury, S.; Tang, A. Deep Learning: An Update for Radiologists. *RadioGraphics* **2021**, *41*, 1427–1445. [CrossRef]
43. Lin, L.; Dou, Q.; Jin, Y.M.; Zhou, G.Q.; Tang, Y.Q.; Chen, W.L.; Su, B.A.; Liu, F.; Tao, C.J.; Jiang, N.; et al. Deep Learning for Automated Contouring of Primary Tumor Volumes by MRI for Nasopharyngeal Carcinoma. *Radiology* **2019**, *291*, 677–686. [CrossRef]
44. Huang, B.; Chen, Z.; Wu, P.M.; Ye, Y.; Feng, S.T.; Wong, C.O.; Zheng, L.; Liu, Y.; Wang, T.; Li, Q.; et al. Fully Automated Delineation of Gross Tumor Volume for Head and Neck Cancer on PET-CT Using Deep Learning: A Dual-Center Study. *Contrast Media Mol. Imaging* **2018**, *2018*, 8923028. [CrossRef]
45. Revailler, W.; Cottereau, A.S.; Rossi, C.; Noyelle, R.; Trouillard, T.; Morschhauser, F.; Casasnovas, O.; Thieblemont, C.; Gouill, S.L.; André, M.; et al. Deep Learning Approach to Automatize TMTV Calculations Regardless of Segmentation Methodology for Major FDG-Avid Lymphomas. *Diagnostics* **2022**, *12*, 417. [CrossRef] [PubMed]
46. Blanc-Durand, P.; Jégou, S.; Kanoun, S.; Berriolo-Riedinger, A.; Bodet-Milin, C.; Kraeber-Bodéré, F.; Carlier, T.; Le Gouill, S.; Casasnovas, R.O.; Meignan, M.; et al. Fully automatic segmentation of diffuse large B cell lymphoma lesions on 3D FDG-PET/CT for total metabolic tumour volume prediction using a convolutional neural network. *Eur. J. Nucl. Med. Mol. Imaging* **2021**, *48*, 1362–1370. [CrossRef] [PubMed]
47. Capobianco, N.; Meignan, M.; Cottereau, A.S.; Vercellino, L.; Sibille, L.; Spottiswoode, B.; Zuehlsdorff, S.; Casasnovas, O.; Thieblemont, C.; Buvat, I. Deep-Learning (18)F-FDG Uptake Classification Enables Total Metabolic Tumor Volume Estimation in Diffuse Large B-Cell Lymphoma. *J. Nucl. Med. Off. Publ. Soc. Nucl. Med.* **2021**, *62*, 30–36. [CrossRef]
48. Jiang, C.; Chen, K.; Teng, Y.; Ding, C.; Zhou, Z.; Gao, Y.; Wu, J.; He, J.; He, K.; Zhang, J. Deep learning-based tumour segmentation and total metabolic tumour volume prediction in the prognosis of diffuse large B-cell lymphoma patients in 3D FDG-PET images. *Eur. Radiol.* **2022**, *32*, 4801–4812. [CrossRef]
49. Jemaa, S.; Paulson, J.N.; Hutchings, M.; Kostakoglu, L.; Trotman, J.; Tracy, S.; de Crespigny, A.; Carano, R.A.D.; El-Galaly, T.C.; Nielsen, T.G.; et al. Full automation of total metabolic tumor volume from FDG-PET/CT in DLBCL for baseline risk assessments. *Cancer Imaging Off. Publ. Int. Cancer Imaging Soc.* **2022**, *22*, 39. [CrossRef]
50. Thieblemont, C.; Tilly, H.; Gomes da Silva, M.; Casasnovas, R.O.; Fruchart, C.; Morschhauser, F.; Haioun, C.; Lazarovici, J.; Grosicka, A.; Perrot, A.; et al. Lenalidomide Maintenance Compared with Placebo in Responding Elderly Patients With Diffuse Large B-Cell Lymphoma Treated With First-Line Rituximab Plus Cyclophosphamide, Doxorubicin, Vincristine, and Prednisone. *J. Clin. Oncol.* **2017**, *35*, 2473–2481. [CrossRef]

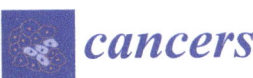

Article

Cancerous Tumor Controlled Treatment Using Search Heuristic (GA)-Based Sliding Mode and Synergetic Controller

Fazal Subhan [1], Muhammad Adnan Aziz [1], Inam Ullah Khan [1,2], Muhammad Fayaz [3], Marcin Wozniak [4,*], Jana Shafi [5] and Muhammad Fazal Ijaz [6,*]

1. Department of Electronic Engineering, School of Engineering and Applied Sciences (SEAS), Isra University Islamabad Campus, Islamabad 44000, Pakistan
2. Department of Engineering, King's College London, London SE1 9NH, UK
3. Department of Computer Science, University of Central Asia, Naryn 722600, Kyrgyzstan
4. Faculty of Applied Mathematics, Silesian University of Technology, 44-100 Gliwice, Poland
5. Department of Computer Science, College of Arts and Science, Prince Sattam bin Abdul Aziz University, Wadi Ad-Dawasir 11991, Saudi Arabia
6. Department of Intelligent Mechatronics Engineering, Sejong University, Seoul 05006, Korea
* Correspondence: marcin.wozniak@polsl.pl (M.W.); fazal@sejong.ac.kr (M.F.I.)

Simple Summary: Cancer is basically a tough condition on a patient's body where cell grows uncontrollably. Normal cells are affected, which destroys the health of the patient. The main problem in cancer is spreading from one part to another. Therefore, the mathematical modeling of cancerous tumors integrates to check overall stability. A novel approach is introduced such as Bernstein polynomial with combination of genetic algorithm, sliding mode controller, and synergetic control. The proposed solution has easily eliminated cancerous cells within five days using synergetic control. In addition, five cases are incorporated to evaluate error function. In addition, a brief comparative study is added to contrast the simulation results with theoretical modeling.

Abstract: Cancerous tumor cells divide uncontrollably, which results in either tumor or harm to the immune system of the body. Due to the destructive effects of chemotherapy, optimal medications are needed. Therefore, possible treatment methods should be controlled to maintain the constant/continuous dose for affecting the spreading of cancerous tumor cells. Rapid growth of cells is classified into primary and secondary types. In giving a proper response, the immune system plays an important role. This is considered a natural process while fighting against tumors. In recent days, achieving a better method to treat tumors is the prime focus of researchers. Mathematical modeling of tumors uses combined immune, vaccine, and chemotherapies to check performance stability. In this research paper, mathematical modeling is utilized with reference to cancerous tumor growth, the immune system, and normal cells, which are directly affected by the process of chemotherapy. This paper presents novel techniques, which include Bernstein polynomial (BSP) with genetic algorithm (GA), sliding mode controller (SMC), and synergetic control (SC), for giving a possible solution to the cancerous tumor cells (CCs) model. Through GA, random population is generated to evaluate fitness. SMC is used for the continuous exponential dose of chemotherapy to reduce CCs in about forty-five days. In addition, error function consists of five cases that include normal cells (NCs), immune cells (ICs), CCs, and chemotherapy. Furthermore, the drug control process is explained in all the cases. In simulation results, utilizing SC has completely eliminated CCs in nearly five days. The proposed approach reduces CCs as early as possible.

Keywords: nonlinear ordinary coupled differential equation (ncode); Bernstein polynomial (bsp); genetic algorithm (ga); sliding mode controller (smc); synergetic controller (sc); chemotherapy; immunotherapy and optimization

Citation: Subhan, F.; Aziz, M.A.; Khan, I.U.; Fayaz, M.; Wozniak, M.; Shafi, J.; Ijaz, M.F. Cancerous Tumor Controlled Treatment Using Search Heuristic (GA)-Based Sliding Mode and Synergetic Controller. *Cancers* **2022**, *14*, 4191. https://doi.org/10.3390/cancers14174191

Academic Editor: Sam Payabvash

Received: 14 July 2022
Accepted: 25 August 2022
Published: 29 August 2022

Publisher's Note: MDPI stays neutral with regard to jurisdictional claims in published maps and institutional affiliations.

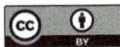

Copyright: © 2022 by the authors. Licensee MDPI, Basel, Switzerland. This article is an open access article distributed under the terms and conditions of the Creative Commons Attribution (CC BY) license (https://creativecommons.org/licenses/by/4.0/).

1. Introduction

Initially, cancer was considered an untreatable disease. Division and uncontrolled cell growth usually occur because of cancer [1]. Unexpected magnification of cells crosses the limit of a normal level, and cells even migrate to neighbor tissues. However, for cancer cells, mathematical models can be applied for treatment or analysis. Tumor development involves a complicated process. During this approach, when the tumor becomes malignant, the tumor can then spread to the overall body to form secondary tumors [2–4]. Globally, cancer is primary cause of death. According to reports from WHO, cancer is the second most dangerous disease in about 112 countries [5]. On the other hand, in 2020, COVID-19 has increased the death rates in comparison to other diseases. Due to current population-based data, the cancer death rate has been reduced since 1990 [6].

The immune system has a direct association in all phases of the tumor lifecycle. Therefore, fast therapy augments the function of a patient's immune system. This whole process is called cancer immunotherapy, which necessitates work on basic and mathematical computational models to formulate an edge-based silico approach. Apart from clinical methods, immunotherapy and computational models help to innovate this field of study [7]. Immunotherapy is typically used to support the human body's natural immune system in the battle against cancerous tumors. Initially, CCs dimensions are usually large in size and can be identified with clinical methods. Chemotherapy investigates tumor stability to maintain tumor-free equilibrium by injecting the chemotherapy dose where the drug is and allowing it to mix with the blood. Therefore, the medication is administered into the circulatory system [8]. Achieving optimal procedure of medicines can be utilized to treat cancerous tumors. The main issue is determining the exact dosing plan as well as a proper medication delivery strategy [7].

Many researchers have provided solutions in the field of cancer to facilitate recovery. Computational techniques are considered a possible solution in designing a novel concept in boosting traditional models. The overall paper is based on a new approach to reduce cancerous cells within the body. Sometimes, reduction of cells affects the body in a negative bad way. Therefore, the concept of controllers in the area of cancer is introduced where other techniques such as SMC and SC are also utilized. This paper presents a theoretical comparison with existing techniques and simulation-based approach as well. Many researchers have utilized the basic model of Depillis et al. [9], which is based on traditional therapies. Initially, there was no concept of controllers in reducing the drug rate or eliminating CCs. The theoretical reasoning lies in having information to reduce CCs with respect to a lesser number of days. Controllers such as steepest descent are utilized but can hardly eliminate CCs in eight days [10]. Online recursive calculation [11] has also given the similar results. Therefore, there is a need for more work regarding mathematical models in CCs elimination.

A solution to the cancer-related problems can likely be determined by establishing mathematical models and understanding their dynamic behaviors. Furthermore, Figure 1 shows the idea of three modes related to cancer, which include immunotherapy, chemotherapy, and SMC and SC as mathematical modeling. Healthy tissue cells consists of immune and host cells that are used in the growth of tumors, which is described in De Pillis [12]. The role of chemotherapy drugs is to have a harmful effect on tumor cells. Thus, a prey–predator model can be used to monitor the growth of tumors within a limited time in immune network [13,14]. Evolutionary computing algorithms are considered the optimal method to address multi-objective engineering problems using spotted hyena optimizer [15]. In addition, for differential evolution, a genetic algorithm can be used to solve the control strategy for cancer treatment drugs [13–23,26]. The main contribution of this research study is as follows:

- This paper introduces a novel drug that eliminates CCs;
- Elimination of CCs but also reduction of the effect of chemotherapy on NCs and ICs was also used to bring NCs up to threshold level.

- A new controller was designed to obtain optimal results where SMC and SC are utilized as drugs;
- The proposed solution eliminates CCs within five days;
- Various methods were incorporated to check the performance of the proposed solution with traditional approaches. Further, two basic approaches such as theoretical and simulation were performed to evaluate the results.

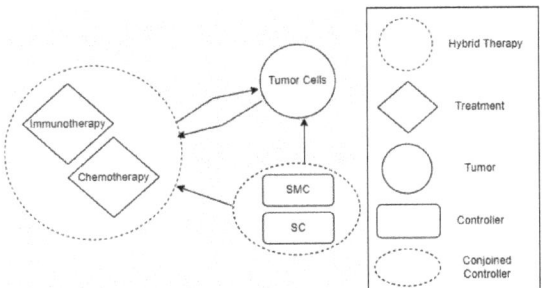

Figure 1. Three different modes for cancer-related problems.

The paper's organization includes Section 2, literature study; Section 3, cancer model with proposed methodology; Section 4, the proposed solution; Section 5, simulation results; Section 6 is comparative discussion, and Section 7 gives the conclusion and future scope.

2. Literature Study

This section is about the literature study performed to extract limitation related to cancer using different techniques, which are as follows:

Sima Sarv et al. described the concept of a mathematical model for cancer immunotherapy. A particle swarm optimization (PSO)-based protocol was designed to deal with cellular immunotherapy. However, tumor interaction needs to be better evaluated by using mathematical modeling. A forward-backward approach is considered contemporary but has problems related with time, which led to convergence issues as well [16]. The immune system responds to cancerous tumors. Therefore, to reduce the tumor's effect on the body overall, immunotherapy is utilized. Due to the human immune system, the fight against cancerous cells is quite easy. In addition, a fixed dose level needs to be deployed to help to reduce CCs. Immunotherapy has attracted researchers with the momentum to utilize antigen T cells, which helps to detect cancerous cells. A special model was designed to reduce cancerous cell growth using chimeric antigen receptor thymus cells (CAR-T cells). Experimentation was performed with in silico tests to select various scenarios. The CAR-T-cell procedure response eliminates cancerous cells and reduces the formation of long-term immuno-memory [17] to maintain the equilibrium that includes cancer cell growth and the immune editing method. Mathematical modeling is quite helpful when it is based on cell population sub-sections. Type 1 interferon receptor (1. IFN) signaling predicts the dominant cancerous cells. For the entire experimentation, triple-negative breast cancer was used [18]. Castrate-resistant prostate cancer (CRPC) with anti-cytotoxic T-lymphocyte-associated protein 4 (anti-CTLA4) was used as a single treatment to estimate results from experimental data. Various constrains were applied to check the performance of CCs, where different drug doses were given to patients to reduce CCs. For better control of CCs, synergy between ipilimumab and sipuleucel-T was utilized [19], giving a possible solution to cancer by using a fractional mathematical model that is based on synergy in between angiogenic and various therapies [20]. Furthermore, a delayed mathematical model of cancerous cells' immune system is needed to effect drug therapies. There is a relevant, pressing need for a drug-free mechanism that can be understood by the dynamics of a multi-therapeutic approach [21].

Kaouthar Moussa et al. introduced injection scheduling to model cancer treatment, which was used to achieve an optimal level under multiplex tasks. However, interaction can be made possible between CCs and ICs. Many applications normally restructure to schedule injection dose. However, uncertainties need to be further investigated on the initial stage of ICs [22].

Virotherapy improves chemotherapy since the ordinary differential equation (ODE)-based mathematical model balances the interaction among ICs, treatment, and oncolytic cells. This method is useful for completely clearing CCs. Sensitivity examination uses forward techniques to access the effect of virotherapy and chemotherapy. Virus reproduction can be balanced to maintain the tumor equilibrium. Pontryagin's maximum approach rectifies prediction modeling during continuous treatment of cost and side effects. Furthermore, stability must be investigated to give proper solutions [23]. Table 1 depicts various treatment methods with limitations.

Table 1. Different treatment methods with limitations.

Treatment and Controller	Behavior	Limitations
Pulsed chemotherapy protocol [9]	Oscillatory behavior of CCs and ICs	CCs not removed completely
Direct collocation as an optimal control with continuous chemotherapy [19]	Oscillation in ICs, slow reduction of CCs	CCs eliminated within 70 days, NCs reduced to dangerous level
Traditional pulse chemotherapy [20]	Reduction of CCs and NCs	CCs still remaining, NCs die down to minimum threshold
Optimal control with chemotherapy [20]	CCs slowly removed	Elimination of CCs within 70 days
Chemo-immunotherapy with optimal control [20]	Oscillatory behavior of NCs and ICs	Treatment destroys the CCs, NCs, and ICs
Multi-objective swarm as an optimal control with chemotherapy [14]	Nonlinear behavior of treatment, NCs and CCs.	NCs reduced to minimum edge, so for the time being, treatment is stopped to recover NCs to a safe level.
Chemo-immunotherapy of triple-negative breast cancer [29]	ICs remain at very low level	CCs eliminated after 60 days
Optimal administration protocols for immunotherapies [22]	Nonlinear behavior of CCs elimination	CCs eliminated after 40 days
Chemo-immunotherapy with SMC [15]	CCs eliminated from the patient's body within 45 days.	The CCs elimination is good but can be enhanced.

The formation of mathematical model is determined to level up the basic reproduction and stability, which is used to conduct numerical demonstration. An epidemic model of cancer with chemotherapy is a non-linear concept using differential equations. Cancer growth cells with parameters must be constant; therefore, increasing drug dose limits the CCs [24]. Giving a solution for overall orbits and bounded coverage utilizes a phase-space mathematical strategy to limit the CCs growth. Control therapy drives a desirable basin where traditional chemotherapy is not well-applicable [25]. In addition, more constraints regarding the mentioned issue are described in Table 1.

Machine learning and other techniques take too much time in comparison to controllers. High-level data sets are involved to give accurate decisions, whereas training and testing is commonly used and do not give quick solution. The rate of error detection and removal is very tough in machine learning. Due to the mentioned problems, controllers will reduce CCs more easily and effectively. When solving higher-order equations using SMC, order rate reduction occurs. The entire system is highly coupled and non-separable, which is quite hard to solve. SMC and SC swap from easily coupled into de-coupled to reduce disturbance. Overall, a synergetic controller is more reliable than SMC. SMC has a chattering phenomenon, which further leads to low accuracy.

The paper is structured as follows: Section 2 is confined to the tumor model based on a system of coupled differential equations, followed by brief introduction of BSP, GA, and SMC. Section 3 presents the proposed methodology and the design of SMC. Section 4 presents the simulation results and discussion. The conclusion is presented in Section 5.

3. Cancer Model with Proposed Methodology

Mathematical models are methods for analyzing the system's behavior, which gives possible solutions to simulate complex systems [13,18,19,23]. A system of nonlinear coupled ordinary differential equations is discussed in this research study. The proposed solution is based on the below-listed assumptions, which include:

1. CCs and NCs follow logistic growth.
2. ICs and drugs must have natural death rates.
3. NCs have controlled growth, but CCs possess uncontrolled behavior; therefore, population growth will be variable.
4. Drug sources can be either constant or exponential.

3.1. Cancer Tumor Model

The cancerous tumor model consists of NCs, CCs, and ICs, where population can be presented by coupled differential equations. Moreover, drug concentration in chemotherapy needs to be monitored using Equation (4). The following Equations (1)–(5) represent NCs, CCs, and ICs with respect to time.

$$\dot{x}_1 = a_2 x_1 (1 - d_2 x_1) - e_4 x_2 x_1 - r_3 C \tag{1}$$

$$\dot{x}_2 = a_1 x_2 (1 - d_1 x_2) - e_2 x_2 x_3 - e_3 x_2 x_1 - r_2 C \tag{2}$$

$$\dot{x}_3 = \alpha + \frac{p x_3 x_2}{s + x_2} - e_1 x_3 x_2 - f_1 x_3 - r_1 C \tag{3}$$

$$\dot{C} = v_c(t) - f_2 C \tag{4}$$

The initial conditions are

$$\begin{aligned} x_1(0) &= 0.9 \\ x_2(0) &= 0.25 \\ x_3(0) &= 0.25 \end{aligned} \tag{5}$$

The mentioned model describes the metrics of cancer with NCs and ICs. However, x_1, x_2, and x_3 are denoted as NCs, CCs,, and ICs respectively. Furthermore, in Equation (4), C is used for chemotherapy treatment, while the remaining model parameters include r_1, r_2, and r_3 coefficients of cell death rate. In addition, d_1 and d_2 drugs carry capacities such as e_1 to e_4. Moreover, f_1 and f_2 are considered natural death rates, and a_1 and a_2 are the growth rates for ICs and drugs, respectively. p is the response rate, and the threshold rate can be symbolized as s [6]. The simulation results utilize chemotherapy drugs, and the maximum effect on body cells are observed within 100 days. The obtained results will not reduce the level of NCs, which is $x_1 \geq 0.75$.

3.2. Bernstein Polynomial (BSP)

Approximation functions can be used in BSP to give an optimal solution. Integral and differential equations are used to solve many complex problems. BSP was introduced by Sergi Natanovich in 1912 [15]. However, polynomials with the order n and with interval $[0, \tau]$ are given in Equations (6)–(12).

$$B_{i,n}(t) = \binom{n}{i} \frac{t^i (\tau - t)^{n-i}}{\tau^n} \tag{6}$$

$0 \leq t \leq 1$, and τ is considering 1.

$$B_{i,n}(t) = \binom{n}{i} t^i (1-t)^{n-i} \tag{7}$$

$$B_{i,n}(t) = \begin{cases} 0 \forall i \neq 0 \\ 1 \forall i = 0 \end{cases} \tag{8}$$

$$B_{i-1,n-1}(1) = \begin{cases} 0 \forall i \neq n \\ 1 \forall i = n \end{cases} \tag{9}$$

$$B_{i,n-1}(1) = \begin{cases} 0 \forall i \neq n \\ 1 \forall i = n-1 \end{cases} \tag{10}$$

Lower-ordered polynomials are represented in Equations (11) and (12), which are considered the properties of BSP:

$$B_{i,n}(t) = (1-t) B_{i,n}(t) + t B_{i,n}(t) \tag{11}$$

$$B_{i,n}(t) = n(B_{i-1,n-1}(t) - B_{i,n-1}(t)) \tag{12}$$

3.3. Heuristic Algorithm

GA is the class of nature-inspired heuristic algorithms. The evolutionary computation technique is based on random population of a candidate solution. This is considered the classical method to optimize complex problems by utilizing pairs of chromosomes' crossover reproduction, mutation, and selection [31]. The genetic algorithm follows the steps below:

i. Random population having unknown length of chromosomes;
ii. Candidate solution and mutation are used in genetic algorithm, which is considered the classical method for optimization;
iii. Fitness function is utilized to check the desired solution;
iv. Crossover, mutation, and selection are found for fitness criteria.

Otherwise, repeat step ii.

3.4. Controllers

Controllers are used to give a solution to complex problems, which can be either linear or nonlinear. Usually, the control system regulates undesired responses with uncertainties to the desired reaction. In nonlinear models, integration of linear control systems can be applied. The proposed model is highly nonlinear, which gives the best possible approach for CCs.

3.5. Sliding Mode Controllers (SMC)

SMC are used to apply a discontinuous control signal, which works on a state feedback control mechanism. SMC is a non-linear system, which is used to give stability in two phases. However, defining sliding surface is the first phase, while managing initial states of the system is the second stage. Moreover, when the system reaches the desire state, it is called sliding mode. Complex systems must control finite time while removing parameter variations, order reduction, and decoupling [25,33].

3.6. Synergetic Controllers (SC)

SC are used to keep correspondence with nonlinearity and open systems. SC subsystems have dynamic interaction during exchange of information. Nonlinear mathematical models have multi-dimensional properties. However, designing a synergetic model utilizes nonlinear control applications. Presently, SC is a type of dynamic nonlinear system [27,34].

4. Proposed Methodology

Cancerous tumor model Equations (1)–(3) are utilized to mimic the error function. For approximation, BSP is demonstrated by using GA, SMC, and SC to the minimize error function of the solution. Linear combination Equations (13)–(16) are evaluated using boundary approaches with different cases.

The below algorithm is considered the proposed solution [24–27], which consists of BSP, genetic computation, SMC, and SC.

Algorithm 1 [24–27]: Model approximation using GA-tuned BSP along with a controller as the proposed drug

1. Model approximation using BSP
2. Coefficients' tuning using GA
    a. Initialization phase
    b. Set parameters for each stage
        i. Approximation
        ii. Assign number of generation
        iii. Generate initial population
            1. While
                a. Calculate fitness
                b. Selection
            2. Do
                a. Crossover
                b. Mutate P(t)
            3. End while
            4. P(t+1) = New Population
3. Applying SMC
    a. Set parameters
    b. Define sliding surface
    c. Design controller to drive initial states to the sliding surface
    d. Applying on model
    e. Repeat step 1 and 2
4. Applying SC
    a. Assume macro-variable
    b. Design sliding manifold
    c. Force the initial states to sliding manifold
    d. Repeat step 1 and 2
5. Compare SMC and SC

Stop

$$x_1(t) = \sum_{i=0}^{n} f_i B_{i,n}(t)$$

$$\dot{x}_1(t) = n\left(\sum_{i=1}^{n} f_i B_{i-1,n-1}(t) - \sum_{i=0}^{n-1} f_i B_{i,n-1}(t)\right) \quad (13)$$

$$x_2(t) = \sum_{i=0}^{n} g_i B_{i,n}(t)$$

$$\dot{x}_2(t) = n\left(\sum_{i=1}^{n} g_i B_{i-1,n-1}(t) - \sum_{i=0}^{n-1} g_i B_{i,n-1}(t)\right) \quad (14)$$

$$x_2(t) = \sum_{n=0}^{n} h_i B_{i,n}(t)$$

$$\dot{x}_2(t) = n\left(\sum_{i=1}^{n} h_i B_{i-1,n-1}(t) - \sum_{i=0}^{n-1} h_i B_{i,n-1}(t)\right) \quad (15)$$

$$x_1(0) = \sum_{i=0}^{n} f_i B_{i,n}(0) = f_0 = 0.9$$
$$x_2(0) = \sum_{i=0}^{n} g_i B_{i,n}(0) = g_0 = 0.25 \qquad (16)$$
$$x_3(0) = \sum_{i=0}^{n} h_i B_{i,n}(0) = h_0 = 0.25$$

However, Equation (16) uses f_i, g_i, and h_i, where ($i = 1, 2, 3, \ldots n$) need to be evaluated through the best possible solution using GA. In addition, x_1, x_2, and x_3 are initiated in Equations (13)–(16). The unknown constants such as f_i, g_i, and h_i easily minimize the objective/error function.

4.1. The Error Function

The error function consists of five cases. In them, case-1 contains only NCs and CCs; ICs are involved in case-2, and in case-3, chemotherapy is added. Meanwhile, the rest of the two cases use the concept of elimination of CCs through chemotherapy using SMC and SC. In addition, a drug control process is involved. Different cases are discussed as follows:

4.1.1. Case-1

The first case describes the growth rate of NCs and CCs. Therefore, Equations (17) and (18) explain the mentioned concept. There is no practice involved, such as immunotherapy, chemotherapy, and controllers.

$$Ex_1 = \frac{1}{11}\sum_{i=0}^{10}\left(\dot{x}_1(t_i) - a_2 x_1(t_i)(1 - d_2 x_1(t_i)) + e_4 x_2(t_i) x_1(t_i)\right)^2 \qquad (17)$$

$$Ex_2 = \frac{1}{11}\sum_{i=0}^{10}\left(\dot{x}_2(t_i) - a_1 x_2(t_i)(1 - d_1 x_2(t_i)) + e_3 x_2(t_i) x_1(t_i)\right)^2 \qquad (18)$$

4.1.2. Case-2

Here, immunotherapy is demonstrated where the body's immune system affects the CCs. However, immunotherapy helps the body defend against CCs. In addition, no concept of chemotherapy and controllers is utilized. Equations (19)–(21) gives the idea of immunotherapy and how it aids in opposing CCs.

$$Ex_1 = \frac{1}{11}\sum_{i=0}^{10}\left(\dot{x}_1(t_i) - a_2 x_1(t_i)(1 - d_2 x_1(t_i)) + e_4 x_2(t_i) x_1(t_i)\right)^2 \qquad (19)$$

$$Ex_2 = \frac{1}{11}\sum_{i=0}^{10}\left(\dot{x}_2(t_i) - a_1 x_2(t_i)(1 - d_1 x_2(t_i)) + e_2 x_3(t_i) x_2(t_i) + e_3 x_2(t_i) x_1(t_i)\right)^2 \qquad (20)$$

$$Ex_3 = \frac{1}{11}\sum_{i=0}^{10}\left(\dot{x}_3(t_i) - \alpha - \frac{p x_3(t_i) x_2(t_i)}{s + x_2(t_i)} + e_1 x_3(t_i) x_2(t_i) + f_1 x_3(t_i)\right)^2 \qquad (21)$$

4.1.3. Case-3

As we know, CCs directly affect the process of immunotherapy. However, we added chemotherapy, which tries to reduce CCs. There is no such controller utilized in Equations (22)–(24). However, the main problem is that using only immunotherapy and chemotherapy does not reduce CCs individually. When chemotherapy and immunotherapy are used together, the CCs are reduced. Moreover, chemotherapy disturbs NCs with cancer and also has an effect on ICs.

$$Ex_1 = \frac{1}{11}\sum_{i=0}^{10}\left(\dot{x}_1(t_i) - a_2 x_1(t_i)(1 - d_2 x_1(t_i)) + e_4 x_2(t_i) x_1(t_i) + r_3 C(t_i)\right)^2 \qquad (22)$$

$$Ex_2 = \frac{1}{11}\sum_{i=0}^{10}\left(\begin{array}{c}\dot{x}_2(t_i) - a_1x_2(t_i)(1-d_1x_2(t_i)) + e_2x_3(t_i)x_2(t_i) + e_3x_2(t_i)x_1(t_i)\\ +r_2C(t_i)\end{array}\right)^2 \quad (23)$$

$$Ex_3 = \frac{1}{11}\sum_{i=0}^{10}\left(\dot{x}_3(t_i) - \alpha - \frac{px_3(t_i)x_2(t_i)}{s+x_2(t_i)} + e_1x_3(t_i)x_2(t_i) + f_1x_3(t_i) + r_1C(t_i)\right)^2 \quad (24)$$

4.1.4. Case-4

In case-4, immunotherapy, chemotherapy, and SMC are used in the investigation. Here, SMC are used to reduce and attempt to quickly eliminate the CCs. Furthermore, a novel error function is designed to speed up the process. The detailed explanation is discussed in Equations (25)–(36).

$$\mu_{x_2}(t) = -\rho_{x_2}sgn(\sigma_{x_2}) - \partial_{x_2}a_1x_2(1-d_1x_2) \quad (25)$$

We added this controller to Equation (2), and after the controller addition ($\mu_{x_2}(t)$), the Equation (2) will be

$$\dot{x}_2 = (1-\partial_{x_2})a_1x_2(1-d_1x_2) - \rho_{x_2}sgn(\sigma_{x_2}) - e_2x_3x_2 - e_3x_2x_1 - r_2C \quad (26)$$

$0 \leq \partial_{x_2} \leq 1$ is a positive constant and is used for sliding surface. Thus, we define a sliding surface as

$$\sigma_{x_2} = m_1x_2 + x_3 \quad (27)$$

m_1 is positive. Next, we differentiate Equation (27)

$$\dot{\sigma}_{x_2} = m_1\dot{x}_2 + \dot{x}_3 \quad (28)$$

We substitute Equations (26) and (3) in Equation (28), multiplying σ_{x_2} on both sides of Equation (28) and following the property $\sigma_{x_2}sgn(\sigma_{x_2}) = |\sigma_{x_2}|$; thus, the Equation (29) is formed. Describing a term η_{x_2} as in Equation (31) and simplifying Equation (30), the Equation (32) will be

$$\sigma_{x_2}\dot{\sigma}_{x_2} = -m_1\rho_{x_2}|\sigma_{x_2}| + \sigma_{x_2}\left(\begin{array}{c}m_1((1-\partial_{x_2})a_1x_2(1-d_1x_2) - e_2x_3x_2 - e_3x_2x_1 - r_2C)\\ +\alpha + \frac{px_3x_2}{s+x_2} - e_1x_3x_2 - f_1x_3 - r_1C\end{array}\right) \quad (29)$$

$$\sigma_{x_2}\dot{\sigma}_{x_2} \leq -|\sigma_{x_2}|\left(m_1\rho_{x_2} - \left|\begin{array}{c}m_1((1-\partial_{x_2})a_1x_2(1-d_1x_2) - e_2x_3x_2 - e_3x_2x_1 - r_2C)\\ +\alpha + \frac{px_3x_2}{s+x_2} - e_1x_3x_2 - f_1x_3 - r_1C\end{array}\right|\right) \quad (30)$$

$$\eta_{x_2} = m_1\rho_{x_2} - \left|\begin{array}{c}m_1((1-\partial_{x_2})a_1x_2(1-d_1x_2) - e_2x_3x_2 - e_3x_2x_1 - r_2C) + \alpha + \frac{px_3x_2}{s+x_2}\\ -e_1x_3x_2 - f_1x_3 - r_1C\end{array}\right| \quad (31)$$

$$\sigma_{x_2}\dot{\sigma}_{x_2} \leq -|\sigma_{x_2}|\eta_{x_2} \quad (32)$$

$$\eta_{x_2} \geq 0$$

According to the stability of the SMC. Estimated ρ_{x_2} from Equation (31) is given in (33) as

$$\rho_{x_2} = \frac{\left|\begin{array}{c}m_1((1-\partial_{x_2})a_1x_2(1-d_1x_2) - e_2x_3x_2 - e_3x_2x_1 - r_2C) + \alpha + \frac{px_3x_2}{s+x_2}\\ -e_1x_3x_2 - f_1x_3 - r_1C\end{array}\right|}{m_1} + \frac{\eta_{x_2}}{m_1} \quad (33)$$

Since $-|\sigma_{x_2}|\eta_{x_2} \leq 0$ by default, the system is therefore asymptotically stable; i.e., $\sigma_{x_2}\dot{\sigma}_{x_2} \leq 0$. In this case, the use of Equations (1), (3), and (31) results in an error function given by Equations (39)–(42).

$$Ex_1 = \frac{1}{11}\sum_{i=0}^{10}\left(\dot{x}_1(t_i) - a_2x_1(t_i)(1-d_2x_1(t_i)) + e_4x_2(t_i)x_1(t_i) + r_3C(t_i)\right)^2 \quad (34)$$

$$Ex_2 = \frac{1}{11}\sum_{j=0}^{10}\left(\begin{array}{c}\dot{x}_2(t_j) - (1-\partial_{x_2})a_1x_2(t_j)(1-d_1x_2(t_j)) \\ +\rho_{x_2}\text{sgn}(\sigma_{x_2}) + e_2x_3(t_j)x_2(t_j) + e_3x_2(t_j)x_1(t_j) + r_2C(t_j)\end{array}\right)^2 \quad (35)$$

$$Ex_3 = \frac{1}{11}\sum_{i=0}^{10}\left(\dot{x}_3(t_i) - \alpha - \frac{px_3(t_i)x_2(t_i)}{s+x_2(t_i)} + e_1x_3(t_i)x_2(t_i) + f_1x_3(t_i) + r_1C(t_i)\right)^2 \quad (36)$$

4.1.5. Case-5

Case-5 is just like the previous experiment but with immunotherapy and chemotherapy, and an updated SC is utilized. Due to this method, CCs are reduced very quickly. From Equations (37)–(53), the mentioned detailed experimentation was performed.

In the case of the controller, the Equation (2) will be

$$\dot{x}_2 = a_1x_2(1-d_1x_2) - e_2x_2x_3 - e_3x_2x_1 - r_2C + \mu_{x_2} \quad (37)$$

Here, μ_{x_2} is a controller

$$\psi = f(x_2) \quad (38)$$

$$\psi = m_2(x_2 - x_{2r}) \quad (39)$$

ψ is a macro variable, and m_2 is a positive constant, while the $x_{2r} = 0$ is the reference of CCs

$$\psi = m_2x_2 \quad (40)$$

We differentiate with respect to time, t

$$\dot{\psi} = m_2\dot{x}_2 \quad (41)$$

and we define a manifold

$$\dot{\psi} + \frac{\psi}{\tau} = 0 \quad (42)$$

Next, we substitute Equations (39) and (40) in Equation (41)

$$m_2(\dot{x}_2 + \frac{x_2}{\tau}) = 0 \quad (43)$$

We substitute Equation (37) in Equation (43), and with some manipulation, we obtain

$$\mu_{x_2} = -a_1x_2(1-d_1x_2) + e_2x_2x_3 + e_3x_2x_1 + r_2C - \frac{x_2}{\tau} \quad (44)$$

Now, we substitute controller Equation (44) in Equation (37), and after simplification, we obtain

$$\dot{x}_2 = -\left(\frac{1}{\tau}\right)x_2 \quad (45)$$

The solution of Equation (45) is

$$x_2 = x_2(0)e^{-\frac{t}{\tau}}x_2(t)_{t\to\infty} = 0 \quad (46)$$

We use the Lyapunov function to check the stability of the controller

$$L = \frac{1}{2}\psi^2 \tag{47}$$

$$\dot{L} = \psi\dot{\psi} \tag{48}$$

We transfer the value of $\dot{\psi}$ from Equation (42) in Equation (48); we arrive at

$$\dot{L} = \frac{-\psi^2}{\tau} \tag{49}$$

$$L = L(0)e^{\frac{-2t}{\tau}} \tag{50}$$

$t \to \infty$; the system approaches zero, so the model is asymptotically stable.

$$Ex_1 = \frac{1}{11}\sum_{i=0}^{10}(\dot{x}_1(t_i) - a_2 x_1(t_i)(1 - d_2 x_1(t_i)) + e_4 x_2(t_i)x_1(t_i) + r_3 C(t_i))^2 \tag{51}$$

$$x_2 = x_2(0)e^{-\frac{t}{\tau}} \tag{52}$$

$$Ex_3 = \frac{1}{11}\sum_{i=0}^{10}\left(\dot{x}_3(t_i) - \alpha - \frac{px_3(t_i)x_2(t_i)}{s + x_2(t_i)} + r_1 C(t_i) + e_1 x_3(t_i)x_2(t_i) + f_1 x_3(t_i)\right)^2 \tag{53}$$

In all the above cases, the error function to be minimized is as follows:

$$E_{optimal} = \text{minimum}(E_N + E_T + E_I) \tag{54}$$

In this section, Table 2 represents different controllers using metric values that vary from either 0 to 1. Therefore, the estimated values and reduction of CCs are incorporated with SMC and SC.

Table 2. Different controllers using parameters with values.

Parameters	Values	Estimated	Description
∂_{x_2}	1	0 to 1	Reduction coefficient of growth rate of CCs
η_{x_2}	0	0 to 0.8	Positive constant
ρ_{x_2}	0	0 to 1	Coefficient of controller nonlinear term
τ_a	0.01	0.01 to 0.2	Convergence time of SC
m_1	1	1	Coefficient of SMC
m_2	1	0 to 1	Coefficient of SMC

5. Numerical Results and Discussion

Previously, two methods were utilized in the literature, which are constant, continuous and pulsed chemotherapy. While trying to reduce cancerous cell using therapies, logic is crucial. To eliminate cancerous cells completely from body, a better approach than using medicines is required. The above figure presents the level of chemotherapy with constant and continuous dose methods. Initially, chemotherapy starts from zero, and then after some time reaches the maximum. On the other hand, the constant approach uses fixed doses throughout the chemotherapy.

Figure 2 depicts the behavior of constant and continuous chemotherapy drugs that are given to a patient with the passage of time. An exponential dose becomes reduced and might be eliminated, while a constant dose is applied regularly. The average value of a constant dose is calculated to be about 0.9942. However, a continuous dose is approximately equal to 0.7499.

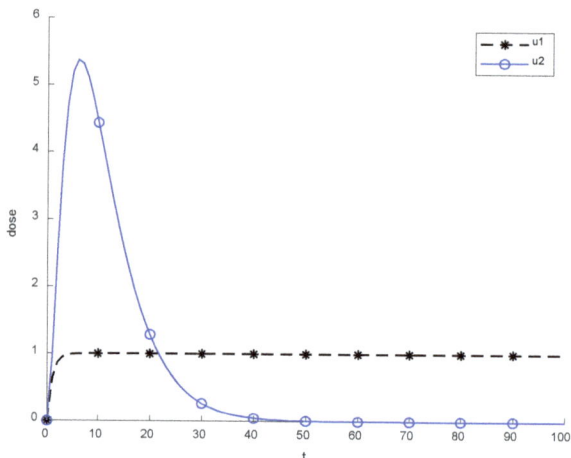

Figure 2. Behavior of constant and continuous chemotherapy.

Figure 3 shows the NCs were reduced and died down, while CCs increased, which is not an optimal case for the body. This figure depicts that no controller or treatment was used; there was only the interaction between normal and cancerous cells, in which NCs were reduced in levels due to cancer. However, CCs increased from their level in comparison with normal cells. During experimentation, the initial value of CCs was 0.25. Therefore, 0.25 is considered the threshold for cancer patients. If the value of CCs is increased from 0.25, then the patient will die on the spot.

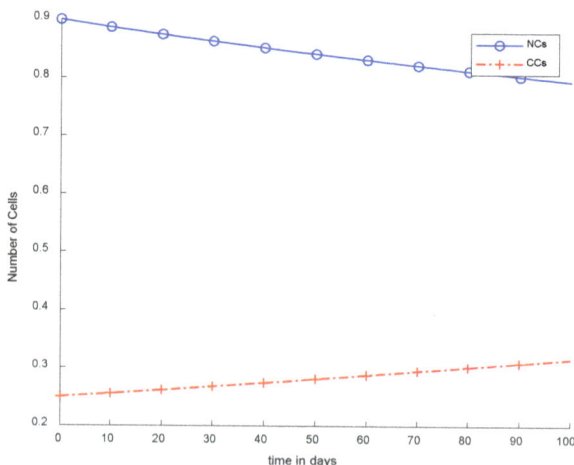

Figure 3. Without ICs, chemotherapy, and controller.

Figure 4 illustrates the concept of case-2, where immunotherapy was added, which reduced the NCs and CCs. Moreover, ICs were in the rising phase, which is shown in case-2. Separately, immunotherapy is not a very appropriate method. In Figure 4, there is clear indication that CCs' growth slowed down but still increased with the passage of time. More interestingly, the result shows that there is a need for other treatments as well with immunotherapy or controllers.

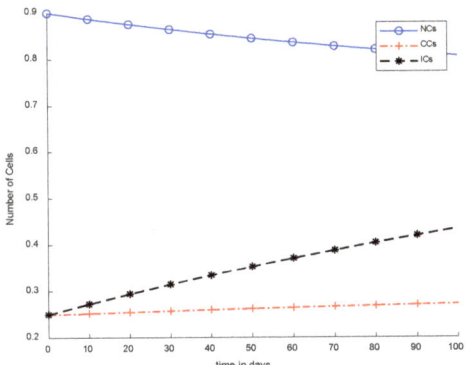

Figure 4. Without chemotherapy and controllers.

In Figure 5, case-3a represents that chemotherapy completely eliminated CCs after one hundred days; there was no such controller utilized, but the dose was constant. In Figure 6, case-3b describes the continuous dose with chemotherapy, where CCs were eliminated within eighty days. However, NCs and ICs became disturbed, which is not good for the body. In Figure 7, case-4a is illustrated, in which SMC were applied, causing CCs to reach the minimum level. Apart from that, ICs and NCs were not disturbed.

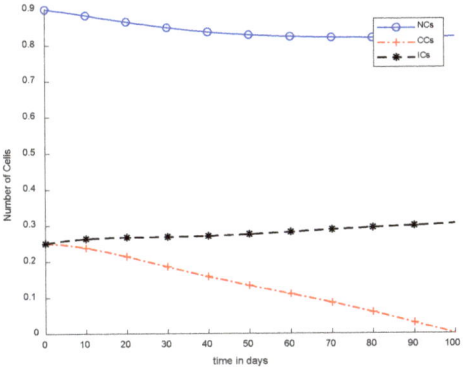

Figure 5. With chemotherapy at a constant dose and without controller.

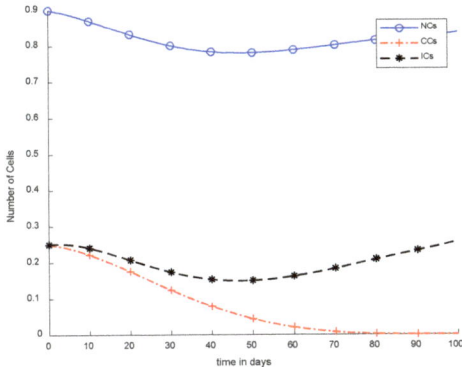

Figure 6. With chemotherapy at a continuous dose and without controller.

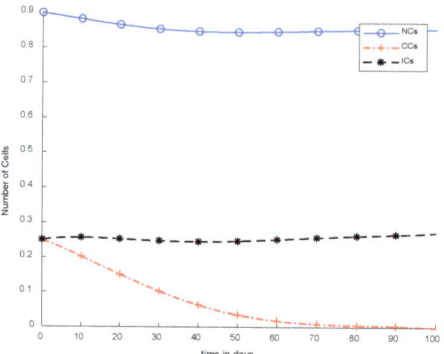

Figure 7. With chemotherapy constant dose and SMC for CCs Killer.

Moreover, in Figure 8, case-4b represents that CCs reduced in about sixty days. Due to the speedy behavior of chemotherapy, CCs and NCs reached the very minimum threshold, which is quite dangerous for the body. In case-5a, whose results are shown in Figure 9, the contemporary SC was applied with chemotherapy at a constant dose. Optimal results were obtained in which NCs and ICs were at maximum level. However, CCs were reduced to level zero within five days. Figure 10 is the result of case-5b, which depicts that using SC, CCs were removed during five days with continuous chemotherapy.

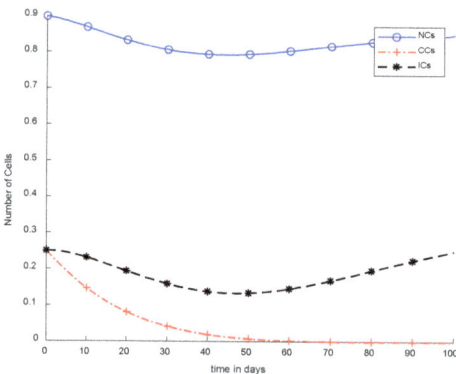

Figure 8. With chemotherapy at a continuous dose and SMC to kill CCs.

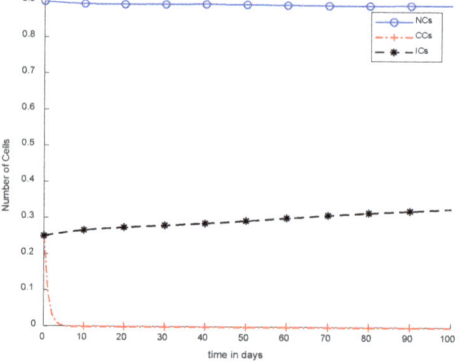

Figure 9. With chemotherapy at a constant dose and SC to kill CCs.

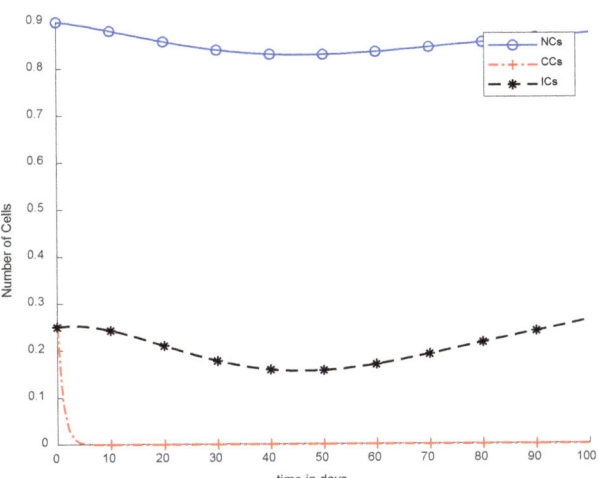

Figure 10. With chemotherapy at a continuous dose and SC to kill CCs.

In Figures 5 and 6, the treatment utilized was the same and was based on chemotherapy. However, Figure 5 shows a fixed-dose treatment. In Figure 6, on the other hand, exponential-dose chemotherapy was used. Further, normal cells were not disturbed too much in Figure 5. Immune cells were at the maximum level, but CCs took a long time to be eliminated from the patient's body.

Figure 6 shows completely different results in comparison with Figure 5. Normal and immune cells showed negative variation. CCs were reduced quickly, in contract with Figure 5.

However, Figure 7 shows results using the SMC controller, whereas in Figures 5 and 6, no such controller was used. A fixed dose of chemotherapy was utilized, which is commonly called constant as well. Comparing Figures 7 and 8, the controller utilized is the same, but Figure 7 shows the optimal results. In addition, normal and immune cells were not disturbed in Figure 7, which is a positive sign for the patient.

It is quite clear in Figure 7 that normal and immune cells show better results. Meanwhile, Figure 8 also utilizes an SMC controller, but CCs were reduced more quickly than in Figure 7. Therefore, Figure 8 shows the main objective was achieved: CCs were eliminated in 50 to 60 days.

However, Figures 9 and 10 both show use of the synergetic controller, which is a completely different approach than SMC, while, Figure 9 presents constant or fixed-dose chemotherapy. Working with the SC approach, ICs and NCs were not affected. In addition, as mentioned, CCs were removed within 5 days. Thus, SC is the only approach that gives better results.

Figure 10 illustrates the same results of CCs reduction in five days, similar to Figure 9. However, in Figure 10, there is a clear negative variation in NCs and ICs using the synergetic controller. In addition, more interestingly, in Figure 10, continuous-dose chemotherapy was utilized.

Figure 11 shows a detailed comparison of CCs with SMC, CCs with SC, and NCs and ICs. The overall results of Figure 11 are based on fixed-dose chemotherapy, while results are quite preferable where CCs are completely eliminated within five days using a synergetic controller. Coupled differential equations are used, and therefore, CCs are shown to have an effect on ICs and NCs using a synergetic controller.

Overall, discussion of Figure 12 is presented in the earlier figures, where chemotherapy with continuous doses of SMC and SC were used. Therefore, in Figure 12, CCs were reduced earlier, but was negative variation normal and immune cells.

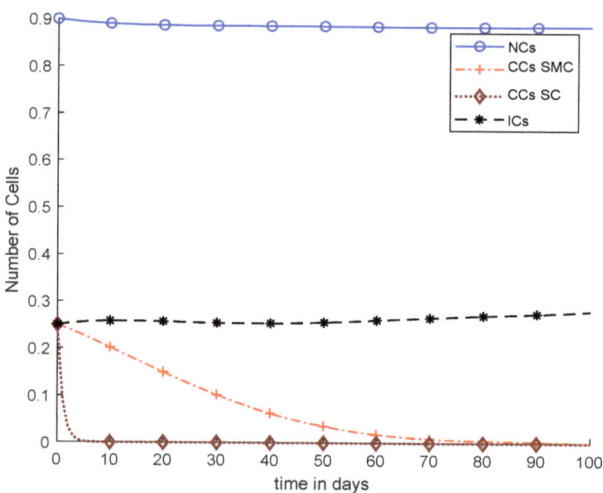

Figure 11. With chemotherapy at a constant dose, SMC on CCs ('+' line) with effect on all equations, and SC on CCs ('−' line).

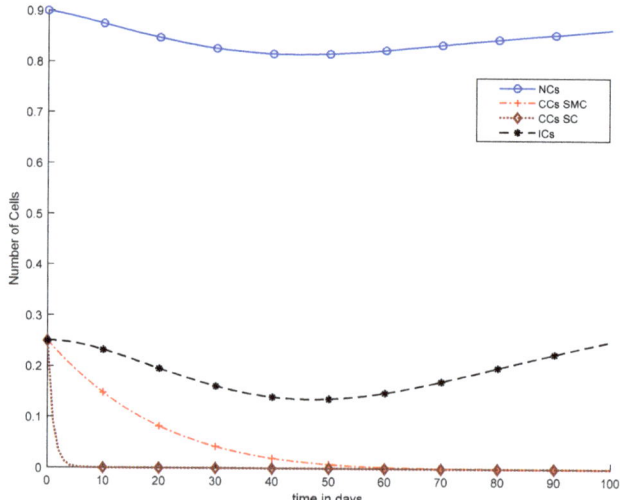

Figure 12. With chemotherapy at a continuous dose and SMC on CCs ('+' line) with effect on all equations and SC on CCs ('−' line).

In Figure 11, case-6a shows the comparison of SMC and SC, in which we utilized constant-dose chemotherapy, and ICs and NCs are at normal level. However, CCs were eliminated in five days with the help of SC. However, using SMC, CCs were minimized in about eighty days. Moreover, in Figure 12, case-6b illustrates an exponential continuous dose with chemotherapy, where using SMC, CCs are reduced nearly in sixty days. However, NCs and ICs are disturbed, which affects the body. In contract with SMC, SC completely removed CCs within five consecutive days. In Figure 13, case-6c shows the idea that SC especially is designed for CCs; later, we utilize the same concept in all other equations. In the above graph, ICs and NCs are at a normal level, while, SMC for CCs showed worse results because CCs survived for about eighty days. The chemotherapy dose is constant in Figure 13. In addition, ICs are at maximum level, which is about 0.25. Furthermore, NCs are near to 0.9, which means NCs are not reduced. This case is basically considered optimal for patients. In Figure 14, case-6d shows similar results as with SC but with SMC, as CCs are reduced in about sixty days using chemotherapy at a continuous dose.

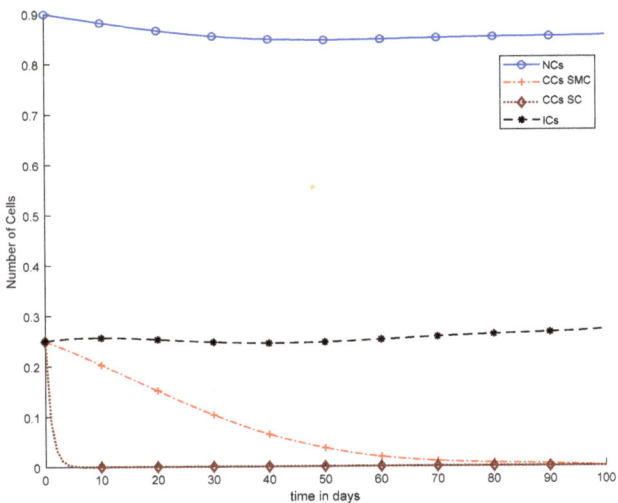

Figure 13. With chemotherapy at a constant dose, SMC on CCs ('+' line), and SC on CCs ('−' line) with effect on all equations.

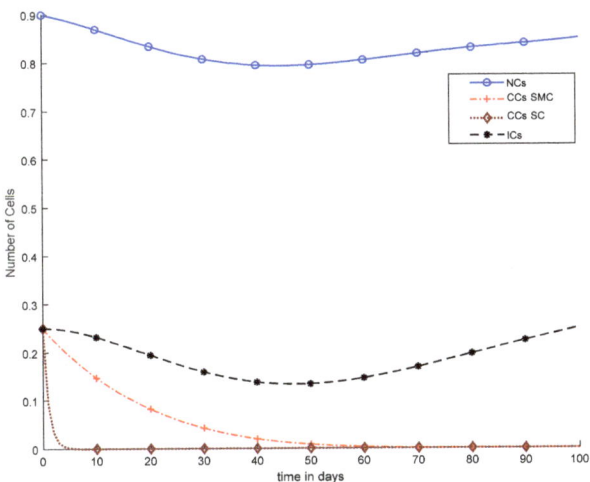

Figure 14. With chemotherapy at a continuous dose, SMC on CCs ('+' line), and SC to kill CCs ('−' line) with effect on all equations.

In Figure 15, Ta is shown where different values are used for SC to remove CCs. Therefore, when Ta = 0.01, CCs are eliminated within five days although if Ta = 0.04, CCs are reduced in about twenty days. In addition, for various values like 0.07, 0.1, and 0.2, SC was evaluated to reduce CCs, which is presented in Figure 14.

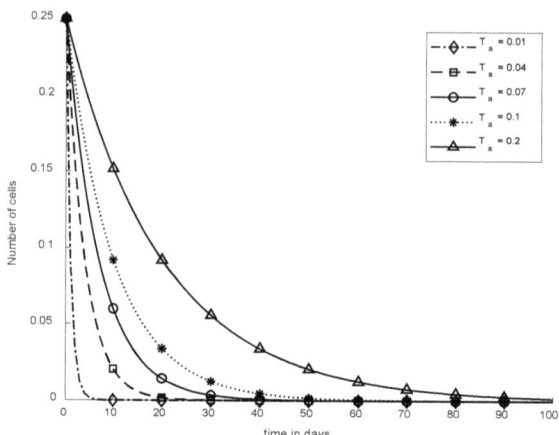

Figure 15. Convergence time of SC.

To reduce the effect of cancerous tumors, chemotherapy and immunotherapy can be utilized. Additionally, hybrid therapies use various types of controllers such as synergetic and sliding mode controllers. Therefore, these controllers can be used as drug treatments to optimize cells of the body. Synergetic controllers are more efficient in comparison with other techniques.

6. Comparative Discussion

Table 3 depicts the comparison of various treatments and controllers used in the study. The proposed approach shows better results in comparison with traditional techniques. Moreover, Depillis et al. [20] demonstrated improved NC levels in contrast with CCs and ICs. However, due to this method, CCs are not eliminated properly. On the other hand, Omar et al. [14] implemented a multi-objective swarm model where NCs cannot exceed the minimum threshold. Apart from that, chemo-immunotherapy with SMC was utilized, which destroyed the CCs in about forty-five days [15], while, in the proposed solution, SC reduced CCs within five days.

However, mathematical modeling for chemotherapy and immunotherapy is rarely used. Normally, immunotherapy is utilized to boost the immune system of the body. The main aim of therapies is to reduce the effect of cancer cells; to target cancerous cells, immunotherapy is quite effective. In comparison with other therapies, mathematical models of cytotoxic chemotherapy were utilized by depillis et al. [9] to eliminate CCs. Formulating a novel chemotherapeutic protocol that improves defense strategies against cancer cells requires a brief understanding of immune system. Therefore, mathematical models of immunotherapies utilize a complex network of cells. Traditional chemotherapies have been studied but without the role of controller. Without the use of a controller, CCs are hardly reduced in about seventy days.

In reference [10], a controller-based model was designed to find the optimal rate of cancer drugs. During therapies, the drug rate is a major factor that can reduce cancer cells. However, due to excess use of the drug, sometimes healthy cells within the body can also experience reduced levels of growth. Therefore, steepest descent technique is utilized to give logical reasoning to improve adaptive controllers. The online recursive calculation approach is used to check the performance of metrics. In the results, NCs improves in a slow way, but CCs are still reduced in about eighty days, which is, again, an alarming condition.

Samira et al. [11] tried to resolve issues related with drug rate and the time needed for giving drugs during immunotherapy. The similar depillis model was implemented by applying the theory of optimal impulsive method, where five differential equations are elaborated with cancer and immune cells. In this study also, CCs were eliminated in about one hundred days, which are not presently better results in comparison with reference [20,28].

Table 3. Comparative study.

Treatment and Controller	Cells	Description
Traditional pulsed chemotherapy without controller [9]	NCs	NCs reduced to minimum level.
	CCs	CCs held at maximum level.
	ICs	Little increase in ICs was observed.
Chemotherapy with optimal control [9]	NCs	NCs hit minimum level and when treatment halted rose to maximum level.
	CCs	Approximately, in 70 days, CCs fell to zero.
	ICs	ICs also increased to a good level.
Chemotherapy and angiotherapy along with adaptive controller [10]	NCs	NCs very slowly increased to a healthy state.
	CCs	More than 80 days needed to decrease to minimum level.
	ECs	During treatment, ECs increased and after that decreased
.Multi immunotherapy [11]	CCs	CCs reduced to minimum level within 100 days but were not completely removed.
	ICs	Also decreased.
Multi objective swarm with optimal control [27]	NCs	When NCs reached minimum threshold, treatment was stopped for a short time for the recovery of NCs.
	CCs	Approximately, in 50 days, CCs fell to zero.
	ICs	ICs increased to a good level.
Chemo-immunotherapy along with SMC controller [15]	NCs	NCs held at maximum level.
	CCs	CCs eliminated within 45 days.
	ICs	ICs achieved a good level.
Multi Chemo-immunotherapy along with Quadratic control [35]	NCs	NCs increased after CCs elimination.
	CCs	CCs eliminated approximately in 40 days.
	ICs	ICs also increased slightly after CCs elimination.
Chemo-immunotherapy along with Quadratic control [28]	CCs	CCs exterminated approximately in 20 days.
	ICs	ICs rose to maximum level after 100 days.
Optimal administration protocols for cancer immunotherapies [36]	CCs	CCs eliminated approximately at 35 to 40 days.
	ICs	ICs also rose after CCs elimination.
Mathematical modelling of CAR-T immunotherapy [32]	CCs	CCs eliminated approximately within 50 days.
	ICs	ICs increased after CCs elimination.
Mathematical modelling of Chemo-immunotherapy in Triple-Negative Breast cancer [21]	CCs	CCs completely removed within 60 days.
	ICs	ICs achieved maximum level after CCs elimination.
Chemo-immunotherapy along with conjoined SMC and SC controller (proposed)	NCs	NCs held to maximum level.
	CCs	CCs eliminated within 5 days.
	ICs	ICs also held to maximum level

Omar et al. [27] presented the concept of combining an optimal control theory with swarm intelligence techniques. Here, in this study, the main focus was drug concentration, where the hybrid approach was far better than other algorithms. To verify the performance, second-order coefficient was used with a multi-objective approach. According to this technique, CCs were easily reduced within fifty days, which presents better results than the above-mentioned study. However, in [35], a new approach of mathematical modeling of CAR-T immunotherapy eliminated cancer cells similarly within fifty days.

Minimizing CCs while injecting drug formulations of Pontryagin's maximum principle established a better balance with cost effectiveness of the control variables. Das et al. [30] eliminated CCs using a quadratic control mechanism in about forty days. However, using an SMC controller, CCs died in forty-five days [28]. Therefore, both cases' results were not optimal and can be further formulated in the near future.

Dehingia et al. [36] recently introduced a technique used to understand the optimality of immune chemotherapy. Feasible domains of various mathematical models are validated using the condition of equilibrium points. This process is used to solve drug toxicity during immune chemotherapy. Further, through this quadratic methodology, CCs were easily reduced in twenty days.

For dealing with cancerous cells, a novel concept of SC was designed in this study. GA, SMC, and SC mathematical models were utilized as a hybrid combination that completely eliminates CCs within five days. This study is compared with existing techniques in the simulation results, where the proposed approach presents superiority. In addition, the theoretical analysis gives a brief overview to compare the proposed solution with previous studies. Therefore, due to both methods, namely simulation and theoretical approach, this study depicts the optimal results of the proposed approach.

This study is limited to the analysis of cancerous tumors and their controlled treatment in the domain of mathematical models at present. Clinical validation of the proposed treatment protocol can be investigated as a prospect study subject to the realization of drugs imitating the effects of SC and SMC utilized in this study.

7. Conclusions

Mathematical models are utilized to evaluate the complex behavior of CCs and NCs, where immune cells are reduced in number due to the fast growth of CCs. Overall, drug dosages need to be exponential with the passage of time. Cancer is considered one of the leading diseases, which arise from uncontrolled division of NCs into CCs. Cancer can be directly reduced or eliminated if CCs can be detected early. For improving the life of cancer patients, various treatment methods such as chemotherapy, immunotherapy, or mathematical modeling need to be utilized for early detection of CCs. This research study consists of using GA, SMC, and SC to reduce the effect and eliminate CCs as soon as possible. However, the proposed work is compared with the existing models to evaluate its performance. The SC easily reduces the CCs in nearly five days and maintains the patient's health state as well. NCs and ICs are improved by using SMC and SC, which is considered an optimal approach for elimination of CCs. SC was determined as the best possible approach as an anti-tumor drug. Figure 13 shows he best optimal result for CCs elimination and also in keeping NCs and ICs at their maximum levels using constant-dose chemotherapy along with SC. In the previous three to four decades, cancer prevention has moved from medicinal studies such as immunotherapy and chemotherapy to mathematical modeling. However, in the future, various evolutionary computational techniques such as ant colony optimization [38], particle swarm optimization [39], differential evolution, and artificial bee colony along with different controllers can be investigated. Additionally machine learning, deep learning, and stochastic Markov chain distribution [40] will envision mathematical modeling not only for CCs but also for different diseases. Further, image classification, data-driven classification models, disease detection, feature classification, and blood vessel segmentation for CCs can be utilized to give possible solutions in the near future [37–43].

Author Contributions: Conceptualization, F.S.; methodology and implementation, F.S.; simulation, F.S.; validation, M.A.A.; data curation, I.U.K.; writing—original draft preparation, I.U.K.; writing—review and editing, M.F., M.W., J.S., and M.F.I.; supervision, M.W., J.S., M.F.I., I.U.K. and M.A.A. All authors have read and agreed to the published version of the manuscript.

Funding: The authors would like to acknowledge contribution to this research from the Rector of the Silesian University of Technology, Gliwice, Poland, under pro-quality grant no. 09/010/RGJ22/0068.

Institutional Review Board Statement: Not applicable.

Informed Consent Statement: Not applicable.

Data Availability Statement: The data presented in this study is available on request from the corresponding author.

Acknowledgments: Jana Shafi would like to thank the Deanship of Scientific Research, Prince Sattam bin Abdul Aziz University, for supporting this work.

Conflicts of Interest: The authors declare that they have no conflicts of interest to report regarding the present study.

Abbreviations

Notation	Description
NCs	Normal cells
CCs	Cancerous tumor cells
ICs	Immune cells
GA	Genetic algorithm
BP	Bernstein polynomial
SMC	Sliding mode controller
SC	Synergetic controller
MOS	Multi-objective swarms
ODE	Ordinary differential equation
NCODE	Nonlinear ordinary coupled differential equation
PSO	Particle swarm optimization
WHO	World health organization
COVID-19	Coronavirus disease of 2019
T-cells	Thymus cells
CAR-T-cells	Chimeric antigen receptor T-cells
1. IFN	Type-1 Interferon receptor
CRPC	Castrate-resistant prostate cancer
Anti-CTLA4	Anti-cytotoxic T-lymphocytes associated protein 4

References

1. Fiore, M.C.; D'Angelo, H.; Baker, T. Effective Cessation Treatment for Patients with Cancer Who Smoke—The Fourth Pillar of Cancer Care. *JAMA Netw. Open* **2019**, *2*, e1912264. [CrossRef] [PubMed]
2. Enderling, H.; Chaplain, A.J.M. Mathematical modeling of tumor growth and treatment. *Curr. Pharm. Des.* **2014**, *20*, 4934–4940. [PubMed]
3. Weidner, N.; Semple, J.P.; Welch, W.R.; Folkman, J. Tumor angiogenesis and metastasis—Correlation in invasive breast carcinoma. *N. Engl. J. Med.* **1991**, *324*, 1–8. [CrossRef] [PubMed]
4. Ganesan, S.; Lingeshwaran, S. Galerkin finite element method for cancer invasion mathematical model. *Comput. Math. Appl.* **2017**, *73*, 2603–2617. [CrossRef]
5. World Health Organization. *WHO Methods and Data Sources for Country Level Causes of Death, 2000–2019. Global Health Estimates Technical Paper WHO/DDI/DNA/GHE/2020.2*; World Health Organization: Geneva, Switzerland, 2020.
6. Siegel, R.L.; Miller, K.D.; Fuchs, H.E.; Jemal, A. Cancer statistics, 2021. *CA. Cancer J. Clin.* **2021**, *71*, 7–33.
7. Konstorum, A.; Vella, A.T.; Adler, A.J.; Laubenbacher, R.C. Addressing current challenges in cancer immunotherapy with mathematical and computational modelling. *J. R. Soc. Interface* **2017**, *14*, 20170150. [CrossRef]
8. Ansarizadeh, F.; Singh, M.; Richards, D. Modelling of tumor cells regression in response to chemotherapeutic treatment. *Appl. Math. Model.* **2017**, *48*, 96–112. [CrossRef]
9. DePillis, L.G.; Eladdadi, A.; Radunskaya, A.E. Modeling cancer-immune responses to therapy. *J. Pharmacokinet. Pharmacodyn.* **2014**, *41*, 461–478. [CrossRef]
10. Khalili, P.; Vatankhah, R. Derivation of an optimal trajectory and nonlinear adaptive controller design for drug delivery in cancerous tumor chemotherapy. *Comput. Biol. Med.* **2019**, *109*, 195–206. [CrossRef]
11. Zouhri, S.; Saadi, S.; Hamdache, A. The Optimal Impulsive Drug Schedule for Cancer Immunotherapy. *Int. J. Sci. Res.* **2017**, *6*, 1643–1652.
12. De Pillis, L.G.; Radunskaya, A. A mathematical tumor model with immune resistance and drug therapy: An optimal control approach. *Comput. Math. Methods Med.* **2001**, *3*, 79–100.
13. Saleem, M.; Agrawal, T. Chaos in a Tumor Growth Model with Delayed Responses of the Immune System. *J. Appl. Math.* **2012**, *2012*, 891095. [CrossRef]
14. Rocha, A.M.A.C.; Costa, M.F.P.; Fernandes, E.M.G.P. On a multiobjective optimal control of a tumor growth model with immune response and drug therapies. *Int. Trans. Oper. Res.* **2018**, *25*, 269–294. [CrossRef]

15. Dhiman, G.; Kumar, V. Multi-objective spotted hyena optimizer: A Multi-objective optimization algorithm for engineering problems. *Knowl. Based Syst.* **2018**, *150*, 175–197. [CrossRef]
16. Ahrabi, S.S. Optimal control in cancer immunotherapy by the application of particle swarm optimization. *arXiv* **2018**, arXiv:1806.04752.
17. Srinivasu, P.N.; Ahmed, S.; Alhumam, A.; Kumar, A.B.; Ijaz, M.F. An AW-HARIS Based Automated Segmentation of Human Liver Using CT Images. *Comput. Mater. Contin.* **2021**, *69*, 3303–3319. [CrossRef]
18. Liu, S.; Yang, B.; Wang, Y.; Tian, J.; Yin, L.; Zheng, W. 2D/3D Multimode Medical Image Registration Based on Normalized Cross-Correlation. *Appl. Sci.* **2022**, *12*, 2828. [CrossRef]
19. Ijaz, M.F.; Attique, M.; Son, Y. Data-Driven Cervical Cancer Prediction Model with Outlier Detection and Over-Sampling Methods. *Sensors* **2020**, *20*, 2809. [CrossRef]
20. Mandal, M.; Singh, P.K.; Ijaz, M.F.; Shafi, J.; Sarkar, R. A Tri-Stage Wrapper-Filter Feature Selection Framework for Disease Classification. *Sensors* **2021**, *21*, 5571. [CrossRef]
21. Srinivasu, P.N.; SivaSai, J.G.; Ijaz, M.F.; Bhoi, A.K.; Kim, W.; Kang, J.J. Classification of skin disease using deep learning neural networks with MobileNet V2 and LSTM. *Sensors* **2021**, *21*, 2852. [CrossRef]
22. Moussa, K.; Fiacchini, M.; Alamir, M. Robust Optimal Control-based Design of Combined Chemo- and Immunotherapy Delivery Profiles. *IFAC-PapersOnLine* **2019**, *52*, 76–81. [CrossRef]
23. Malinzi, J.; Ouifki, R.; Eladdadi, A.; Torres, D.F.M.; White, K.A.J. Enhancement of chemotherapy using oncolytic virotherapy: Mathematical and optimal control analysis. *arXiv* **2018**, arXiv:1807.04329. [CrossRef] [PubMed]
24. Lestari, D.; Sari, E.R.; Arifah, H. Dynamics of a mathematical model of cancer cells with chemotherapy. *J. Physics Conf. Ser.* **2019**, *1320*, 012026. [CrossRef]
25. De Pillis, L.; Radunskaya, A. The dynamics of an optimally controlled tumor model: A case study. *Math. Comput. Model.* **2003**, *37*, 1221–1244. [CrossRef]
26. Lobato, F.S.; Machado, V.S.; Steffen, V., Jr. Determination of an optimal control strategy for drug administration in tumor treatment using multi-objective optimization differential evolution. *Comput. Methods Programs Biomed.* **2016**, *131*, 51–61. [CrossRef]
27. Shindi, O.; Kanesan, J.; Kendall, G.; Ramanathan, A. The combined effect of optimal control and swarm intelligence on optimization of cancer chemotherapy. *Comput. Methods Programs Biomed.* **2020**, *189*, 105327. [CrossRef]
28. Subhan, F.; Aziz, M.A.; Shah, J.A.; Kadir, K.A.; Qureshi, I.M. Tumor Treatment Protocol by Using Genetic Algorithm Based Bernstein Polynomials and Sliding Mode Controller. *IEEE Access* **2021**, *9*, 152503–152513. [CrossRef]
29. Mehdizadeh, R.; Shariatpanahi, S.P.; Goliaei, B.; Peyvandi, S.; Rüegg, C. Dormant Tumor Cell Vaccination: A Mathematical Model of Immunological Dormancy in Triple-Negative Breast Cancer. *Cancers* **2021**, *13*, 245. [CrossRef]
30. Coletti, R.; Pugliese, A.; Lunardi, A.; Caffo, O.; Marchetti, L. A Model-Based Framework to Identify Optimal Administration Protocols for Immunotherapies in Castration-Resistance Prostate Cancer. *Cancers* **2021**, *14*, 135. [CrossRef]
31. Subhan, F.; Malik, S.A.; Khan, M.A.; Aziz, M.A.; Uddin, M.I.; Ullah, I. Numerical Investigation of Thin Film Flow of a Third-Grade Fluid on a Moving Belt Using Evolutionary Algorithm-Based Heuristic Technique. *J. Circuits Syst. Comput.* **2021**, *31*, 2250011. [CrossRef]
32. Utkin, V. Discontinuous Control Systems: State of Art in Theory and Applications. *IFAC Proc.* **1987**, *20*, 25–44. [CrossRef]
33. Skruch, P.; Długosz, M. Design of Terminal Sliding Mode Controllers for Disturbed Non-Linear Systems Described by Matrix Differential Equations of the Second and First Orders. *Appl. Sci.* **2019**, *9*, 2325. [CrossRef]
34. Kolesnikov, A.A. Introduction of synergetic control. In Proceedings of the 2014 American control conference, Portland, OR, USA, 4–6 June 2014; pp. 3013–3016.
35. Das, P.; Das, S.; Upadhyay, R.K.; Das, P. Optimal treatment strategies for delayed cancer-immune system with multiple therapeutic approach. *Chaos Solitons Fractals* **2020**, *136*, 109806. [CrossRef]
36. Dehingia, K.; Sarmah, H.K.; Hosseini, K.; Sadri, K.; Salahshour, S.; Park, C. An optimal control problem of immuno-chemotherapy in presence of gene therapy. *AIMS Math.* **2021**, *6*, 11530–11549. [CrossRef]
37. Barros, L.R.C.; Paixão, E.A.; Valli, A.M.P.; Naozuka, G.T.; Fassoni, A.C.; Almeida, R.C. CART math—A Mathematical Model of CAR-T Immunotherapy in Preclinical Studies of Hematological Cancers. *Cancers* **2021**, *13*, 2941. [CrossRef]
38. Khan, I.U.; Qureshi, I.M.; Aziz, M.A.; Cheema, T.A.; Shah, S.B.H. Smart IoT Control-Based Nature Inspired Energy Efficient Routing Protocol for Flying Ad Hoc Network (FANET). *IEEE Access* **2020**, *8*, 56371–56378. [CrossRef]
39. Abbasi, A.; Sultan, K.; Aziz, M.A.; Khan, A.U.; Khalid, H.A.; Guerrero, J.M.; Zafar, B.A. A Novel Dynamic Appliance Clustering Scheme in a Community Home Energy Management System for Improved Stability and Resiliency of Microgrids. *IEEE Access* **2021**, *9*, 142276–142288. [CrossRef]
40. Khan, I.U.; Abdollahi, A.; Alturki, R.; Alshehri, M.D.; Ikram, M.A.; Alyamani, H.J.; Khan, S. Intelligent Detection System Enabled Attack Probability Using Markov Chain in Aerial Networks. *Wirel. Commun. Mob. Comput.* **2021**, *2021*, 1542657. [CrossRef]
41. Dash, S.; Verma, S.; Kavita; Khan, S.; Wozniak, M.; Shafi, J.; Ijaz, M.F. A Hybrid Method to Enhance Thick and Thin Vessels for Blood Vessel Segmentation. *Diagnostics* **2021**, *11*, 2017. [CrossRef]
42. Vulli, A.; Srinivasu, P.N.; Sashank, M.S.K.; Shafi, J.; Choi, J.; Ijaz, M.F. Fine-Tuned DenseNet-169 for Breast Cancer Metastasis Prediction Using FastAI and 1-Cycle Policy. *Sensors* **2022**, *22*, 2988. [CrossRef]
43. Cao, Z.; Wang, Y.; Zheng, W.; Yin, L.; Tang, Y.; Miao, W.; Liu, S.; Yang, B. The algorithm of stereo vision and shape from shading based on endoscope imaging. *Biomed. Signal Process. Control* **2022**, *76*, 103658. [CrossRef]

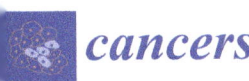 cancers

Article

Chaotic Sparrow Search Algorithm with Deep Transfer Learning Enabled Breast Cancer Classification on Histopathological Images

K. Shankar [1], Ashit Kumar Dutta [2], Sachin Kumar [1], Gyanendra Prasad Joshi [3,*] and Ill Chul Doo [4,*]

1. Big Data and Machine Learning Laboratory, South Ural State University, 454080 Chelyabinsk, Russia; drkshankar@ieee.org (K.S.); kumars@susu.ru (S.K.)
2. Department of Computer Science and Information System, College of Applied Sciences, AlMaarefa University, Riyadh 11597, Saudi Arabia; adotta@mcst.edu.sa
3. Department of Computer Science and Engineering, Sejong University, Seoul 05006, Korea
4. Artificial Intelligence Education, Hankuk University of Foreign Studies, Dongdaemun-gu, Seoul 02450, Korea
* Correspondence: joshi@sejong.ac.kr (G.P.J.); dic@hufs.ac.kr (I.C.D.)

Citation: Shankar, K.; Dutta, A.K.; Kumar, S.; Joshi, G.P.; Doo, I.C. Chaotic Sparrow Search Algorithm with Deep Transfer Learning Enabled Breast Cancer Classification on Histopathological Images. *Cancers* **2022**, *14*, 2770. https://doi.org/10.3390/cancers14112770

Academic Editors: Marcin Woźniak and Muhammad Fazal Ijaz

Received: 18 April 2022
Accepted: 30 May 2022
Published: 2 June 2022

Publisher's Note: MDPI stays neutral with regard to jurisdictional claims in published maps and institutional affiliations.

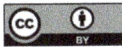

Copyright: © 2022 by the authors. Licensee MDPI, Basel, Switzerland. This article is an open access article distributed under the terms and conditions of the Creative Commons Attribution (CC BY) license (https://creativecommons.org/licenses/by/4.0/).

Simple Summary: Cancer is considered the most significant public health issue which severely threatens people's health. The occurrence and mortality rate of breast cancer have been growing consistently. Initial precise diagnostics act as primary factors in improving the endurance rate of patients. Even though there are several means to identify breast cancer, histopathological diagnosis is now considered the gold standard in the diagnosis of cancer. However, the difficulty of histopathological image and the rapid rise in workload render this process time-consuming, and the outcomes might be subjected to pathologists' subjectivity. Hence, the development of a precise and automatic histopathological image analysis method is essential for the field. Recently, the deep learning method for breast cancer pathological image classification has made significant progress, which has become mainstream in this field. Therefore, in this work, we focused on the design of metaheuristics with deep learning based breast cancer classification process. The proposed model is found to be an effective tool to assist physicians in the decision making process.

Abstract: Breast cancer is the major cause behind the death of women worldwide and is responsible for several deaths each year. Even though there are several means to identify breast cancer, histopathological diagnosis is now considered the gold standard in the diagnosis of cancer. However, the difficulty of histopathological image and the rapid rise in workload render this process time-consuming, and the outcomes might be subjected to pathologists' subjectivity. Hence, the development of a precise and automatic histopathological image analysis method is essential for the field. Recently, the deep learning method for breast cancer pathological image classification has made significant progress, which has become mainstream in this field. This study introduces a novel chaotic sparrow search algorithm with a deep transfer learning-enabled breast cancer classification (CSSADTL-BCC) model on histopathological images. The presented CSSADTL-BCC model mainly focused on the recognition and classification of breast cancer. To accomplish this, the CSSADTL-BCC model primarily applies the Gaussian filtering (GF) approach to eradicate the occurrence of noise. In addition, a MixNet-based feature extraction model is employed to generate a useful set of feature vectors. Moreover, a stacked gated recurrent unit (SGRU) classification approach is exploited to allot class labels. Furthermore, CSSA is applied to optimally modify the hyperparameters involved in the SGRU model. None of the earlier works have utilized the hyperparameter-tuned SGRU model for breast cancer classification on HIs. The design of the CSSA for optimal hyperparameter tuning of the SGRU model demonstrates the novelty of the work. The performance validation of the CSSADTL-BCC model is tested by a benchmark dataset, and the results reported the superior execution of the CSSADTL-BCC model over recent state-of-the-art approaches.

Keywords: breast cancer; histopathological images; computer aided diagnosis; cancer; medical imaging; deep learning

1. Introduction

Cancer is considered the most significant public health issue which severely threatens people's health. The occurrence and mortality rate of breast cancer (BC) have been growing consistently. Initial precise diagnostics act as primary factors in improving the endurance rate of patients [1]. A mammogram is the starting stage of initial prognosis; hence, it becomes hard to detect cancer in the denser breasts of teenage women. X-ray radiation warns radiologists of the patient's health [2]. The golden standard for BC prognosis is only pathological examination. Pathological examinations generally attain tumor samples via excision, puncture, etc. [3]. Hematoxylin combines deoxyribonucleic acid (DNA), and eosin combines proteins. The precise prognosis of BC demands proficient histopathologists, and it needs more time and endeavor to finish this work. Moreover, the prognosis outcomes of distinct histopathologists are dissimilar and heavily based on histopathologists' earlier experience [4].

Recently, BC prognosis is dependent on the histopathological image, and this is confronted by three major difficulties. At first, there is a shortcoming of proficient histopathologists across the globe, particularly in quite a few undeveloped regions and small hospitals [5]. Next, the prognosis of histopathologists is subjective, and evaluation is not performed on an objective basis. Whether prognosis is right or not is wholly based on the histopathologists' earlier knowledge [6]. Lastly, the prognosis of BC depends on the histopathological image, which is time consuming, highly complex, and labor-intensive, and it is considered ineffective during the era of big data. Despite such issues, an objective and effective BC prognosis technique is essential for mitigating the pressure of the workload of histopathologists [7]. The speedy advancement of computer-aided diagnosis (CAD) was slowly employed in the clinical domain. The CAD system will not act as a substitute for the physician; however, it can be utilized as a "second reader" in assisting the physician in recognizing diseases [8]. However, there are false-positive areas identified by the computer that will consume time for the physician in evaluating the outcomes induced by the computer, again leading to a decline in effectiveness and preciseness. Thus, methods for improving the sensitiveness of computer-aided tumor identification methodologies while greatly minimizing the incorrect positive identification rate and enhancing the efficiency of the identification technique constitute a potential research area [9].

Currently, deep learning (DL) methods have become popular in computer vision (CV), particularly in biomedical image processing. These methods were able to investigate complex and enhanced characteristics from images automatically. At the same time, these methods greatly require the attention of several authors in using such techniques to categorize BC histopathology images [10]. In particular terms, convolutional neural networks (CNNs) are broadly utilized in image-based works because of their capabilities to efficiently distribute variables over several layers inside a DL method.

This study introduces a novel chaotic sparrow search algorithm with a deep transfer learning-enabled breast cancer classification (CSSADTL-BCC) model applied on histopathological images. The presented CSSADTL-BCC model applies the Gaussian filtering (GF) approach to eradicate the occurrence of noise. In addition, a MixNet-based feature extraction model was employed to generate a useful set of feature vectors. Furthermore, a CSSA with a stacked gated recurrent unit (SGRU) classification approach was exploited to allot class labels. The CSSADTL-BCC model does not exist in the literature to the best of our knowledge. The design of the CSSA for optimal hyperparameter tuning of the SGRU model demonstrates the novelty of the work. The performance validation of the CSSADTL-BCC model was verified using benchmark data collection, and the outcomes were inspected under different evaluation measures.

The remaining sections of the paper are planned as follows. Section 2 indicates the existing works related to BC classification. Next, Section 3 elaborates the proposed model, and Section 4 offers the performance validation. At last, Section 5 draws the conclusions.

2. Literature Review

In [11], the authors proposed a real time data augmentation-related transfer learning method to resolve existing limitations. Two popular and well-established image classification methods, such as Xception and InceptionV3 frameworks, have been trained on a freely accessible BC histopathological image data named BreakHis. Alom et al. [12] presented a technique for classifying BC using the Inception Recurrent Residual Convolution Neural Network (IRRCNN) framework. The proposed method is an effective DCNN system that integrates the strength of the Recurrent Convolution Neural Network (RCNN), Inception Network (Inception-v4), and the Residual Network (ResNet). The experiment result illustrates better performance against RCNN, Inception Network, and ResNet for object-detection tasks.

Vo et al. [13] presented a technique that employs the DL method with a convolution layer for extracting the visual feature for BC classification. It has been found that the DL model extracts the most useful feature when compared to the handcrafted feature extraction approach. In [14], the authors proposed a BC histopathological image categorization related to deep feature fusion and enhanced routing (FE-BkCapsNet) to exploit CapsNet and CNN models. Firstly, a new architecture with two channels could simultaneously extract capsule and convolutional features and incorporate spatial and sematic features into the new capsule to obtain a discriminative dataset.

The researchers in [15] proposed a patch-based DL method named Pa-DBN-BC for classifying and detecting BC on histopathology images with the Deep Belief Network (DBN). The feature is extracted by supervised finetuning and unsupervised pre-training phases. The network extracts feature automatically from image patches. Logistic regression is utilized for classifying the patches from histopathology images. In [16], the authors proposed a robust and novel technique based convolution-LSTM (CLSTM) learning method, the pre-processing method with the optimized SVM classifier, and the marker-controlled watershed segmentation algorithm (MWSA) for automatically identifying BC. Saxena et al. [17] presented a hybrid ML method for solving class imbalance problems. The presented method uses the kernelized weighted ELM and pre-trained ResNet50 for CAD of BC using histopathology.

Several automated breast cancer classification models are available in the literature. However, the models still contains a challenging problem. Because of the continual deepening of models, the number of parameters of DL models also increases quickly, which results in model overfitting. At the same time, different hyperparameters have a significant impact on the efficiency of the CNN model, particularly in terms of the learning rate. Modifying the learning rate parameter for obtaining better performance is also required. Therefore, in this study, we employ the CSSA technique for the hyperparameter tuning of the SGRU model.

3. The Proposed Model

In this study, a new CSSADTL-BCC model was developed to classify BC on histopathological images. The presented CSSADTL-BCC model mainly focused on the recognition and classification of BC. At the primary stage, the CSSADTL-BCC model employed the GF technique to eradicate the occurrence of noise. It was then followed by using a MixNet-based feature extraction model employed to produce a useful set of feature vectors. Then, the CSSA-SGRU classifier was exploited to allot class labels. Figure 1 illustrates the overall process of the CSSADTL-BCC technique.

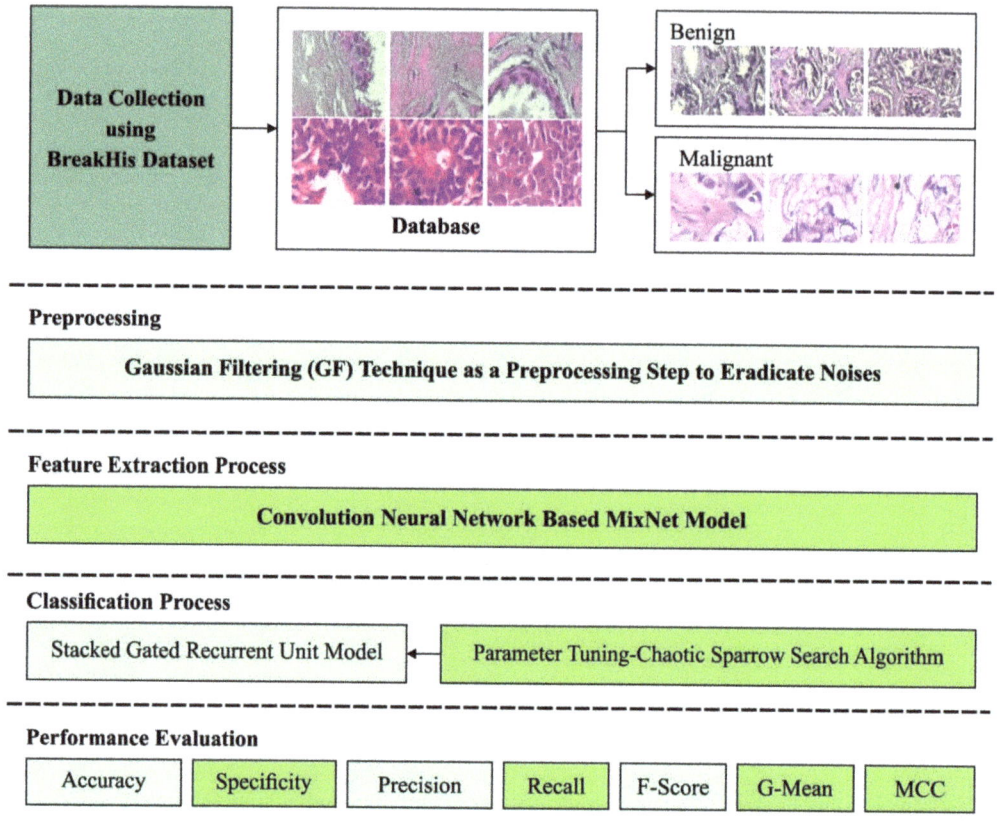

Figure 1. The overall process of the CSSADTL-BCC technique.

3.1. Image Pre-Processing

At the primary stage, the CSSADTL-BCC model employed the GF technique to eradicate the occurrence of noise. GF is a bandpass filter, viz., efficiently implemented in machine vision and image processing applications [18]. A two-dimensional Gabor purpose was oriented by sinusoidal grates controlled by two dimensional Gaussian envelopes. In the two-dimensional coordinate (a, b) model, the GF comprising an imaginary and real one is illustrated by the following:

$$G_{\delta,\theta,\psi,\sigma,\gamma}(a,b) = \exp\left(-\frac{a'^2 + \gamma^2 b'^2}{2\sigma^2}\right) \times \exp\left(j\left(2\pi\frac{a'}{\delta} + \psi\right)\right) \quad (1)$$

where they are described as follows.

$$a' = a \cos\theta + b \sin\theta \quad (2)$$

$$b' = -a \sin\theta + b \cos\theta \quad (3)$$

Now θ implies the orientation separation angle of the Gabor kernel, and δ signifies the wavelength of sinusoidal features. Notably, it is essential to consider θ from the range $[0°, 180°]$ as symmetry generates another redundant direction. ψ denotes the stage offset, σ indicates the standard derivation of the Gaussian envelope, and γ represents the ratio of spatial features for identifying the ellipticity of the Gabor role. $\psi = 0$ and $\psi = \pi/2$ return the real and imaginary parts of GF. Variable 0 can be determined as 6 and spatial frequency bandwidth bw is given by the following.

$$\sigma = \frac{\delta}{pi}\sqrt{\frac{ln2}{2}}\frac{2^{bw}+1}{2^{bw}-1} \quad (4)$$

3.2. MixNet-Based Feature Extractor

Next, for image pre-processing, a MixNet-based feature extraction model is employed to generate a useful set of feature vectors. A CNN algorithm created by the traditional convolutional operation is difficult to use for mobile terminals due to its complicated calculations and excessive parameters. In order to improve its effectiveness on mobile terminals and to guarantee the accuracy of the model, a sequence of lightweight convolutional operators has been presented. Amongst them, one of the most commonly utilized is a depthwise separable convolution layer. A depthwise separable convolutional layer splits the convolution into pointwise and depthwise convolution. In the initial phase, it convolves a single channel at a time using convolutional kernels at size = 3. In the second phase, it uses a feature map with the 1×1 convolutional kernel. Assume that N $D_k \times D_k$ feature view and 1 convolutional sliding step are utilized to convolve a feature map with $D_F \times D_F \times M$ dimensions, including the output feature map with dimensions of $D_F \times D_F \times N$. The parameter amount of traditional convolutional operations is provided as follows.

$$D_k \times D_k \times M \times N \quad (5)$$

The parameters involved in the depthwise separable convolutional operation is provided below.

$$D_k \times D_k \times M + 1 \times 1 \times M \times N \quad (6)$$

The computation involved in traditional convolutional operation is provided as follows.

$$D_k \times D_k \times M \times N \times D_F \times D_F \quad (7)$$

The computation involved in depthwise separable convolutional operation is defined in Equation (8).

$$D_k \times D_k \times M \times D_F \times D_F \times M \times N \times D_F \times D_F \quad (8)$$

The ratio of the two operations is provided as follows.

$$\frac{D_k \times D_k \times M \times D_F \times D_F \times M \times N \times D_F \times D_F}{D_k \times D_k \times M \times N \times D_F \times D_F} \quad (9)$$

A depthwise separable convolutional layer uses a similar size 3×3 convolutional kernel in the computation method; however, a network with larger convolutional kernels of 5×5 or 7×7 confirms that a larger convolutional kernel improves the efficiency and accuracy of the model. However, the experiment shows that the case where a larger convolutional kernel is better is rare; simultaneously, a large convolutional kernel minimizes the model's accuracy. Here, MDConv splits the input channel with M size into C groups, later convolving all the groups with distinct kernel sizes. The standard depthwise separable convolution splits the input channel with M size into M groups and later implements convolutional calculations for all groups with a similar kernel size.

3.3. Image Classification Using SGRU Model

At this stage, the generated feature vectors are passed into the SGRU classifier to allot class labels. SGRU is made up of various GRU units. For time series t, the input series $\{e_1, e_2, \ldots, e_t\}$ first enters into hidden layer $\{h_1^1, h_2^1, \ldots, h_t^1\}$ to attain all data from the previous time step. Next, the upper hidden layer takes the output from the lower hidden layers at a similar time step as the input for extracting features [19]. In particular, the upper layer of the hidden layer is $\{h_1^2, h_2^2, \ldots, h_t^2\}$. For all layers, a hidden layer h_t^i, as provided in Equation (13), is shown by Equations (10)–(12) to attain the candidate value, update, and reset gates. It should be noted that in Equations (10)–(12), we have included embedding vector e_t in the initial layer. Starting from the next layer upward, we employ the hidden state from the current time step in the previous layer, h_t^{i-1}, rather than e_t in (10)–(12). Figure 2 depicts the framework of SGRU.

$$u_t^i = \sigma\left(W_u^i h_{t-1}^i + U_u^i e_t + b_u^i\right) \tag{10}$$

$$r_t^i = \sigma\left(W_r^i h_{t-1}^i + U_r^i e_t + b_r^i\right) \tag{11}$$

$$\tilde{C} = \tanh\left(W_c^i \cdot \left[r_t^i \times h_{t-1}^i\right] + U_c^i e_t + b_c^i\right) \tag{12}$$

$$h_t^i = u_t^i \times \tilde{C}_t^i + \left(1 - u_t^i\right) \times h_{t-1}^i \tag{13}$$

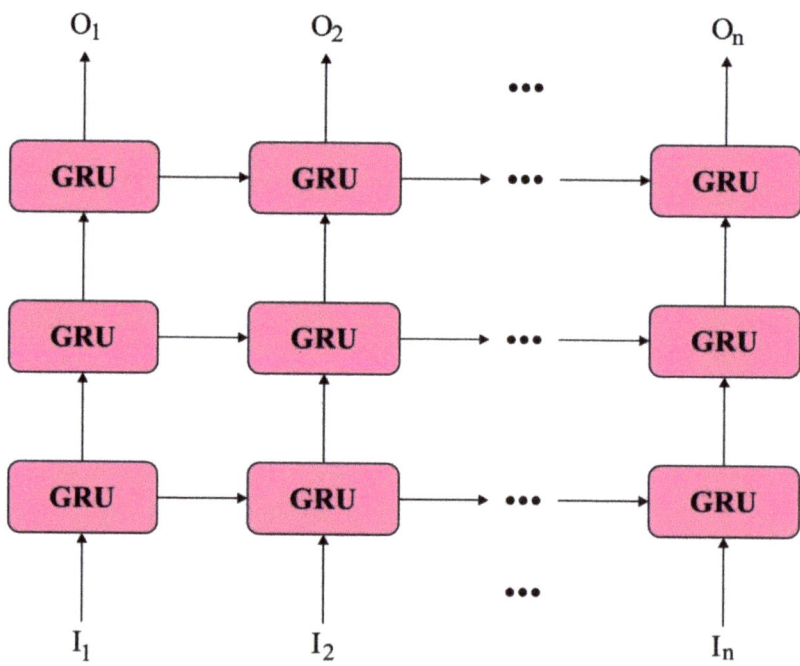

Figure 2. Framework of SGRU model.

3.4. Hyperparameter Optimization

Finally, CSSA is implied to optimally modify the hyperparameters included in the MixNet model. SSA attains the best possible solution by mimicking certain behaviors of sparrows [20]. Firstly, the discoverer–joiner sparrow population models are established, and then the sparrow is arbitrarily chosen as a guard. The joiner snatches food from the discoverer, observes the discoverer, and follows the discoverer for food. The discoverer takes the responsibility to provide foraging direction and areas for the sparrow population. Once the vigilante realizes the threat, the population implements anti-predation behavior immediately. Lastly, with various iterations of the location of the discoverer and joiner, the adoptive position for the entire population can be found. The sparrow population is within the space of $N \times D$, where N indicates the overall amount of sparrows, D represents the spatial dimension. Next, the location of the i-th sparrow in space represents $X_i = (x_{i1}, x_{i2}, \cdots, x_{id})$, $i \in [1, N]$, $d \in [1, D]$, and x_{id} characterizes the location of i-th sparrow in d-dimension. The position update equation of the discoverer can be shown in the following Equation (14).

$$x_{id}^{t+1} = \begin{cases} x_{id}^t \cdot exp.\left(\frac{-i}{\alpha \cdot T}\right) & R_2 < ST \\ x_{id}^t + Q \cdot L, & R_2 \geq ST \end{cases} \quad (14)$$

In the equation, t signifies the existing amount of iterations; T indicates the maximal amount of iterations; α represents an arbitrary value within $[0, 1]$; Q implies an arbitrary value with standard distribution; L indicates a matrix in that element is 1, and its size is $1 \times d$; $R_2 \in [0, 1]$ signifies the warning values; $ST \in [0.5, 1]$ denotes the safety values. If $R_2 < ST$, this implies that the population is not at risk and the discoverer continues searching. If $R_2 \geq ST$, this implies that the vigilante discovered the predator and instantly delivered an alarm to the others. The sparrow population implements anti-predation behavior immediately any fly to a safer region for food. The position update equation of the joiner can be shown in the following Equation (15).

$$x_{id}^{t+1} = \begin{cases} Q \cdot exp\left(\frac{x_{worstd}^t - x_{id}^t}{i^2}\right) & i > \frac{N}{2} \\ x_{best\ d}^{t+1} + \frac{1}{D}\sum_{d=1}^{D}(rand(-1,1) \cdot \left|x_{id}^t - x_{best\ d}^{t+1}\right| & i \leq \frac{N}{2} \end{cases} \quad (15)$$

Here, x_{worstd}^t signifies the global worst place in tth iteration; x_{bestd}^{t+1} signifies the global optimal location at the tth iteration. If $i > \frac{N}{2}$, it implies that the i-th joiner has not attained food and that it needs to fly toward another location in order to search for food. If $i \leq \frac{N}{2}$, this implies that the i-th joiner is closer to the world's best location and is arbitrarily foraging around. The vigilant location upgrade equation is provided as follows:

$$x_{id}^{r+1} = \begin{cases} x_{worst\ d}^t + \beta(x_{id}^t - x_{worst\ d}^t), & f_i \neq f_g \\ x_{id}^t + K\left(\frac{x_{id}^t - x_{worst\ d}^t}{|f_i - f_w| + e}\right) & f_i = f_g \end{cases} \quad (16)$$

where β signifies the step length control variable that is an arbitrary value subjected to a regular distribution with a variance of 1 and means value of 0; K denotes the movement direction of sparrow, and arbitrary values lie within $[1, 1]$; e indicates a constant with smaller value; f_i characterizes the fitness of i-th sparrow; f_g signifies the optimum fitness of the existing population; f_w denotes the worst fitness of existing population. If $f_i \neq f_g$, this implies that the i-th sparrow is at the edge of the population and can be attacked easily by the predator. If $f_i = f_g$, this implies that i-th sparrow is within center of the population, and it is aware of danger; it relocates closer to other sparrows in order to reduce the threat of becoming caught.

With the addition of a global optimum sparrow neighborhood in all iterations, the searching ability of SSA can be enhanced. Additionally, this could assist the sparrow group in attaining the best location through the search process. The chaotic local searching technique can be employed in the iteration process of SSA for improving the capability of exploitation and maintaining a better harmony among the core search processes. Moreover, the logical chaotic function is employed to calculate chaotic SSA. This can be obtained as follows.

$$\rho_{k+1} = \mu \rho_k (1 - \rho_k), k = 1, 2, \ldots, N - 1 \quad (17)$$

On the other hand, $\rho_1 \in (0, 1)$ and $\rho_1 \neq 0.25, 0.5, 0.75,$ and 1 once the control parameter μ is set to 4, and the logistic function is converted to a chaotic state. Therefore, the chaotic local searching function is shown below.

$$P_i = b + \rho_i \times (b - a), i = 1, 2, \ldots, N \quad (18)$$

Here, $[a, b]$ indicates the searching space, and the chaotic function was produced by mapping chaotic parameters ρ_i into the chaotic vector P_i. Furthermore, chaotic vector P_i was linearly integrated with targeted position TP for generating candidate location CL, which is expressed as follows.

$$CL = (1 - SC) \times TP + SC \times P_i \tag{19}$$

$$SC = (T - t + 1)/T \tag{20}$$

The CSSA approach resolves an FF for obtaining higher classification performances. It defines a positive integer for demonstrating the optimal performance of candidate solutions. During this case, the minimized classifier error rate was regarded as FF, as offered in Equation (21).

$$fitness(x_i) = ClassifierErrorRate(x_i) = \frac{number\ of\ misclassified\ samples}{Total\ number\ of\ samples} \times 100 \tag{21}$$

4. Performance Validation

In this section, the experimental validation of the CSSADTL-BCC model is tested using a benchmark dataset [21], and the details are provided in Table 1. The CSSADTL-BCC model is simulated using the Python 3.6.5 tool. The parameter settings are provided as follows: learning rate—0.01; dropout—0.5; batch size—5; epoch count—50; activation—ReLU. A few sample images are demonstrated in Figure 3.

Table 1. Dataset details.

Category	Class Names	Labels	No. of Images	Total
Benign	Adenosis	A	106	588
	Fibroadenoma	F	237	
	Phyllodes Tumor	PT	115	
	Tubular Adenoma	TA	130	
Malignant	Carcinoma	DC	788	1232
	Lobular Carcinoma	LC	137	
	Mucinous Carcinoma	MC	169	
	Papillary Carcinoma	PC	138	
	Total Number of Images			1820

Figure 4 illustrates the confusion matrices produced by the CSSADTL-BCC model under distinct epochs. With 500 epochs, the CSSADTL-BCC model has identified 65 samples in class A, 205 samples in class F, 81 samples in class PT, 84 samples in class TA, 760 samples in class DC, 93 samples in class LC, 117 samples in class MC, and 96 samples in class PC. Along with that, with 2000 epochs, the CSSADTL-BCC approach has identified 89 samples in class A, 228 samples in class F, 109 samples in class PT, 112 samples in class TA, 779 samples in class DC, 116 samples in class LC, 160 samples in class MC, and 121 samples in class PC.

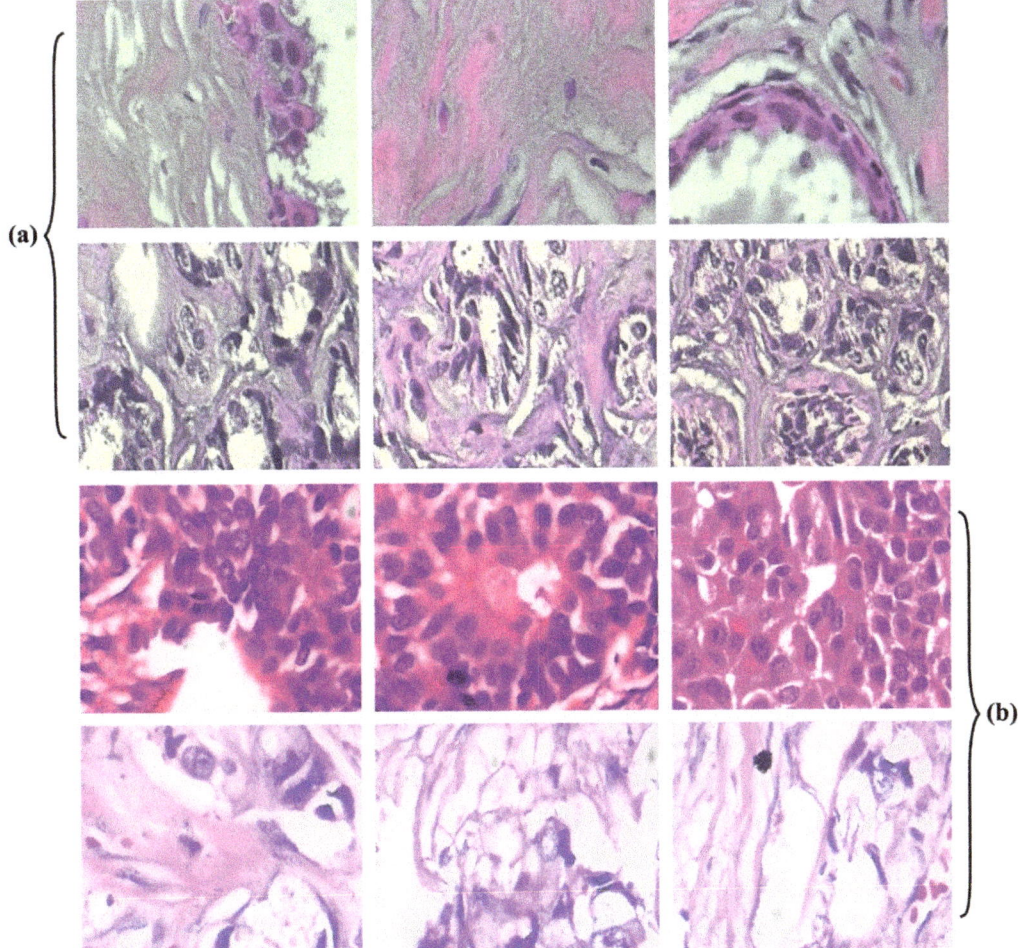

Figure 3. Sample images: (**a**) benign (**b**) malignant.

Table 2 and Figure 5 highlight the overall classification outcomes of the CSSADTL-BCC model under distinct epochs and class labels. The experimental outcomes implied that the CSSADTL-BCC model has resulted in ineffectual outcomes over other models in terms of different measures such as accuracy ($accu_y$), precision ($prec_n$), recall ($reca_l$), specificity ($spec_y$), F-score (F_{score}), MCC, and G-mean (G_{mean}). For instance, with 500 epochs, the CSSADTL-BCC model provided the averages of $accu_y$, $prec_n$, $reca_l$, $spec_y$, F_{score}, MCC, and G_{mean} at 95.62%, 78.78%, 73.25%, 97.09%, 75.71%, 73.18%, and 84.01%, respectively. Moreover, with 1000 epochs, the CSSADTL-BCC method obtained the averages of $accu_y$, $prec_n$, $reca_l$, $spec_y$, F_{score}, MCC, and G_{mean} at 97.10%, 85.21%, 82.09%, 98.16%, 83.52%, 81.84%, and 89.62%, respectively. In addition, with 1500 epochs, the CSSADTL-BCC methodology provided averages of $accu_y$, $prec_n$, $reca_l$, $spec_y$, F_{score}, MCC, and G_{mean} at 98.61%, 92.80%, 91.48%, 99.14%, 92.10%, 91.29%, and 95.19%, respectively. At last, with 2000 epochs, the CSSADTL-BCC technique obtained the averages of $accu_y$, $prec_n$, $reca_l$, $spec_y$, F_{score}, MCC, and G_{mean} at 98.54%, 92.58%, 90.87%, 99.08%, 91.66%, 90.82%, and 94.84%, respectively.

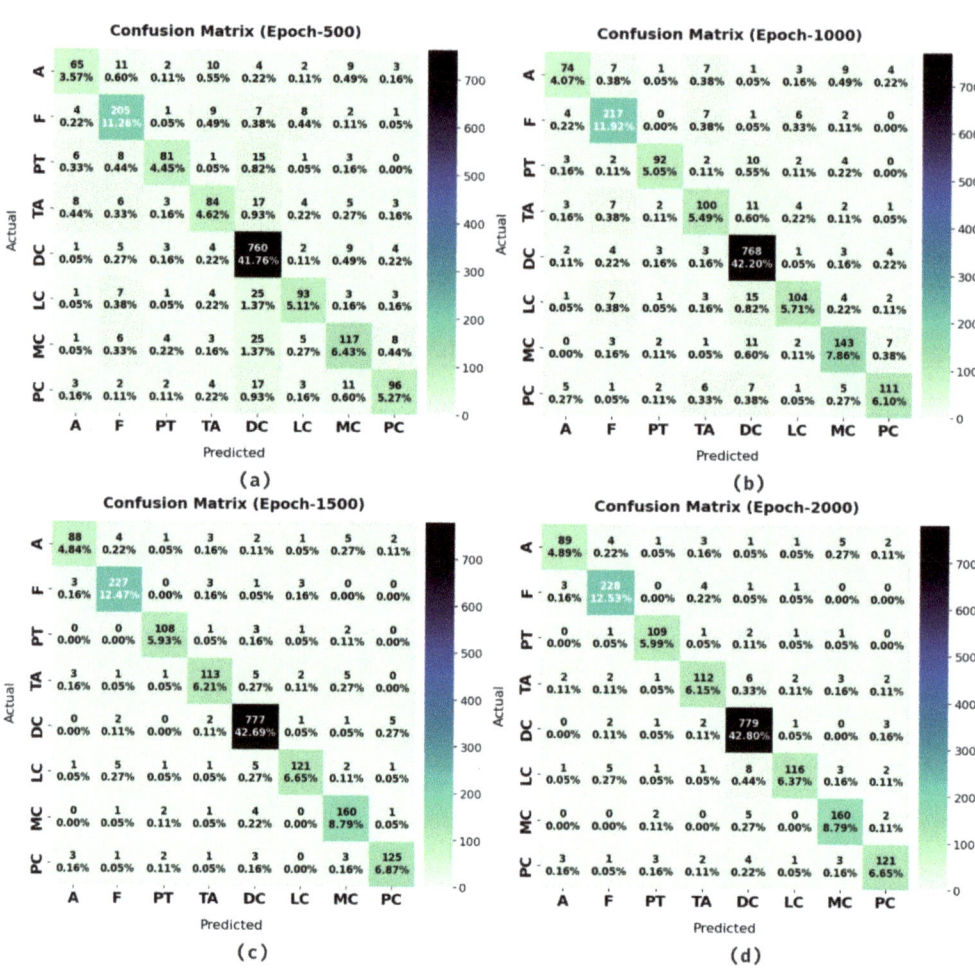

Figure 4. Confusion matrix of CSSADTL-BCC technique under various epochs: (**a**) 500 epochs, (**b**) 1000 epochs, (**c**) 1500 epochs, and (**d**) 2000 epochs.

Table 2. Result analysis of CSSADTL-BCC technique with various measures and epochs.

Class Labels	Accuracy	Precision	Recall	Specificity	F-Score	MCC	G-Mean
				Epoch-500			
A	96.43	73.03	61.32	98.60	66.67	65.07	77.76
F	95.77	82.00	86.50	97.16	84.19	81.79	91.67
PT	97.25	83.51	70.43	99.06	76.42	75.27	83.53
TA	95.55	70.59	64.62	97.93	67.47	65.16	79.55
DC	92.42	87.36	96.45	89.34	91.68	85.10	92.83
LC	96.21	78.81	67.88	98.51	72.94	71.14	81.78
MC	94.84	73.58	69.23	97.46	71.34	68.54	82.14
PC	96.48	81.36	69.57	98.69	75.00	73.38	82.86
Average	95.62	78.78	73.25	97.09	75.71	73.18	84.01

Table 2. *Cont.*

Class Labels	Accuracy	Precision	Recall	Specificity	F-Score	MCC	G-Mean
				Epoch-1000			
A	97.25	80.43	69.81	98.95	74.75	73.51	83.11
F	97.20	87.50	91.56	98.04	89.48	87.90	94.75
PT	98.13	89.32	80.00	99.35	84.40	83.56	89.15
TA	96.76	77.52	76.92	98.28	77.22	75.48	86.95
DC	95.82	93.20	97.46	94.57	95.29	91.61	96.01
LC	97.14	84.55	75.91	98.87	80.00	78.60	86.63
MC	96.98	83.14	84.62	98.24	83.87	82.21	91.18
PC	97.53	86.05	80.43	98.93	83.15	81.87	89.20
Average	97.10	85.21	82.09	98.16	83.52	81.84	89.62
				Epoch-1500			
A	98.46	89.80	83.02	99.42	86.27	85.53	90.85
F	98.68	94.19	95.78	99.12	94.98	94.22	97.43
PT	99.23	93.91	93.91	99.59	93.91	93.50	96.71
TA	98.41	90.40	86.92	99.29	88.63	87.79	92.90
DC	98.13	97.12	98.60	97.77	97.86	96.21	98.19
LC	98.68	93.80	88.32	99.52	90.98	90.31	93.76
MC	98.52	89.89	94.67	98.91	92.22	91.44	96.77
PC	98.79	93.28	90.58	99.46	91.91	91.27	94.92
Average	98.61	92.80	91.48	99.14	92.10	91.29	95.19
				Epoch-2000			
A	98.57	90.82	83.96	99.47	87.25	86.57	91.39
F	98.68	93.83	96.20	99.05	95.00	94.25	97.62
PT	99.18	92.37	94.78	99.47	93.56	93.13	97.10
TA	98.30	89.60	86.15	99.23	87.84	86.95	92.46
DC	98.02	96.65	98.86	97.38	97.74	96.00	98.12
LC	98.46	94.31	84.67	99.58	89.23	88.55	91.83
MC	98.68	91.43	94.67	99.09	93.02	92.31	96.86
PC	98.46	91.67	87.68	99.35	89.63	88.82	93.33
Average	98.54	92.58	90.87	99.08	91.66	90.82	94.84

The training accuracy (TA) and validation accuracy (VA) attained by the CSSADTL-BCC model on test dataset are demonstrated in Figure 6. The experimental outcomes implied that the CSSADTL-BCC model has gained maximum values of TA and VA. In particular, VA appeared to be higher than TA.

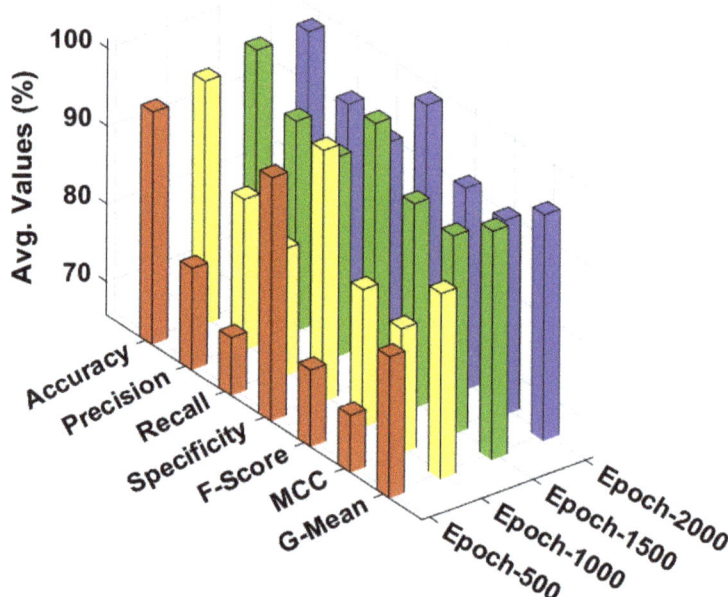

Figure 5. Result analysis of CSSADTL-BCC technique with distinct epochs.

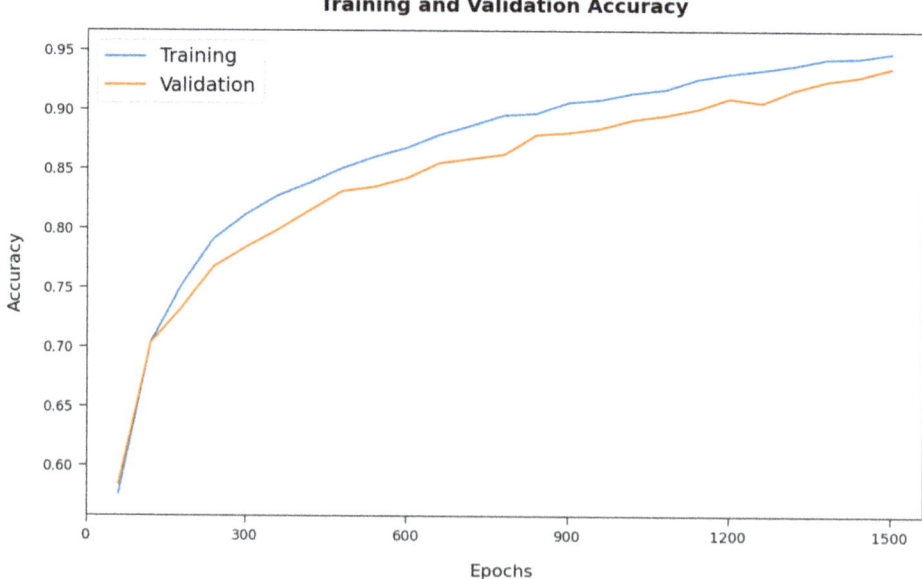

Figure 6. TA and VA analysis of CSSADTL-BCC technique.

The training loss (TL) and validation loss (VL) achieved by the CSSADTL-BCC method on test dataset are established in Figure 7. The experimental outcome inferred that the CSSADTL-BCC model obtained the lowest values of TL and VL. In particular, VL seemed to be lower than TL. Next, a brief precision–recall examination performed on the CSSADTL-

BCC method on the test dataset is displayed in Figure 8. By observing the figure, it can be observed that the CSSADTL-BCC approach has established maximal precision–recall performance under all classes.

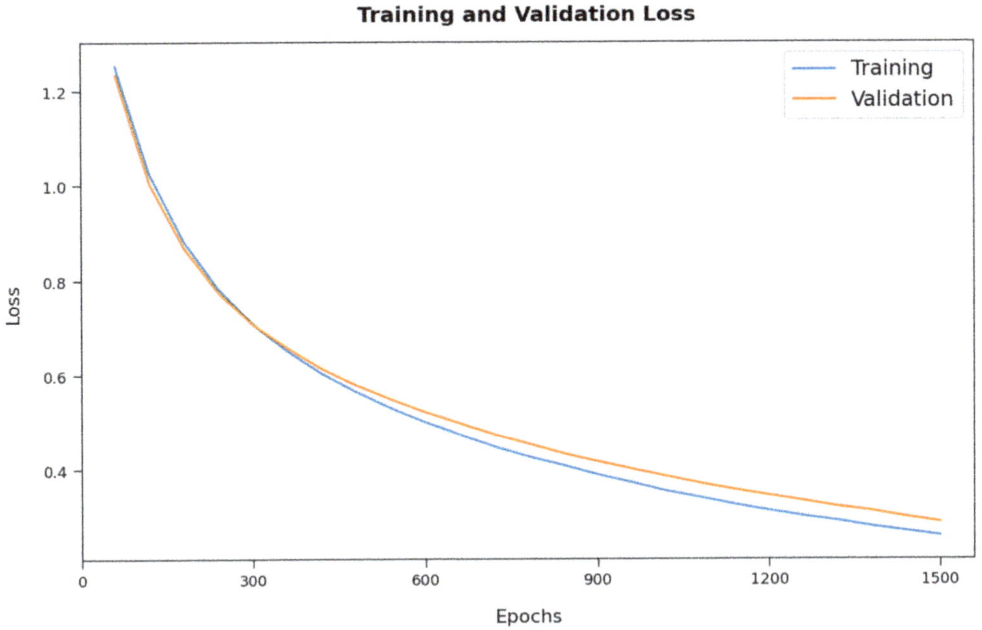

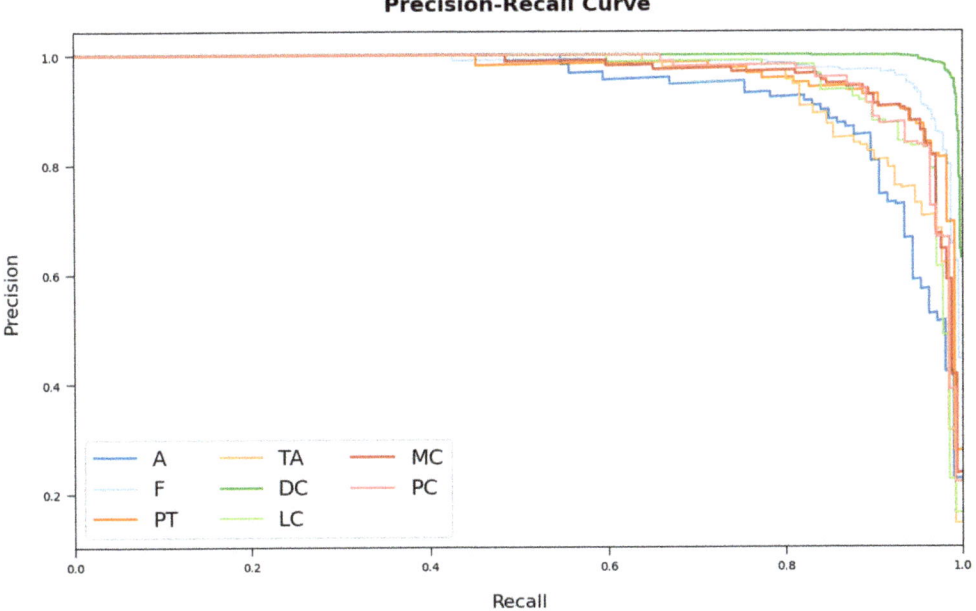

Figure 7. TL and VL analysis of CSSADTL-BCC technique.

Figure 8. Precision–recall curve analysis of CSSADTL-BCC technique.

Figure 9 portrays a clear ROC investigation of the CSSADTL-BCC model on the test dataset. The figure portrayed that the CSSADTL-BCC model has resulted in proficient results with maximum ROC values under distinct class labels.

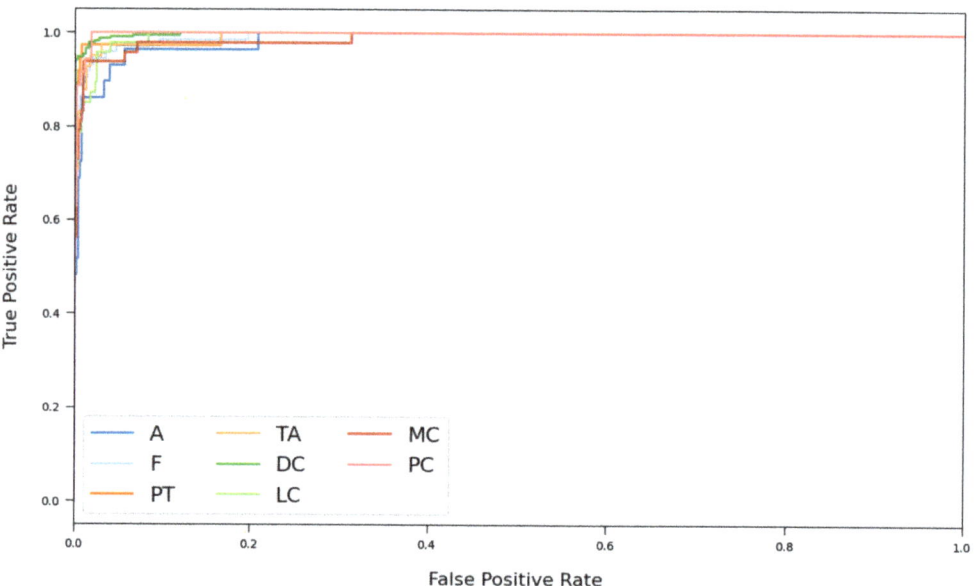

Figure 9. ROC curve analysis of the CSSADTL-BCC technique.

Figure 10 reports detailed classification accuracy outcomes of the CSSADTL-BCC model under distinct iterations and runs. The figures highlighted that CSSADTL-BCC has showcased effectual classifier results under every epoch.

To highlight the enhanced outcomes of the CSSADTL-BCC model, a brief comparison study with recent models is shown in Table 3 [22]. Figure 11 investigates a detailed $accu_y$ and F_{score} analysis of the CSSADTL-BCC with existing models. The results indicated that GLCM-KNN and GLCM-NB models obtained lower values of $accu_y$ and F_{score}. At the same time, the GLCM-discrete transform, GLCM-SVM, and Deep learning-IRV2 models have attained moderately closer values of $accu_y$ and F_{score}. Next to that, the GLCM-DL and Deep learning INV3 models have resulted in reasonable $accu_y$ and F_{score} values. However, the CSSADTL-BCC model has gained an effectual outcome with maximum $accu_y$ and F_{score} at 98.61% and 92.80%, respectively.

Figure 12 examines a detailed $prec_n$ and $reca_l$ examination of CSSADTL-BCC with existing techniques. The outcomes represented that the GLCM-KNN and GLCM-NB approaches have gained lesser values of $prec_n$ and $reca_l$. Moreover, the GLCM-discrete transform, GLCM-SVM, and Deep learning-IRV2 algorithms have attained moderately closer values of $prec_n$ and $reca_l$. Along with that, the GLCM-DL and Deep learning INV3 approaches have resulted in reasonable $prec_n$ and $reca_l$ values. However, the CSSADTL-BCC technique has gained effectual outcomes with maximum values of $prec_n$ and $reca_l$ at 92.80% and 91.48%, respectively. After observing the results and discussion, it is apparent that the CSSADTL-BCC model has showcased enhanced outcomes over other methods. The enhanced performance of the CSSADTL-BCC model is due to the effectual hyperparameter tuning process of the SGRU classifier. Thus, the proposed model can be applied to assist physicians in the disease diagnosis process.

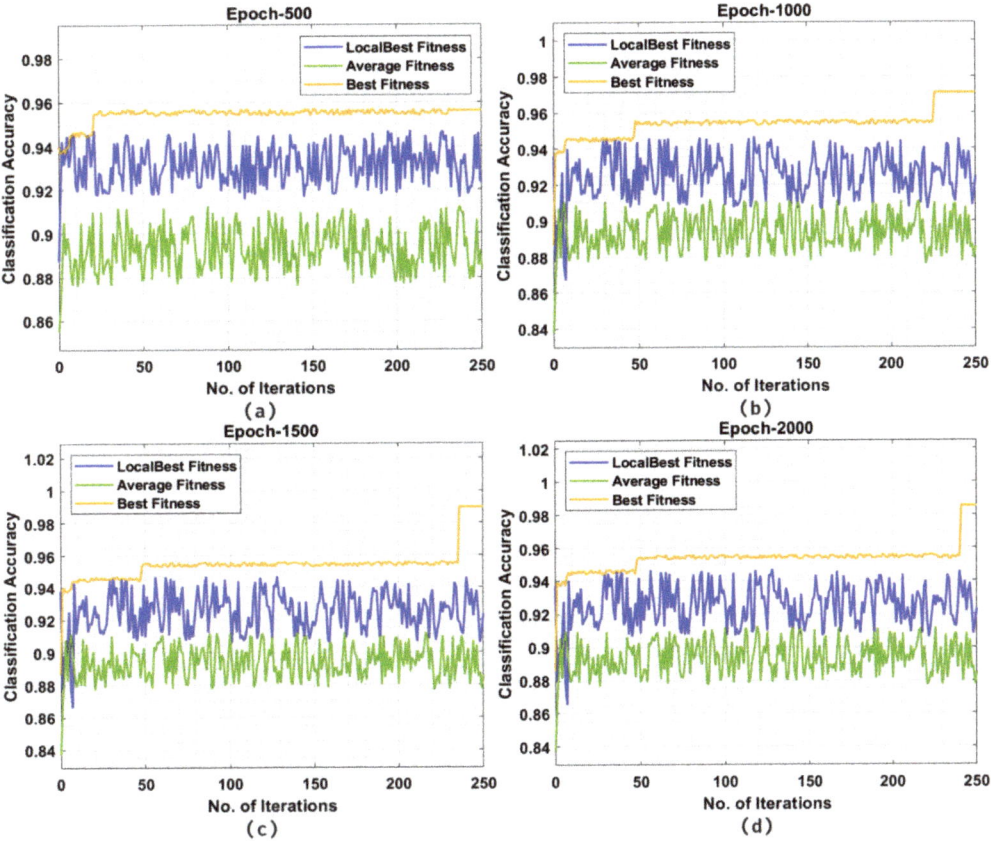

Figure 10. Classification accuracy of CSSADTL-BCC technique under distinct iterations: (**a**) 500 epochs, (**b**) 1000 epochs, (**c**) 1500 epochs, and (**d**) 2000 epochs.

Table 3. Comparative analysis of the CSSADTL-BCC technique with existing algorithms.

Methods	Accuracy	Precision	Recall	F-Score
GLCM-KNN Model	76.17	62.40	83.60	82.22
GLCM-NB Model	78.45	82.16	83.45	86.97
GLCM-Discrete transform	85.00	83.56	81.66	84.69
GLCM-SVM Model	85.00	87.32	87.61	81.62
GLCM-DL Model	92.44	86.89	80.24	87.92
Deep Learning-INV3	94.71	87.57	87.07	81.86
Deep Learning-IRV2	88.12	81.70	81.44	86.42
CSSADTL-BCC	98.61	92.80	91.48	92.10

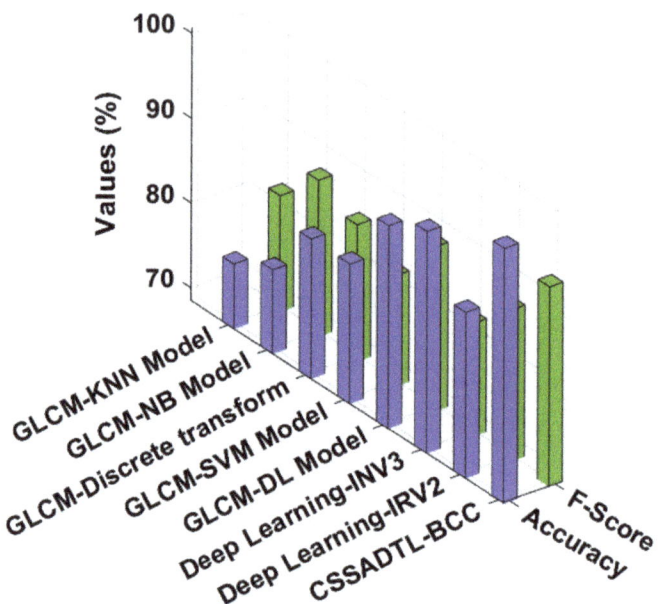

Figure 11. $Accu_y$ and F_{score} analysis of CSSADTL-BCC technique with existing algorithms.

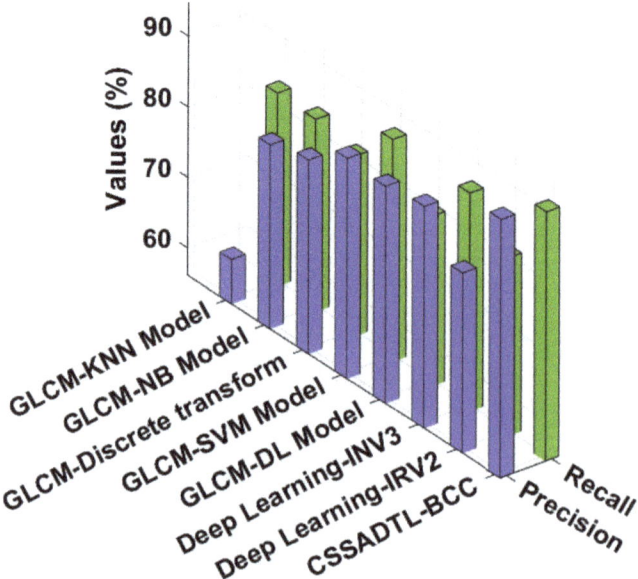

Figure 12. $Reca_l$ and $Prec_n$ analysis of the CSSADTL-BCC technique with existing algorithms.

5. Conclusions

In this study, a new CSSADTL-BCC method was advanced for classifying BC on histopathological images. The presented CSSADTL-BCC model mainly focused on the recognition and classification of BC. At the primary stage, the CSSADTL-BCC model employed the GF technique to eradicate the occurrence of noise. Moreover, a MixNet-based feature extraction model was employed for producing a useful collection of feature vectors. Then, the SGRU classifier was exploited to allot class labels. Furthermore, CSSA is applied to optimally modify the hyperparameters involved in the MixNet model. The performance validation of the CSSADTL-BCC model can be tested by using a benchmark dataset, and the results reported the superior efficiency of the CSSADTL-BCC method over the current existing approaches with a maximum accuracy of 98.61%. In the future, deep instance segmentation approaches can be included to enhance classification performance. In addition, the classifier's results can be boosted by designing deep fusion-based ensemble models.

Author Contributions: Conceptualization, K.S.; methodology, K.S., A.K.D.; software, S.K.; validation, S.K., I.C.D.; formal analysis, K.S.; investigation, I.C.D.; resources, G.P.J.; data curation, A.K.D.; writing—original draft preparation, K.S.; writing—review and editing, G.P.J.; visualization, S.K.; supervision, I.C.D.; project administration, I.C.D. funding acquisition, G.P.J., I.C.D. All authors have read and agreed to the published version of the manuscript.

Funding: This work was supported by Hankuk University of Foreign Studies Research Fund (of 2022) and the Ministry of Science and Higher Education of the Russian Federation (Government Order FENU-2020-0022).

Institutional Review Board Statement: Not applicable.

Informed Consent Statement: Not applicable.

Data Availability Statement: Data sharing not applicable to this article as no datasets were generated during the current study.

Conflicts of Interest: The authors declare no conflict of interest.

References

1. Das, A.; Nair, M.S.; Peter, S.D. Computer-aided histopathological image analysis techniques for automated nuclear atypia scoring of breast cancer: A review. *J. Digit. Imaging* **2020**, *33*, 1091–1121. [CrossRef] [PubMed]
2. Krithiga, R.; Geetha, P. Breast cancer detection, segmentation and classification on histopathology images analysis: A systematic review. *Arch. Comput. Methods Eng.* **2021**, *28*, 2607–2619. [CrossRef]
3. Carvalho, E.D.; Antonio Filho, O.C.; Silva, R.R.; Araujo, F.H.; Diniz, J.O.; Silva, A.C.; Paiva, A.C.; Gattass, M. Breast cancer diagnosis from histopathological images using textural features and CBIR. *Artif. Intell. Med.* **2020**, *105*, 101845. [CrossRef] [PubMed]
4. Xie, J.; Liu, R.; Luttrell, J., IV; Zhang, C. Deep learning based analysis of histopathological images of breast cancer. *Front. Genet.* **2019**, *10*, 80. [CrossRef]
5. Kaushal, C.; Bhat, S.; Koundal, D.; Singla, A. Recent trends in computer assisted diagnosis (CAD) systems for breast cancer diagnosis using histopathological images. *IRBM* **2019**, *40*, 211–227. [CrossRef]
6. Yan, R.; Ren, F.; Wang, Z.; Wang, L.; Zhang, T.; Liu, Y.; Rao, X.; Zheng, C.; Zhang, F. Breast cancer histopathological image classification using a hybrid deep neural network. *Methods* **2020**, *173*, 52–60. [CrossRef]
7. Mehra, R. Breast cancer histology images classification: Training from scratch or transfer learning? *ICT Express* **2018**, *4*, 247–254.
8. Alkassar, S.; Jebur, B.A.; Abdullah, M.A.; Al-Khalidy, J.H.; Chambers, J.A. Going deeper: Magnification-invariant approach for breast cancer classification using histopathological images. *IET Comput. Vis.* **2021**, *15*, 151–164. [CrossRef]
9. Sohail, A.; Khan, A.; Wahab, N.; Zameer, A.; Khan, S. A multi-phase deep CNN based mitosis detection framework for breast cancer histopathological images. *Sci. Rep.* **2021**, *11*, 6215. [CrossRef]
10. Ahmad, N.; Asghar, S.; Gillani, S.A. Transfer learning-assisted multi-resolution breast cancer histopathological images classification. *Vis. Comput.* **2021**, 1–20. [CrossRef]
11. Rai, R.; Sisodia, D.S. Real-time data augmentation based transfer learning model for breast cancer diagnosis using histopathological images. In *Advances in Biomedical Engineering and Technology*; Springer: Singapore, 2021; pp. 473–488.
12. Alom, M.Z.; Yakopcic, C.; Nasrin, M.; Taha, T.M.; Asari, V.K. Breast cancer classification from histopathological images with inception recurrent residual convolutional neural network. *J. Digit. Imaging* **2019**, *32*, 605–617. [CrossRef] [PubMed]
13. Vo, D.M.; Nguyen, N.Q.; Lee, S.W. Classification of breast cancer histology images using incremental boosting convolution networks. *Inf. Sci.* **2019**, *482*, 123–138. [CrossRef]
14. Wang, P.; Wang, J.; Li, Y.; Li, P.; Li, L.; Jiang, M. Automatic classification of breast cancer histopathological images based on deep feature fusion and enhanced routing. *Biomed. Signal Process. Control.* **2021**, *65*, 102341. [CrossRef]
15. Hirra, I.; Ahmad, M.; Hussain, A.; Ashraf, M.U.; Saeed, I.A.; Qadri, S.F.; Alghamdi, A.M.; Alfakeeh, A.S. Breast cancer classification from histopathological images using patch-based deep learning modeling. *IEEE Access* **2021**, *9*, 24273–24287. [CrossRef]
16. Demir, F. DeepBreastNet: A novel and robust approach for automated breast cancer detection from histopathological images. *Biocybern. Biomed. Eng.* **2021**, *41*, 1123–1139. [CrossRef]

17. Saxena, S.; Shukla, S.; Gyanchandani, M. Breast cancer histopathology image classification using kernelized weighted extreme learning machine. *Int. J. Imaging Syst. Technol.* **2021**, *31*, 168–179. [CrossRef]
18. Wang, Y.; Yan, J.; Yang, Z.; Zhao, Y.; Liu, T. Optimizing GIS partial discharge pattern recognition in the ubiquitous power internet of things context: A MixNet deep learning model. *Int. J. Electr. Power Energy Syst.* **2021**, *125*, 106484. [CrossRef]
19. Al Wazrah, A.; Alhumoud, S. Sentiment Analysis Using Stacked Gated Recurrent Unit for Arabic Tweets. *IEEE Access* **2021**, *9*, 137176–137187. [CrossRef]
20. Yuan, J.; Zhao, Z.; Liu, Y.; He, B.; Wang, L.; Xie, B.; Gao, Y. DMPPT control of photovoltaic microgrid based on improved sparrow search algorithm. *IEEE Access* **2021**, *9*, 16623–16629. [CrossRef]
21. Spanhol, F.; Oliveira, L.S.; Petitjean, C.; Heutte, L. A Dataset for Breast Cancer Histopathological Image Classification. *IEEE Trans. Biomed. Eng. (TBME)* **2016**, *63*, 1455–1462. [CrossRef]
22. Reshma, V.K.; Arya, N.; Ahmad, S.S.; Wattar, I.; Mekala, S.; Joshi, S.; Krah, D. Detection of Breast Cancer Using Histopathological Image Classification Dataset with Deep Learning Techniques. *BioMed Res. Int.* **2022**. [CrossRef] [PubMed]

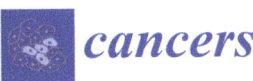

Article

Lightweight Deep Learning Model for Assessment of Substitution Voicing and Speech after Laryngeal Carcinoma Surgery

Rytis Maskeliūnas [1], Audrius Kulikajevas [1], Robertas Damaševičius [1,*], Kipras Pribuišis [2], Nora Ulozaitė-Stanienė [2] and Virgilijus Uloza [2]

[1] Faculty of Informatics, Kaunas University of Technology, 51368 Kaunas, Lithuania; rytis.maskeliunas@ktu.lt (R.M.); audrius.kulikajevas@ktu.edu (A.K.)
[2] Department of Otorhinolaryngology, Lithuanian University of Health Sciences, 50061 Kaunas, Lithuania; Kipras.pribuisis@lsmuni.lt (K.P.); Nora.ulozaite@lsmuni.lt (N.U.-S.); Virgilijus.ulozas@lsmuni.lt (V.U.)
* Correspondence: robertas.damasevicius@ktu.lt

Simple Summary: A total laryngectomy involves the full and permanent separation of the upper and lower airways, resulting in the loss of voice and inability to interact vocally. To identify, extract, and evaluate replacement voicing following laryngeal oncosurgery, we propose employing convolutional neural networks for categorization of speech representations (spectrograms). With an overall accuracy of 89.47 percent, our technique has the greatest true-positive rate of any of the tested state-of-the-art methodologies.

Abstract: Laryngeal carcinoma is the most common malignant tumor of the upper respiratory tract. Total laryngectomy provides complete and permanent detachment of the upper and lower airways that causes the loss of voice, leading to a patient's inability to verbally communicate in the postoperative period. This paper aims to exploit modern areas of deep learning research to objectively classify, extract and measure the substitution voicing after laryngeal oncosurgery from the audio signal. We propose using well-known convolutional neural networks (CNNs) applied for image classification for the analysis of voice audio signal. Our approach takes an input of Mel-frequency spectrogram (MFCC) as an input of deep neural network architecture. A database of digital speech recordings of 367 male subjects (279 normal speech samples and 88 pathological speech samples) was used. Our approach has shown the best true-positive rate of any of the compared state-of-the-art approaches, achieving an overall accuracy of 89.47%.

Keywords: laryngeal carcinoma; substitution voicing; voice analysis; convolutional neural networks; deep learning

1. Introduction

Laryngeal carcinoma remains the most common malignant tumor of the upper respiratory tract worldwide as reported by Steuer et al. [1]. Literature reports an incidence of around 5 cases per 100,000 inhabitants but National Cancer Institute's Cancer registry reported 18.3 cases per 100,000 Lithuanian citizens [2]. The most current American Cancer Society estimates for laryngeal cancer in the United States for 2022 are: estimated 12,470 new cases of laryngeal cancer, and predicted 3820 deaths from laryngeal cancer [3]. Although the overall incidence is declining, laryngeal cancer is one of the few oncological diseases in which the 5-year survival rate has decreased over the past 40 years, from 66% to 63%. This may be attributed to more conservative treatment protocols, as well as factors that might delay the patient's follow-up, mainly—the lack of medical care availability near the patient's place of residence as described by the report in Journal of Clinical Oncology [4]. Programs that require less specialized medical care and provide patients with reliable follow-up means might help to improve the 5-year survival rate, as well as, increase patient safety during the pandemics [5]. Software that reduces the need for specialized medical care might free up medical facilities for COVID-19 patients. Additionally, this software might reduce the workload of specialized medical personnel and make them available for COVID-19 related tasks. Fewer nonessential trips to outpatient facilities lead to a lower risk of infection during pandemics [6]. This can potentially be achieved without incurring additional costs to the healthcare system.

Chemoradiotherapy and surgery are usually feasible treatment choices for patients with early (stage I-II) laryngeal cancer. The extent of surgery is primarily determined by the tumor's spread. Depending on the tumor stage, surgical treatment results in locoregional cancer control comparable to that provided by laryngeal radiation or chemoradiation therapy or even higher survival rates, cancer can be achieved for patients who undergo surgical treatment for advanced-stage laryngeal [1].

After laryngeal oncosurgery that may include extended cordectomy (removal of the vocal fold), partial or total laryngectomy patients lose one or even both vocal folds. As a consequence, the voice is generated by a single vocal fold oscillating with the remaining laryngeal and pharyngeal structures or alaryngeal (oesophageal or tracheoesophageal) speech is used. These conditions can be considered as substitution voicing (SV), which is defined as the voicing without two true vocal folds [7]. In SV, involuntary aphonic (unvoiced) segments of speech coexist with rough-voiced ones. Various degrees of speech impairment or even a complete inability to speak after laryngeal oncosurgery are the most important complaints expressed by patients and may lead to their social isolation [8].

During the current pandemic, a lot of specialized medical care facilities and personnel have been dedicated to fighting COVID-19 [9]. This in turn led to delayed diagnostics for primary laryngeal cancer patients and follow-up for patients after treatment [10]. This resulted in the need of more radical cancer treatments and increased patient mortality which otherwise could have been avoided. More than half of laryngeal cancer patients present with stage III or higher at the first appointment. For patients with those stages, total laryngectomy is usually advised for favorable locoregional cancer control and an optimal 5-year survival rate [11]. Total laryngectomy is also performed when the patient is not eligible for conservative techniques like chemotherapy and radiotherapy or in case of their failure. Total laryngectomy provides complete and permanent detachment of the upper and lower airways. This separation causes the loss of voice, smell, xerostomia, and altered taste. Total laryngectomy leads to a patient's inability to verbally communicate in the postoperative period. Patients after laryngectomy often have to rely on pen and paper or other forms of written text to communicate anywhere from 2 weeks to 6 months after the initial surgery. This is especially troubling during the COVID -19 pandemic when patients have to rely on text messaging to contact their families and have trouble receiving basic social or telemedicine care simply because they can not use the phone by themselves [12].

According to Pereira da Silva et al., loss of voice has a significant influence on the quality of life of laryngeal cancer patients [13]. It has an impact on their communication, social life, and even their ability to keep a job. Furthermore, failure to communicate effectively generates worry, and 40–57% of these people develop a serious depressive condition [14]. As a result, it is critical to give trustworthy voice and speech rehabilitation choices to laryngectomized patients. Because of its ease of use, high success rate in generating speech, and quick training period, vocal prosthesis has become a popular way of rehabilitation [15]. Although effective, all established speech restoration techniques provide patients with distinctly distorted speech patterns, which are perceived as unhealthy by both the patient and society. This is due to the fact that substitution voicing generated speech features high irregularity, frequency shifts, and aperiodicity, together with frequent speech phonatory breaks [16]. This problem often becomes more apparent when the patient has to speak in a loud environment or over the phone [17]. Practitioners often rely on expert opinion on the perceived voice quality measurements, classification, and diagnosis of voice pathology. The problem is that often the procedure is time consuming and can be subject to parameter sensitivity [18]. Latest digitization trends have pushed towards a major improvement in computer-assisted medical techniques. Thus, following established practice, the acoustic prosodic properties of the speech signal have to be modulated by a variety of health-related effects [19], leading to changes in a human voice and the automated detection of pathologies using machine learning has attracted significant medical attention [20].

Many approaches for detecting voice pathology have been proposed in recent research in the above-mentioned literature [21]. However, these systems only attempted to distinguish normal voices from diseased sounds, indicating that there is a research gap in terms of voice illness detection in relation to laryngeal cancer. There are circumstances in machine learning algorithms when speech signals cannot ensure high accuracy and cause time consumption in pathology monitoring systems. As a result, there is an urgent need for a research that highlights the most essential concerns and challenges confronting vocal pathology systems, as well as the importance of illness identification in voice pathology. To our knowledge, not much data on the application of artificial intelligence (AI) technologies for SV assessment exists in the literature (see Section 2). As a result, implementing AI-based models for objective assessment and classification of SV could potentially open up new avenues in research and clinical practice, paving the way for the development of a useful and reliable tool for evaluating SV following laryngeal oncosurgery. Existing deep learning voice analysis approaches generally tend to apply some form of recurrent gates for temporal voice signal analysis, these methods tend to suffer from poor performance and are notoriously difficult to train. It is noticeable, that there is no working AI prototype for SV assessment. As a result, using an AI-based models to objectively assess and classify SV could possibly open up new avenues for study and clinical use. To begin with, a well-designed algorithm might standardize SV evaluation across numerous oncology canters, allowing data sets in different patient groups to be simply compared. The same data sets could be used to improve the algorithm in the future. Instead of the existing methods, but not very efficient already applied methods, requiring prior medical knowledge for signal analysis, we aim to exploit modern areas of machine learning (deep learning) research to extract, measure and objectively classify substitution voicing and speech after laryngeal oncosurgery from the audio signal. The objective estimates obtained can be simplified and used by general practitioners and patients. This would be especially valuable when movement is limited or specialized medical centers are difficult to find, as it was during the peak of the COVID-19 pandemic. Last but not least, AI saves time and does not retire—the knowledge gained via its use is always available and does not expire.

In this paper, we propose using convolutional neural networks (CNNs), generally applied for image classification for the analysis of audio signals by transforming the audio signals waveform into Mels spectrogram and using it as an input in a re-purposed lightweight image classification network. This approach allowed us to achieve the overall accuracy of 89.47% with a simpler network architecture, allowing the approach to be used on computing devices having only Central Processing Unit (CPU) but without a dedicated Graphical Processing Unit (GPU) for the classification of subjects voice pathology.

The paper is structured as follows: Section 2 discusses the state-of-the-art works. The dataset used in this study and the deep neural architecture are described in Section 3. The experimental results are presented and analyzed in Section 4. Finally, the results of this study are discussed in Section 5. The paper concludes with Section 6.

2. State of the Art Analysis

A chaotic nature of the substitution voicing signal makes evaluation of substitution voicing improper or even impossible with standard methods of acoustic voice analysis used in clinical settings. Multiparametric models for evaluating voice quality and dysphonia severity are sufficiently reliable and valid because of their correlations to auditory-perceptual evaluation and high reliability and validity in voice pathology detection [22]. Currently, two multiparametric acoustic indices based on sustained vowels and on continuous speech analysis have gained popularity in research and clinical settings to objectively estimate dysphonia: i.e., the Cepstral Spectral Index of Dysphonia (CSID) and the Acoustic Voice Quality Index (AVQI) [23,24]. Both indices may provide reasonable estimates of dysphonia severity and represent valid acoustic metrics for objectifying abnormal overall voice quality [25,26]. However, the use of these indices for assessing SV could be unreliable or technically impossible due to irregular and rather chaotic origin of SV signal. There is no data in the literature about the use of CSID for SV assessment. Only the recent study by van Sluis et al. [27] employed the AVQI to evaluate acoustic voice quality in patients who had undergone total laryngectomy. However, the authors noted that a specific AVQI cut-off value and the discriminative power of this index for SV (tracheoesophageal speech) after laryngeal oncosurgery have to be determined in future research studies. The AMPEX algorithm developed by Van Immerseel and Martens allows automatic reliable analysis of running speech, recognizing regularity patterns for pitch values <100 Hz and differentiating between noise and voicing at low frequencies [28]. Despite the feasibility of AMPEX as a tool for evaluating highly irregular speech has been supported by several studies, this algorithm has not yet gained wider clinical recognition [7,29].

Consequently, to perform automatic voice pathology classification and diagnosis, it is important to obtain reliable signal properties, which is essential for the reliability of the result. The clinical interpretation of vocal features is often conducted before the process of pathology detection [30]. Judging from the analysis of other studies, it is clear that from a technological point of view, many researchers distinguish signal processing functions such as Mel Frequency Coefficients, waveform packet transformations, others use multiple voice analysis tools for a variety of physiological and etiological reasons [31–33]. Multiple parameters are used to determine speech roughness, including height, vibration, and flicker, and other methods are often used, such as Harmonic to Noise Ratio, Normalized Noise Energy, and Smooth-to-Noise Ratio [34].

There are two types of possible features to analyze disease impact on voice/speech signal: temporal and spectral [35]. The temporal features (time-domain features) are used to extract and have an easy physical interpretation of a signal (energy, zero-crossing rate, maximum amplitude, minimum energy, time of the ending transient or Log-Attack-Time Descriptor) and are sensitive to articulation. The spectral features (frequency-based features) are obtained by converting the time-based signal into the frequency domain using the Fourier Transform. They might be more efficient for automatic classification because they are not dependent on articulation [36]. The most popular frequency descriptors are fundamental frequency, frequency components, spectral centroid, spectral flux, spectral density, irregularity of spectrum, brightness, etc. [37]. These features can be used to identify changing features in human speech, where the Mel Frequency Cepstral Coefficients are often used in human voice analysis [38]. Methodology from standard speech analysis could be adapted, i.e., using OpenSMILE features [39,40], Essential descriptors, MPEG7 descriptors, jAudio, YAAFE, Tsanas features [41], Wavelet Time Scattering features [42] and Random Forest supervised learning algorithms to detect the symptoms [43] and also to fuse information in the form of soft decisions, obtained using various audio feature sets from separate modalities [44]. In addition, Cepstral Separation Difference could be applied for quantification of speech impairment [45]. Feature extraction using signal-to-noise ratio, harmonic-to-noise ratio, glottal to noise excitation, vocal fold excitation ratio, and empirical mode decomposition excitation ratio methods with Random Forests and support vector machines for classification algorithms can also be used [46].

Alternative approaches could be adopted through Syllable-level Features, Low-Level Descriptor Features, Formant Features, Phonotactic Features with SVM classifier, features extracted using Principal Component Analysis and Linear Discriminant Analysis), SVM, Adaptive Boosting (AdaBoost), K-Nearest Neighbor (KNN) and Adaptive Resonance Theory-Kohonen Neural Network classifiers and the likes. In addition, dimensional reduction techniques such as linear discriminant analysis, principal component analysis, kernel PCA, feeder discriminant ratio, singular value decomposition, and so on are used to find suitable latent variables for classification [47]. Other researchers have taken into account the characteristics of human voice and hearing systems. Aicha et al. [48] used glottal waveform with feature selection using PCA and classification using SVM. Fontes et al. proposed a low-complexity approach using correntropy spectral density [49]. MPEG-7 features are most commonly used for indexing video and audio media and were investigated for this purpose [50]. Hossain et al. have demonstrated that the low-level functions of MPEG-7 sound are effective in diagnosing pathological voice using support vector machines [51]. Vaziri et al. distinguished between a healthy voice and a pathological voice using nonlinear dynamics performance and voice acoustic disturbances [52].

A wide variety of statistical, machine learning based, and other types of algorithms are now widely used for the detection of pathological voice based on the computed acoustic features of the input signal [53]. Pathology classification methods can be sorted into two categories [54]. The first category is "classical" methods, often based on k-nearest neighbor methods and Hilbert-Huang Transforms [55], random forests [56], support vector machines [57], Gaussian mixture models [58], latent Markov models [59], Dynamic time warping [60], discriminative paraconsistent machines [61] and so on. Often these methods are used in combination with traditional features, as illustrated by Ghulam et al., who singled out MFCC from long-term voice voice samples as characteristics and found a significant increase in accuracy in diagnosing pathological voices using the Gaussian mixture model [62]. Other researchers treated voice signals as normal vibration signals when classifying, e.g., Cordeiro et al. calculated the spectral envelope peaks of the voice signal as a function of the classification of pathological voices [63]. Alternatively, Saeedi et al. proposed a pathological voice recognition method based on wave transformation, which calculated the parameters of a wave filter bank using a genetic algorithm [64].

"Modern" side of pathology detection is often related to traditional dense neural networks [65], the more advanced CNNs [66] and very popular recurrent neural networks [67]. Deep learning, which transforms intelligent signal analysis so that algorithms can under certain conditions, theoretically might reach near-medical (expert) capabilities in a variety of voice pathology classification tasks. Chen et al. used 12 Mel frequency cepstral coefficients of each voice sample as row features for their deep learning implementation [68]. Miliaresi et al. suggest to analyze various properties of the voice signal window as low-level descriptors (LLDs) by extracting and analyzing variable-length fragments from the speech signal using the prisms of the main tone, energy, and spectrum [69] and using this data to train the deep learning models. Furthermore, a number of functional elements, such as moments, extremes, percentiles, and regression parameters, will then be applied to each LLD [70], to form a set of aggregate features for a healthy and unhealthy human voice. These statistical summaries can also be combined to form tensors for the training of AI (deep learning) algorithms, where multipath learning and learning transfer could be applied according to the multifunctional LSTM-RNN paradigm [71]. Kim et al. [72] collected features from voice samples of a vowel sound of /a:/ and computed the Mel-frequency cepstral coefficients (MFCCs) using the software package for speech analysis in phonetics (PRAAT), which were used identify between patients with laryngeal cancer and healthy controls. Depending on the features extracted, some authors suggest to an investigation of [53]. Alternatively, it is possible to try to introduce kernel-based extreme learning machines [73] and data preprocessing [74]. Or involves a combination of the k-means clustering-based feature weighting method and a complex-valued artificial neural network [75].

3. Materials and Methods

3.1. Clinical Evaluation and Equipment

All participants of the study were evaluated by clinical voice specialists performing video laryngostroboscopy (VLS) at the Department of Otorhinolaryngology of the Lithuanian University of Health Sciences (LUHS), Kaunas, Lithuania. VLS was performed using the XION EndoSTROB DX device (XION GmbH, Berlin, Germany) with a 70° rigid endoscope. VLS is routine in clinical practice and did not cause any additional discomfort or delays for the participants.

Speech recordings of the phonetically balanced Lithuanian sentence 'Turėjo senelė žilą oželį' ('The grandmother had a little grey goat') were obtained using a T-series silent room for hearing testing (T-room, CA Tegner AB, Bromma, Sweden) via a D60S Dynamic Vocal (AKG Acoustics, Vienna, Austria) microphone placed 10.0 cm from the mouth with an about 90° microphone-to-mouth angle. Speech recordings were made at a rate of 44,100 samples per second and exported as uncompressed 16-bit deep WAV audio files.

3.2. Dataset

A database of digital speech recordings of 367 male subjects (279 normal speech samples and 88 pathological speech samples) was used. Subjects' age ranged from 18 to 80 years. The control group comprised 279 healthy male volunteers (mean age 38.1 ± 12.7 years) with the voices evaluated as healthy by the clinical voice specialists. The control group (class 0) subjects had no present or preexisting speech, neurological, hearing, or laryngeal disorders and were free of common cold or upper respiratory infection at the time of speech recording. Furthermore, no pathological alterations in the larynx of the subjects of the normal voice subgroup group were found during VLS. The pathological speech subgroup consisted of 88 (64.1 ± 6.9 years) male patients who used substitution voicing (SV) after oncosurgery. This subgroup included 43 patients after extended cordectomy (class 1), 17 patients after partial vertical laryngectomy (class 2), and 28 patients after total laryngectomy who used tracheoesophageal prosthesis (TEP) (class 3). The pathological speech subgroup patients were recruited from consecutive patients who were diagnosed with the before-mentioned conditions. Speech recordings were obtained at least 6 months after the surgery to ensure a reasonable amount of time for the laryngeal tissue to heal and speech rehabilitation programs to end. A comparison cochleagrams of each class are illustrated in Figure 1. We use the cochleagrams of sound signals for time-frequency analysis and feature extraction instead of the more traditional spectrograms. The signal is initially passed via a gammatone filter, which is designed to mimic the auditory filters found in the human cochlea. The filtered signal is then divided into small windows, with the energy in each window summed and normalized to produce the cochleagram image's intensity values.

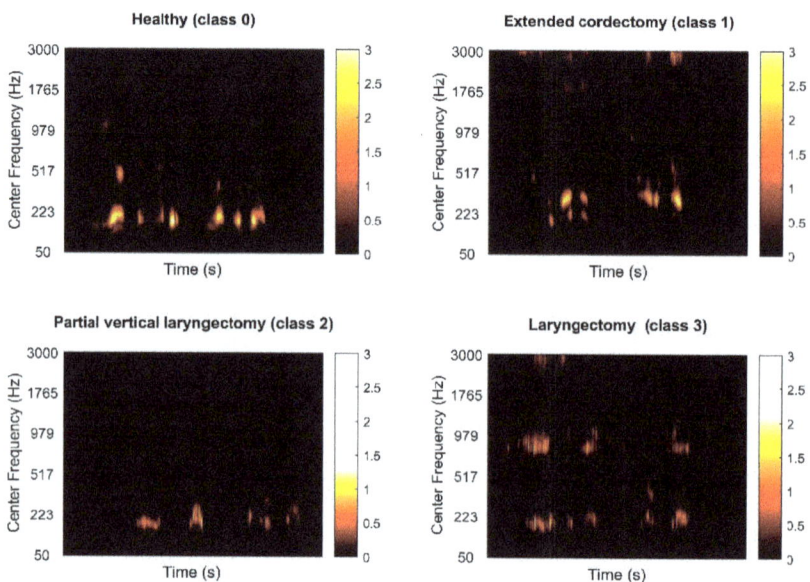

Figure 1. Cochleagrams of each class.

3.3. Data Analysis

Table 1 summarizes the voice features captured in the dataset.

Table 1. Summary of voice features.

Feature	Description
PVF	Percentage of voiced frames
PVS	Percentage of voiced speech frames
AVE	Mean voicing evidence of voiced frames
PVFU	Percentage of unreliable voiced frames
MD	Average F0 modulation
MDc	MD only in frames with a "reliable" F0 estimate. Vocal frequency estimate F0 is considered reliable if it deviates less than 25% from the average over all voiced frames.
Jitter	F0-jitter in all voiced frame pairs (=2 consecutive frames)

Figure 2 shows the histograms of database feature value distributions among classes. The analysis was supported by one-way ANOVA statistical test, which revealed statistically significant differences between classes in PVF ($p < 0.001$), PVS ($p < 0.001$), AVE ($p < 0.001$), PVFU ($p < 0.001$), MD ($p < 0.001$), MDc ($p < 0.01$), and Jitter ($p < 0.001$) values. There was no statistically significant difference in Tmax values.

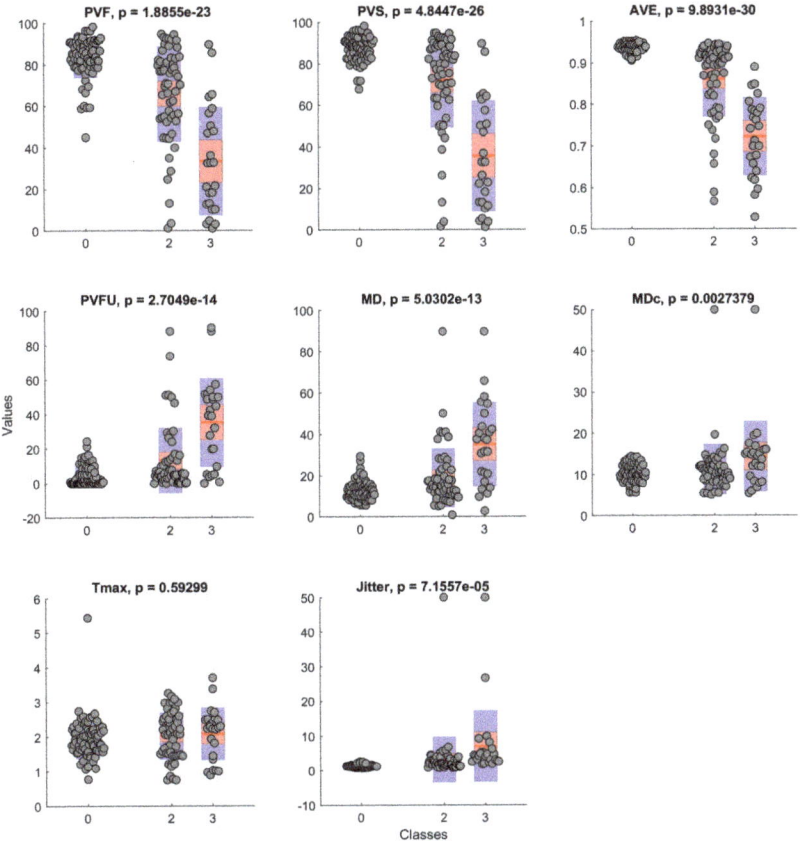

Figure 2. Histogram of feature value distribution among classes with p-value from ANOVA test.

Figure 3 shows the correlation between feature values among classes in database. The strong correlation was found between PVS and PVF ($R = 0.963, p < 0.001$), PVS and AVE ($R = 0.942, p < 0.001$), and MD and PVFU ($R = 0.898, p < 0.001$). This shows a strong co-linearity property in the database, which makes it difficult to use for training classical machine learning models [76].

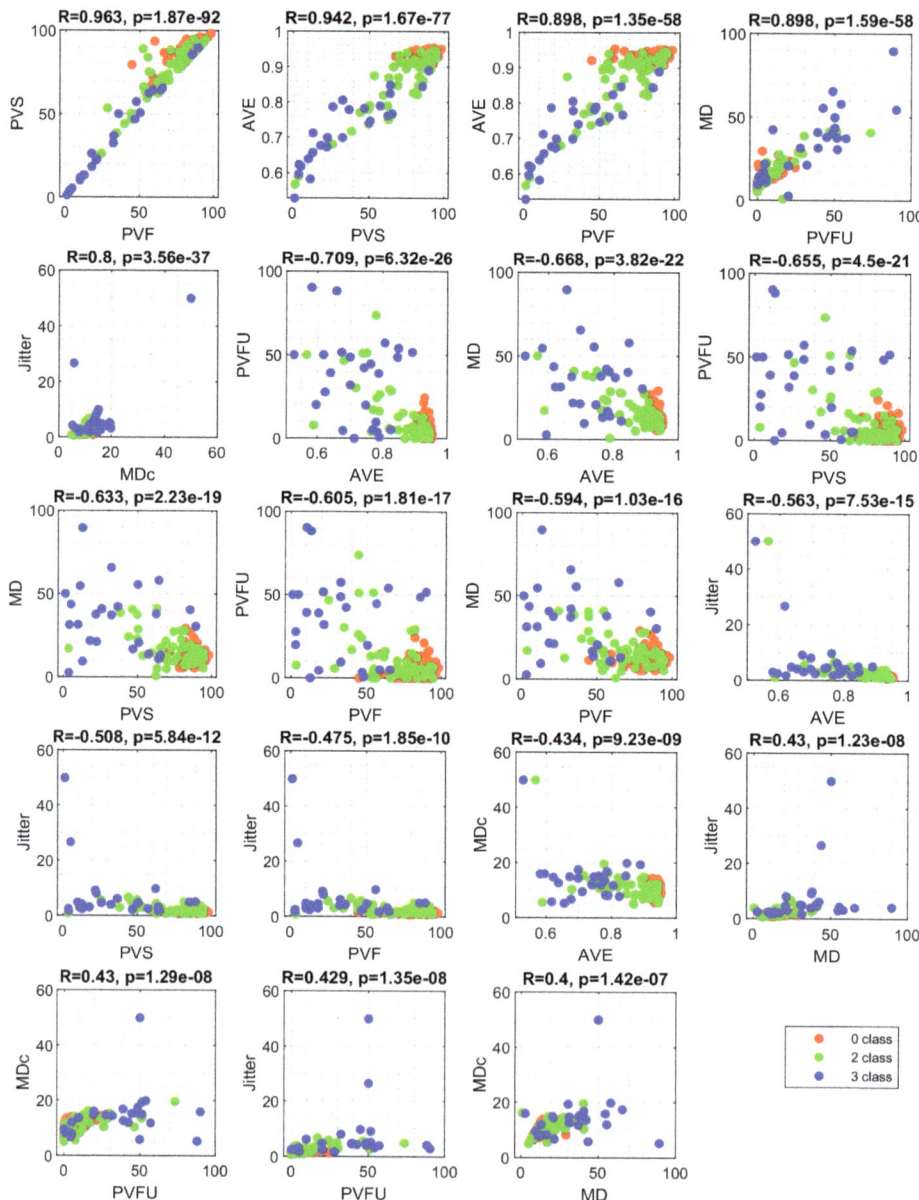

Figure 3. Correlation between feature values among classes. Correlation value (R) and its significance (p) are given. The plots are arranged by decreasing statistical significance of the determination coefficient (R^2). Only plots with significant correlations are shown.

3.4. Architecture

Figure 4 shows our approach deep neural network architecture. Our approach takes an input of Mel-frequency spectrogram (MFCC) as an input with a total of 80 coefficients. Therefore, given a waveform, the converted MFCC spectroctrogram gives an input of $N \times 80 \times 1$ where N is the sequence length. Each of the layer blocks starts with a convolutional network with stride 2, this reduces the input dimensionality by half. Layers 2, 3 and 4 internally contain skip connections (dashed lines), these allow for a better gradient flow. The fourth and final layer is then connected to fully-connected that has 4 neuron output, each of the neurons is belongs to one of four voice classes. The network is trained using initial learning rate of $lr = 10^{-4}$ with the batch size of $n = 16$, to reduce memory requirements training was performed on half-precision floating points. Because the sequence length between the audio files was not equal the each of the batch audio files have been padded with zeroes to equalize the sequence length. The network was trained for 3000 epochs using Adam optimizer [77] and cosine annealing with warm restarts every 500 epochs, which would adjust the learning rate in the range of $lr = [10^{-7}; 10^{-4}]$, cosine annealing was chosen for it has demonstrated the ability to achieve better recall rates due to potentially jumping out of local minimums [78]. The hyper-parameter values were chosen during empirical experiments. Over-fitting was avoided by employing an early stopping process and batch normalization.

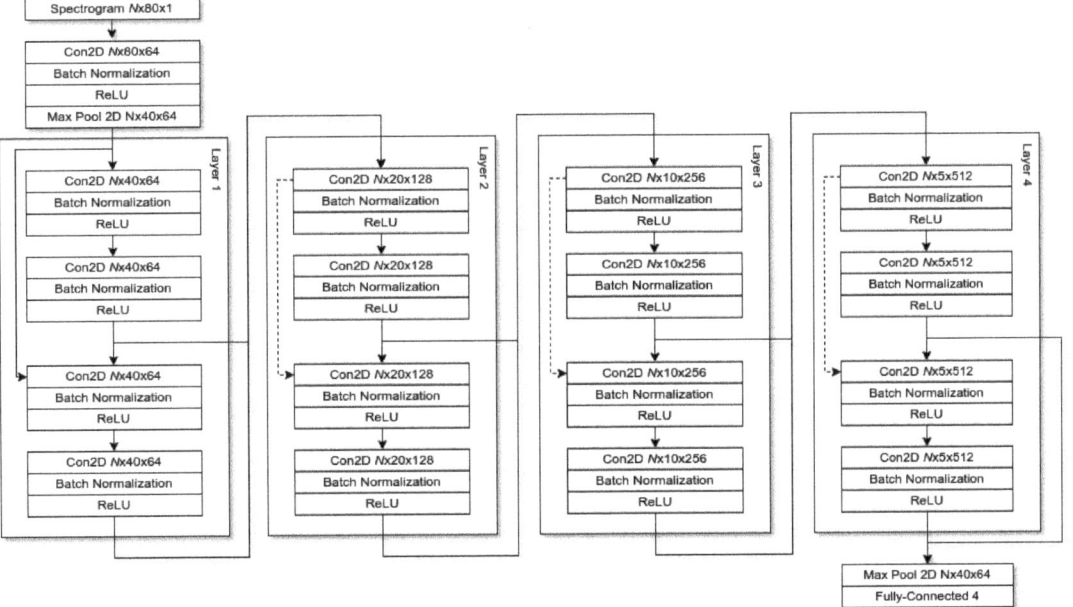

Figure 4. Our approach, here N is the sequence length, dashed lines are skip connections.

3.5. Implementation

In Figures 5–7 we can see how our approach works for evaluating subject's voice class. In order for the subject to evaluate their voice, firstly they need to make a voice recording using their microphone, the audio waveform is sampled using mono-channel 8000 Hz sampling rate (as 8 kHz still retains voice information (as stipulated by most standards, including telephony), a down-sampling (from 44 kHz to 8 kHz) was performed to optimize the required quantity of data and reduce network overhead while taking VRAM limits into account.). After the voice waveform is recorded, it is then converted into Mels-frequency diagram using 80 coefficients. Normally, this would be around 40 MFCC samples, however the system kept too little information in our situation (as substitution voicing loses a lot of information in relation to "healthy" speech), therefore 80 MFCC samples was the best determined option. The MFCC spectrogram is then used as an input in our neural network, where one of four classes are predicted: healthy, one-voice fold pathology, two-voice fold pathology, and finally nonspecific voice pathology.

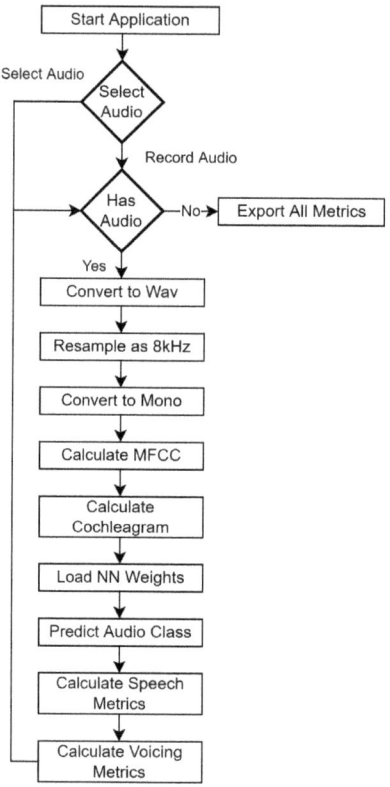

Figure 5. Architecture of the system.

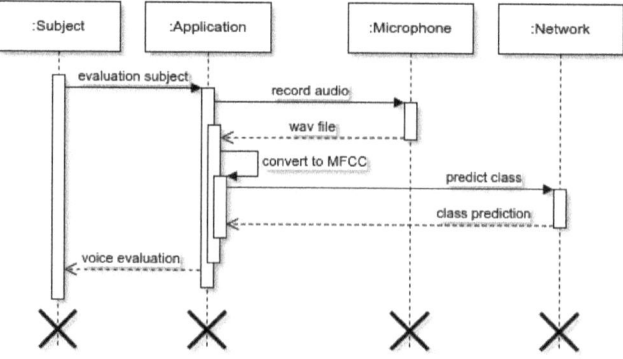

Figure 6. Voice evaluation sequence diagram.

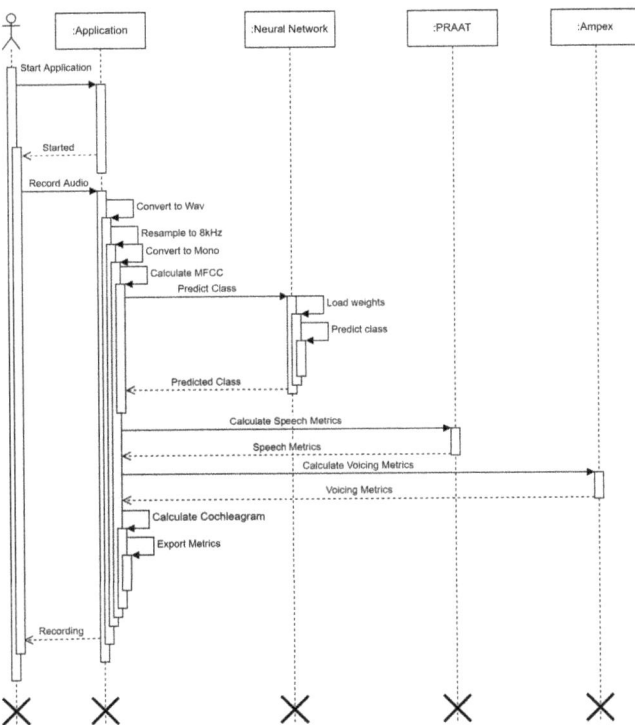

Figure 7. Composition of the voice evaluation sequence processes.

4. Experimental Evaluation and Results

4.1. Setup

To test our minimalistic CPU optimized approach, we have used augmented the dataset and used 147 recordings containing no voice pathology (normal voice), 111 voice recordings of mass lesions of one single vocal fold, 57 recordings of mass lesions in both vocal folds, and finally 67 recordings containing nonspecific voice pathology from the dataset collected in Lithuanian University of Health Sciences (see Section 3.2). The training set is divided using 80:20 rule, where 80% of the recordings of each class separately are used for training, and the remaining are used for validation. Additionally, because the dataset is highly unbalanced, we have dropped the data points in classes that have an excess of data, this allows all classes to have an identical amount of data samples, reducing the probability that the network will overfit using any of the underlying classes. To evaluate and compare our approach versus state of the art, we have used confusion matrices as they best reflect the results in multiclass problems by allowing us to evaluate true-positive versus false-positive rates.

4.2. Metrics

We used accuracy, precision, recall and F1-score as fitness measures. These are defined as follows:

$$Accuracy = \frac{TP + TN}{TP + TN + FP + FN} \times 100\% \quad (1)$$

$$Recall = \frac{TP}{TP + FN} \quad (2)$$

$$Precision = \frac{TP}{TP + FP} \quad (3)$$

$$F1 = 2 * \frac{Precision * Recall}{Precision + Recall}. \tag{4}$$

where TP (true positives) is the number of voice pathology samples that were labeled correctly, TN (true negatives) is the number of non-pathotology voice samples that were labeled correctly. FP (false positives) is the number of voice pathology samples that were labeled incorrectly as being not voice pathology samples, and FN (false negatives) is the number of not-pathology samples that were miss classified as pathology samples.

4.3. Results

In addition to our approach, we have tested three additional approaches, ResNet-101 [79], a state-of-the-art image classification network, Wav2Letter [80] and M5 [81] as state-of-the-art audio classification networks using the identical training procedure and datasets. The confusion matrices for our approach can be seen in Figure 8, for ResNet-101 can be seen in Figure 9, Wav2Letter in Figure 10, and finally M5 confusion matrix can be seen in Figure 11. Here Class 0 represents normal voice; Class 1 represents SV after cordectomy; Class 2 represents SV after partial laryngectomy; Class 3 represents SV using TEP. As we can see, our approach has shown the best true positive rate of any of the compared state-of-the-art approaches. Giving an overall accuracy of 89.47%.

	Predicted 0	Predicted 1	Predicted 2	Predicted 3
True 0	93.10%	3.45%	0.00%	3.45%
True 1	8.70%	82.61%	8.70%	0.00%
True 2	0.00%	9.09%	90.91%	0.00%
True 3	7.69%	0.00%	0.00%	92.31%

Figure 8. Confusion Matrix for our approach.

	Predicted 0	Predicted 1	Predicted 2	Predicted 3
True 0	86.21%	10.34%	0.00%	3.45%
True 1	21.74%	78.26%	0.00%	0.00%
True 2	0.00%	45.45%	54.55%	0.00%
True 3	15.38%	0.00%	0.00%	84.62%

Figure 9. Confusion Matrix for ResNet-101 model.

	Predicted 0	Predicted 1	Predicted 2	Predicted 3
True 0	34.48%	62.07%	3.45%	0.00%
True 1	8.70%	91.30%	0.00%	0.00%
True 2	9.09%	36.36%	54.55%	0.00%
True 3	0.00%	100.00%	0.00%	0.00%

Figure 10. Confusion Matrix for Wav2Letter model.

	Predicted 0	Predicted 1	Predicted 2	Predicted 3
True 0	55.17%	20.69%	0.00%	24.14%
True 1	8.70%	56.52%	8.70%	26.09%
True 2	0.00%	54.55%	45.45%	0.00%
True 3	23.08%	7.69%	0.00%	69.23%

Figure 11. Confusion Matrix for M5 model.

In Figure 12 we can see the model accuracy comparison side-by-side for each of the approaches broken down by class, additionally we can see our approach result breakdown in Table 2, as we can see, the accuracy for all of each of the individual classes is above 90%.

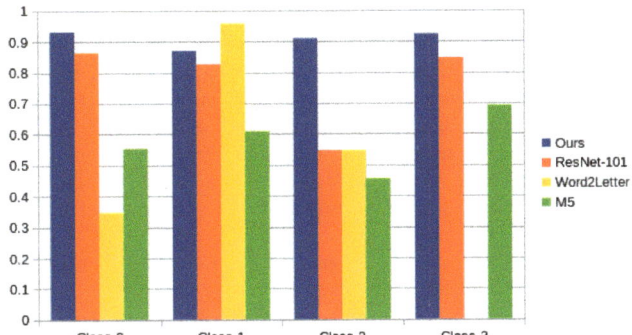

Figure 12. Comparison of performance between different models: ResNet-101, Word2Letter, M5 and our model.

Table 2. Our result approach breakdown by class.

Class	n (Truth)	n (Classified)	Accuracy	Precision	Recall	F1 Score
0—normal voice	30	29	93.42%	0.93	0.9	0.92
1—SV after cordectom	21	23	92.11%	0.83	0.9	0.86
2—SV after partial laryngectomy	12	11	96.05%	0.91	0.83	0.87
3—SV using TEP	13	13	97.37%	0.92	0.92	0.92

To analyze the predictions of models more precisely, we used t-distributed stochastic neighbor embedding (t-SNE), a statistical method for visualizing high-dimensional data by mapping it to a two-dimensional embedding. The results are presented in Figure 13. It shows that the classes are well separated while the miss-classifications using the best model (resnet18) are few.

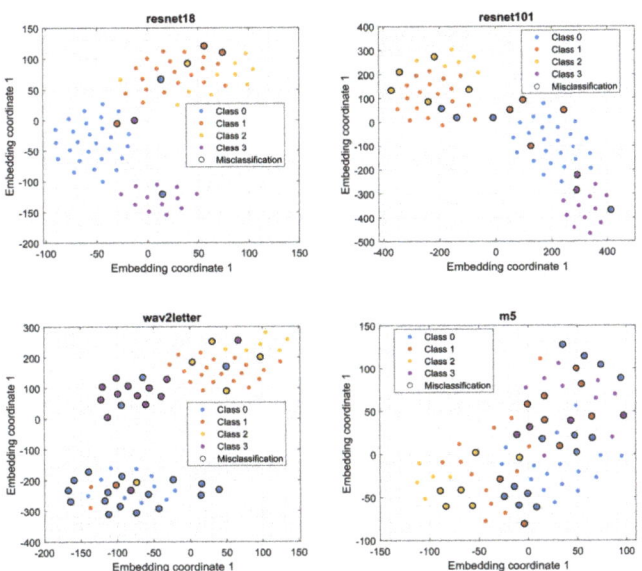

Figure 13. Comparison between t-SNE embeddings of different model predictions.

5. Discussion

This work provides a technique for automatically assessing if a voice is healthy or whether its quality has changed owing to a pathological condition. Because these spread swiftly, automatic detection is necessary, yet it is frequently underestimated. Machine learning is making a significant contribution to illness diagnosis and early detection in cardiology, pulmonology, liver tumor segmentation, and other fields of healthcare. As a consequence, machine learning might be employed effectively in a computer or mobile healthcare system to automatically identify and detect irregularities in a person's speech for early diagnosis.

For the study of speech audio signals, we propose employing well-known CNN models that have been used for image classification. Our method uses a Mel-frequency spectrogram (MFCC) as an input to a deep neural network architecture while achieving very good classification results. Our outcomes demonstrate that a deep learning model after training using a pathological speech database, voice alone might be utilized for common vocal fold illness identification using a deep learning technique. This AI-based technique might be therapeutically effective for screening general vocal fold illness using the voice. A brief assessment and a general health examination are part of the strategy. It can be used during telemedicine in places where primary care facilities do not have laryngoscopic capabilities. It might aid physicians in pre-screening patients by allowing invasive exams to be done only in situations involving issues with automatic recognition or listening, as well as expert evaluations of other clinical examination findings that raise concerns about the existence of diseases.

The biggest issue that each patient suffers, especially those who live in distant areas, is the lack of physicians and care in emergency circumstances. As a result, there is a need to provide a new framework in such remote locations by utilizing telecommunication means and artificial intelligence methods for automated voice analysis in the context of remotely-provided telehealth services [82]. Telehealth is a successful paradigm for diagnosing and treating voice issues in remote locations, as an alternative to face-to-face consultations. Telehealth consultations have been found to contribute to medical diagnosis for a variety of vocal problems, with diagnostic decision outcomes comparable to in-person consultations [83]. There are several instances in which patients require long-term monitoring. In this sense, the provision of continuous monitoring is critical. Because laryngeal cancer is a potentially fatal disease, new and effective methods for laryngeal cancer early detection are desperately needed. The method provided in this study enables an effective and noninvasive way for diagnosing laryngeal carcinoma.

6. Conclusions

In this paper we used cutting-edge deep learning research to objectively categorize, extract, and assess substitution voicing after laryngeal oncosurgery from audio signals. For the study of speech audio signals, we propose employing well-known CNNs that have been used for image classification. Our method uses a Mel-frequency spectrogram as an input to a deep neural network architecture. A database of 367 male participants' digital voice recordings (279 normal speech samples and 88 abnormal speech samples) was employed. Our method has the highest true-positive rate of any of the assessed state-of-the-art methods, with an overall accuracy of 89.47%.

Author Contributions: All authors have contributed equally to this manuscript. All authors have read and agreed to the published version of the manuscript.

Funding: This research has received funding from European Regional Development Fund (project No. 13.1.1-LMT-K-718-05-0027) under grant agreement with the Research Council of Lithuania (LMTLT). Funded as European Union's measure in response to COVID-19 pandemic.

Institutional Review Board Statement: The study was conducted in accordance with the Declaration of Helsinki, and approved by the Institutional Review Board.

Informed Consent Statement: Informed consent was obtained from all subjects involved in the study.

Data Availability Statement: The dataset used in this study is available from the corresponding author upon reasonable request.

Conflicts of Interest: The authors declare no conflict of interest.

References

1. Steuer, C.E.; El-Deiry, M.; Parks, J.R.; Higgins, K.A.; Saba, N.F. An update on larynx cancer. *CA A Cancer J. Clin.* **2017**, *67*, 31–50. [CrossRef] [PubMed]
2. Sass, V.; Gadeyne, S. Social Disparities in Survival from Head and Neck Cancers in Europe. In *Social Environment and Cancer in Europe*; Launoy, G., Zadnik, V., Coleman, M.P., Eds.; Springer International Publishing: Berlin/Heidelberg, Germany, 2021; pp. 141–158. [CrossRef]
3. American Cancer Society. Key Statistics for Laryngeal and Hypopharyngeal Cancers. *Cancer.org* **2022**. Available online: https://www.cancer.org/cancer/laryngeal-and-hypopharyngeal-cancer/about/key-statistics.html (accessed on 20 January 2022).
4. Groome, P.A.; O'Sullivan, B.; Irish, J.C.; Rothwell, D.M.; Schulze, K.; Warde, P.R.; Schneider, K.M.; Mackenzie, R.G.; Hodson, D.I.; Hammond, J.A.; et al. Management and Outcome Differences in Supraglottic Cancer Between Ontario, Canada, and the Surveillance, Epidemiology, and End Results Areas of the United States. *J. Clin. Oncol.* **2003**, *21*, 496–505. [CrossRef] [PubMed]
5. Anthony Jnr, B. Implications of telehealth and digital care solutions during COVID-19 pandemic: A qualitative literature review. *Inf. Health Soc. Care* **2021**, *46*, 68–83. [CrossRef] [PubMed]
6. Sharifi, M.; Asadi-Pooya, A.A.; Mousavi-Roknabadi, R.S. Burnout among Healthcare Providers of COVID-19; a Systematic Review of Epidemiology and Recommendations. *Arch. Acad. Emerg. Med.* **2021**, *9*, e7. [CrossRef]
7. Moerman, M.; Martens, J.P.; Dejonckere, P. Multidimensional assessment of strongly irregular voices such as in substitution voicing and spasmodic dysphonia: A compilation of own research. *Logop. Phoniatr. Vocol.* **2015**, *40*, 24–29. [CrossRef]
8. Semple, C.; Parahoo, K.; Norman, A.; McCaughan, E.; Humphris, G.; Mills, M. Psychosocial interventions for patients with head and neck cancer. *Cochrane Database Syst. Rev.* **2013**. [CrossRef]
9. Kumar, V.; Singh, D.; Kaur, M.; Damaševičius, R. Overview of Current State of Research on the Application of Artificial Intelligence Techniques for COVID-19. *PeerJ Comput. Sci.* **2021**, *7*, 1–34. [CrossRef]
10. Thomas, A.; Manchella, S.; Koo, K.; Tiong, A.; Nastri, A.; Wiesenfeld, D. The impact of delayed diagnosis on the outcomes of oral cancer patients: A retrospective cohort study. *Int. J. Oral Maxillofac. Surg.* **2021**, *50*, 585–590. [CrossRef]
11. Noel, C.W.; Li, Q.; Sutradhar, R.; Eskander, A. Total Laryngectomy Volume During the COVID-19 Pandemic: Looking for Evidence of Stage Migration. *JAMA Otolaryngol. Neck Surg.* **2021**, *147*, 909. [CrossRef]
12. Singh, A.; Bhardwaj, A.; Ravichandran, N.; Malhotra, M. Surviving COVID-19 and multiple complications post total laryngectomy. *BMJ Case Rep. CP* **2021**, *14*, e244277. doi: 10.1136/bcr-2021-244277. [CrossRef]
13. Pereira da Silva, A.; Feliciano, T.; Vaz Freitas, S.; Esteves, S.; Almeida e Sousa, C. Quality of Life in Patients Submitted to Total Laryngectomy. *J. Voice* **2015**, *29*, 382–388. [CrossRef] [PubMed]
14. Zilcha-Mano, S.; Goldstein, P.; Dolev-Amit, T.; Ben David-Sela, T.; Barber, J.P. A randomized controlled trial for identifying the most suitable treatment for depression based on patients' attachment orientation. *J. Consult. Clin. Psychol.* **2021**, *89*, 985–994. [CrossRef] [PubMed]
15. Brook, I.; Goodman, J.F. Tracheoesophageal Voice Prosthesis Use and Maintenance in Laryngectomees. *Int. Arch. Otorhinolaryngol.* **2020**, *24*, e535–e538. [CrossRef] [PubMed]
16. Mattys, S.L.; Davis, M.H.; Bradlow, A.R.; Scott, S.K. Speech recognition in adverse conditions: A review. *Lang. Cogn. Process.* **2012**, *27*, 953–978. [CrossRef]
17. Uscher-Pines, L.; Sousa, J.; Raja, P.; Mehrotra, A.; Barnett, M.L.; Huskamp, H.A. Suddenly Becoming a "Virtual Doctor": Experiences of Psychiatrists Transitioning to Telemedicine During the COVID-19 Pandemic. *Psychiatr. Serv.* **2020**, *71*, 1143–1150. [CrossRef] [PubMed]
18. Hossain, M.S.; Muhammad, G.; Alamri, A. Smart healthcare monitoring: A voice pathology detection paradigm for smart cities. *Multimed. Syst.* **2019**, *25*, 565–575. [CrossRef]
19. Cummins, N.; Baird, A.; Schuller, B.W. Speech analysis for health: Current state-of-the-art and the increasing impact of deep learning. *Methods* **2018**, *151*, 41–54. [CrossRef]
20. Lee, J.Y. Experimental Evaluation of Deep Learning Methods for an Intelligent Pathological Voice Detection System Using the Saarbruecken Voice Database. *Appl. Sci.* **2021**, *11*, 7149. [CrossRef]
21. Al-Dhief, F.T.; Latiff, N.M.A.; Malik, N.N.N.A.; Salim, N.S.; Baki, M.M.; Albadr, M.A.A.; Mohammed, M.A. A Survey of Voice Pathology Surveillance Systems Based on Internet of Things and Machine Learning Algorithms. *IEEE Access* **2020**, *8*, 64514–64533. [CrossRef]
22. Barsties, B.; De Bodt, M. Assessment of voice quality: Current state-of-the-art. *Auris Nasus Larynx* **2015**, *42*, 183–188. [CrossRef]
23. Awan, S.N.; Roy, N.; Dromey, C. Estimating dysphonia severity in continuous speech: Application of a multi-parameter spectral/cepstral model. *Clin. Linguist. Phon.* **2009**, *23*, 825–841. [CrossRef] [PubMed]
24. Maryn, Y.; De Bodt, M.; Roy, N. The Acoustic Voice Quality Index: Toward improved treatment outcomes assessment in voice disorders. *J. Commun. Disord.* **2010**, *43*, 161–174. [CrossRef] [PubMed]

25. Barsties v. Latoszek, B.; Mathmann, P.; Neumann, K. The cepstral spectral index of dysphonia, the acoustic voice quality index and the acoustic breathiness index as novel multiparametric indices for acoustic assessment of voice quality. *Curr. Opin. Otolaryngol. Head Neck Surg.* **2021**, *29*, 451–457. [CrossRef]
26. Lee, J.M.; Roy, N.; Peterson, E.; Merrill, R.M. Comparison of Two Multiparameter Acoustic Indices of Dysphonia Severity: The Acoustic Voice Quality Index and Cepstral Spectral Index of Dysphonia. *J. Voice* **2018**, *32*, 515-e1. [CrossRef] [PubMed]
27. van Sluis, K.E.; van Son, R.J.J.H.; van der Molen, L.; MCGuinness, A.J.; Palme, C.E.; Novakovic, D.; Stone, D.; Natsis, L.; Charters, E.; Jones, K.; et al. Multidimensional evaluation of voice outcomes following total laryngectomy: A prospective multicenter cohort study. *Eur. Arch.-Oto-Rhino-Laryngol.* **2020**, *278*, 1209–1222. [CrossRef]
28. Manfredi, C.; Giordano, A.; Schoentgen, J.; Fraj, S.; Bocchi, L.; Dejonckere, P. Validity of jitter measures in non-quasi-periodic voices. Part II: The effect of noise. *Logop. Phoniatr. Vocol.* **2011**, *36*, 78–89. [CrossRef]
29. Dejonckere, P.H.; Moerman, M.B.J.; Martens, J.P.; Schoentgen, J.; Manfredi, C. Voicing quantification is more relevant than period perturbation in substitution voices: An advanced acoustical study. *Eur. Arch.-Oto-Rhino-Laryngol.* **2012**, *269*, 1205–1212. [CrossRef]
30. Muhammad, G.; Alhamid, M.; Hossain, M.; Almogren, A.; Vasilakos, A. Enhanced Living by Assessing Voice Pathology Using a Co-Occurrence Matrix. *Sensors* **2017**, *17*, 267. [CrossRef]
31. Jiang, J.; Li, Y. Review of active noise control techniques with emphasis on sound quality enhancement. *Appl. Acoust.* **2018**, *136*, 139–148. [CrossRef]
32. Avila, A.R.; Gamper, H.; Reddy, C.; Cutler, R.; Tashev, I.; Gehrke, J. Non-intrusive Speech Quality Assessment Using Neural Networks. In Proceedings of the ICASSP 2019–2019 IEEE International Conference on Acoustics, Speech and Signal Processing (ICASSP), Brighton, UK, 12–17 May 2019; pp. 631–635. [CrossRef]
33. Gamper, H.; Reddy, C.K.A.; Cutler, R.; Tashev, I.J.; Gehrke, J. Intrusive and Non-Intrusive Perceptual Speech Quality Assessment Using a Convolutional Neural Network. In Proceedings of the 2019 IEEE Workshop on Applications of Signal Processing to Audio and Acoustics (WASPAA), New Paltz, NY, USA, 20–23 October 2019; pp. 85–89. [CrossRef]
34. v. Latoszek, B.B.; Maryn, Y.; Gerrits, E.; Bodt, M.D. A Meta-Analysis: Acoustic Measurement of Roughness and Breathiness. *J. Speech Lang. Hear. Res.* **2018**, *61*, 298–323. [CrossRef]
35. Muhammad, G.; Melhem, M. Pathological voice detection and binary classification using MPEG-7 audio features. *Biomed. Signal Process. Control* **2014**, *11*, 1–9. [CrossRef]
36. Yin, D.; Luo, C.; Xiong, Z.; Zeng, W. PHASEN: A Phase-and-Harmonics-Aware Speech Enhancement Network. *AAAI Conf. Artif. Intell.* **2020**, *34*, 9458–9465. [CrossRef]
37. Yuanbo, W.; Changwei, Z.; Ziqi, F.; Yihua, Z.; Xiaojun, Z.; Zhi, T. Voice Pathology Detection and Multi-classification Using Machine Learning Classifiers. In Proceedings of the 2020 International Conference on Sensing, Measurement Data Analytics in the Era of Artificial Intelligence (ICSMD), Xi'an, China, 15–17 October 2020; pp. 319–324. [CrossRef]
38. Fang, S.H.; Tsao, Y.; Hsiao, M.J.; Chen, J.Y.; Lai, Y.H.; Lin, F.C.; Wang, C.T. Detection of Pathological Voice Using Cepstrum Vectors: A Deep Learning Approach. *J. Voice* **2019**, *33*, 634–641. [CrossRef] [PubMed]
39. Guimaraes, M.T.; Medeiros, A.G.; Almeida, J.S.; Falcao Y Martin, M.; Damasevicius, R.; Maskeliunas, R.; Cavalcante Mattos, C.L.; Reboucas Filho, P.P. An Optimized Approach to Huntington's Disease Detecting via Audio Signals Processing with Dimensionality Reduction. In Proceedings of the International Joint Conference on Neural Networks, Glasgow, UK, 3 October 2020.
40. Narendra, N.; Alku, P. Automatic assessment of intelligibility in speakers with dysarthria from coded telephone speech using glottal features. *Comput. Speech Lang.* **2021**, *65*, 101117. [CrossRef]
41. Arora, S.; Tsanas, A. Assessing Parkinson's Disease at Scale Using Telephone-Recorded Speech: Insights from the Parkinson's Voice Initiative. *Diagnostics* **2021**, *11*, 1892. [CrossRef]
42. Lauraitis, A.; Maskeliunas, R.; Damaševičius, R.; Krilavičius, T. Detection of Speech Impairments Using Cepstrum, Auditory Spectrogram and Wavelet Time Scattering Domain Features. *IEEE Access* **2020**, *8*, 96162–96172. [CrossRef]
43. Braga, D.; Madureira, A.M.; Coelho, L.; Ajith, R. Automatic detection of Parkinson's disease based on acoustic analysis of speech. *Eng. Appl. Artif. Intell.* **2019**, *77*, 148–158. [CrossRef]
44. Qian, Y.; Chen, Z.; Wang, S. Audio-Visual Deep Neural Network for Robust Person Verification. *IEEE/ACM Trans. Audio Speech Lang. Process.* **2021**, *29*, 1079–1092. [CrossRef]
45. Patil, A.T.; Patil, H.A.; Khoria, K. Effectiveness of energy separation-based instantaneous frequency estimation for cochlear cepstral features for synthetic and voice-converted spoofed speech detection. *Comput. Speech Lang.* **2022**, *72*, 101301. [CrossRef]
46. Jalali-najafabadi, F.; Gadepalli, C.; Jarchi, D.; Cheetham, B.M. Acoustic analysis and digital signal processing for the assessment of voice quality. *Biomed. Signal Process. Control* **2021**, *70*, 103018. [CrossRef]
47. Jothi, K.R.; Sivaraju, S.S.; Yawalkar, P.J. AI based Speech Language Therapy using Speech Quality Parameters for Aphasia Person: A Comprehensive Review. In Proceedings of the 2020 4th International Conference on Electronics, Communication and Aerospace Technology (ICECA), Coimbatore, India, 5–7 November 2020; pp. 1263–1271. [CrossRef]
48. Aicha, A.B. Noninvasive Detection of Potentially Precancerous Lesions of Vocal Fold Based on Glottal Wave signal and sVM Approaches. *Procedia Comput. Sci.* **2018**, *126*, 586–595. [CrossRef]
49. Fontes, A.I.R.; Souza, P.T.V.; Neto, A.D.D.; Martins, A.d.M.; Silveira, L.F.Q. Classification System of Pathological Voices Using Correntropy. *Math. Probl. Eng.* **2014**, *2014*, 1–7. [CrossRef]
50. Alías, F.; Socoro, J.; Sevillano, X. A Review of Physical and Perceptual Feature Extraction Techniques for Speech, Music and Environmental Sounds. *Appl. Sci.* **2016**, *6*, 143. [CrossRef]

51. Hossain, M.S.; Muhammad, G. Healthcare Big Data Voice Pathology Assessment Framework. *IEEE Access* **2016**, *4*, 7806–7815. [CrossRef]
52. Vaziri, G.; Giguère, C.; Dajani, H.R. Evaluating noise suppression methods for recovering the Lombard speech from vocal output in an external noise field. *Int. J. Speech Technol.* **2019**, *22*, 31–46. [CrossRef]
53. Hegde, S.; Shetty, S.; Rai, S.; Dodderi, T. A Survey on Machine Learning Approaches for Automatic Detection of Voice Disorders. *J. Voice* **2019**, *33*, 947.e11–947.e33. [CrossRef]
54. Zhang, D.; Wu, K. *Pathological Voice Analysis*; Springer: Singapore, 2020. [CrossRef]
55. Chen, L.; Wang, C.; Chen, J.; Xiang, Z.; Hu, X. Voice Disorder Identification by using Hilbert-Huang Transform (HHT) and K Nearest Neighbor (KNN). *J. Voice* **2021**, *35*, 932.e1–932.e11. [CrossRef]
56. Uloza, V.; Padervinskis, E.; Vegiene, A.; Pribuisiene, R.; Saferis, V.; Vaiciukynas, E.; Gelzinis, A.; Verikas, A. Exploring the feasibility of smart phone microphone for measurement of acoustic voice parameters and voice pathology screening. *Eur. Arch. Oto-Rhino* **2015**, *272*, 3391–3399. [CrossRef]
57. Amami, R.; Smiti, A. An incremental method combining density clustering and support vector machines for voice pathology detection. *Comput. Electr. Eng.* **2017**, *57*, 257–265. [CrossRef]
58. Lee, J.Y. A two-stage approach using Gaussian mixture models and higher-order statistics for a classification of normal and pathological voices. *EURASIP J. Adv. Signal Process.* **2012**, *2012*, 252. [CrossRef]
59. Pham, M.; Lin, J.; Zhang, Y. Diagnosing Voice Disorder with Machine Learning. In Proceedings of the 2018 IEEE International Conference on Big Data (Big Data), Seattle, WA, USA, 10–13 December 2018; pp. 5263–5266. [CrossRef]
60. Hammami, I.; Salhi, L.; Labidi, S. Voice Pathologies Classification and Detection Using EMD-DWT Analysis Based on Higher Order Statistic Features. *IRBM* **2020**, *41*, 161–171. [CrossRef]
61. Fonseca, E.S.; Guido, R.C.; Junior, S.B.; Dezani, H.; Gati, R.R.; Mosconi Pereira, D.C. Acoustic investigation of speech pathologies based on the discriminative paraconsistent machine (DPM). *Biomed. Signal Process. Control* **2020**, *55*, 101615. [CrossRef]
62. Muhammad, G.; Alhussein, M. Convergence of Artificial Intelligence and Internet of Things in Smart Healthcare: A Case Study of Voice Pathology Detection. *IEEE Access* **2021**, *9*, 89198–89209. [CrossRef]
63. Cordeiro, H.T.; Ribeiro, C.M. Spectral envelope first peak and periodic component in pathological voices: A spectral analysis. *Procedia Comput. Sci.* **2018**, *138*, 64–71. [CrossRef]
64. Erfanian Saeedi, N.; Almasganj, F.; Torabinejad, F. Support vector wavelet adaptation for pathological voice assessment. *Comput. Biol. Med.* **2011**, *41*, 822–828. [CrossRef]
65. Vásquez-Correa, J.; Klumpp, P.; Orozco-Arroyave, J.R.; Nöth, E. Phonet: A Tool Based on Gated Recurrent Neural Networks to Extract Phonological Posteriors from Speech. In Proceedings of the Interspeech 2019, ISCA, Graz, Austria, 15–19 September 2019; pp. 549–553. [CrossRef]
66. Wu, H.; Soraghan, J.; Lowit, A.; Di Caterina, G. Convolutional Neural Networks for Pathological Voice Detection. In Proceedings of the 2018 40th Annual International Conference of the IEEE Engineering in Medicine and Biology Society (EMBC), Honolulu, HI, USA, 18–21 July 2018; pp. 1–4. [CrossRef]
67. Areiza-Laverde, H.J.; Castro-Ospina, A.E.; Peluffo-Ordóñez, D.H. Voice Pathology Detection Using Artificial Neural Networks and Support Vector Machines Powered by a Multicriteria Optimization Algorithm. In *Applied Computer Sciences in Engineering*; Figueroa-García, J.C., López-Santana, E.R., Rodriguez-Molano, J.I., Eds.; Springer International Publishing: Berlin/Heidelberg, Germany, 2018; Volume 915, pp. 148–159. [CrossRef]
68. Chen, L.; Chen, J. Deep Neural Network for Automatic Classification of Pathological Voice Signals. *J. Voice* **2020**, *36*, 288.E15–288.E24. [CrossRef]
69. Miliaresi, I.; Poutos, K.; Pikrakis, A. Combining acoustic features and medical data in deep learning networks for voice pathology classification. In Proceedings of the 2020 28th European Signal Processing Conference (EUSIPCO), Amsterdam, The Netherlands, 18–21 January 2021; pp. 1190–1194. [CrossRef]
70. Gómez García, J.A. Contributions to the Design of Automatic Voice Quality Analysis Systems Using Speech Technologies. Ph.D. Thesis, Universidad Politécnica de Madrid, Madrid, Spain, 2018. [CrossRef]
71. Syed, S.A.; Rashid, M.; Hussain, S.; Zahid, H. Comparative Analysis of CNN and RNN for Voice Pathology Detection. *BioMed Res. Int.* **2021**, *2021*, 1–8. [CrossRef]
72. Kim, H.; Jeon, J.; Han, Y.J.; Joo, Y.; Lee, J.; Lee, S.; Im, S. Convolutional Neural Network Classifies Pathological Voice Change in Laryngeal Cancer with High Accuracy. *J. Clin. Med.* **2020**, *9*, 3415. [CrossRef]
73. Wahengbam, K.; Singh, M.P.; Nongmeikapam, K.; Singh, A.D. A Group Decision Optimization Analogy-Based Deep Learning Architecture for Multiclass Pathology Classification in a Voice Signal. *IEEE Sens. J.* **2021**, *21*, 8100–8116. [CrossRef]
74. Raj, J.R.; Jabez, J.; Srinivasulu, S.; Gowri, S.; Vimali, J.S. Voice Pathology Detection Based on Deep Neural Network Approach. *IOP Conf. Ser. Mater. Sci. Eng.* **2021**, *1020*, 012001. [CrossRef]
75. Fan, Z.; Wu, Y.; Zhou, C.; Zhang, X.; Tao, Z. Class-Imbalanced Voice Pathology Detection and Classification Using Fuzzy Cluster Oversampling Method. *Appl. Sci.* **2021**, *11*, 3450. [CrossRef]
76. Tolosi, L.; Lengauer, T. Classification with correlated features: Unreliability of feature ranking and solutions. *Bioinformatics* **2011**, *27*, 1986–1994. [CrossRef] [PubMed]
77. Kingma, D.P.; Ba, J. Adam: A Method for Stochastic Optimization. 2017. Available online: http://xxx.lanl.gov/abs/1412.6980 (accessed on 20 January 2022).

78. Loshchilov, I.; Hutter, F. SGDR: Stochastic Gradient Descent with Warm Restarts. 2017. Available online: http://xxx.lanl.gov/abs/1608.03983 (accessed on 20 January 2022).
79. He, K.; Zhang, X.; Ren, S.; Sun, J. Deep Residual Learning for Image Recognition. 2015. Available online: http://xxx.lanl.gov/abs/1512.03385 (accessed on 20 January 2022).
80. Collobert, R.; Puhrsch, C.; Synnaeve, G. Wav2Letter: An End-to-End ConvNet-Based Speech Recognition System. 2016. Available online: http://xxx.lanl.gov/abs/1609.03193 (accessed on 20 January 2022).
81. Dai, W.; Dai, C.; Qu, S.; Li, J.; Das, S. Very Deep Convolutional Neural Networks for Raw Waveforms. 2016. Available online: http://xxx.lanl.gov/abs/1610.00087 (accessed on 20 January 2022).
82. Vanagas, G.; Engelbrecht, R.; Damaševičius, R.; Suomi, R.; Solanas, A. EHealth Solutions for the Integrated Healthcare. *J. Healthc. Eng.* **2018**, *2018*, 3846892. [CrossRef] [PubMed]
83. Payten, C.L.; Nguyen, D.D.; Novakovic, D.; O'Neill, J.; Chacon, A.M.; Weir, K.A.; Madill, C.J. Telehealth voice assessment by speech language pathologists during a global pandemic using principles of a primary contact model: An observational cohort study protocol. *BMJ Open* **2022**, *12*, e052518. [CrossRef]

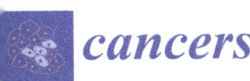

Review

Artificial Intelligence in Urooncology: What We Have and What We Expect

Anita Froń [1,*], Alina Semianiuk [1], Uladzimir Lazuk [1], Kuba Ptaszkowski [2], Agnieszka Siennicka [3], Artur Lemiński [4], Wojciech Krajewski [1], Tomasz Szydełko [1] and Bartosz Małkiewicz [1,*]

1. Department of Minimally Invasive and Robotic Urology, University Center of Excellence in Urology, Wroclaw Medical University, 50-556 Wroclaw, Poland; alina.semianiuk@student.umw.edu.pl (A.S.); uladzimir.lazuk@student.umw.edu.pl (U.L.); wojciech.krajewski@umw.edu.pl (W.K.); tomasz.szydelko@umw.edu.pl (T.S.)
2. Department of Physiotherapy, Wroclaw Medical University, 50-368 Wroclaw, Poland; kuba.ptaszkowski@umw.edu.pl
3. Department of Physiology and Pathophysiology, Wroclaw Medical University, 50-556 Wroclaw, Poland; agnieszka.siennicka@umw.edu.pl
4. Department of Urology and Urological Oncology, Pomeranian Medical University, 70-111 Szczecin, Poland; artur.leminski@pum.edu.pl
* Correspondence: anita.fron@student.umw.edu.pl (A.F.); bartosz.malkiewicz@umw.edu.pl (B.M.); Tel.: +48-660083243 (A.F.); +48-506158136 (B.M.)

Simple Summary: Our study provides an overview of the current state of artificial intelligence applications in urooncology and explores potential future advancements in this field. With remarkable progress already achieved, artificial intelligence has revolutionized urooncology by facilitating image analysis, grading, biomarker research, and treatment planning. We also discuss types of artificial intelligence and their possible applications in the management of cancers such as prostate, kidney, bladder, and testicular. As artificial intelligence technology continues to evolve, it holds immense promise for further advancing urooncology and enhancing the care of patients with cancer.

Abstract: Introduction: Artificial intelligence is transforming healthcare by driving innovation, automation, and optimization across various fields of medicine. The aim of this study was to determine whether artificial intelligence (AI) techniques can be used in the diagnosis, treatment planning, and monitoring of urological cancers. Methodology: We conducted a thorough search for original and review articles published until 31 May 2022 in the PUBMED/Scopus database. Our search included several terms related to AI and urooncology. Articles were selected with the consensus of all authors. Results: Several types of AI can be used in the medical field. The most common forms of AI are machine learning (ML), deep learning (DL), neural networks (NNs), natural language processing (NLP) systems, and computer vision. AI can improve various domains related to the management of urologic cancers, such as imaging, grading, and nodal staging. AI can also help identify appropriate diagnoses, treatment options, and even biomarkers. In the majority of these instances, AI is as accurate as or sometimes even superior to medical doctors. Conclusions: AI techniques have the potential to revolutionize the diagnosis, treatment, and monitoring of urologic cancers. The use of AI in urooncology care is expected to increase in the future, leading to improved patient outcomes and better overall management of these tumors.

Keywords: artificial intelligence; machine learning; urooncology; prostate cancer

Citation: Froń, A.; Semianiuk, A.; Lazuk, U.; Ptaszkowski, K.; Siennicka, A.; Lemiński, A.; Krajewski, W.; Szydełko, T.; Małkiewicz, B. Artificial Intelligence in Urooncology: What We Have and What We Expect. *Cancers* **2023**, *15*, 4282. https://doi.org/10.3390/cancers15174282

Academic Editors: Muhammad Fazal Ijaz and Marcin Woźniak

Received: 17 July 2023
Revised: 15 August 2023
Accepted: 24 August 2023
Published: 26 August 2023

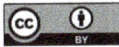

Copyright: © 2023 by the authors. Licensee MDPI, Basel, Switzerland. This article is an open access article distributed under the terms and conditions of the Creative Commons Attribution (CC BY) license (https://creativecommons.org/licenses/by/4.0/).

1. Introduction

Medicine has changed over the decades. Due to better access to medical care, the number of patients has increased, indicating an increase in data that must be acquired and processed. Over the years, science has made numerous discoveries that can be applied to several medical issues, even in unexpected fields. It is necessary to determine how to apply these solutions to issues that seem unsuitable and even irrelevant.

The journey of Artificial Intelligence (AI) in medicine began in the 1950s and 1960s with early attempts at developing machines capable of making decisions and mimicking human conversation [1]. During the 1970s to 2000s, despite periods of reduced funding and interest, collaborations among pioneers in AI continued, leading to prototypes like the CASNET—model for glaucoma consultation. This causal-associational network included model-building, consultation, and a database, enabling personalized advice for physicians on patient management. Another milestone was the "backward chaining" AI system called MYCIN. It used patient information provided by physicians and a knowledge base of about 600 rules to suggest potential bacterial pathogens and recommend antibiotic treatments adjusted for the patient's body weight.

The early 2000s saw a revival of interest in Machine Learning (ML) and AI with the development of the question-answering system Watson by IBM, an open-domain question-answering system. Watson harnessed the power of DeepQA technology, utilizing natural language processing and data analysis to generate probable answers from unstructured content. This breakthrough allowed for evidence-based clinical decision-making by drawing information from patients' electronic medical records.

With improved computer hardware and software, digitalized medicine rapidly advanced, including the use of chatbots like Siri and Alexa. Deep Learning (DL) emerged as a game-changer, allowing AI systems to classify data autonomously and process large datasets more efficiently.

Today, AI assists medical professionals in establishing diagnoses, making therapeutic decisions, and predicting the outcome. It supports every procedure that involves data processing and knowledge and is used by healthcare professionals in their everyday duties. Currently, AI can perform all these tasks with the same efficiency as skilled physicians [2]. Sometimes, it can even outperform expert clinicians [3].

AI is capable of a broad range of tasks, including separating cancer cells from healthy tissue, determining whether lymph node metastases have occurred, discovering biomarkers, predicting outcomes, and making therapeutic decisions [4]. In this review, we explore AI applications in urogenital system cancers, drawing from the latest research. Providing a comprehensive view of urooncology while focusing on individual cancer types, this study fosters a detailed and integrated understanding of the subject.

2. Materials and Methods

For this narrative review, we conducted comprehensive English-language literature research for original and review articles published until 31 December 2022 in the PUBMED/Scopus database. We searched for the following terms, alone or in combination: artificial intelligence, machine learning, deep learning, neural networks, computer-aided diagnosis, urooncology, prostate cancer, kidney cancer, testicular cancer, bladder cancer, and upper tract urothelial carcinoma. We found 249 related articles. The relevant studies were identified by evaluating the abstracts, and complete articles were obtained in cases where abstracts were unavailable. Duplicate papers were removed, and the data were screened to exclude irrelevant works. Case reports, comments, conference papers, commentaries, surveys, and animal studies were all excluded from the full-text publications. After applying the exclusion criteria, 99 full-text manuscripts were assessed for eligibility with the consensus of the authors.

3. Definition and Types of AI

Artificial intelligence (AI) is a broad term encompassing computer systems capable of performing tasks that traditionally require human cognition [5]. It involves programmed machines that can learn, identify patterns, and establish relationships between inputs and outputs [6]. Utilizing diverse mathematical and algorithmic methods, AI sits at the convergence of neurocomputing, statistical inference, pattern recognition, data mining, knowledge discovery, and machine learning (ML) [7]. In recent times, AI has emerged as a powerful tool, making remarkable strides in addressing numerous medical challenges.

Artificial intelligence (AI) encompasses several fields with the common goal of computationally simulating human intelligence:

1. Machine learning (ML) is one of the most important types of artificial intelligence. This technology involves prediction by identifying patterns in data using mathematical algorithms. Machine learning includes three methods: deep learning, logistic regression, and neural network architecture. ML algorithms can help automate the process of detecting and diagnosing cancer.

Deep learning (DL) predicts using multilayer neural network algorithms inspired by the neurological architecture of the brain. Deep learning (DL) can automatically extract features and assimilate and evaluate large amounts of complex data. Using large amounts of medical data and state-of-the-art computing technologies, DL can improve cancer diagnosis and treatment. DL has found widespread application in oncology research, encompassing early cancer detection, diagnosis, classification, and grading. Additionally, it has been instrumental in molecular tumor characterization, predicting patient outcomes and treatment response, facilitating personalized treatment approaches, automating radiation therapy workflows, and even aiding in the discovery of new anticancer drugs. Furthermore, DL plays a crucial role in streamlining clinical trials, revolutionizing how oncology research and patient care are conducted [8,9].

2. Neural networks (NNs) are increasingly being applied to complex ML data and include artificial neural networks (ANNs), multilayer perceptrons (MLPs), recurrent neural networks (RNNs), and convolutional neural networks (CNNs).

Artificial Neural Networks (ANNs) are computational tools inspired by the structure of the human nervous system. These networks comprise interconnected computer processors, often referred to as "neurons", which can process data and represent knowledge through parallel computations. ANNs consist of multiple layers of neurons, including an input layer, one or more hidden layers, and an output layer. Each neuron is connected to others in the network through links, and each link possesses a numerical weight. One notable aspect of ANNs is their capacity to learn from their experiences in a training environment, making them adaptive and capable of improving their performance over time. Thanks to their analytical abilities, ANNs can compare various interactions among clinical, biological, and pathological variables and identify relationships between these variables. Researchers actively use ANNs to diagnose, treat, and predict outcomes in challenging clinical situations [9,10].

Convolutional neural networks (CNNs) are widely regarded as the most popular and effective deep learning architectures. They are particularly adept at handling large and intricate image data and extracting essential features through convolutional filters. By adjusting these filters based on learned parameters, CNNs can identify the most relevant features for specific tasks. The use of CNNs is not limited to image data; they have also been adapted to analyze non-image data, like genomic data represented in vector, matrix, or tensor formats [6,9,11]. MLPs, on the other hand, are simpler neural networks that process input data sequentially through layers, making general predictions but being susceptible to overfitting [12,13]. RNNs are designed to handle sequential data, capturing past elements in hidden "state vectors" and making predictions based on current and previous elements [12]. While some neural network models have already been approved and accepted in clinical settings, the routine clinical application of neural networks is still somewhat limited. Nevertheless, their potential for revolutionizing healthcare continues to grow, especially in fields such as cancer diagnosis and prediction [14,15].

3. NLP systems address a wide range of important clinical and research tasks. NLP is capable of processing free clinical text and generating structured output. There has been extensive focus on applying NLP techniques to identify and extract key data (information) from unstructured text so that it can be transformed into structured data that can later be analyzed and stored in a database. The steps for extracting information are as follows:

named entity recognition, relationship extraction, event and temporal expression extraction, and entity merging and normalization [16].

4. Computer vision, a vital branch of artificial intelligence (AI), empowers computers and systems to derive valuable insights from digital images, videos, and visual data. By understanding and interpreting visual input, computers gain the ability to take action and provide informed recommendations. This field employs advanced deep learning technologies, particularly convolutional neural networks (CNNs), to process and analyze visual information. The primary goal of computer vision is to develop algorithms, data representations, and computer architectures that emulate human-like visual capabilities. Through computer vision, machines can "see", observe, and comprehend the world around them, opening up new possibilities for numerous applications [16].

The discussed subfields of artificial intelligence are presented in Figure 1.

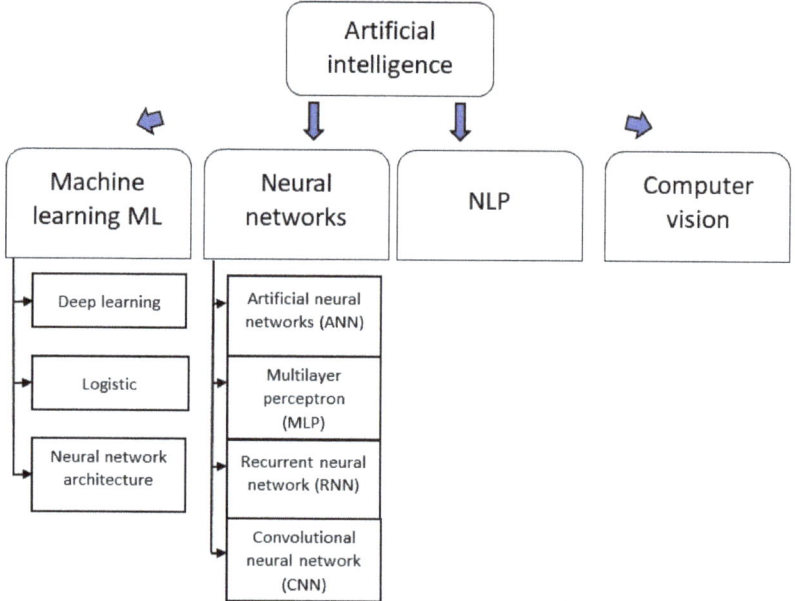

Figure 1. Subfields of Artificial Intelligence.

4. Application of AI in Urological Oncology

4.1. Prostate Cancer

Prostate cancer (PCa) is one of the main causes of cancer-related morbidity and mortality across the world. It is a complex and diverse disease with various diagnostic methods, including biopsy, PSA testing, and MRI. The majority of prostate cancer cases are adenocarcinomas, originating from luminal or basal epithelial cells in the peripheral regions of the prostate. Risk factors like family history, ethnicity, age, and obesity contribute to its variation across populations. Treatment options such as active surveillance, chemotherapy, radiation therapy, and surgery are tailored to individual tumor characteristics. Understanding these factors is crucial for the effective management and treatment of prostate cancer [17,18].

Given the large increase in life expectancy over the past few decades, it is reasonable to assume that the number of patients with prostate cancer will grow. Unfortunately, there are still many uncertainties surrounding the diagnosis and treatment of PCa. Consequently, it is necessary to develop new methods for managing this condition [19,20].

4.1.1. Imaging and Diagnosis

AI systems can automate the detection of cases in which prostate cancer is highly suspected. In a study by Cao et al. [21], the deep learning algorithm FocalNet was trained using 3T T2-weighted imaging and diffusion-weighted imaging of 553 patients who later underwent radical prostatectomy. Lesion detection sensitivity vs. the number of false-positive detections at various thresholds on suspicion scores was used to compare the PCa recognition rates of FocalNet and radiologists. For clinically important and index lesions, respectively, FocalNet performed 5.1% and 4.7% worse than radiologists. However, the differences were not statistically significant ($p = 0.413$ and $p = 0.282$, respectively) [21].

Giannini et al. proposed a computer-aided diagnosis (CAD) tool that can help manage patients suspected of having PCa and determine the target for an MRI-guided biopsy. CAD is a two-stage system. First, a map of the probability that prostate voxels will develop cancer is made. Next, to evaluate the sensitivity of the system and the quantity of false-positive (FP) regions recognized by the system, a candidate segmentation phase is carried out to highlight questionable areas. In a study by Giannini et al. [22], the area under the curve (AUC) for a cohort of 56 patients (i.e., 65 lesions) acquired during the voxel-wise phase was 0.91, and the second stage resulted in a per-patient sensitivity of 97%, with a median number of FP equal to 3, in the entire prostate sample [22].

CAD's ability to detect more challenging cancers in the gland's center may increase specificity and the radiologists' level of experience. The objective of Gaur's study was to compare the effectiveness of CAD to that of traditional multiparametric MRI (mpMRI) interpretation in prostate cancer identification. Index lesion sensitivities of CAD were 76% ($p = 0.39$) for the whole prostate, 77% ($p = 0.07$) for the peripheral zone, and 79% ($p = 0.15$) for the transition zone compared to those of mpMRI at 79%, 84%, and 76%, respectively [23].

In a study by Pantanowitz et al., an AI-based algorithm was created using samples of prostate core needle biopsies stained with hematoxylin and eosin. It was trained with 1,357,450 visual patches from 549 slides and tested with 2501 samples internally and with 1627 samples externally. The AUC of the algorithm was 0.997 in the internal test set and 0.991 in the external test set. The AUC for identifying Gleason pattern 5 was 0.971, and the AUC for differentiating between low-grade (Gleason score 6 or ASAP) cancer and high-grade (Gleason score 7–10) cancer was 0.941, along with 0.957 for perineural invasion. This study also provided the first instance of undetected cancer that the algorithm managed to identify [3].

Wang's [24] prospective multi-center randomized comparative trial aimed to compare the prostate cancer (PCa) detection rate using different biopsy methods. Four hundred patients were divided into three groups: TRUS-guided 12-core standard systematic biopsy (TRUS-SB), cognitive fused mpMRI-guided 12-core biopsy (mpMRI), and artificial intelligence ultrasound of the prostate (AIUSP)-targeted biopsy. The AIUSP group showed the highest PCa detection rate (49.6%) compared to TRUS-SB (34.6%) and mpMRI (35.8%). The detection rate of clinically significant PCa (csPCa) was also highest in the AIUSP group (32.3%). The overall biopsy core positive rate was significantly lower in the TRUS-SB and mpMRI groups than in the AIUSP group. These findings suggest that AIUSP may serve as a promising alternative to systematic biopsy for PCa diagnosis in the future.

Furthermore, Stojadinović et al. demonstrated that AI can predict the risk of PCa and minimize overdiagnosis and overtreatment. They created a classification and regression tree (CART) model that, regardless of the prostate specific antigen (PSA) level, could be applied to patients referred for an abnormal PSA level, a digital rectal examination (DRE), or both in order to recognize patients with severe prostate cancer (PCa) on prostate biopsy. The CART analysis was performed using each predictor identified by the univariate logistic regression analysis. A variety of clinical utility and predictive performance aspects of risk projections were investigated. The model identified PCa in 92 (41.6%; AUC = 0.833) of 221 patients. To conclude, CART analysis prevents any major PCa from being missed while reducing unnecessary biopsies [25].

There have also been attempts to use machine learning for prostate cancer localization using transrectal ultrasound [26] and classifier ensembles using T_2-weighted MRI alone [27].

4.1.2. Gleason Grading

The ability of AI to localize, detect, and grade prostate cancer in biopsy samples can be comparable to that of prominent prostate pathology experts. Marginean et al. [28] used 698 prostate biopsy samples from 174 patients to train an AI algorithm and then tested it on 37 biopsy sections from 21 patients. AI achieved high accuracy in detecting the cancer areas, with a sensitivity of 100% and a specificity of 68%. The Gleason patterns were assigned correctly, with an intraclass correlation coefficient (ICC) of 0.96 for Gleason patterns 3 and 4, and with an ICC of 0.82 for Gleason pattern 5. Furthermore, the algorithm was comparable with pathologists in detecting cancer areas (ICC = 0.99). This discovery can undoubtedly simplify the diagnosis of prostate cancer [28].

Ström et al. conducted a study in which deep neural networks were trained with 6682 biopsy slides from 976 patients and tested with 1631 samples from 246 men. The assignment was to determine the occurrence, extent, and Gleason grade of malignant tissue with the help of AI. The AUC for the AI was 0.997 for differentiating benign and malignant biopsy slides. Moreover, the cancer length assigned by the reporting pathologist and predicted by the AI had a 0.96 correlation [29].

Here, the PANDA challenge ought to be mentioned. In this largest histopathology trial, 1290 developers competed to create repeatable AI algorithms for Gleason grading using 10,616 digitalized prostate samples. On external validation sets from the United States and Europe, the algorithms met expert uropathologists' agreement levels of 0.862 (95% confidence interval (CI), 0.840–0.884) and 0.868 (95% CI, 0.835–0.900), respectively. This indicates that AI tools were capable of identifying and grading cancers with pathologist-level accuracy, achieving professional reference criteria. Furthermore, it was discovered that the algorithms missed fewer tumors than the pathologists in the US external validation set [30].

4.1.3. Nodal Staging

In a study by Hartenstein et al. [31], convolutional neural networks (CNNs) were trained to establish lymph node status in patients with PCa using only computer tomography images. Three CNNs were trained with ^{68}Ga-PSMA-PET/CT imaging of 549 patients, with 2616 lymph nodes segmented. The CNNs were conducted with an AUC of 0.86. The expert clinician's AUC was 0.81, which confirms that CNNs can adequately determine the lymphatic spread. Moreover, CNNs demonstrated the ability to "learn" since they predicted the chances of infiltration based on the anatomical regions, which positively affected their performance [31].

4.1.4. Biomarkers

AI may be valuable in analyzing and verifying potential PCa biomarkers. Green et al. attempted to determine whether the potential biomarkers Ki67 and DLX2 could be reliable indicators of PCa progression. First, they investigated the connection between tumor protein levels of Ki67 and DLX2 in transurethral resected prostatectomy samples and time to death and metastasis. Artificial neural network (ANN) analysis showed that Ki67, which was found only in 6.8% of the patients, can be predictive of reduced survival and increased probability of metastasis ($p = 0.025$), independent of the PSA level and Gleason score. Moreover, DLX2 was detected in 73% of the patients, and DLX2 was co-expressed with high Ki67 levels in 8.2% of the patients. According to ANN, DLX2 is a potential marker of increased metastasis risk. In conclusion, Ki67 and DLX2 can assist physicians in identifying patients who need to be actively monitored [32].

As a predictor of the presence of biomarkers, AI is faster and more objective than manual quantification. Calle et al. [33] tested the AI algorithm to identify anti-Ki67 and ERG antibodies in 648 samples. Results differed from those of manual detection by only

5% and were 100% accurate in identifying the positive tumors. Interestingly, the algorithm was also able to increase its accuracy following each round of adjustments and input from the training set [33].

AI may also identify promising prostate cancer biomarkers. The genetic algorithm-optimized artificial neural network (GA-ANN) was developed in order to create a diagnostic prediction model and filter potential genes obtained by meta-analysis of the openly accessible microarray data by RankProd. The expression of three genes was considered. C1QTNF3 was proven to be significantly correlated with PCa patient recurrence-free survival (RFS; $p < 0.001$, AUC = 0.57). This procedure can be used to identify other oncogenes or biomarkers in various urooncology diseases [34].

Proteomic analysis can also be used to discover possible biomarkers. To explore new potential proteomic signatures for prostate cancer, Kim et al. [35] created a unique method that combines targeted proteomics with computational biology. First, they identified 133 different expressed proteins in patients with PCa. Next, using synthetic peptides, they assessed these proteins in a group of 74 patients. Next, machine learning methods were used to create clinical predictive models of the diagnosis and prognosis of prostate cancer. The findings suggest that precise, noninvasive biomarkers can be found via computationally guided proteomics [35]. Furthermore, AI can predict different indicators, e.g., the 10-year cancer-specific survival (CSS) and overall survival (OS) of patients with PCa. Two gradient-boosting models using the data of patients diagnosed with PCa were trained on 7021 cases and tested on 1755 cases. The accuracy was 0.87 for the CSS and 0.98 for the OS. The ability of AI to interpret data offers clinicians and patients a new approach for predicting prostate cancer and its outcome [36].

4.1.5. Treatment

AI can determine the most appropriate treatment plan for patients. Auffenberg et al. [37] showed AI as a tool that can assist patients with PCa who have just received a diagnosis by predicting therapy choices on the basis of information from a registry of patients with comparable conditions. A prospective database of patients with PCa was built using information from 45 units of the Michigan Urological Surgery Improvement Collaborative (MUSIC). Then, a random forest machine learning model was applied, which was trained with a sample containing two-thirds of the patients and evaluated with the remaining one-third of the patients. The individualized prediction was exact (AUC = 0.81). Patients can use this online tool to obtain a better understanding of the various treatment options offered by their physicians, as well as physicians advice to seek a different therapy approach from their first choice. Indubitably, both sides can benefit from this instrument [37].

To predict and understand late genitourinary (GU) toxicity after radiation therapy in patients with prostate cancer, Lee et al. [38] used bioinformatics tools and machine learning techniques on genome-wide data. First, the patterns in genome-wide single-nucleotide polymorphisms (SNPs) were recognized and gathered. Next, a preconditioned random forest regression method was used to speculate on the risk on the basis of that data. The system was tested on 234 patients who had undergone radiation treatment two years earlier. The patients performed a self-assessment for four urinary symptoms using the International Prostate Symptom Score. Across the symptoms, the prediction accuracy of the method varied. It only managed to achieve a significant AUC of 0.70 for the weak stream endpoint. Nevertheless, as a result of their research, a more accurate predictive model could be created, and probable biomarkers and biological processes connected to GU toxicity could be identified [38].

Using megavoltage (MV) pictures for image-guided radiation therapy (IGRT) in prostate cancer patients would undoubtedly be advantageous. It eliminates the need for additional equipment and imaging doses. It additionally provides motion data with treatment beam alignment. For this purpose, Chrystall et al. [39] developed a novel real-time marker tracking system using a convolutional neural network (CNN) classifier. The CNN demonstrated high accuracy in identifying implanted prostate markers with an AUC of 0.99, a sensitivity of 98.31%, and a specificity of 99.87%. The marker tracking system achieved sub-millimeter accuracy, making it suitable for real-time applications in IGRT and providing a promising approach for accurate and efficient treatment.

AI-based treatment planning systems are efficient and save time. In a study by Nicolae et al. [40], 41 patients who had received ^{125}I low-dose-rate brachytherapy were divided into two groups randomly. The treatment of 21 patients was planned using a machine-learning-based prostate implant planning algorithm (PIPA) system, while the treatment of the remaining patients was planned using the conventional method. After the radiation oncologist modified the plan, the first evaluation was carried out by determining the dice coefficient of the prostate V150% isodose volume between PIPA and the standard method. Additional comparisons between groups focused on dosimetric results at preimplant and Day 30, as well as the amount of planning time. Results indicated that the plans of more patients' in the PIPA group did not require modification, and compared to the conventional technique (43.13 $\pm$ 58.70 min), the planning time for PIPA was significantly shorter (2.38 $\pm$ 0.96 min). In addition, no discernible differences between these two groups were discovered [40].

Deng et al. showed a similar strategy. Docetaxel, the medication used to treat metastatic castration-resistant prostate cancer, is only effective in 20% of patients. AI can accurately divide patients into docetaxel-tolerant and docetaxel-intolerant groups, which can help select adequate treatment and avoid early therapeutic failure [41].

Table 1 summarizes the most important studies examining AI applications in prostate cancer.

Table 1. Studies looking at applications of AI in prostate cancer.

Study	Objective	Algorithm/Method	Study Design	Results
Cao et al. [21]	Detection of prostate cancer using 3 T multiparametric magnetic resonance imaging	Deep learning algorithm	• development cohort: 427 patients • evaluation cohort: 126 patients	Detection sensitivity: 5.1% and 4.7% below the radiologists for clinically significant and index lesions, respectively
Giannini et al. [22]	Setting of the MRI-guided biopsy target	Computer-aided diagnosis	• 56 patients • 65 lesions	Accuracy—97%
Gaur et al. [23]	Detection of prostate cancer using mpMRI	Computer-aided diagnosis	• 144 case patients • 72 control patients	Improved patient-level specificity (72%) compared to mpMRI-alone (45%)
Wildeboer et al. [42]	Detection of prostate cancer using B-mode, shear-wave elastography, and contrast-enhanced ultrasound radiomics	Machine learning	• 48 patients	AUC-ROC of 0.75 for detecting PCa and 0.9 for detecting Gleason score greater than 3 + 4
Viswanath et al. [27]	Detection of peripheral zone prostate tumors using T$_2$-weighted MRI	Computer-aided diagnosis	• 85 prostate cancer datasets acquired from across 3 different institutions (1 for discovery, 2 for independent validation)	AUC of 0.744 for detecting PCa
Marginean et al. [28]	Standardization of Gleason grading in prostate biopsies	Machine learning and convolutional neural networks	• 698 prostate biopsy sections from 174 patients for training • 37 biopsy sections from 21 patients for test	Sensitivity in detecting cancer (100%) and identifying the correct Gleason pattern (80–91%) depending on the Gleason pattern, and specificity (68–98%) depending on the Gleason pattern.

Table 1. Cont.

Study	Objective	Algorithm/Method	Study Design	Results
Ström et al. [29]	Detection and grading of prostate cancers in prostate biopsies	Deep neural networks	• 6953 prostate biopsy samples from 1063 patients for training • 1943 biopsy samples from 391 patients for evaluations	AUC-ROC of 0.997 in distinguishing the malignancy, comparable performance to expert pathologists in assigning Gleason grades.
Bulten et al. [30]	Detection and grading of prostate cancers in prostate biopsies	Multiparametric algorithms	• 10,616 digitized prostate biopsies	Agreements of 0.862 and 0.868 with expert uropathologists
Hartenstein et al. [31]	Prostate cancer nodal staging using CT imaging	Convolutional neural networks (CNNs)	• 2616 lymph node samples from 546 patients were segmented	AUC of 0.95 and 0.86 compared to an AUC of 0.81 for experienced radiologists
Green et al. [32]	Identification and validation new biomarkers	Artificial neural network (ANN)	• 192 tissue microarrays (TMA) constructed from transurethral resected prostatectomy histology samples	High Ki67 is predictive of reduced survival and increased risk of metastasis, independent of PSA and Gleason score. DLX2 shows increased metastasis risk and co-expression with a high Ki67 score
Calle et al. [33]	Automation analysis of biomarkers	Deep learning algorithm	• 648 samples of tissue microarrays (TMA)	5% variance compared to manually generated results; 100% accuracy in identifying positive tumors
Hou et al. [34]	Identification and validation of new biomarkers	Genetic algorithm-optimized artificial neural network (GA-ANN)	• Meta-analysis using RankProd from microarray data	AUC of 0.953 for diagnostic accuracy and AUC of 0.808 for prognostic capability
Auffenberg et al. [37]	Development of a web-based system to provide newly diagnosed men with predicted treatment decisions	Random forest ML model	• Registry data from 45 MUSIC urology practices from 2015 to 2017	AUC of 0.81 for personalized prediction
Lee et al. [38]	Prediction of late GU toxicity after prostate radiation therapy	Preconditioned random forest regression method	• 324 patients at 2 years post-radiation therapy	Accuracy—70%

4.2. Kidney Cancer

Renal cell carcinoma is a diverse group of cancers with various genetic and molecular alterations, including clear-cell, papillary, and chromophobe subtypes. Established risk factors include tobacco smoking, hypertension, and obesity. Renal carcinoma can often remain clinically silent until reaching an advanced stage. Classic symptoms, such as pain, haematuria, and flank mass, occur in only a small percentage of cases. Routine imaging has become instrumental in identifying renal cell carcinoma incidentally. The most crucial staging technique is computed tomography (CT) of the abdomen. Survival rates are more favorable when tumors are confined to the kidney. However, renal carcinoma is notoriously resistant to chemotherapy, making radical nephrectomy the standard treatment [43,44].

Machine learning models and deep learning algorithms are used to diagnose renal tumors, differentiate benign and malignant renal tumors, and differentiate renal cell carcinoma (RCC) types. Table 2 summarizes the research looking at applications of AI in kidney cancer.

Table 2. Studies looking at applications of AI in kidney cancer.

Study	Objective	Algorithm/Method	Study Design	Results
Santoni et al. [45]	Prediction of new cases of RCC	ANN	• Statistics on US population numbers	24.7% increase in new RCC cases, rising from 44,400 in 2020 to 55,400 in 2050
Houshyar et al. [46]	Development of a surgical planning aid	CNN	• CT images of 319 patients	Median Dice coefficients for kidney and tumor segmentation were 0.970 and 0.816, respectively.
Erdim et al. [47]	Distinguishing between benign and malignant solid renal masses	ML	• 21 patients with benign renal masses • 63 patients with malignant renal masses • 271 texture features extracted from CT images	Best predictive performance with an accuracy of 90.5% and an AUC of 0.915
Uhlig et al. [48]	Distinguishing between benign and malignant clinical T1 renal masses	Random forest algorithm	• 48 patients	AUC of 0.83 compared to radiologists' 0.68, sensitivity 0.88 vs. 0.80, $p = 0.045$, specificity 0.67 vs. 0.50, $p = 0.083$
Uhm et al. [49]	Differentiation of RCC types	DL	• Dataset of 1035 CT images from 308 patients containing five major types of renal tumors	AUC of 0.855, comparable diagnostic performance to that of radiologists
Nikpanah et al. [50]	Distinguishing clear cell renal cell carcinoma from renal oncocytoma	Deep neural network (AlexNet)	• 74 patients with 243 renal masses	Overall accuracy of 91% and an AUC of 0.9
Tabibu et al. [51]	Differentiation of RCC types	CNN	• Histopathological images from patients with RCC subtypes	Accuracy of 93.39% for distinguishing clear cell and chromophobe RCC from normal tissue; accuracy of 94.07% for distinguishing clear cell, chromophobe, and papillary RCC subtypes
Ding et al. [52]	Differentiation grade of ccRCC	CT-based radiomic models	• 14 patients with ccRCC who underwent partial or radical nephrectomy	AUC of 0.826, 0.878, and 0.843 for models 1, 2, and 3, respectively
Kocak et al. [53]	Detection PBRM1 mutations through CT texture analysis	ANN and RF	• 45 patients with clear-cell RCC, among whom 16 had the PBRM1 mutation	ANN algorithm's AUC of 0.925, RF algorithm's AUC of 0.987
Tian et al. [54]	Screening for kidney cancer prognosis biomarkers	RF	• Kidney cancer RNA sequencing data from the Gene Expression Omnibus (GEO) database	In tumor tissue, RNASET2 and FXYD5 were found to be highly expressed, while NAT8 was observed to be lowly expressed at both the protein and transcription levels
Buchner et al. [55]	Prediction of the metastatic RCC outcome	ANN	• 175 patient records with available follow-up data for a median of 36 months	95% overall accuracy, outperforming logistic regression models (78% accuracy)

Table 2. *Cont.*

Study	Objective	Algorithm/Method	Study Design	Results
Barkan et al. [56]	Predicting OS for mRCC patients	ML	• 322 patients	AUC of 0.786 for three-year OS and 0.771 for five-year OS

4.2.1. Prediction and Detection of Kidney Cancer

The incidence of kidney cancer is increasing every year. In 2020, the number of cases of RCC registered in the United States was 44,400. Researchers predict that, by 2050, the number of RCC cases will rise to 55,400. Consequently, several studies are attempting to counter this trend with new ways to predict and detect kidney cancer. Santoni et al. [45] attempted to implement an artificial neural network to predict new cases in the population. They used data such as population index, obesity, smoking prevalence, uncontrolled hypertension, and life expectancy data in the United States. The study involved collecting statistics on the US population and assessing how various factors affect the incidence of kidney cancer. MATLAB R2018 (MathWorks) software was used to implement an artificial neural network. As per the results, hypertension prevention has the greatest impact on reducing the incidence of kidney cancer. The study estimated that, by preventing hypertension, it will be possible to reduce the incidence of kidney cancer by 575 cases per year by 2030. Other factors had a more limited impact [45]. A group of researchers led by Houshyar [46] retrospectively analyzed CT images of 319 patients. They created two separate CNNs. The first CNN focused on localizing the bounding cube of the right and left kidney hemispheres, while the second CNN focused on segmenting the renal parenchyma and tumors within each cube. The performance of the CNNs was evaluated in a cohort of 269 patients. The median Sorensen-Dice coefficients for kidney and tumor segmentation were 0.970 and 0.816, respectively, indicating accurate delineation. Moreover, the Pearson correlation coefficients between the CNN-generated and human-annotated estimates of kidney and tumor volumes were 0.998 and 0.993, respectively ($p < 0.001$), confirming the reliability of the CNN approach.

These preliminary findings demonstrate the potential of automated deep learning AI techniques for rapid and precise segmentation of kidneys and renal tumors on single-phase contrast-enhanced CT scans. Additionally, CNNs can accurately calculate tumor and kidney volumes, offering valuable assistance in clinical practice [46].

4.2.2. Differentiation of Benign and Malignant Renal Tumors

Distinguishing between benign and malignant tumors is crucial, as benign tumors, like adiposarcoma (AML) and oncocytoma, are sometimes misclassified as RCC. This differentiation is essential to avoiding unnecessary medical procedures. Recent advancements in machine learning and deep learning using radiomics have shown promise in accurately differentiating these tumors [57]. Erdim et al. [47] conducted a study where they analyzed CT images of benign and malignant tumors, extracting texture features to create a predictive model with machine learning algorithms. The random forest algorithm, utilizing five selected contrast-enhanced CT texture features, demonstrated the best predictive performance with an accuracy of 90.5% and an area under the curve (AUC) of 0.915.

Another study by Uhlig et al. [48] compared the diagnostic accuracy of two experienced radiologists with the random forest algorithm in evaluating renal masses from CT imaging. The results showed that the random forest algorithm outperformed the radiologists in correctly identifying and classifying renal masses.

These findings highlight the potential of machine learning algorithms in accurately differentiating between benign and malignant renal tumors, providing valuable assistance in clinical decision-making, and optimizing patient care.

4.2.3. Differentiation of RCC Types

Radiomics analysis has led to the development of machine learning and deep learning models to distinguish between the five types of RCC, including oncocytoma, AML, clear cell RCC, papillary RCC, and chromophobe RCC. CT texture analysis is utilized by ML and DL algorithms to differentiate various renal masses [43–45]. ML and DL algorithms can predict nuclear class and identify specific genetic mutations, which affect the prediction of prognosis, recurrence, and survival outcomes [58].

In their study, Kocak et al. [59] used 275 textural features from CT images to predict and identify the nuclear class of ccRCC. The machine learning models performed well in differentiating different forms of renal cell carcinoma (RCC), but their identification of the three basic types was poor. SVM showed the highest predictive value for nuclear grades in ccRCC cases (85.1%). Cortico-subcortical CT images provided more texture parameters than nonenhanced images.

Uhm et al. [49] Uhm et al. developed a dataset of 1035 CT images from 308 patients containing five major types of renal tumors. They compared the diagnostic performance of their deep learning model with that of six radiologists. The AI outperformed radiologists in diagnosing most types of RCC and benign tumors, showing significantly better results in diagnosing oncocytoma and liposarcoma AML tumors. However, the results were similar for the diagnosis of clear-cell RCC.

Nikpanah et al. [50] conducted a retrospective study involving 74 patients with 243 renal masses to assess a deep convolutional neural network's diagnostic efficacy in distinguishing clear-cell renal cell carcinoma from renal oncocytoma. MR imaging was performed before pathologic confirmation, and a deep neural network (AlexNet) was fine-tuned for this task. The AI system achieved an overall accuracy of 91% and an area under the curve of 0.9 in distinguishing ccRCC from oncocytoma using fivefold cross-validation. Utilizing features extracted from 20,000 CT images, Pedersen et al. [60] created convolutional neural networks that exhibited a remarkable 93.3% accuracy and a specificity of 93.5% in effectively differentiating oncocytoma from RCC.

A group of researchers led by Tabibu et al. [51] conducted a study that explored the application of a deep learning method to identify and classify different RCC types, achieving an impressive classification accuracy of 94.07%. They introduced a novel support vector machine-based approach to enhance model performance in multiclass classification (pan-RCC), resulting in a remarkable 93% accuracy in cancer detection. Furthermore, the researchers utilized morphological features extracted from tumor regions identified by CNNs to predict survival outcomes for patients with the prevalent clear-cell RCC.

4.2.4. Differentiation Grade of Clear Renal Cell Carcinoma (Fuhrman Grade)

The Fuhrman grading system [61] evaluates nuclear size, shape, and nucleolar prominence, categorizing tumors into four nuclear grades (1–4) based on increasing testicular size, irregularity, and prominence. This grading system is a robust predictor of distant metastasis after nephrectomy. Metastasis rates correlate with nuclear grade, with grade 1 tumors exhibiting significantly lower rates compared to grades 2 to 4. Survival outcomes are also stratified into three categories: grade 1, grade 4, and grades 2 and 3.

Ding et al. [52] illustrated enhanced precision in staging the classification of clear cell renal cell carcinoma by preoperatively distinguishing between high-grade (Fuhrman III–IV) and low-grade (Fuhrman I–II) tumors. Their algorithm integration encompassed six key non-textural features: pseudocapsule, round mass, maximum tumor diameter (Diametermax), intracellular artery (Arteritumor), tumor enhancement value (TEV), and relative TEV (rTEV), alongside texture features. Extracted from CT images of the segment with the largest renal mass area in the corticospinal and nephrographic phases, these texture features underwent selection through the least absolute shrinkage and selection operator (LASSO) to calculate a texture score for each patient. In their approach, a logistic regression model utilizing three iterations—model 1 with all non-texture features, model 2 with all non-texture features and texture score, and model 3 with only texture score—distinguished high-grade ccRCC from low-grade ccRCC during nephrectomy. These models exhibited strong discrimination in the training cohort, yielding area under the receiver operating characteristic curve (AUC) values of 0.826, 0.878, and 0.843 for models 1, 2, and 3, respectively. Notably, a significant difference in AUC was observed between model 1 and model 2.

Tian et al. [62] developed a CAD system for Fuhrman classification in ccRCC using 395 whole-mount images. Their model, incorporating 26 features, predicted tumor grade with 84.6% sensitivity and 81.3% specificity. Their results were significantly related to overall survival. Holdbrook et al. [63] concentrated on nuclear pleomorphic patterns, creating a binary CAD system for renal cell carcinoma grading. This system demonstrated high accuracy (F-score = 0.78–0.83) and predicted survival with similar precision as an established scoring system based on multigene testing.

A different approach was shown by Wen-Zi [64]. The study utilized deep learning algorithms to predict the pathological staging and grading of tumors in 878 patients based on preoperative clinical variables. The proposed models, including BiLSTM, CNN-BiLSTM, and CNN-BiGRU, achieved impressive accuracy in predicting tumor pathological staging, with AUC values of 0.933, 0.947, and 0.948, respectively. For tumor pathological grading, the models yielded AUC values of 0.754, 0.720, and 0.770, respectively.

4.2.5. Genetic Mutation

Li et al. [65] harnessed gene expression, machine learning (utilizing random forest variable hunting), and Cox regression analysis to construct a risk score model based on 15 genes. This model aimed to predict the survival of ccRCC patients in the Cancer Genome Atlas dataset (N = 533). Remarkably, the higher-risk group demonstrated significantly worse prognosis and survival compared to the lower-risk group. A similar pattern was observed in recurrence-free survival. Interestingly, the risk scores were not correlated with patient characteristics such as gender or age but were linked to hemoglobin levels and tumor characteristics like size and grade. Notably, radiation therapy had no influence on the predictive value of the risk score. Multivariate Cox regression underlined the importance of the risk score as an indicator of prognosis in ccRCC. Ultimately, this risk score model, driven by the expression of 15 selected genes, exhibited the ability to predict the survival of ccRCC patients.

In their research, Kocak et al. [53] employed both an artificial neural network (ANN) algorithm and a random forest (RF) algorithm to detect PBRM1 mutations through CT texture analysis. The ANN demonstrated accurate identification of 88% of ccRCCs with a PBRM1 mutation status, while the RF algorithm showed even higher performance, correctly classifying 95.0% of ccRCCs with a PBRM1 mutation status.

Machine learning has demonstrated high accuracy in distinguishing CD117 (c-KIT) oncocytomas from the chromophobe subtype of renal cell carcinoma using the peak early enhancement rate (PEER), with a 95% accuracy for tumor type classification (100% sensitivity and 89% specificity) [66].

In their study, Tian et al. [54] investigated mRNA expression profiles in the GSE53757 dataset and their relation to the clinical prognosis of renal cell carcinoma. They developed a seven-gene independent prognostic model that showed significant correlations with the prognosis of renal cell carcinoma. The researchers carefully selected renal cancer differentiation genes from the dataset and performed functional enrichment analysis, revealing enriched biological functions related to catabolic processes of small molecules, T-cell activation, and other aspects.

Tian et al. [54] employed RF and SVM models to refine their prognostic model, identifying seven hub mRNAs through Cox LASSO analysis as robust predictors of kidney cancer prognosis. Subsequent measurement of these seven genes in kidney cancer and normal tissue pairs revealed higher expression of RNASET2 and FXYD5 in cancer tissue, while NAT8 exhibited relatively lower expression. However, no significant differences were observed in the expression of EZH2, KLF18A, CDCA7, or WNT7B between tumor tissue and adjacent tissue.

Tian et al. [54] utilized bioinformatics technology to integrate genomic data and identify differentially expressed genes (DEGs) associated with renal cell carcinoma prognosis. Their developed prognostic mRNA model outperformed single mRNA models, effectively distinguishing patients at high risk of recurrence from those at low risk. The model's prognostic performance remained independent of age and stage. The study suggests that a nomogram combining seven gene signatures can accurately depict the risk level and overall survival based on the patient's clinical stage, age, and other factors.

4.2.6. Treatment of Kidney Cancer

In 2003, Kattan et al. [67] published experiments with AI. The authors compared AI and Cox regression to predict disease recurrence after surgery. In their experiments, Cox regression models showed better performance. For kidney cancer, they used ANN and Cox regression to predict behavior (median accuracy of 71% for ANN and 75% for Cox). Khene and a group of collaborating researchers studied the response of patients to nivolumab therapy. Nivolumab serves as an effective immunotherapy with checkpoint inhibition in mRCC [68]. They showed that pretreatment imaging radiomics could accurately identify those responding to nivolumab. The model could achieve an accuracy of more than 90% in predicting treatment response [69]. Buchner et al. [55] examined the potential of AI in predicting the outcome of patients with metastatic renal cell carcinoma who were about to start systemic therapy. The AI model was trained using data from 175 patients who had undergone radical or partial nephrectomy of the primary tumor prior to commencing systemic therapy. The main objective was to predict overall survival at the 3-year mark based on parameters available at the initiation of first-line therapy. AI was able to achieve an accuracy of 95%.

The Barkan et al. [56] study aimed to assess the capabilities of emerging AI technologies in predicting three- and five-year overall survival (OS) for patients with advanced metastatic renal cell carcinoma (mRCC) undergoing their first-line systemic treatment. The retrospective analysis included 322 Italian patients treated between 2004 and 2019. An ensemble of three AI predictive models was developed, outperforming existing prognostic systems and providing better clinical support for decision-making. The model achieved high accuracy and specificity, with AUC values of 0.786 and 0.771 for 3-year OS and 5-year OS, respectively. The AI models demonstrate promising potential for enhancing patient management in mRCC treatment, but larger studies are needed to validate their effectiveness further.

The objective of Le et al.'s [70] study was to develop and validate predictive models using machine learning algorithms for patients with bone metastases (BM) from clear cell renal cell carcinoma (ccRCC) and to identify suitable models for clinical decision-making. The researchers obtained data from the Surveillance, Epidemiology, and End Results (SEER) database for 1490 ccRCC-BM patients and collected clinicopathological information for 42 patients at their hospital. Four ML algorithms (extreme gradient boosting, logistic regression, random forest, and Naive Bayes model) were employed to predict overall survival (OS) in ccRCC-BM patients. The patients were divided into training and validation cohorts for evaluation. The models performed well in predicting 1-year and 3-year OS, suggesting that ML can be a valuable tool in clinical decision-making for ccRCC-BM patients.

AI can also be used to assess recurrence risk following surgical resection of RCC. Khene et al.'s [71] study explored the effectiveness of machine learning models, including Random Survival Forests, Survival Support Vector Machines, and Extreme Gradient Boosting, in predicting recurrence after surgical resection of nonmetastatic renal cell carcinoma. Conducted across 21 French medical centers with over 4000 patients, the ML models outperformed traditional prognostic models in predicting disease-free survival. ML models demonstrated higher concordance index values, good calibration, and superior net benefit in decision curve analysis.

From this research, it can be concluded that artificial intelligence methods are futureproof. Tests using new technologies can, taking into account predisposing behavioral factors, not only detect the disease at an early stage but also help actively control predisposed individuals. Deep learning methods reduce the waiting time for histopathology results and can help differentiate types of kidney cancer. With the help of AI, it is possible to assess the response to gene therapy and, taking into account genetic mutations, to evaluate prognosis and survival time.

4.3. Bladder Cancer

Bladder cancer is a prevalent malignancy affecting both men and women, with the most common type being transitional cell carcinoma arising from urothelial cells in the bladder. Its primary symptoms include hematuria and lower urinary tract issues. Thanks to advanced imaging and diagnostic tools, bladder cancers are now more likely to be detected in their early stages. About 75% of cases are non-muscle-invasive and treated with transurethral resection of the tumor, while the remaining have invaded deeper layers or formed metastases, necessitating radical cystectomy [72–74].

4.3.1. Diagnosis

Cystoscopy is considered the gold standard for diagnosing and monitoring non-muscle-invasive bladder cancer (NMIBC). However, this procedure is not a perfect test. In addition to being user-dependent, white-light cystoscopy can also have various limitations; small tumors, carcinoma in situ, and other nonobvious lesions in certain anatomic locations can be easily missed. Due to the increasing number of different upgrades, such as blue-light cystoscopy (BLC) and artificial intelligence, the procedure is becoming more accurate [75].

Various researchers of AI methods have evaluated the effectiveness of machine learning in overcoming human mistakes and ensuring that diseases are not missed. Some of the main algorithms used to improve cystoscopic diagnosis in addition to survival and prognosis prediction in bladder cancer are convolutional neural networks (CNNs), multilayer perceptrons (MLPs), support vector machines (SVMs), and genetic algorithms (GAs). Ikeda et al. [76] aimed to support the cystoscopic diagnosis of bladder cancer using a convolutional neural network. They created a CNN-based tumor classification. The trained classifier dataset consisted of 2102 cystoscopic images (1671 images of normal tissue and 431 images of tumor lesions). Its effectiveness was evaluated using test data (87 tumor images and 335 normal images). In the result, 78 images were true positives, 315 were true negatives, 20 were false positives, and nine were false negatives (i.e., sensitivity was 89.7% and specificity was 94.0%). Eminaga et al. [77] applied the same kind of AI technology, creating various deep CNN models and assessing them using the F1-score. The greatest F1-score, 99.52%, was obtained for the XCeption-based model. Other models that could identify all cystoscopic images with bladder were based on ResNet50 and the harmonic series concept, which achieved F1-scores of 99.48% and 99.45%, respectively.

The multilayer perceptron (MLP)-based method, presented by Lorencin et al. [78], uses image resizing and a Laplacian edge detector for the preprocessing of input images. The method provides an alternative strategy for diagnosing bladder cancer. AI was trained with the data of 1997 and 986 images with and without bladder cancer, respectively. Results were encouraging, with an AUC value of up to 0.99. Hashemi et al. [79] applied the local binary pattern (LBP) method to extract the features in bladder cystoscopy images. Then, they used the MLP neural network to train and evaluate the classifier for images from a bladder cystoscopy. In order to enhance the performance of this method, the researchers applied an adaptive learning rate and a genetic algorithm. The simulated results revealed a significant 7% reduction in error and improved convergence speed compared to other competing methods. The findings underscore the immense potential of deep learning for accurately diagnosing cystoscopic images.

4.3.2. Metastasis Detection

A particularly important thing in determining the patient's condition is to confirm the presence of metastases in the lymph nodes. In Gresser et al.'s [80] study, a radiomics signature was developed using machine learning to detect lymph node metastases in bladder cancer patients who underwent radical cystectomy with lymphadenectomy. Out of 1354 patients screened, 391 with pathological nodal staging were included and divided into training and test cohorts. Radiomics features were extracted from each lymph node, and an ML model was trained using histopathology labels. Manual and automated lymph node segmentations were compared to radiologist assessments for detecting metastases. The results showed that the radiomics-based analysis using manual lymph node segmentation achieved an AUC of 0.80, while the fully automated approach achieved an AUC of 0.70. Combining the manually segmented radiomic signature with radiologist assessment improved the AUC to 0.81.

In Wu et al.'s [81] study, researchers developed a lymph node metastases diagnostic model (LNMDM) using whole slide images and assessed the clinical impact of an artificial intelligence-assisted (AI) workflow. The LNMDM was developed using data from 998 bladder cancer patients who underwent radical cystectomy and pelvic lymph node dissection. The model demonstrated high diagnostic sensitivity, with an area under the curve (AUC) ranging from 0.978 to 0.998 in five internal validation sets. Comparisons between the LNMDM and pathologists showed that the model outperformed both junior and senior pathologists in detecting lymph node metastases. AI assistance improved sensitivity for pathologists, enhancing diagnostic accuracy. Notably, the model identified tumor micrometastases that had been missed by pathologists in some cases.

Another study [82] aimed to develop and validate a machine-learning-based approach using [^{18}F]FDG PET/CT criteria to accurately identify pelvic lymph node involvement in patients with muscle-invasive bladder cancer (MIBC). The study consisted of 173 patients. The developed machine-learning-based combination of criteria, which included features from pelvic lymph nodes and the primary bladder tumor, showed comparable diagnostic performance (AUC = 0.59) to the consensus of experts (AUC = 0.64) in the validation set. The interrater agreement was also good (K = 0.66) for both the machine-learning approach and the experts.

4.3.3. Prediction and Prognosis

Machine learning algorithms can be used to improve more than just cystoscopy. The other aspects of bladder urooncology where artificial intelligence may be employed are the prediction and prognosis of mortality, postcystectomy recurrence and survival, and therapy response. Deep learning systems (DLSs) are also being developed for clinical cytology in order to detect the malignant potential of urothelial carcinoma cells.

Wang et al. [83] employed a least squares support vector machine (SVM) to predict the 5-year overall and cancer-specific mortality of patients who underwent radical cystectomy. The model achieved an accuracy of over 75% in this prognostic prediction. [4]. To predict the prognosis over the next 5 years using various combinations of image, clinical, and spatial features, Gavriel et al. [84] proposed an ensemble system that consists of ML-based algorithms. The method demonstrated a 71.4% accuracy in correctly identifying patients who experienced unfavorable outcomes and succumbed to muscle-invasive bladder cancer (MIBC) within a 5-year timeframe. This value is impressive considering that it is significantly higher than the 28.6% of the TNM staging system, the current clinical gold standard.

4.3.4. Disease Progression and Chemotherapy Efficacy

ML-based algorithms and models have been used in several articles to identify genes that can potentially foretell the recurrence or future progression of disease. Slides from patients with MIBC were marked with immunofluorescence (IF) and then applied to measure the tumor buds. In this way, the efficacy of neoadjuvant chemotherapy was evaluated, and the patients who did not respond to the therapy were identified, with the aim being to stop the treatment midway in such patients to avoid the harmful effects of chemotherapy [4,85–87]. Nojima et al. [88] developed a DLS to detect high-grade urothelial carcinoma (HGUC) cells in urine cytology specimens using a pretrained VGG16 model. The DLS demonstrated exceptional performance when trained on high-power field images of both malignant and benign cases. It accurately diagnosed invasive UC lesions with an AUC of 0.8628 and an F1-score of 0.8239. Moreover, it successfully identified high-grade UC lesions with an AUC of 0.8661 and an F1-score of 0.8218.

The results indicated that the DLS exhibited the potential to more accurately determine the malignant potential of tumors compared to classical cytology. Considering this possibility, along with improvements in prognosis and prediction, urologists may be better able to develop therapeutic strategies that will ultimately benefit patients.

Table 3 summarizes the studies examining the use of AI in bladder cancer.

Table 3. Studies looking at applications of AI in bladder cancer.

Study	Objective	Algorithm/Method	Study Design	Results
Ikeda et al. [76]	Improvement of the quality of bladder cancer diagnosis by supporting cystoscopic diagnosis using AI	Convolutional neural network (CNN)	• 1671 cystoscopic images of normal tissue • 431 cystoscopic images of tumor lesions	AUC-ROC of 0.98 in distinguishing normal and tumor tissue
Eminaga et al. [77]	Exploration of the potential of AI for the diagnostic classification of cystoscopic images	Convolutional neural network (CNN)	• 18,681 cystoscopic images from 479 patients	CNN achieved F1 scores of 99.52%, 99.48%, and 99.45%
Lorencin et al. [78]	Investigation of the MLP implementation possibility for the detection of urinary bladder cancer	Multi-Layer Perceptron (MLP)	• 1997 images of bladder cancer • 986 images of noncancer tissue	AUC of up to 0.99
Wu et al. [81]	Development of LNMDM	(AI-assisted workflow	• 998 patients	AUC from 0.978 to 0.998
Girard et al. [82]	Developing criteria to identify pelvic lymph node involvement in MIBC patients	ML-based combination of criteria	• 129 MIBC patients for training • 44 patients for test	AUC of 0.59 in diagnostic performance compared to the experts (AUC = 0.64)
Gavriel et al. [84]	Development of an AI tool for predicting the 5-year prognosis of MIBC patients	ML-based algorithms	• 78 patients	71.4% accuracy in classification of patients who succumbed to MIBC
Nojima et al. [88]	Developing DLS as a diagnosis support tool for clinical cytology in urinary cytology	Deep Learning System (DLS)	• Cytology images from Papanicolaou-stained urinary cytology glass slides obtained from 232 patients.	AUC of 0.9890 and an F1 score of 0.9002

4.4. Upper Tract Urothelial Carcinoma (UTUC)

Upper tract urothelial cancer (UTUC), a specific type of urothelial cancer, occurs in the ureter and renal pelvis. It is a relatively rare cancer, accounting for 5–10% of all urothelial carcinomas. A significant number of UTUC tumors are invasive at the time of diagnosis, and the 5-year cancer-specific survival rates for advanced stages are low. The standard treatment for high-risk UTUC is radical nephroureterectomy (RNU) with bladder-cuff removal. However, kidney-sparing surgery (KSS) is gaining popularity to preserve renal function, akin to managing parenchymal renal cancer. Neoadjuvant chemotherapy shows potential benefits for high-risk UTUC patients [89].

Currently, the gold standard for UTUC diagnosis and conservative treatment is flexible ureteroscopy (URS). URS allows for a thorough examination of the urinary system tissue, identification of tumors, assessment of their size, and biopsy of suspicious lesions [90]. The procedure is performed with the assistance of an endoscopic camera to provide visual guidance [91].

Similar to other endoscopic procedures, in this procedure, too, artificial intelligence can be used to enhance the outcomes.

Primary research on this subject, presented by Lazo et al. [92], provided an automated method based on convolutional neural networks to produce an accurate segmentation of the hollow lumen. The described method included an ensemble of four parallel CNNs (U-Net-based, Mask-RCNN, and two modifications of the former ones) to process both single-frame and multi-frame data simultaneously. Using a unique dataset of 11 recordings (2673 frames) that were gathered from six patients and manually annotated, they evaluated the proposed method, which outperformed earlier state-of-the-art techniques with an F1-score of 80%. Although the results demonstrated that the ensemble model may successfully enhance hollow lumen segmentation in ureteroscopic images, the development of the submitted method might further the UTUC finding, particularly if it works effectively even when there is limited visibility, occasional bleeding, or specular reflections.

4.5. Testicular Tumors

Testicular cancer is a prevalent solid malignancy affecting young adult men, and its occurrence has been on the rise globally. Testicular cancer accounts for about 1% of newly diagnosed cancers in men globally and is most common in men aged 14 to 44 in Western countries. Cryptorchidism, a birth defect where one or both testicles are not in the scrotum, is a significant risk factor for testicular cancer, increasing the risk nearly fivefold. Other potential risk factors include hypospadias and a low sperm count. The precursor lesion to malignant testicular germ cell tumors is germ cell neoplasia in situ (GCNIS). Germ cell tumors (GCT) constitute the majority of testicular cancers and are divided into seminoma and nonseminoma subtypes. Seminomas are homogeneous tumors of embryonic germ cells, while nonseminomas comprise various histologic subtypes. Advances in testicular cancer management have led to remarkable success, with a cure rate exceeding 70% for the first metastatic solid tumor [93,94].

Lymphovascular invasion (LVI) holds significant prognostic value, particularly in stage 1 non-seminomatous tumors and germ cell tumors of the testis. LVI refers to tumors found within endothelium-lined lymphatic or vascular channels. To automate the identification of suspected LVI areas in digital whole-slide images of testicular tumors, Ghosh et al. [95] developed an artificial intelligence algorithm using deep learning. They trained the algorithm with 184 histology slides stained with hematoxylin and eosin (H&E) from 19 patients with testicular germ cell tumors. The algorithm successfully identified areas of potential LVI in a validation set of 118 whole-slide images from 10 patients, with a precision of 0.68 for suitable areas and 0.56 for definite LVI areas. This proof-of-concept study demonstrates the feasibility of an artificial intelligence tool that aids reporting pathologists in highlighting areas for potential LVI assessment [95].

Distant metastasis in testicular cancer patients, beyond non-regional lymph nodes and lungs, presents a significant concern. Ding et al. addressed this issue by developing a machine learning (ML) algorithm to predict the risk of patients with germ cell testicular cancer (GCTC) progressing to the M1b stage, enabling early intervention. The predictive model was constructed using data from 4323 GCTC patients obtained from the Surveillance, Epidemiology, and End Results (SEER) database. Six ML algorithms were utilized to build the model, demonstrating high accuracy, stability, and computational efficiency. These promising results have valuable implications for clinical decision-making and provide a potential tool for timely interventions in GCTC patients [96].

Linder et al. [97] developed a deep learning approach to identify and count tumor-infiltrating lymphocytes (TILs) in primary testicular cancer patients. They analyzed H&E-stained whole slides from 113 patients and found a significant association between low TIL numbers and disease recurrence. A higher TIL density was correlated with a lower clinical tumor stage, seminoma histology, and absence of lymphovascular invasion at presentation.

Baessler et al. [98] used ML-based CT radiomics to distinguish between malignant and benign lymph nodes in patients with retroperitoneal LN metastases from NSTGCT, aiming to reduce overtreatment in young patients. The model achieved an accuracy of 81%, a sensitivity of 88%, and a specificity of 72%.

Another study [99] compared custom-designed and commercial ANNs for staging testicular cancer using pathological parameters. The custom ANN outperformed the commercial ANN (92% vs. 80% accuracy), highlighting the importance of individual network refinement by investigators, which currently limits widespread commercial adoption of these methods.

5. Conclusions

Less than 20 years after the dawn of computing, AI has been applied to clinical decision-making. However, only recently, with the development of machine learning, has it been integrated into clinical practice. AI methods for analyzing big data cohorts seem more precise and exploratory than conventional regression statistics. Additionally, they provide specific health behavior predictions. Each artificial intelligence method has features that make it effective for various tasks. Understanding the basics of AI approaches and their potential, especially the flexibility of certain systems, will enable these innovative methods to be developed further and play a significant role in urologists' work with patients with cancer.

Author Contributions: Conceptualization, B.M. and A.F.; methodology, B.M., A.F. and W.K.; validation, A.F., A.S. (Alina Semianiuk) and U.L.; formal analysis, A.F., A.S. (Alina Semianiuk), U.L. and A.L.; investigation, A.F., A.S. (Alina Semianiuk) and U.L.; writing—original draft preparation, A.F., A.S. (Alina Semianiuk) and U.L.; writing—review and editing, B.M., A.S. (Agnieszka Siennicka) and K.P.; visualization, A.F. and A.S. (Alina Semianiuk); supervision, T.S. and B.M.; project administration, B.M. All authors have read and agreed to the published version of the manuscript.

Funding: This research received no external funding.

Institutional Review Board Statement: Not applicable.

Informed Consent Statement: Not applicable.

Data Availability Statement: The data can be shared up on request.

Conflicts of Interest: The authors declare no conflict of interest.

References

1. Hamet, P.; Tremblay, J. Artificial intelligence in medicine. *Metabolism* **2017**, *69*, S36–S40. [CrossRef] [PubMed]
2. van der Laak, J.; Litjens, G.; Ciompi, F. Deep learning in histopathology: The path to the clinic. *Nat. Med.* **2021**, *27*, 775–784. [CrossRef] [PubMed]
3. Pantanowitz, L.; Quiroga-Garza, G.M.; Bien, L.; Heled, R.; Laifenfeld, D.; Linhart, C.; Sandbank, J.; Shach, A.A.; Shalev, V.; Vecsler, M.; et al. An artificial intelligence algorithm for prostate cancer diagnosis in whole slide images of core needle biopsies: A blinded clinical validation and deployment study. *Lancet Digit. Health* **2020**, *2*, e407–e416. [CrossRef] [PubMed]
4. Shah, M.; Naik, N.; Somani, B.K.; Hameed, B.Z. Artificial intelligence (AI) in urology-Current use and future directions: An iTRUE study. *Turk. J. Urol.* **2020**, *46*, S27–S39. [CrossRef] [PubMed]
5. Rodrigues, J.A.; Krois, J.; Schwendicke, F. Demystifying artificial intelligence and deep learning in dentistry. *Braz. Oral Res.* **2021**, *35*, e094. [CrossRef] [PubMed]
6. Chen, Z.; Lin, L.; Wu, C.; Li, C.; Xu, R.; Sun, Y. Artificial intelligence for assisting cancer diagnosis and treatment in the era of precision medicine. *Cancer Commun.* **2021**, *41*, 1100–1115. [CrossRef]

7. Gruson, D.; Helleputte, T.; Rousseau, P.; Gruson, D. Data science, artificial intelligence, and machine learning: Opportunities for laboratory medicine and the value of positive regulation. *Clin. Biochem.* **2019**, *69*, 1–7. [CrossRef]
8. Shimizu, H.; Nakayama, K.I. Artificial intelligence in oncology. *Cancer Sci.* **2020**, *111*, 1452–1460. [CrossRef]
9. Tran, K.A.; Kondrashova, O.; Bradley, A.; Williams, E.D.; Pearson, J.V.; Waddell, N. Deep learning in cancer diagnosis, prognosis and treatment selection. *Genome Med.* **2021**, *13*, 1–17. [CrossRef]
10. Ramesh, A.; Kambhampati, C.; Monson, J.; Drew, P. Artificial intelligence in medicine. *Ann. R Coll. Surg. Engl.* **2004**, *86*, 334. [CrossRef]
11. Eraslan, G.; Avsec, Ž.; Gagneur, J.; Theis, F.J. Deep learning: New computational modelling techniques for genomics. *Nat. Rev. Genet.* **2019**, *20*, 389–403. [CrossRef] [PubMed]
12. LeCun, Y.; Bengio, Y.; Hinton, G. Deep learning. *Nature* **2015**, *521*, 436–444. [CrossRef] [PubMed]
13. Dias, R.; Torkamani, A. Artificial intelligence in clinical and genomic diagnostics. *Genome Med.* **2019**, *11*, 1–12. [CrossRef] [PubMed]
14. Massion, P.P.; Antic, S.; Ather, S.; Arteta, C.; Brabec, J.; Chen, H.; Declerck, J.; Dufek, D.; Hickes, W.; Kadir, T.; et al. Assessing the Accuracy of a Deep Learning Method to Risk Stratify Indeterminate Pulmonary Nodules. *Am. J. Respir. Crit. Care Med.* **2020**, *202*, 241–249. [CrossRef] [PubMed]
15. Kanan, C.; Sue, J.; Grady, L.; Fuchs, T.J.; Chandarlapaty, S.; Reis-Filho, J.S.O.; Salles, P.G.; da Silva, L.M.; Gil Ferreira, C.; Pereira, E.M. Independent validation of paige prostate: Assessing clinical benefit of an artificial intelligence tool within a digital diagnostic pathology laboratory workflow. *J. Clin. Oncol.* **2020**, *38*, e14076. [CrossRef]
16. Bitterman, D.S.; Miller, T.A.; Mak, R.H.; Savova, G.K. Clinical Natural Language Processing for Radiation Oncology: A Review and Practical Primer. *Int. J. Radiat. Oncol. Biol. Phys.* **2021**, *110*, 641–655. [CrossRef]
17. Wasim, S.; Lee, S.-Y.; Kim, J. Complexities of Prostate Cancer. *Int. J. Mol. Sci.* **2022**, *23*, 14257. [CrossRef]
18. Sekhoacha, M.; Riet, K.; Motloung, P.; Gumenku, L.; Adegoke, A.; Mashele, S. Prostate Cancer Review: Genetics, Diagnosis, Treatment Options, and Alternative Approaches. *Molecules* **2022**, *27*, 5730. [CrossRef]
19. Eggener, S. Prostate Cancer. *Sci. World J.* **2011**, *11*, 749–750. [CrossRef]
20. Schatten, H. Brief Overview of Prostate Cancer Statistics, Grading, Diagnosis and Treatment Strategies. *Adv. Exp. Med. Biol.* **2018**, *1095*, 1–14. [CrossRef]
21. Cao, R.; Zhong, X.; Afshari, S.; Felker, E.; Suvannarerg, V.; Tubtawee, T.; Vangala, S.; Scalzo, F.; Raman, S.; Sung, K. Performance of Deep Learning and Genitourinary Radiologists in Detection of Prostate Cancer Using 3-T Multiparametric Magnetic Resonance Imaging. *J. Magn. Reson. Imaging* **2021**, *54*, 474–483. [CrossRef] [PubMed]
22. Giannini, V.; Mazzetti, S.; Vignati, A.; Russo, F.; Bollito, E.; Porpiglia, F.; Stasi, M.; Regge, D. A fully automatic computer aided diagnosis system for peripheral zone prostate cancer detection using multi-parametric magnetic resonance imaging. *Comput. Med. Imaging Graph.* **2015**, *46*, 219–226. [CrossRef] [PubMed]
23. Gaur, S.; Lay, N.; Harmon, S.A.; Doddakashi, S.; Mehralivand, S.; Argun, B.; Barrett, T.; Bednarova, S.; Girometti, R.; Karaarslan, E.; et al. Can computer-aided diagnosis assist in the identification of prostate cancer on prostate MRI? a multi-center, multi-reader investigation. *Oncotarget* **2018**, *9*, 33804–33817. [CrossRef]
24. Wang, X.; Xie, Y.; Zheng, X.; Liu, B.; Chen, H.; Li, J.; Ma, X.; Xiang, J.; Weng, G.; Zhu, W.; et al. A prospective multi-center randomized comparative trial evaluating outcomes of transrectal ultrasound (TRUS)-guided 12-core systematic biopsy, mpMRI-targeted 12-core biopsy, and artificial intelligence ultrasound of prostate (AIUSP) 6-core targeted biopsy for prostate cancer diagnosis. *World J. Urol.* **2022**, *41*, 653–662. [CrossRef]
25. Stojadinović, M.M.; Stojadinović, M.M.; Pantić, D.N. Decision tree analysis for prostate cancer prediction. *Srp. Arh. Celok. Lek.* **2019**, *147*, 52–58. [CrossRef]
26. Wildeboer, R.R.; van Sloun, R.J.; Wijkstra, H.; Mischi, M. Artificial intelligence in multiparametric prostate cancer imaging with focus on deep-learning methods. *Comput. Methods Programs Biomed.* **2020**, *189*, 105316. [CrossRef] [PubMed]
27. Viswanath, S.E.; Chirra, P.V.; Yim, M.C.; Rofsky, N.M.; Purysko, A.S.; Rosen, M.A.; Bloch, B.N.; Madabhushi, A. Comparing radiomic classifiers and classifier ensembles for detection of peripheral zone prostate tumors on T2-weighted MRI: A multi-site study. *BMC Med. Imaging* **2019**, *19*, 1–12. [CrossRef]
28. Marginean, F.; Arvidsson, I.; Simoulis, A.; Overgaard, N.C.; Åström, K.; Heyden, A.; Bjartell, A.; Krzyzanowska, A. An Artificial Intelligence–based Support Tool for Automation and Standardisation of Gleason Grading in Prostate Biopsies. *Eur. Urol. Focus* **2021**, *7*, 995–1001. [CrossRef]
29. Ström, P.; Kartasalo, K.; Olsson, H.; Solorzano, L.; Delahunt, B.; Berney, D.M.; Bostwick, D.G.; Evans, A.J.; Grignon, D.J.; Humphrey, P.A.; et al. Artificial intelligence for diagnosis and grading of prostate cancer in biopsies: A population-based, diagnostic study. *Lancet Oncol.* **2020**, *21*, 222–232. [CrossRef]
30. Bulten, W.; Kartasalo, K.; Chen, P.-H.C.; Ström, P.; Pinckaers, H.; Nagpal, K.; Cai, Y.; Steiner, D.F.; van Boven, H.; Vink, R.; et al. Artificial intelligence for diagnosis and Gleason grading of prostate cancer: The PANDA challenge. *Nat. Med.* **2022**, *28*, 154–163. [CrossRef]
31. Hartenstein, A.; Lübbe, F.; Baur, A.D.J.; Rudolph, M.M.; Furth, C.; Brenner, W.; Amthauer, H.; Hamm, B.; Makowski, M.; Penzkofer, T. Prostate Cancer Nodal Staging: Using Deep Learning to Predict 68Ga-PSMA-Positivity from CT Imaging Alone. *Sci. Rep.* **2020**, *10*, 3398. [CrossRef] [PubMed]

32. Green, W.J.; Ball, G.; Hulman, G.; Johnson, C.; Van Schalwyk, G.; Ratan, H.L.; Soria, D.; Garibaldi, J.M.; Parkinson, R.; Hulman, J.; et al. KI67 and DLX2 predict increased risk of metastasis formation in prostate cancer–a targeted molecular approach. *Br. J. Cancer* **2016**, *115*, 236–242. [CrossRef]
33. de la Calle, C.M.; Nguyen, H.G.; Hosseini-Asl, E.; So, C.; Socher, R.; Xiong, C.; Xue, L.; Carroll, P.; Cooperberg, M.R. Artificial intelligence for streamlined immunofluorescence-based biomarker discovery in prostate cancer. *J. Clin. Oncol.* **2020**, *38*, 279. [CrossRef]
34. Hou, Q.; Bing, Z.-T.; Hu, C.; Li, M.-Y.; Yang, K.-H.; Mo, Z.; Xie, X.-W.; Liao, J.-L.; Lu, Y.; Horie, S.; et al. RankProd Combined with Genetic Algorithm Optimized Artificial Neural Network Establishes a Diagnostic and Prognostic Prediction Model that Revealed C1QTNF3 as a Biomarker for Prostate Cancer. *EBioMedicine* **2018**, *32*, 234–244. [CrossRef]
35. Kim, Y.; Jeon, J.; Mejia, S.; Yao, C.Q.; Ignatchenko, V.; Nyalwidhe, J.O.; Gramolini, A.O.; Lance, R.S.; Troyer, D.A.; Drake, R.R.; et al. Targeted proteomics identifies liquid-biopsy signatures for extracapsular prostate cancer. *Nat. Commun.* **2016**, *7*, 11906. [CrossRef]
36. Bibault, J.; Xing, L. Predicting Survival in Prostate Cancer Patients with Interpretable Artificial Intelligence. *SSRN Electron. J.* **2020**. [CrossRef]
37. Auffenberg, G.B.; Ghani, K.R.; Ramani, S.; Usoro, E.; Denton, B.; Rogers, C.; Stockton, B.; Miller, D.C.; Singh, K. askMUSIC: Leveraging a Clinical Registry to Develop a New Machine Learning Model to Inform Patients of Prostate Cancer Treatments Chosen by Similar Men. *Eur. Urol.* **2018**, *75*, 901–907. [CrossRef]
38. Lee, S.; Kerns, S.; Ostrer, H.; Rosenstein, B.; Deasy, J.O.; Oh, J.H. Machine Learning on a Genome-wide Association Study to Predict Late Genitourinary Toxicity After Prostate Radiation Therapy. *Int. J. Radiat. Oncol. Biol. Phys.* **2018**, *101*, 128–135. [CrossRef] [PubMed]
39. Chrystall, D.M.; Mylonas, A.; Hewson, E.; Martin, J.; Keall, P.J.; Booth, J.T.; Nguyen, D.T. Deep learning enables MV-based real-time image guided radiation therapy for prostate cancer patients. *Phys. Med. Biol.* **2023**, *68*, 095016. [CrossRef]
40. Nicolae, A.; Semple, M.; Lu, L.; Smith, M.; Chung, H.; Loblaw, A.; Morton, G.; Mendez, L.C.; Tseng, C.-L.; Davidson, M.; et al. Conventional vs machine learning–based treatment planning in prostate brachytherapy: Results of a Phase I randomized controlled trial. *Brachytherapy* **2020**, *19*, 470–476. [CrossRef]
41. Deng, K.; Li, H.; Guan, Y. Treatment Stratification of Patients with Metastatic Castration-Resistant Prostate Cancer by Machine Learning. *iScience* **2020**, *23*, 100804. [CrossRef]
42. Wildeboer, R.R.; Mannaerts, C.K.; van Sloun, R.J.; Budaus, L.; Tilki, D.; Wijkstra, H.; Salomon, G.; Mischi, M. Automated multiparametric localization of prostate cancer based on B-mode, shear-wave elastography, and contrast-enhanced ultrasound radiomics. *Eur. Radiol.* **2020**, *30*, 806–815. [CrossRef]
43. Corgna, E.; Betti, M.; Gatta, G.; Roila, F.; De Mulder, P.H. Renal cancer. *Crit. Rev. Oncol. Hematol.* **2007**, *64*, 247–262. [CrossRef]
44. Capitanio, U.; Montorsi, F. Renal cancer. *Lancet* **2016**, *387*, 894–906. [CrossRef] [PubMed]
45. Santoni, M.; Piva, F.; Porta, C.; Bracarda, S.; Heng, D.Y.; Matrana, M.R.; Grande, E.; Mollica, V.; Aurilio, G.; Rizzo, M.; et al. Artificial Neural Networks as a Way to Predict Future Kidney Cancer Incidence in the United States. *Clin. Genitourin. Cancer* **2020**, *19*, e84–e91. [CrossRef]
46. Houshyar, R.; Glavis-Bloom, J.; Bui, T.-L.; Chahine, C.; Bardis, M.D.; Ushinsky, A.; Liu, H.; Bhatter, P.; Lebby, E.; Fujimoto, D.; et al. Outcomes of Artificial Intelligence Volumetric Assessment of Kidneys and Renal Tumors for Preoperative Assessment of Nephron-Sparing Interventions. *J. Endourol.* **2021**, *35*, 1411–1418. [CrossRef]
47. Erdim, C.; Yardimci, A.H.; Bektas, C.T.; Kocak, B.; Koca, S.B.; Demir, H.; Kilickesmez, O. Prediction of Benign and Malignant Solid Renal Masses: Machine Learning-Based CT Texture Analysis. *Acad. Radiol.* **2020**, *27*, 1422–1429. [CrossRef]
48. Uhlig, J.; Biggemann, L.; Nietert, M.M.; Beißbarth, T.; Lotz, J.; Kim, H.S.; Trojan, L.; Uhlig, A. Discriminating malignant and benign clinical T1 renal masses on computed tomography: A pragmatic radiomics and machine learning approach. *Medicine* **2020**, *99*, e19725. [CrossRef] [PubMed]
49. Uhm, K.-H.; Jung, S.-W.; Choi, M.H.; Shin, H.-K.; Yoo, J.-I.; Oh, S.W.; Kim, J.Y.; Kim, H.G.; Lee, Y.J.; Youn, S.Y.; et al. Deep learning for end-to-end kidney cancer diagnosis on multi-phase abdominal computed tomography. *npj Precis. Oncol.* **2021**, *5*, 1–6. [CrossRef]
50. Nikpanah, M.; Xu, Z.; Jin, D.; Farhadi, F.; Saboury, B.; Ball, M.W.; Gautam, R.; Merino, M.J.; Wood, B.J.; Turkbey, B.; et al. A deep-learning based artificial intelligence (AI) approach for differentiation of clear cell renal cell carcinoma from oncocytoma on multi-phasic MRI. *Clin Imaging.* **2021**, *77*, 291–298. [CrossRef] [PubMed]
51. Tabibu, S.; Vinod, P.K.; Jawahar, C.V. Pan-Renal Cell Carcinoma classification and survival prediction from histopathology images using deep learning. *Sci. Rep.* **2019**, *9*, 1–9. [CrossRef] [PubMed]
52. Ding, J.; Xing, Z.; Jiang, Z.; Chen, J.; Pan, L.; Qiu, J.; Xing, W. CT-based radiomic model predicts high grade of clear cell renal cell carcinoma. *Eur. J. Radiol.* **2018**, *103*, 51–56. [CrossRef] [PubMed]
53. Kocak, B.; Durmaz, E.S.; Ates, E.; Ulusan, M.B. Radiogenomics in Clear Cell Renal Cell Carcinoma: Machine Learning–Based High-Dimensional Quantitative CT Texture Analysis in Predicting PBRM1 Mutation Status. *Am. J. Roentgenol.* **2019**, *212*, W55–W63. [CrossRef]
54. Tian, M.; Wang, T.; Wang, P. Development and Clinical Validation of a Seven-Gene Prognostic Signature Based on Multiple Machine Learning Algorithms in Kidney Cancer. *Cell Transplant.* **2021**, *30*. [CrossRef]

55. Buchner, A.; Kendlbacher, M.; Nuhn, P.; Tüllmann, C.; Haseke, N.; Stief, C.G.; Staehler, M. Outcome Assessment of Patients with Metastatic Renal Cell Carcinoma Under Systemic Therapy Using Artificial Neural Networks. *Clin. Genitourin. Cancer* **2012**, *10*, 37–42. [CrossRef]
56. Barkan, E.; Porta, C.; Rabinovici-Cohen, S.; Tibollo, V.; Quaglini, S.; Rizzo, M. Artificial intelligence-based prediction of overall survival in metastatic renal cell carcinoma. *Front. Oncol.* **2023**, *13*, 1021684. [CrossRef] [PubMed]
57. Lambin, P.; Leijenaar, R.T.H.; Deist, T.M.; Peerlings, J.; de Jong, E.E.C.; van Timmeren, J.; Sanduleanu, S.; Larue, R.T.H.M.; Even, A.J.G.; Jochems, A.; et al. Radiomics: The bridge between medical imaging and personalized medicine. *Nat. Rev. Clin. Oncol.* **2017**, *14*, 749–762. [CrossRef] [PubMed]
58. Kim, H.; Hong, S.-H. Use of artificial intelligence to characterize renal tumors. *Investig. Clin. Urol.* **2022**, *63*, 123–125. [CrossRef] [PubMed]
59. Kocak, B.; Yardimci, A.H.; Bektas, C.T.; Turkcanoglu, M.H.; Erdim, C.; Yucetas, U.; Koca, S.B.; Kilickesmez, O. Textural differences between renal cell carcinoma subtypes: Machine learning-based quantitative computed tomography texture analysis with independent external validation. *Eur. J. Radiol.* **2018**, *107*, 149–157. [CrossRef]
60. Pedersen, M.; Andersen, M.B.; Christiansen, H.; Azawi, N.H. Classification of renal tumour using convolutional neural networks to detect oncocytoma. *Eur. J. Radiol.* **2020**, *133*, 109343. [CrossRef]
61. Fuhrman, S.A.; Lasky, L.C.; Limas, C. Prognostic significance of morphologic parameters in renal cell carcinoma. *Am. J. Surg. Pathol.* **1982**, *6*, 655–664. [CrossRef]
62. Tian, K.; Rubadue, C.A.; Lin, D.I.; Veta, M.; Pyle, M.E.; Irshad, H.; Heng, Y.J. Automated clear cell renal carcinoma grade classification with prognostic significance. *PLoS ONE* **2019**, *14*, e0222641. [CrossRef] [PubMed]
63. Holdbrook, D.A.; Singh, M.; Choudhury, Y.; Kalaw, E.M.; Koh, V.; Tan, H.S.; Kanesvaran, R.; Tan, P.H.; Peng, J.Y.S.; Tan, M.-H.; et al. Automated Renal Cancer Grading Using Nuclear Pleomorphic Patterns. *JCO Clin. Cancer Inform.* **2018**, *2*, 1–12. [CrossRef]
64. Wen-Zhi, G.; Tai, T.; Zhixin, F.; Huanyu, L.; Yanqing, G.; Yuexian, G.; Xuesong, L. Prediction of pathological staging and grading of renal clear cell carcinoma based on deep learning algorithms. *J. Int. Med Res.* **2022**, *50*. [CrossRef] [PubMed]
65. Li, P.; Ren, H.; Zhang, Y.; Zhou, Z. Fifteen-gene expression based model predicts the survival of clear renal cell carcinoma. *Medicine* **2018**, *97*, e11839. [CrossRef]
66. Baghdadi, A.; Aldhaam, N.A.; Elsayed, A.S.; Hussein, A.A.; Cavuoto, L.A.; Kauffman, E.; Guru, K.A. Automated differentiation of benign renal oncocytoma and chromophobe renal cell carcinoma on computed tomography using deep learning. *BJU Int.* **2020**, *125*, 553–560. [CrossRef]
67. Kattan, M.W.; Kantoff, P.W.; Nelson, J.B.; Carroll, P.R.; Roach, M.; Higano, C.S. Comparison of Cox Regression with Other Methods for Determining Prediction Models and Nomograms. *J. Urol.* **2003**, *170*, S6–S10. [CrossRef]
68. Zarrabi, K.; Wu, S. An evaluation of nivolumab for the treatment of metastatic renal cell carcinoma. *Expert Opin. Biol. Ther.* **2018**, *18*, 695–705. [CrossRef]
69. Khene, Z.; Mathieu, R.; Peyronnet, B.; Kokorian, R.; Gasmi, A.; Khene, F.; Rioux-Leclercq, N.; Kammerer-Jacquet, S.-F.; Shariat, S.; Laguerre, B.; et al. Radiomics can predict tumour response in patients treated with Nivolumab for a metastatic renal cell carcinoma: An artificial intelligence concept. *World J. Urol.* **2021**, *39*, 3707–3709. [CrossRef] [PubMed]
70. Le, Y.; Xu, W.; Guo, W. The Construction and Validation of a new Predictive Model for Overall Survival of Clear Cell Renal Cell Carcinoma Patients with Bone Metastasis Based on Machine Learning Algorithm. *Technol. Cancer Res. Treat.* **2023**, *22*. [CrossRef]
71. Khene, Z.-E.; Bigot, P.; Doumerc, N.; Ouzaid, I.; Boissier, R.; Nouhaud, F.-X.; Albiges, L.; Bernhard, J.-C.; Ingels, A.; Borchiellini, D.; et al. Application of Machine Learning Models to Predict Recurrence After Surgical Resection of Nonmetastatic Renal Cell Carcinoma. *Eur. Urol. Oncol.* **2023**, *6*, 323–330. [CrossRef]
72. Lenis, A.T.; Lec, P.M.; Chamie, K. Bladder cancer: A review. *JAMA* **2020**, *324*, 1980–1991. [CrossRef] [PubMed]
73. Ng, K.L.; Mbbs, D.P. Frcs The Etiology of Bladder Cancer. *Urol. Cancers* **2022**, 23–28. [CrossRef]
74. Dobruch, J.; Oszczudłowski, M. Bladder Cancer: Current Challenges and Future Directions. *Medicina* **2021**, *57*, 749. [CrossRef] [PubMed]
75. Shkolyar, E.; Jia, X.; Xing, L.; Liao, J. LBA-20 automated cystoscopic detection of bladder cancer using deep-learning. *J. Urol.* **2019**, *201*, e1000–e1001. [CrossRef]
76. Ikeda, A.; Nosato, H.; Kochi, Y.; Kojima, T.; Kawai, K.; Sakanashi, H.; Murakawa, M.; Nishiyama, H. Support System of Cystoscopic Diagnosis for Bladder Cancer Based on Artificial Intelligence. *J. Endourol.* **2020**, *34*, 352–358. [CrossRef] [PubMed]
77. Eminaga, O.; Semjonow, A.; Breil, B. Diagnostic classification of cystoscopic images using deep convolutional neural networks. *Eur. Urol. Suppl.* **2018**, *17*, e1232. [CrossRef]
78. Lorencin, I.; Anđelić, N.; Španjol, J.; Car, Z. Using multi-layer perceptron with Laplacian edge detector for bladder cancer diagnosis. *Artif. Intell. Med.* **2020**, *102*, 101746. [CrossRef]
79. Hashemi, S.M.R.; Hassanpour, H.; Kozegar, E.; Tan, T. Cystoscopic Image Classification Based on Combining MLP and GA. *Int. J. Nonlinear Anal. Appl.* **2020**, *11*, 93–105. [CrossRef]
80. Gresser, E.; Woźnicki, P.; Messmer, K.; Schreier, A.; Kunz, W.G.; Ingrisch, M.; Stief, C.; Ricke, J.; Nörenberg, D.; Buchner, A.; et al. Radiomics Signature Using Manual Versus Automated Segmentation for Lymph Node Staging of Bladder Cancer. *Eur. Urol. Focus* **2023**, *9*, 145–153. [CrossRef]

81. Wu, S.; Hong, G.; Xu, A.; Zeng, H.; Chen, X.; Wang, Y.; Luo, Y.; Wu, P.; Liu, C.; Jiang, N.; et al. Artificial intelligence-based model for lymph node metastases detection on whole slide images in bladder cancer: A retrospective, multicentre, diagnostic study. *Lancet Oncol.* **2023**, *24*, 360–370. [CrossRef] [PubMed]
82. Girard, A.; Dercle, L.; Vila-Reyes, H.; Schwartz, L.H.; Girma, A.; Bertaux, M.; Radulescu, C.; Lebret, T.; Delcroix, O.; Rouanne, M. A machine-learning-based combination of criteria to detect bladder cancer lymph node metastasis on [^{18}F]FDG PET/CT: A pathology-controlled study. *Eur. Radiol.* **2023**, *33*, 2821–2829. [CrossRef]
83. Wang, G.; Zhang, G.; Choi, K.-S.; Lam, K.-M.; Lu, J. Output based transfer learning with least squares support vector machine and its application in bladder cancer prognosis. *Neurocomputing* **2020**, *387*, 279–292. [CrossRef]
84. Gavriel, C.G.; Dimitriou, N.; Brieu, N.; Nearchou, I.P.; Arandjelovic, O.; Schmidt, G.; Harrison, D.J.; Caie, P.D. Identification of immunological features enables survival prediction of muscle-invasive bladder cancer patients using machine learning. *bioRxiv* **2020**. [CrossRef]
85. Bartsch, G.; Mitra, A.P.; Mitra, S.A.; Almal, A.A.; Steven, K.E.; Skinner, D.G.; Fry, D.W.; Lenehan, P.F.; Worzel, W.P.; Cote, R.J. Use of Artificial Intelligence and Machine Learning Algorithms with Gene Expression Profiling to Predict Recurrent Nonmuscle Invasive Urothelial Carcinoma of the Bladder. *J. Urol.* **2016**, *195*, 493–498. [CrossRef]
86. Wu, E.; Hadjiiski, L.M.; Samala, R.K.; Chan, H.-P.; Cha, K.H.; Richter, C.; Cohan, R.H.; Caoili, E.M.; Paramagul, C.; Alva, A.; et al. Deep Learning Approach for Assessment of Bladder Cancer Treatment Response. *Tomography* **2019**, *5*, 201–208. [CrossRef]
87. Hasnain, Z.; Mason, J.; Gill, K.; Miranda, G.; Gill, I.S.; Kuhn, P.; Newton, P.K. Machine learning models for predicting post-cystectomy recurrence and survival in bladder cancer patients. *PLoS ONE* **2019**, *14*, e0210976. [CrossRef]
88. Nojima, S.; Terayama, K.; Shimoura, S.; Hijiki, S.; Nonomura, N.; Morii, E.; Okuno, Y.; Fujita, K. A deep learning system to diagnose the malignant potential of urothelial carcinoma cells in cytology specimens. *Cancer Cytopathol.* **2021**, *129*, 984–995. [CrossRef]
89. Freifeld, Y.; Krabbe, L.-M.; Clinton, T.N.; Woldu, S.L.; Margulis, V. Therapeutic strategies for upper tract urothelial carcinoma. *Expert Rev. Anticancer. Ther.* **2018**, *18*, 765–774. [CrossRef] [PubMed]
90. Rojas, C.P.; Castle, S.M.; Llanos, C.A.; Cortes, J.A.S.; Bird, V.; Rodriguez, S.; Reis, I.M.; Zhao, W.; Gomez-Fernandez, C.; Leveillee, R.J.; et al. Low biopsy volume in ureteroscopy does not affect tumor biopsy grading in upper tract urothelial carcinoma. *Urol. Oncol. Semin. Orig. Investig.* **2013**, *31*, 1696–1700. [CrossRef]
91. Motiwala, F.; Kucheria, R. Ureteroscopy. *Surg. Proced. Core Urol. Trainees* **2020**, 19–31. [CrossRef]
92. Lazo, J.F.; Marzullo, A.; Moccia, S.; Catellani, M.; Rosa, B.; de Mathelin, M.; De Momi, E. Using spatial-temporal ensembles of convolutional neural networks for lumen segmentation in ureteroscopy. *Int. J. Comput. Assist. Radiol. Surg.* **2021**, *16*, 915–922. [CrossRef]
93. Cheng, L.; Albers, P.; Berney, D.M.; Feldman, D.R.; Daugaard, G.; Gilligan, T.; Looijenga, L.H.J. Testicular cancer. *Nat. Rev. Dis. Prim.* **2018**, *4*, 29. [CrossRef]
94. King, J.; Adra, N.; Einhorn, L.H. Testicular Cancer: Biology to Bedside. *Cancer Res.* **2021**, *81*, 5369–5376. [CrossRef]
95. Ghosh, A.; Sirinukunwattana, K.; Alham, N.K.; Browning, L.; Colling, R.; Protheroe, A.; Protheroe, E.; Jones, S.; Aberdeen, A.; Rittscher, J.; et al. The Potential of Artificial Intelligence to Detect Lymphovascular Invasion in Testicular Cancer. *Cancers* **2021**, *13*, 1325. [CrossRef] [PubMed]
96. Ding, L.; Wang, K.; Zhang, C.; Zhang, Y.; Wang, K.; Li, W.; Wang, J. A Machine Learning Algorithm for Predicting the Risk of Developing to M1b Stage of Patients with Germ Cell Testicular Cancer. *Front. Public Health* **2022**, *10*, 916513. [CrossRef]
97. Linder, N.; Taylor, J.C.; Colling, R.; Pell, R.; Alveyn, E.; Joseph, J.; Protheroe, A.; Lundin, M.; Lundin, J.; Verrill, C. Deep learning for detecting tumour-infiltrating lymphocytes in testicular germ cell tumours. *J. Clin. Pathol.* **2019**, *72*, 157–164. [CrossRef] [PubMed]
98. Baessler, B.; Nestler, T.; dos Santos, D.P.; Paffenholz, P.; Zeuch, V.; Pfister, D.; Maintz, D.; Heidenreich, A. Radiomics allows for detection of benign and malignant histopathology in patients with metastatic testicular germ cell tumors prior to post-chemotherapy retroperitoneal lymph node dissection. *Eur. Radiol.* **2020**, *30*, 2334–2345. [CrossRef] [PubMed]
99. Abbod, M.F.; Catto, J.W.; Linkens, D.A.; Hamdy, F.C. Application of Artificial Intelligence to the Management of Urological Cancer. *J. Urol.* **2007**, *178*, 1150–1156. [CrossRef]

Disclaimer/Publisher's Note: The statements, opinions and data contained in all publications are solely those of the individual author(s) and contributor(s) and not of MDPI and/or the editor(s). MDPI and/or the editor(s) disclaim responsibility for any injury to people or property resulting from any ideas, methods, instructions or products referred to in the content.

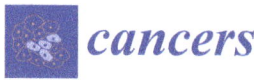

Review

AI-Powered Diagnosis of Skin Cancer: A Contemporary Review, Open Challenges and Future Research Directions

Navneet Melarkode [1], Kathiravan Srinivasan [1,*], Saeed Mian Qaisar [2,3] and Pawel Plawiak [4,5,*]

1. School of Computer Science and Engineering, Vellore Institute of Technology, Vellore 632014, India
2. Electrical and Computer Engineering Department, Effat University, Jeddah 22332, Saudi Arabia
3. LINEACT CESI, 69100 Lyon, France
4. Department of Computer Science, Faculty of Computer Science and Telecommunications, Cracow University of Technology, Warszawska 24, 31-155 Krakow, Poland
5. Institute of Theoretical and Applied Informatics, Polish Academy of Sciences, Bałtycka 5, 44-100 Gliwice, Poland
* Correspondence: kathiravan.srinivasan@vit.ac.in (K.S.); plawiak@pk.edu.pl (P.P.)

Simple Summary: The proposed research aims to provide a deep insight into the deep learning and machine learning techniques used for diagnosing skin cancer. While maintaining a healthy balance between both Machine Learning as well as Deep Learning, the study also discusses open challenges and future directions in this field. The research includes a comparison on widely used datasets and prevalent review papers discussing skin cancer diagnosis using Artificial Intelligence. The authors of this study aim to set this review as a benchmark for further studies in the field of skin cancer diagnosis by also including limitations and benefits of historical approaches.

Abstract: Skin cancer continues to remain one of the major healthcare issues across the globe. If diagnosed early, skin cancer can be treated successfully. While early diagnosis is paramount for an effective cure for cancer, the current process requires the involvement of skin cancer specialists, which makes it an expensive procedure and not easily available and affordable in developing countries. This dearth of skin cancer specialists has given rise to the need to develop automated diagnosis systems. In this context, Artificial Intelligence (AI)-based methods have been proposed. These systems can assist in the early detection of skin cancer and can consequently lower its morbidity, and, in turn, alleviate the mortality rate associated with it. Machine learning and deep learning are branches of AI that deal with statistical modeling and inference, which progressively learn from data fed into them to predict desired objectives and characteristics. This survey focuses on Machine Learning and Deep Learning techniques deployed in the field of skin cancer diagnosis, while maintaining a balance between both techniques. A comparison is made to widely used datasets and prevalent review papers, discussing automated skin cancer diagnosis. The study also discusses the insights and lessons yielded by the prior works. The survey culminates with future direction and scope, which will subsequently help in addressing the challenges faced within automated skin cancer diagnosis.

Keywords: artificial intelligence; computer-aided diagnostics; deep learning; dermatologists; dermatology; digital dermatology; machine learning; man-machine systems; skin cancer; skin neoplasms

Citation: Melarkode, N.; Srinivasan, K.; Qaisar, S.M.; Plawiak, P. AI-Powered Diagnosis of Skin Cancer: A Contemporary Review, Open Challenges and Future Research Directions. *Cancers* **2023**, *15*, 1183. https://doi.org/10.3390/cancers15041183

Academic Editors: Muhammad Fazal Ijaz and Marcin Woźniak

Received: 3 December 2022
Revised: 7 February 2023
Accepted: 8 February 2023
Published: 13 February 2023

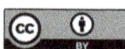

Copyright: © 2023 by the authors. Licensee MDPI, Basel, Switzerland. This article is an open access article distributed under the terms and conditions of the Creative Commons Attribution (CC BY) license (https://creativecommons.org/licenses/by/4.0/).

1. Introduction

Skin cancer is the abnormal growth of skin cells. The cancerous growth may affect both the layers—dermis and epidermis, but this review is concerned primarily with epidermal skin cancer; the two types of skin cancers that can arise from the epidermis are carcinomas and melanomas, depending on their cell type—keratinocytes or melanocytes, respectively [1–75]. It is a challenge to estimate the incidence of skin cancer due to various reasons, such as the multiple sub-types of skin cancer [76–99]. This poses as a problem while collating data, as non-melanoma is often not tracked by registries or are left incomplete because most cases are treated via surgery. As of 2020, the World Cancer Research Fund International reported a total of 300,000 cases of melanoma in skin, and a total of 1,198,073 cases of non-melanoma skin cancer [100–131]. The reasons for the occurrence of skin cancer cannot be singled out, but they include and are not limited to exposure to ultraviolet rays, family history, or a poor immune system [126]. The affected spot on the skin is called a lesion, which can be further segregated into multiple categories depending on its origin [1]. A comparison between different lesion types is usually accompanied by the presence or the absence of certain dermoscopic features.

There are three stages associated with an automated dermoscopy image analysis system, namely pre-processing, image segmentation, and feature extraction [2,4]. Segmentation plays a vital role, as the succeeding steps are dependent on this stage's output. Segmentation can be carried out in a supervised manner by considering parameters such as shapes, sizes, and colors, coupled with skin texture and type. Melanoma development that takes place horizontally or radially along the epidermis is called "single cancer melanoma", which carries critical importance in the early diagnosis of skin cancer [3]. Dermoscopy is a non-invasive diagnostic method which allows for a closer examination of the pigmented skin lesion. It is performed with the help of an instrument called a dermatoscope. The procedure of dermoscopy allows for a visualization of the skin structure in the epidermis that would not otherwise be possible to the naked eye. Studies [127] suggest that a growing number of practitioners are incorporating dermoscopy into their daily practices. Dermoscopy can be categorized into three modes—polarized contact, polarized non-contact, and nonpolarized contact (unpolarized dermoscopy). Polarized and nonpolarized dermoscopy are complementary, and utilizing both to acquire clinical images increases the diagnostic accuracy [128]. These images can then be processed with the help of AI methods to assist in the diagnosis of skin cancer [132–134].

Even though the mortality rate of skin cancer is significantly high, early detection helps to bolster the survival rate to over 95% [5]. Deep learning models are generalizations of multi-layer perceptron models and are widely used due to their high accuracy in visual imaging tasks. There are two major promising paths for skin cancer detection in this research. The first is employing machine learning techniques and strategies to assist in the detection of skin lesions, and classifying them accordingly. The second, as this article discusses, is deep learning frameworks and model-based approaches being implemented in the recent advancements concerning skin cancer diagnosis. Table A1 in Appendix A contains a list of abbreviations used in this review, as well as their definitions.

1.1. Contribution of this Survey

We provide a comprehensive study of the various machine learning and deep learning models used for skin cancer diagnosis. Brief explanations of several machine learning and deep learning methodologies are included.

- This survey comprehensively discusses the application of various machine learning and deep learning methods in the implementation of skin cancer diagnosis.
- There is a discussion of new techniques in skin lesion detection such as deep belief networks and extreme learning machines, along with the traditional Computational Intelligence techniques such as random forests, recurrent neural networks, and k-nearest neighbors, etc.
- There is a designated tabular summary of works on the deep learning and machine learning techniques used for skin cancer diagnosis and detection. The tabulated summary also includes key contributions and limitations for the same.
- There is a classification of various types of skin cancer based on tumor characteristics that have been elucidated for a deeper understanding of the problem statement.
- The study also describes various open challenges present and future research directions for further improvements in the field of skin cancer diagnosis.

Table 1 presents a comparison between the current review and the previous review articles of machine-learning-based and deep-learning-based techniques in skin cancer diagnosis. The depth of the discussion in Table 1 has been used as a criterion for comparing different review articles. A high or H depth of the discussion indicates that the article contains a dedicated session for the said topic. A moderate or M depth of the discussion denotes that the review article has a subsection or a paragraph corresponding to the topic. A low or L depth of the discussion implies that the article has mentioned the topic, but not explained it comprehensively. A not discussed or N depth of the discussion indicates that the topic has not been covered in the article.

Table 1. Comparison of the current review with the previous reviews in AI-powered skin cancer diagnosis.

Reference	Year	One-Phrase Summary	Machine Learning Models in Skin Cancer Diagnosis	Deep Learning in Skin Cancer Diagnosis	Open Challenges in Skin Cancer Diagnosis	Future Directions for Skin Cancer Diagnosis
Our review	-	A comprehensive survey on machine learning and deep learning techniques used to diagnose skin cancer	H	H	H	H
[11]	2022	A review on cancer diagnosis using Artificial Intelligence	H	H	M	N
[12]	2022	A research article on the recent advancements in cancer diagnosis using machine learning and deep learning techniques	H	H	L	M
[6]	2021	A review of machine learning and its applications in the field of skin cancer	H	L	M	H
[7]	2021	A minireview on deep learning and its use in cancer diagnosis and prognosis prediction	N	H	M	H
[10]	2021	A review on skin disease diagnosis with deep learning	N	H	N	H
[14]	2021	A review on skin cancer classification via convolution neural networks	N	M	M	N
[15]	2021	A survey on deep learning techniques for skin lesion analysis and melanoma cancer detection	N	H	M	N
[9]	2020	A review article on Artificial-Intelligence-based methods for diagnosis of skin cancer	M	M	H	N
[13]	2020	A review on malignant melanoma classification using deep learning	N	H	M	H
[16]	2020	A survey in cancer detection using machine learning	H	N	H	H
[8]	2019	A bibliographic review on cancer diagnosis using deep learning	N	H	M	N

Depth of discussion: L—low, M—moderate, H—high, N—not discussed.

1.2. Survey Methodology

1.2.1. Search Strategy and Literature Sources

Repositories and databases such as IEEE, ScienceDirect, and PubMed, etc., were used to find relevant research studies and articles. The relevancy was determined based on the paper's context (the central theme of the paper being the diagnosis of skin cancer based on AI/ML/DL models), the research paper's title, abstract screening, keyword matching, and the conclusion of the study. The keywords employed were cancer diagnosis, skin cancer, deep learning, machine learning, skin lesion, melanoma cancer, and cancer detection, etc. A total of 1057 non-duplicate articles were found initially. Table 2 includes the search terms and the corresponding set of keywords associated with these terms.

Table 2. Search terms.

Search Term	Set of Keywords
Skin	skin cancer, skin disease, skin cancer diagnosis, skin cancer detection, skin lesion
Cancer	cancer type, cancer diagnosis
Deep	deep learning, deep neural networks
Melanoma	melanoma skin cancer, melanoma cancer
Machine	machine learning
Machine learning techniques	artificial neural network, naïve Bayes, decision tree, k-nearest neighbors, k-means clustering, random forest, support vector machines, ensemble learning
Deep learning techniques	recurrent neural networks, deep autoencoders, long short-term memory, deep neural network, deep belief network, deep convolutional neural network, deep Boltzmann machine, deep reinforcement learning, extreme learning machine

1.2.2. Inclusion Criteria

The articles included were primarily filtered based on their relevance. Apart from relevancy, only articles written in English were selected. Furthermore, only articles published after 2014 were considered for inclusion.

1.2.3. Elimination Criteria

The elimination of articles was based on abstract and introduction screening. Articles were then eliminated based on the quality of their research and the lack of references. The parameters used to judge the research quality were the reputation of the journal the article was published in, using metrics such as the h-index and impact factor, the date of publication (the older the date, the less relevant the article may be in present day), and the number of citations the research study had. In addition, any missing relevancy and the redundancy of the research were also considered in the elimination process.

1.2.4. Results

Out of the 1057 non-duplicate articles filtered out from the various research repositories, 826 articles were excluded during the abstract and title screening. From the remaining 231 articles, 62 articles were excluded during the redundancy check and 48 articles were excluded during the full text screening. Finally, 121 articles were obtained after applying the inclusion/exclusion criteria. Figure 1 shows the PRISMA method implementation for the same. Figure 2 indicates the number of reference papers published in each year. Figure 3 demonstrates the various methods that this study encapsulates, and the number of papers cited corresponding to each methodology.

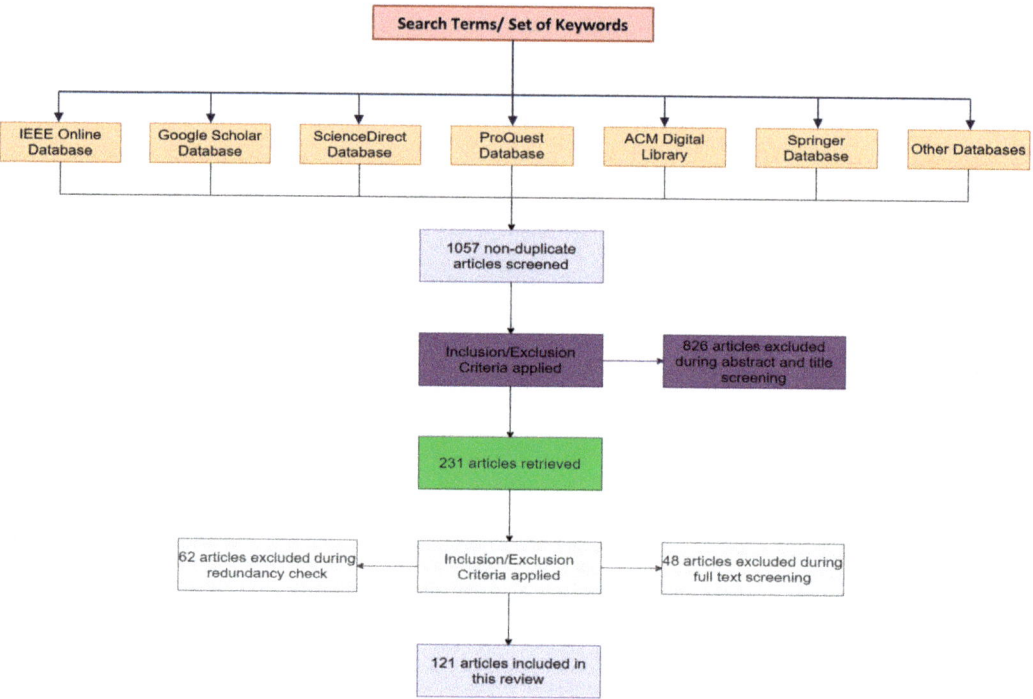

Figure 1. Flow diagram for the selection process of research articles using PRISMA method.

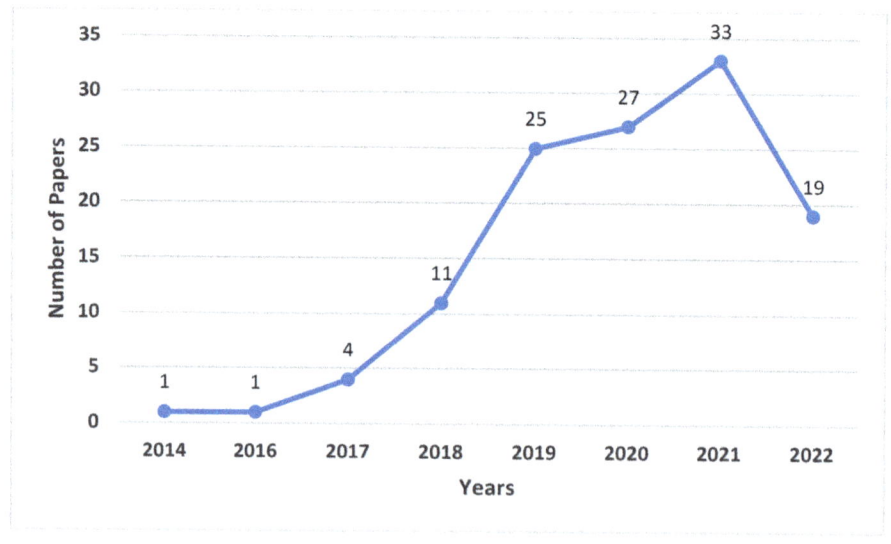

Figure 2. Number of papers per year, used in the review.

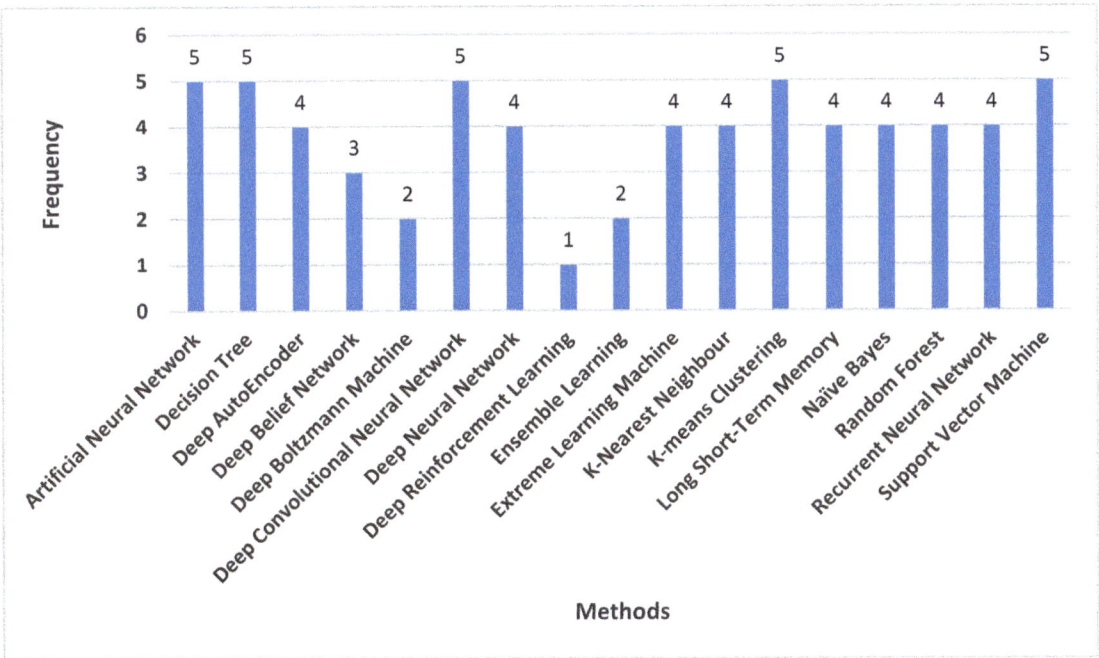

Figure 3. ML and DL methods versus frequency of papers used in this work.

1.3. Structure of this Review

This paper is organized as follows. A comparison with previous reviews on skin cancer diagnosis and survey methodology for the same is covered in Section 1. Section 2 provides an overview of skin cancer, as well as the datasets commonly used in various studies in the field of skin cancer diagnosis. Section 3 is divided into two major subsections. The subsections describe the techniques used to diagnose skin cancer using machine learning and deep learning frameworks and algorithms, respectively. Section 4 talks about the open challenges faced in the field of skin cancer diagnosis, while Section 5 gives an insight into future research directions. The conclusion is given in Section 6, followed by the references used for this research. Figure 4 visualizes the structure of this study.

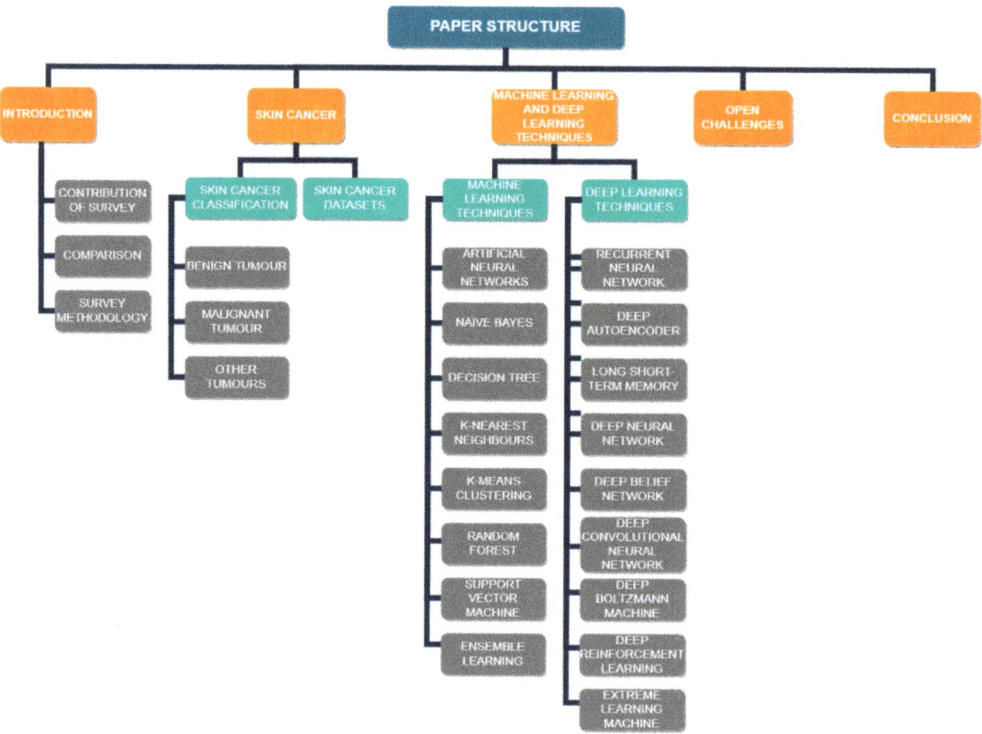

Figure 4. Structure of this review.

2. Skin Cancer

Skin cancer is associated with the abnormal growth of skin cells that are found either in the epidermis or the dermis. The skin cells are usually those that are exposed to sunlight, but skin cancer can also occur in those cells that are not ordinarily exposed [129]. This research focuses on the skin cancer that occurs in the epidermal cells, namely keratinocytes and melanocytes. Skin cancer can be largely divided into three subcategories.

1. Basal cell carcinoma: this type of cancer affects and originates from the basal cells. Basal cell carcinoma comes from keratinocytes, which are found in the epidermis. These may invade the entire epidermal thickness.
2. Squamous cell carcinoma: this subdivision deals with the uncontrollable growth of the abnormal squamous cells present in the root. Squamous cells are flat cells that are found in the tissue that constitutes the surface of the skin, and the lining of vital organs such as the respiratory organs, digestive tracts, and hollow organs of the body.
3. Melanoma: this form of cancer develops when melanocytes start to grow abnormally. Melanocytes are the cells that can become melanoma. Melanoma can develop anywhere in the skin, while it can also form in other parts of the body such as the eyes, mouth, and genitals, etc.

Figures 5 and 6 include images from the International Skin Imaging Collaboration (ISIC) dataset to demonstrate the different types of skin cancer images that are available for training and testing. Figure 5 shows dermoscopic images, while Figure 6 displays clinical images from the skin cancer dataset.

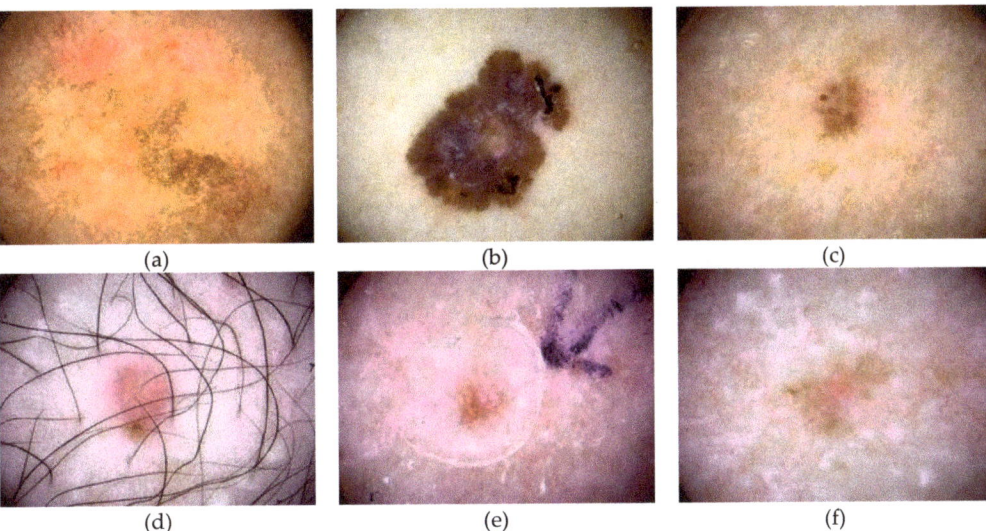

Figure 5. Dermoscopic sample images of skin cancer: (**a**) squamous cell carcinoma, (**b**) basal cell carcinoma, (**c**) benign dermatofibroma, (**d**) benign seborrheic keratosis, (**e**) benign actinic keratosis, and (**f**) malignant melanoma.

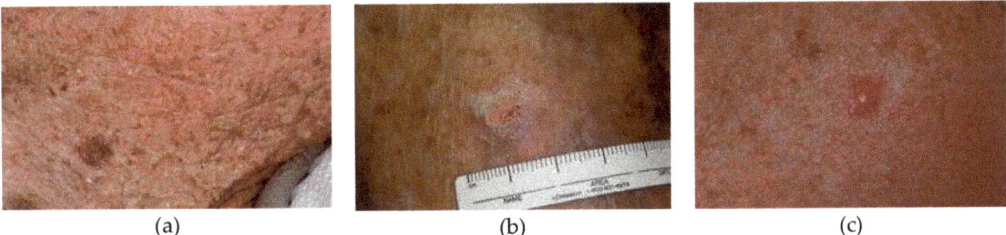

Figure 6. Clinical sample images of skin cancer: (**a**) malignant melanoma, (**b**) squamous cell carcinoma, and (**c**) basal cell carcinoma.

Branching out of skin cancer are skin tumors, which are chiefly responsible for the mortality rate once diagnosed with the same [17]. Skin tumors can be categorized into two types, namely melanoma and non-melanoma. Irrespective of the technological advancements made in the field of curing cancer, to date, the early detection and diagnosis of any tumor combined with enough therapy leads the way to a successful treatment [18]. There are multiple ways to classify and categorize skin cancer. Most of them employ the use of deep learning techniques such as convolution neural networks in [19], while the others use specialized tools such as non-invasive imaging tools [20].

2.1. Skin Cancer Classification

When cells become cancerous, they start to grow uncontrollably due to various reasons, one such reason being a damaged cell DNA. This random behavior of the cell may lead to uneven accumulation and form a solid mass or lump, called a tumor. Tumors are often associated with uncontrollable growth in solid tissues such as muscles and bones. Tumors are further subdivided into two major categories, as described in the following section.

2.1.1. Benign Tumor

Benign tumors are a collection of these cells that grow abnormally but are non-cancerous. According to [21], these tumors are generally classified according to their level of origin within the skin. The skin has three levels of subclassification in this regard, the epidermal layer, the dermal layer, and the subcutaneous layer. Another common taxonomy followed for benign tumors is based on the cell of their origin. Certain well-known examples are the melanocyte or the keratinocyte [22].

2.1.2. Malignant Tumor

Malignant tumors are tumors that are cancerous. The affected cells metastasize through the bloodstream and the lymph nodes. In the context of skin cancer, malignant tumors emerging from the surface epithelium of the skin and the epidermis include cutaneous melanoma and non-melanoma cancers such as basal cell carcinoma [23]. Cutaneous melanomas constitute only 4% of all skin cancers, but they are by far the most significant ones, due to their lethality [24]. Ref. [25] conducted a study on developing deep learning techniques to help classify tumors as benign or malignant. False positives and negatives lead to a substandard prognosis of skin cancer. Article [26] discusses the challenges of detecting malignant tumors, which include, but are not limited to, noisy images, irregular tumor boundaries, and uneven image sizes. Hence, the need for deep learning and machine learning methods to detect malignant tumors is paramount.

2.1.3. Other Tumors

The last subclassification of tumors is loosely classified as pre-malignant tumors. These cells are not cancerous at that moment of time, but they have the potential to become malignant. The major problem faced by the authors of [27] while detecting pre-malignant tumors was the scarcity of images. This led to them use the same dataset for training and validation. This does not come a surprise, as the study conducted in [28] also faced difficulty in recording pre-malignant lesion data. Pre-malignant tumors are often clubbed with certain malignant subtypes such as actinic keratosis, which is a squamous cell carcinoma despite being premalignant as well [25]. This makes it difficult to distinguish between the different classes of tumors.

2.2. Skin Cancer Datasets

Table 3 describes the various datasets used in previous studies and analyzes the constituents of each dataset. Furthermore, the table also identifies the skin cancer image categories available in the respective datasets.

Table 3. List of various skin cancer datasets employed by previous studies.

Reference	Creator and Year of Dataset	Skin Cancer Categories	Dataset Used	Dataset Size	Type of Data	Details About the Dataset
[132]	International Skin Imaging Collaboration, 2020	Actinic keratosis, basal cell carcinoma, dermatofibroma, melanoma, nevus, seborrheic keratosis, squamous cell carcinoma, vascular lesion	ISIC	2357 images	Dermoscopic images	Contains images of malignant and benign oncological diseases. Melanoma and mole images are slightly dominant in the dataset
[133]	Nilsel Ilter, H. Altay Guvenir, 1998	Melanoma and non-melanoma	DermIS, DermQuest	72 images in DermIS and 274 images in DermQuest	Not reported	Contains lesion images. They are subject to various artifacts such as drastic shadow effect and differing illumination.

Table 3. Cont.

Reference	Creator and Year of Dataset	Skin Cancer Categories	Dataset Used	Dataset Size	Type of Data	Details About the Dataset
[134]	Tschandl, P., 2018	Actinic keratoses and intraepithelial carcinoma, basal cell carcinoma, benign keratosis-like lesions, dermatofibroma, melanoma, melanocytic nevi, and vascular lesions	HAM10000	10015 images	Dermoscopic images	More than half of lesion images are validated through histopathology. Remaining images are confirmed through expert consensus or in-vivo confocal microscopy.
[35]	Dongtan Sacred Heart Hospital, Hallym University, and Sanggye Paik Hospital, Inje University, 2016	Basal cell carcinoma	Hallym	152 images	Dermoscopic images	Country of origin is South Korea and a total of 106 members participated in the creation of this dataset
[35]	Department of Dermatology at Asan Medical Center, 2017	Basal cell carcinoma, squamous cell carcinoma, intraepithelial carcinoma, and melanoma	Asan Dataset	17125 images and 1276 test images	Clinical images	While the thumbnails were available for free downloading, the full-size images required external permission and it came at a cost of US $200 or £145.
[34]	Mitko Veta et al., 2016	Not reported	TUPAC 2016 Dataset	500 training and 321 test images	Whole slide images	Images to predict tumor proliferation scores from whole slide images.

3. Machine Learning and Deep Learning Models for Skin Cancer Diagnosis

3.1. Need for Machine Learning and Deep Learning Models for Skin Cancer Diagnosis

Artificial Intelligence has laid the foundation for integrating computers into the medical field seamlessly [30]. It provides an added dimension to diagnosis, prognosis, and therapy [36]. Recent studies have indicated that machine learning and deep learning models for skin cancer screening have been on the rise. This is primarily because these models, as well as other variants of Artificial Intelligence, use a concoction of algorithms, and when provided with data, accomplish tasks. In the current scenario, the tasks include, but are not limited to, the diagnosis of the patient, the prognosis of the patient, or predicting the status governing the ongoing treatment [37]. Diagnosis is the process of understanding the prevailing state of the patient, while prognosis refers to the process of predicting the future condition of the patient by extrapolating all the current parameters and their corresponding outputs. AI has now progressed to the point where it can be successfully used to detect cancer earlier than the traditional methods [6]. As early detection is key for a fruitful treatment and better outcome of skin cancer, the need for machine learning and deep learning models in the field of skin cancer is paramount.

3.2. Machine Learning Techniques

3.2.1. Artificial Neural Networks

Artificial neural networks (ANNs) are systems that draw inspiration from the animal brain. ANNs have been used to predict non-melanoma skin cancer by inputting a certain set of tried and tested parameters fit for training, such as gender, vigorous exercise habits, hypertension, asthma, age, and heart disease etc. [38] The ANN takes the entire dataset as the input. To improve the accuracy of the model, the network inputs are normalized to values between 0 and 1. The outputs are treated as typical classification outputs, which return fractional values between 0 and 1. ANNs can also be used to detect skin cancer by taking an image input and subjecting it through hidden layers [39]. This process is carried out in four sequential steps, the first of which is to initialize random weights in the ANN system. Next, each of the activation values are calculated. Consequently, the magnitude of the error is also known as the loss change. The weights are updated proportionately, with respect to the loss. Until the loss reaches a certain lower bound or a floor value, the three steps are repeated. In this field that pertains to skin cancer detection, visual inspection is the introductory stage. This is due to the similarities shared between various subcategories of tumors, such as color, area, and distribution. Owing to this reason, the use of ANNs is encouraged to enhance multi-class skin lesion detection [40]. The trained network models are used with a logistic regression model to successfully detect skin lesions while reducing the false positives and negatives in the process. The choice of activation function for the ANN is completely dependent on the user, and it is to be noted that each function carries its own sets of advantages and disadvantages with respect to the convergence of the model and the computational load [40]. ANNs have been used to simultaneously predict various symptoms that generally occur in cancer-affected patients, as seen in [41]. The risk of symptoms predicted were that of pain, depression, and poor well-being. The input to the ANN was a list of 39 distinct covariates. The input features can be classified into five subcategories, such as demographic characteristics such as age and sex, clinical characteristics such as the cancer type and stage, treatment characteristics such as the radiation treatment and cancer surgery, baseline patient reported measures such as the performance status and symptom burden status, and finally, health care utilization measures such as whether the patient has been hospitalized or if they have a live-in caregiver. ANNs play an important role in predicting skin cancer and the presence of a tumor, due to their flexible structure and data-driven nature, owing to which they are considered as a potential modeling approach [42].

The model proposed by [38] reports a sensitivity of 88.5% and a specificity of 62.2% on the training set, while the validation set showed a comparable sensitivity of 86.2% and a specificity of 62.7%. Similarly, the ANN model in [39] was tested over multiple sets, each using an increasing number of training and testing image ratios. The accuracy returned by the model falls between 80% and 88.88%.

In [38–40], emphasis is put on the need for optimizing predictors, increased model parameters, and the conduction of more clinical testing to improve the sensitivity and specificity of the model. Despite being easy to implement and cost effective, ANN models require further development in future studies for skin cancer diagnosis.

3.2.2. Naïve Bayes

Naïve Bayes classifiers are probabilistic classifiers that work by employing the use of Bayes' theorem. Naïve Bayes classifiers have been used in the field of skin cancer to classify clinical and dermatological images with high precision [43]. The model has reached an accuracy of 70.15%, as it makes use of important pieces of data to develop a strong judgement and assists physicians in the diagnosis and precise detection of the disease. Naïve Bayes classifiers extend their applications by providing a means to detect and segment skin diseases [44]. For each output class of the classifier, a posterior probability distribution is obtained. This process is performed iteratively, which implies that the method requires lesser computational resources, as it avoids the need for multiple training sessions. The Bayesian approach has also been used to probabilistically predict the nature of a data point to a high degree of accuracy, as seen in [45]. The final classification made in this case combines the existing knowledge of data points to use in the Bayesian analysis. The Bayesian sequential framework has also been put into use to aid models that help to detect a melanoma invasion into human skin. A total of three model parameters were estimated with the help of the model, namely, the melanoma cell proliferation rate, the melanoma cell diffusivity, and ultimately, a constant that determines the degradation rate of melanoma cells in the skin tissue. The algorithm learns data through the following, in a sequential manner: a spatially uniform cell assay, a 2D circular barrier assay, and finally, a 3D invasion assay. This Bayesian framework can be extracted and used in other biological contexts due to its versatile nature. This is chiefly possible in situations where detailed quantitative biological measurements, such as skin lesion extraction from scientific images, is not easy; hence, the extraction method must incorporate simple measurements from the images provided, like the Bayesian framework does [46].

Naïve Bayes classifiers, as discussed in [43], achieve an accuracy of 70.15% and a specificity of 73.33%. At the same time, the classifiers do not breach the 70% mark in sensitivity and precision. The accuracy appears to follow a similar pattern in naïve Bayes classifiers from other studies such as [44], where the diagnostic accuracies reported are 72.7%.

The recurring scope of improvement in [43–45] revolves around experimenting with different color models, as well as using different types of dermal cancer datasets in the training. In [44,46], they elucidate the pressing need for further pre-processing before training naïve Bayes classifiers for skin cancer diagnosis.

3.2.3. Decision Tree

Decision trees are a supervised learning method which are primarily used for classification problems and are occasionally extended to fit regression problem statements as well. Decision trees have been used to provide an intuitive algorithm that helps quantify the long-term risk of non-melanoma skin cancer after a liver transplant. This is done by utilizing the variables closely associated with the peri-transplant period [47]. The classifier is used as a view for the patients which provides personalized solutions such as chemoprophylaxis. A slight variation of decision trees can also be employed, as seen in [48]. The article proposes a random decision tree algorithm to detect breast surgery infection. The risk factors that came along with the algorithm in this case were obesity, diabetes, and kidney failure, etc. While the study investigates breast cancer, skin cancer is most closely associated with breast cancer due to the presence of the dangerous melanoma type. Decision trees showcase its versatility in the way it is used. In [49], decision trees are used as a mode for the visual representation of problem by dividing each branch into the different outcomes possible during a clinical procedure. The decision tree model was used to gauge the cost effectiveness of the sentinel lymph node biopsy, a new standard technique used in the treatment of melanoma and breast cancer. The cost effectiveness was measured with respect to head and neck cutaneous squamous cell carcinoma, a subsection of skin cancer. The decision tree presented outputs to determine whether the treatment was cost effective for a particular set of tumors, or if it could be used generally. Decision trees can also be used as an intermediate layer instead of keeping them as a standalone classifier. In [50], they demonstrate the effectiveness of this architecture in extracting regions and classifying skin cancer, using deep convolution neural networks. Most of the features are classified using decision trees and other counterpart algorithms such as support vector machines and k-nearest neighbors. Decision trees are also used to attain clarity in the classification of breast cancer, as can be seen from [51]. The error analysis of the proposed model reveals that the foundational decision tree models provide users with easy-to-use outcomes and a very high degree of clinical detection and diagnostic performance, as compared to its predecessors.

The decision tree model from [47] reports a specificity of 42% and a sensitivity of 91%. Similarly, the models presented in [48] return a sensitivity, specificity, and accuracy greater than 90%. This trend follows suit in the model proposed by [50], where all the three parameters cross 94%. On the contrary, models like those in [49] return a slightly lower sensitivity of 77% but report a 100% specificity.

Decision trees' model predictions are heavily dependent on the quality of the datasets. The common pitfalls encountered by [47,50] are that the model testing and training datasets had an identical distribution of variables; hence, this eliminates the prospect of training the model on entirely independent cohorts.

3.2.4. K-Nearest Neighbors

The k-nearest neighbors algorithm, also referred to as the KNN, is a parametric supervised classification algorithm that uses distance and proximity as metrics to classify the data points. KNNs were used as an evaluation algorithm to detect skin cancer and melanomas. The KNN model was then used to produce a confusion matrix which helps with visualizing the accuracy of the entire model [52]. Apart from this case of use, KNNs have also been used extensively by extending the model as per requirement. In [53], they extend KNN to use the Radius Nearest Neighbors classifier to classify breast cancer and calculate the evaluation metrics such as accuracy and specificity. The reason for augmenting the KNN solely lay in the limitations posed by an extreme value of k. For a small k, the KNN classifier is highly sensitive to outliers, and for a large value of k, the classifier underfits on the training data points. This problem is overcome by normalizing the radius value of each point to recognize outliers effectively. The applications of KNNs have been expanded by using them for detecting the anomalous growth of skin lesions [54]. KNNs are hybridized with Firefly to provide quantitative information about a skin lesion without having to perform any unnecessary skin biopsies. The hybrid classifier built upon KNN is used to predict and classify using two primary methods: threshold-based segmentation and ABCD feature extraction. The Firefly optimization coupled with KNN helps to recognize skin cancer much more effectively than its predecessors, while keeping computational and temporal complexity to a minimum. To classify and discriminate between melanoma and benign skin lesion in clinical images, ref. [55] made use of multiple classifiers, out of which the KNN classifier returned competent results. The article also makes use of different color spaces and tests the classifiers on each of them to demonstrate the feasibility of the algorithms to detect melanomas in various color spaces.

The KNN classifiers of [52], with the number of neighbors set to 15, returned an accuracy of 66.8%, with a precision and recall for positive predictions of 71% and 46%, respectively. The recall value increases almost twofold for negative predictions, while the precision score for the same lingers around 65%. The values in [53] provide a different perspective to the modified KNN classifiers, as they report an accuracy of over 96%. Fuzzy KNN classifiers, as shown in [54], have an accuracy of 93.33%, with a sensitivity of 88.89% and a specificity of 100%.

Despite being a viable approach to diagnosing skin cancer, KNN classifiers require the provision to be trained continually, as suggested by [52]. Furthermore, with the dearth of feasible datasets, the size of suitable training data proves to be a limitation for [52,53]. To mitigate the adverse effects of minimal training data, the KNN classifier can fit into an online learning method that builds over time and keeps learning as and when the classifier acquires more data.

3.2.5. K-Means Clustering

K-means clustering is a clustering method that is grouped under unsupervised learning. By employing a fuzzy logic with the existing k-means clustering algorithm, studies have been conducted on segmenting the skin melanoma at its earliest stage [56]. Fuzzy k-means clustering is applied to the pre-processed clinical images to delineate the affected regions. This aids the process to subsequently be used in melanoma disease recognition. K-means clustering has widespread cases of use and can be used to segment skin lesions, as seen in [57]. The algorithm groups objects, thereby ensuring that the variance within each group is at minimum. This enables the classifier to return high-feature segmented images. Each image pixel is assigned a randomly initialized class center. The centers are recalculated based on every data point added. The process is repeated until all the data points have been assigned clusters. Unlike a binary classifier like k-means, where each data point can belong to only one cluster, fuzzy c-means clustering enables the data points to be a part of any number of clusters, with a likelihood attached to hit. The fuzzy c-means algorithm outputs comparatively better results in comparison with the legacy k-means clustering algorithm. Fuzzy c-means provide a probability for data points that depends on the distance between the cluster center and the point itself. In [58], fuzzy c-means were used in place of the k-means algorithm to detect skin cancer, inspired by a differential evolution artificial neural network. The simulated results indicated that the proposed method outperformed traditional approaches in this regard. The k-means algorithm can also be used as an intermediate layer to produce outputs, as trained on by deep learning methods. In [59], they demonstrated an algorithm where k-means were used to segment the input images based on the variation of intensities. The clusters thus formed were then subjected to further processing to aid in the detection of melanoma cancer. The traditional k-means algorithm can also be used to detect skin lesions. To augment the quality of the results, it can be used with a gray level co-event matrix, a local binary pattern, and red, green, and blue color modes [60]. K-means clustering is heavily dependent on external factors being extracted successfully, such as color features, lesion orientation, and image contrast [56,58,59]. This engenders the need for coherency in the diagnosis pipeline that utilizes the k-means clustering. The pipeline must accurately extract external features before the clustering algorithms take them as input.

K-means clustering models tend to return a high detection accuracy. For instance, the model that extends fuzzy logic, like in [56], returns an accuracy of over 95%. Other k-means clustering models, like those in [58] and [59], also report a detection accuracy of 90%.

3.2.6. Random Forest

Random forests are an extension of decision trees. They are an ensemble learning method commonly used for classification problems. Random forests extend their applications to detect skin cancer and classify skin lesions, as done in [61]. Random forests permit the evaluation of sampling allocation. The steps followed in the proposed method are to initialize a training set. The training set is then bootstrapped to generate multiple sub-training sets. By calculating the Gini index for each of the sub-training sets, the model is then populated with decision values. The individual decision values are then combined to generate a model that classifies by voting on the test samples. Skin cancer can also be classified by characterizing the Mueller matrix elements using the random forest algorithm [62]. The random forest algorithm builds various sub-decision trees as the foundation for classification and categorization tasks. Every individual decision tree is provided with a unique logic that constitutes the binary question framework used in the entirety of the system. In comparison with the original decision tree, the random forest provides enhanced results while reducing the variance bias. This helps to prevent the overfitting of the data, which was otherwise seen in decision trees. Other studies in the classification of skin cancer involve classifying the dermoscopic images into seven sub-types. This has been implemented with the help of random forests [63]. The procedure to create a random forest is slightly unconventional in this study. After preparing a dataset to train on, the random forest is then amassed by arranging a relapse tree. The ballot casting is conducted after the forest architecture is built. The different types of sub-classifications that the random forest was trained on were basal cell carcinoma, benign keratosis lesion, dermatofibroma, melanocytic nevi, melanoma, and vascular types. Similarly, skin lesion classification has also been performed with the help of random forests and decision trees in [64]. Using random forests are key since predecessor algorithms lack the reliability aspect of skin image segmentation and classification. The random forest is generated by selecting a subset of random samples in the skin lesion dataset. For each feature in the subsets, a decision tree is created to get a prediction. A voting process is then established for each of the prior outputs, and a forecast result with the most votes is selected as the final step.

Random forest classifiers, as seen in [61], report an accuracy, sensitivity, and specificity of around 70%, regardless of the features incorporated to segment the required area, such as ABCD rule or GLCM features. Depending on the dataset used, random forest classifiers can also have a high accuracy while detecting skin cancer. The models in [62] achieved an average accuracy of 93%.

The features of a random forest classification algorithm are invariant to image translation and rotation [61,64]. This allows future research to be more liberal with its datasets and extend them to a variety of geographies to discern the consistency in results returned by skin cancer classification.

3.2.7. Support Vector Machine

Support vector machines (SVMs) are supervised learning models that help classify, predict, and extrapolate data by analyzing them. SVMs can be used to classify different types of skin lesions. In [65], ABCD features are used for extracting the characteristic features like shape, color, and size from the clinical images provided. After selecting the features, the skin lesion is classified with the help of SVMs into melanoma, seborrheic keratosis, and lupus erythematosus. This method of using ABCD along with SVM generates great results while delivering significant information. For a narrower classification, SVMs have also been used to classify skin lesions as melanoma or non-melanoma [66]. The process was divided into six phases: acquiring the image, pre-processing the image, segmentation, extracting the features, classifying the image, and viewing the result. From the experiment, the features extracted were texture, color, and shape. To extend the nature of the above model, SVMs have also been employed to identify and detect carcinoma or infection in the early stages before it aggravates [67]. The chief difference in the extension and itself lies in the feature extraction procedure. In [67], they pre-process the input image by employing grey scale conversion and then chaining the resultant image with noise removal and binarization subprocesses. The region of interest is removed in segmentation to help with accurate classification. Similarly, for the early detection and diagnosis of skin cancer, a bag-of-features method was used, which included spatial information. The SVM was developed with the help of a histogram of an oriented gradient optimized set. This resulted in encouraging results when compared to state-of-the-art algorithms [68]. By using Bendlet Transform (BT) as features of the SVM classifier, unwanted features such as hair and noise are discarded. These are removed using the preliminary step of median filtering. BT outperforms representation systems such as wavelets, curvelets, and contourlets, as it can classify singularities in images much more precisely [69].

The average accuracy of the SVM classifier models presented in [65] was about 98%, while the sensitivity and specificity averaged to 95%. The SVM model in [66] also had all three parameters greater than 90%.

3.2.8. Ensemble Learning

Ensemble learning is a machine learning model that combines the predictions of two or more models. The constituent models are also called ensemble members. These models can be trained on the same dataset or can be suited to something completely different. The ensemble members are grouped together to output a prediction for the problem statement. Ensemble classifiers have been used for diagnosing melanoma as malignant or benign [70]. The ensemble members for the same are trained individually on balanced subspaces, thereby reducing the redundant predictors. The remaining classifiers are grouped using a neural network fuser. The presented ensemble classifier model returns statistically better results than other individual dedicated classifier models. Furthermore, ensemble learning has also been used in the multi-class classification of skin lesions to assist clinicians in early detection [71]. The ensemble model made use of five deep neural network models: ResNeXt, SeResNeXt, ResNet, Xception, and DenseNet. Collectively, the ensemble model performed better than all of them individually.

3.2.9. Summary of Machine Learning Techniques

Analyzing the various implementations of machine learning models in the field of skin cancer diagnosis indicates that simple vector machines are undoubtedly the most precise and accurate models. The main caveat of using SVMs is the need for the meticulous pre-processing of input data. In terms of user flexibility, k-means clustering and k-nearest neighbors lead the way, without compromising much on accuracy and performance. KNNs, however, require to be trained continuously as more data points are added. This might prove to be quite tedious as the volume of input data is highly irregular and cannot be predicted. Naïve Bayes models have the lowest accuracy of all the machine learning techniques studied in this paper, and understandably so, as various techniques make use of the fundamentals of the naïve Bayes theorem and develop it further, such as decision trees and random forests. Decision trees perform decently but are highly dependent on the quality of the dataset, which is an uncontrollable variable in the system. Random forests do not have the provision to learn image rotation and translation on the fly, reflecting the same in their classification accuracy. Depending on the dataset used, random forests can either perform really well, or get only around 50% of classifications correct. ANNs, being the steppingstone for various techniques to develop, suggest that while the results may be good, they cannot be increased further. ANNs have reached a saturation point in terms of the modifications made, and other techniques must be employed if any improvement is expected. Ensemble models, although complicated and tough to implement, return accuracies higher than the models taken individually for the multi-class classification.

Table 4 provides an executive summary of the machine learning techniques used in the diagnosis of skin cancer. Figure 7 conceptualizes the machine learning models in skin cancer diagnosis discussed in this study.

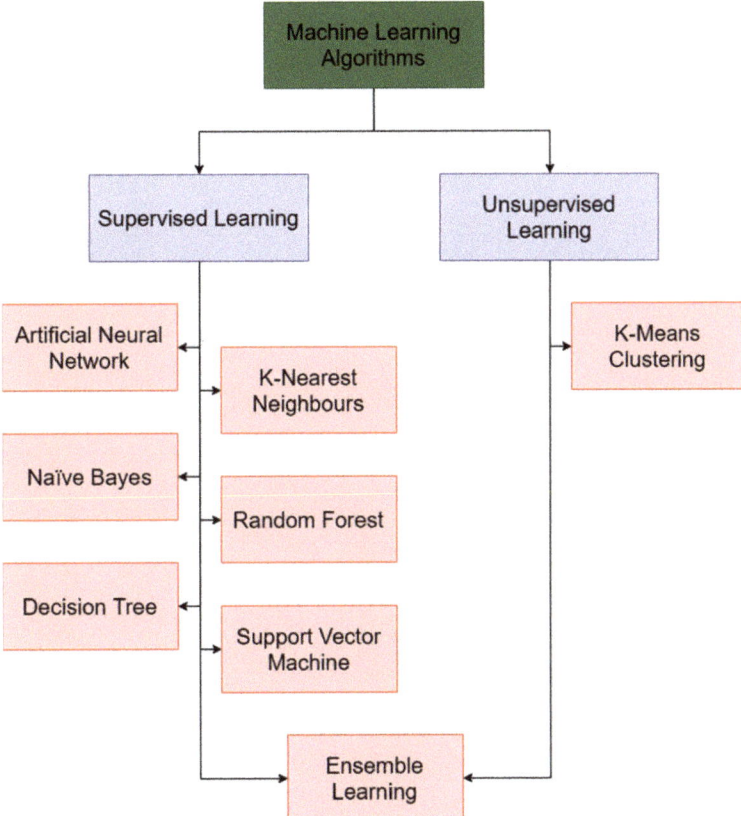

Figure 7. Current machine learning models in skin cancer diagnosis: tree illustration.

Table 4. Summary of works on machine learning techniques in skin cancer diagnosis.

Reference	Skin Cancer Category	Machine Learning Model	Description of Approach Used	Dataset	Key Contribution	Limitations	Performance Evaluation Metrics and Results
[38]	Non-melanoma skin cancer	Artificial neural network	12 neurons in each layer, inputs normalized to fall between 0 and 1, sigmoid activation function	National Health Interview Survey Dataset (NHIS 2016)	Multi-parametrized artificial neural network	Model does not include ultraviolet radiation exposure and family history data while making predictions	AUC is area under ROC curve. Training AUC—0.8058, validation AUC—0.8099
[44]	Skin disease detection and segmentation	Naïve Bayes classifier	Skin lesion segmentation using a dynamic graph cut algorithm followed by a naïve bayes classifier for skin disease classification	ISIC 2017	Flexible group minimizing for alike functions, making them decipherable in polynomial time	Cannot differentiate between certain colors	Diagnostic accuracy–72.7%, sensitivity– 91.7%, specificity-70.1%
[47]	Non-melanoma skin cancer	Decision tree	Cox regression analysis to identify variables that enter the decision tree analysis	Oregon Procurement Transplant Network STAR 2016	Confirms importance of known risk factors and also identifies new variables establishing risk of getting non melanoma skin cancer	Model building and validation sets were not from independent cohorts	Cumulative incidence rate highest risk group: 7.4%, intermediate risk group: 3.1–5.5%, lowest risk group: 0.8%
[54]	Skin lesion	K-nearest neighbor classifier	Firefly with k-nearest neighbor algorithm to predict and classify skin cancer using threshold-based segmentation	-	Recognize skin cancer without performing unnecessary skin biopsies	Image pre-processing and segmentation is heavily dependent on threshold values	False predictive value: 0.0, false negative rate: 11.11%, sensitivity: 88.89%, specificity: 100%
[56]	Melanoma skin cancer	K-means clustering	Region-based convolutional neural networks along with fuzzy k-means clustering.	ISIC 2016, ISIC 2017, PH2	Fully automated skin lesion segmentation at its earliest stage	Model is heavily reliant on successful segmentation from the R-CNN stage	Sensitivity: 90%, specificity: 97.1%, accuracy: 95.4%
[61]	Melanoma skin Cancer	Random forest	Watershed segmentation used for feature extraction and then classified with random forest	ISIC	Section lesions on skin with increased precision	Same classification can be carried out with higher accuracy using a simple vector machine	Accuracy: 74.32%, sensitivity: 76.85%, specificity: 71.79%
[66]	Melanoma skin cancer	Simple vector machine	Extracted features such as texture, color, shape are inputs to the SVM classifier for skin lesion classification	University Medical Center Groningen (UMCG) database	Computer Aided Diagnosis support system for image acquisition, pre-processing, segmentation, extraction, classification, and result viewing	No support for hair removal and image cropping techniques, classification model can be improved further	Confusion matrix: [3,7,62,64], where [true positive, true negative, false positive, false negative] sensitivity: 90%, specificity: 96%
[71]	Multi-class skin cancer	Ensemble learning	Weighted average ensemble learning based model using 5 deep learning models	Human Against Machine (HAM10000), ISIC 2019	Significantly improved result as compared to models individually and existing systems	Trained over a highly imbalanced dataset leading to compromised results while testing and validation	Confusion matrix, ROC-AUC score

3.3. Deep Learning Techniques

3.3.1. Recurrent Neural Network

A recurrent neural network (RNN) is categorized as a subdivision of artificial neural networks. RNNs have been used in the detection of melanoma skin cancer [72]. The classification phase of the proposed model employs deep learning techniques by combining the optimization notion into an RNN. The existing region growing algorithm and RNN have been improved by using them alongside the modified deer hunting optimization algorithm (DHOA). Apart from standalone models, RNNs have also been used in ensemble models alongside convolution neural networks, as seen in [73], to classify skin diseases. Predecessor models were unable to use the long-term dependence connection between key image features and image classes. This served as the motivation for the proposed model. Deep features are extracted from the clinical images, after which the features are fed into the dual bidirectional long short-term memory network to learn the features. Ultimately, a SoftMax activation function is used to classify the images. Similarly, ensemble models can also be used to automate the detection of mammogram breast cancer [74]. Just like in [73], the first step involves feature extraction through the grey level co-occurrence matrix and the grey level run-length matrix. These two are then given to the RNN layer as inputs, and the tumor segmented binary image is provided as input to the convolution neural network layer. The two independent classifiers' results show an improved diagnostic accuracy. RNNs have also been used in the segmentation of various dermoscopic images [75]. The reason for incorporating a recurrent model is primarily due to its ability to train deeper and bigger models. Furthermore, recurrent models ensure better feature representation and ultimately, better performance for the same number of parameters.

Modified RNNs, as proposed in [72], have an average accuracy of slightly over 90%, with an F1-score of 0.865. By varying the variable value in the equation used, the accuracy follows a linear trend by increasing as the value increases. Like the previous result, the RNNs in [74] have an accuracy of 98% but an F1-score of 0.745. The model in [75] reports a testing accuracy of 87.09% and an average F1-score of 0.86.

3.3.2. Deep Autoencoder

Deep autoencoders are neural networks that are trained to emulate the input as the output. They consist of two symmetrical deep belief networks. In the field of skin cancer, deep autoencoders have been used for reconstructing the dataset, which is then used to detect melanocytes by employing spiked neural networks [76]. The structure of the autoencoder model consists of three main layers: the input layer, hidden layers, and the output layer. The model is run on the foundational principle that every feature is not independent of each other, otherwise it would compromise the efficiency of the model. Autoencoders have also been used to recognize and detect melanoma skin disease [77]. The various autoencoders used were Deeplabv3+, Inception-ResNet-v2-unet, mobilenetv2_unet, Resnet50_unet, and vgg19_unet. Quantitative evaluation metrics showed that the Deeplabv3+ was a significant upgrade from the other architectures used in the study to detect melanoma skin. Skin cancer detection has also been carried out with the help of custom algorithms involving autoencoders, such as the social bat optimization algorithm [78]. The detection process takes place in three steps. Firstly, the clinical images are pre-processed to remove the noise and artefacts present. The pre-processed images are then fed to the feature extraction stage through a convolution neural network and a local pixel pattern-based texture feature. Right after this stage, the classification is completed using a deep stacked autoencoder, much like the evaluation in [77,79] of different autoencoders for skin lesion detection. The five architectures evaluated in this study are u-net, resu-net, vgg16unet, desnenet121, and efficientnetb0. Among the evaluated architectures, the densenet121 architecture showed the highest accuracy.

The autoencoder-based dataset used in [76] returned an average accuracy of 87.32%, with the sensitivity and specificity within one point of accuracy as well. The study in [77] concluded that using autoencoders consistently increased the accuracy and F1-score in various datasets, as opposed to the models that did not employ deep autoencoders. The average accuracy of the models in [77] after using autoencoders is around 94%. In a similar fashion, the deep stacked autoencoder presented in [78] returned an average accuracy of 93%, sensitivity of 84%, and specificity of 96%.

3.3.3. Long Short-Term Memory

Long short-term memory, or LSTM, is an artificial neural network that uses feedback connections to enable the processing of not only single data points, but also sequential data. LSTM has helped in classifying skin diseases by efficiently maintaining stateful information for accurate predictions [80]. The robustness of the proposed algorithm helps to recognize target regions faster, while using almost half the number of computations compared to predecessor algorithms. The use of LSTM further bolsters the accuracy of prediction due to its previous timestamp retention properties. Other than plain recognition, LSTMs can also be used to predict cancer and tumors in irregular medical data [81]. This is made possible by the enhanced overall performance of LSTMs in screening time series data. The risk groups being dealt with in the proposed study correlated well to the temporal cancer data (time to cancer diagnosis). Skin disease classification models have been designed using deep learning approaches like LSTM with the assistance of hybrid optimization algorithms such as the Hybrid Squirrel Butterfly Search Optimization algorithm (HSBSO) [82]. The modified LSTM is developed by implementing the HSBSO and the optimized parameters of an LSTM model to maximize the classification accuracy. LSTMs help in improving the overall efficiency of the proposed skin disease classification model. Deep learning models are not only limited to the clinical images of tumors. Certain studies demonstrate the usage of convolutional LSTMs to detect aneurysms on angiography images [83]. The angiography images are obtained from the 2D digital subtraction angiography, thereby making it hard to distinguish cerebral aneurysms from the overlapping vessels. The convolutional LSTM (C-LSTM) is a variant of the LSTM. Each LSTM cell has a convolutional operation associated with it. C-LSTM inherits the advantages of LSTM while being very suitable for the analysis of spatiotemporal data due to its internal convolution architecture. In real-life diagnoses, physicians combine lateral and frontal sequences to aid the decision-making process. Employing a similar concept, the C-LSTM is fed with two inputs: frontal and lateral images to increase the spatial information, consequently improving the performance of the entire system.

The incorporation of LSTM components to pretrained models such as the MobileNet V2, as seen in [81], outperforms some state-of-the-art models, with a training accuracy of 93.89% and validation accuracy of 90.72%. The study conducted in [82] demonstrated that LSTM performs better than most machine learning models, with an average sensitivity of 53% and specificity of 80%.

3.3.4. Deep Neural Network

Deep neural networks are those neural networks that expand to a certain level of complexity and depth. Vaguely, the certain level is decided to be two or more layers. Deep nets have been used to estimate the uncertainty lying in skin cancer detection [84]. The motivation behind the model lies in the ineptness of publicly available skin cancer detection software for providing confident estimates of the predictions. The study proposes the Deep Uncertainty Estimation for Skin Cancer (DUNEScan) that provides an in-depth and intuitive analysis of the uncertainty involved in each prediction. Deep nets have also been used to classify skin cancer at a dermatological level [85]. The classification of skin lesions, with the help of images alone, is an arduous task due to the minute variations in the visual appearance of lesions. Deep nets show immense potential for varied tasks that constitute multiple fine subcategories. The performance of the model is evaluated using biopsy-proven clinical images that were classified into two binary classification problems: keratinocyte carcinomas and benign seborrheic keratoses, and malignant melanomas and benign nevi. The deep net model achieves a performance that matches and, in some cases, outperforms all the experts associated with the evaluation program. For instance, the confusion matrix comparison between deep nets and dermatologists (experts) exhibits similarities in the misclassification of tumors [85]. The distribution demonstrates the difficulty in classifying malignant dermal tumors for both experts as well as deep nets, but also shows that experts noticeably confuse benign and malignant melanocytic lesions with each other, while the deep net classifies it with a higher degree of accuracy. Deep nets are usually implemented as a single-stream network. Two-stream deep nets, on the other hand, combine two recognition streams to handle the separate features associated with the input data. Two-stream deep nets have been used to design intelligent systems that classify skin cancer [86]. The two streams in the proposed method are a fusion-based contrast enhancement technique coupled with a pretrained DenseNet201 architecture, and down sample the extracted features using the proposed selection framework. The evaluation parameters suggest that the proposed method returns an improved performance upgrade over the predecessor models. Deep net models have also been deployed in real world applications, empowering medical professionals by assisting the process of diagnosing skin cancer and employing a prediction model for over 100 skin disorders [87]. The deep learning algorithms have proven to be a successful method with which to diagnose malignant tumors, as well as suggest treatment if trained with a dataset consisting of substantial numbers of Asian and Caucasian populations. Using a convolution neural network as the ancillary tool, the performance is elevated and can be used to diagnose cutaneous skin diseases.

3.3.5. Deep Belief Network

Deep belief networks (DBN) are generative graphical models that are composed of multiple layers of latent variables. DBNs have been used for cancer prediction, as can be seen in [88]. They perform the model training in two steps. Firstly, each layer is separately trained in an unsupervised manner. This is done to retain the maximum feature information. Subsequently, the output features are taken and used to train the entity relationship classifier in a supervised manner. DBNs have been designed to automatically detect regions of breast mass and diagnose them as benign, malignant, or neither [89]. The proposed DBN performs comparatively better than its conventional counterparts. This is because the conventional approaches depend on the output of selection feature algorithms. On the contrary, all the features were directly used without any reduction in their dimensions for the DBN model. To improve the diagnosis of skin melanoma by using DBNs in place of the traditional approach, dermoscopy has been studied [90]. The deep belief learning network architecture disperses the weights and hyperparameters to every position in the clinical image. By doing so, this makes it possible to scale the algorithm to varying sizes. The images are first use a Gaussian filter to remove the high and low intensities from the images. Subsequently, the pre-processed images are segmented using the k-means algorithm. The resultant images are then classified as per the output format of the proposed DBN.

The DBN presented in [88] reports a diagnostic accuracy of 81.48%. According to the study, for the evaluation criteria tested, the DBN outperformed the RNNs and CNNs, which had an accuracy of 73% and 68%, respectively. DBNs that are used to complement computer-aided diagnosis, as seen in [89], report an average accuracy of around 91%. For unsegmented images, the DBN model in [90] achieves an accuracy of 73% while the same model, when subjected to segmented images, achieves an accuracy of 90%. This suggests that DBNs might accurately predict if the input is segmented and pre-processed correctly.

3.3.6. Deep Convolutional Neural Network

Convolutional neural networks (CNNs) are artificial neural networks that are primarily used in image processing and recognition. Deep convolutional neural networks have been implemented to classify skin cancer into four different categories: basal cell carcinoma, squamous cell carcinoma, actinic keratosis, and melanoma [91]. The methodology involves two methods, an error-correcting output codes simple vector machine (ECOC SVM) classifier, and a deep CNN. The authors use accuracy, sensitivity, and specificity as evaluation parameters. A slight variation from the previous method introduces a LeNet-5 architecture along with a deep CNN to classify the image data [92]. The model aids the diagnosis of melanoma cancer. The experiment results indicate that training data and number of epochs for training are integral to the process of the detection and diagnosis of melanoma cancer. Results suggest that training the model for over 100 epochs may lead to overfitting while training it for below 100 epochs leads to underfitting. In addition, there are several parameters which account for the accuracy of the results, such as the learning rate, number of layers, and dimensions of the input image. Since dermatologists use patient data along with deep CNNs for an increased diagnostic accuracy, recent studies have investigated the influence of integrating image feature data into the deep CNN model [93]. The commonly used patient data were sex, age, and lesion location. To accommodate the patient data, one-hot encoding was performed. The key differentiator between fusing the image features was the complexity associated with each classification, respectively. The studies indicate the potential benefits and advantages of amalgamating patient data into a deep CNN algorithm. Region-based CNNs have been employed to detect keratinocytic skin cancer on the face [94]. The algorithm aims to automatically locate the affected and suspected areas by returning a probabilistic value of a malignant lesion. The deep CNN was trained on over one million image crops to help locate and diagnose cancer. While the algorithm demonstrated great potential, certain pitfalls were highlighted: skin markings were mistaken as lesions by the deep CNN model. Secondly, the testing data usually made use of the physician's evaluation data, rather than the clinical photographs alone, which ultimately led to the need for a multimodal approach. The developments of recent studies have enabled newly designed models to outperform expert dermatologists and contemporary deep learning methods in the field of multi-class skin cancer classification, using deep CNNs [95]. The model was fine-tuned over seven classes in the HAM10000 dataset. While ensemble models increase the accuracy for classification problems, they do not have a major role in refining the performance of the finely-tuned hyperparameter setup for deep CNNs.

The deep CNNs, as seen in [91], could classify skin cancer with an accuracy of 94.2%. Furthermore, the sensitivity and specificity of the model were also above 90%. Region-based CNN that is used to classify skin cancer on the face [94] returns an average accuracy of 91.5%. The study further emphasized the benefits of using a CNN-based model as a screening tool to improve public health, as the sensitivity of the general public was merely 50%. The model, on the other hand, averaged a sensitivity of 85%.

3.3.7. Deep Boltzmann Machine

Deep Boltzmann machines (DBM) are probabilistic, unsupervised, and generative models that possess undirected connections between multiple layers within the model. Multi-modal DBMs have been proposed to monitor and diagnose cancer before the mortality rate rises [96]. The multi-modal DBM learns the correlation between an instance's genetic structure. The testing and evaluation phase use the same to predict the genes that are cancer-causing mutations specific to the specimen. By combining restricted Boltzmann machines (RBM) and a skin lesion classification model through optimal segmentation, the OS-RBM model helps to detect and classify the presence of skin lesions in clinical images [97]. The OS-RBM model carries out certain steps sequentially: image acquisition, pre-processing using Gaussian filters, segmenting the pre-processed images, extracting the features, and classifying the images. Segmenting images is executed through the Artificial Bee Colony algorithm.

3.3.8. Deep Reinforcement Learning

Reinforcement learning (RL) is a training method often associated with rewarding and punishing the desired and undesired behaviors, respectively. Reinforcement learning algorithms have been incorporated into the medical scene to automatically detect skin lesions [98]. This is done by initially proceeding from coarse segmentation to sharp and fine results. The model is trained on the popular ISIC 2017 dataset and HAM10000 dataset. The regions are initially delineated. By tuning the hyperparameters appropriately, the segmentation accuracy is also boosted. As deep RL methods have the capability to detect and segment small irregular shapes, the potential for deep RLs in the medical background is immense.

3.3.9. Extreme Learning Machine

Extreme learning machines (ELM) are essentially feedforward neural networks. While they provide a good generalization performance, the major difference arises in the learning speed. ELM models have been proposed to tackle the existing problem of skin cancer detection [99]. This detection takes place by differentiating between benign and malignant lesions. Upon pre-processing the clinical images, the regions are segmented using the Otsu method. The model optimizes and learns with the help of a deep belief network which introduces a Thermal Exchange Optimization algorithm. Using hybrid pretrained models along with ELMs for diagnosing skin cancer has also been researched [100]. The proposed diagnostic model makes use of the SqueezeNet model for the batch normalization layers. The layers towards the end of the model are replaced by ELMs. The ELMs are usually linked with a metaheuristic, for instance, the Bald Eagle Search Optimization metaheuristic, that enable the model to converge much faster than its contemporary counterparts. Instead of pretrained models, hybrid deep learning models have also been combined with extreme learning machines to classify skin lesions into multiple classes [101]. While majority of the steps remain the same, the major differences lie in the deep feature extraction that uses transfer learning and feature selection, which makes use of hybrid whale optimization and entropy-mutual information algorithms. Extreme learning machines can also be modified and used as an extreme gradient boosting method for the remote diagnosis of skin cancer [102]. Apart from diagnosis, the model also helps in the process of health triage. The major problem faced by the authors were the unbalanced categories in the dataset. To overcome this imbalance, data augmentation was incorporated. Integrating the skin lesions with the clinical data reinforced the accuracy and efficacy of the model.

ELM models that are used for multi-class skin lesion classification [101] produce high-quality predictions with an accuracy of over 94%. ELM models have been shown to consistently outperform respective benchmark studies, as seen in [102]. Even though the accuracy of the model in [102] hovers around 77%, it is significantly higher than the benchmark studies for the same set of data and conditions. When coupled with data augmentation, ELMs can avoid the risk of overfitting.

3.3.10. Summary of Deep Learning Models

Deep learning models provide robust solutions for skin cancer detection. Recurrent neural networks can accurately predict the incidence of skin cancer to a fairly high degree, but they come with the limitation of being efficient only when using large datasets. For smaller data points, RNNs will not have enough data to learn the features and predict as accurately. Autoencoders serve as a recourse for insufficient data. Deep autoencoder-based datasets, used with pretrained models, return highly accurate results. The major drawback involved in deep autoencoders is the parameter value initialization. Most of the studies employ a preliminary trial method to settle for the initial parameter values, which may prove to be infeasible for large models. Long short-term memory models outperform other deep learning techniques in terms of classification and tumor growth progress analysis, but the accuracy of the model sharply drops to below 80% when the quality of the images is substandard, such as poor illumination or conditions different from those in the testing dataset. Deep neural networks produce good results but cannot match the versatility of other deep learning techniques such as RNNs or LSTMs. DNN models find it tough to distinguish between blurry shadows or irregular borders unless they have been trained on such data. To be widely adopted, DNNs require training images with adequate quality, making it a cause of concern, as clinical data may not emulate the training dataset conditions. Deep belief network models return highly accurate results, but in similar conditions, are often outperformed by convolutional neural networks. CNNs provide users with the flexibility to extend the model with different learning techniques, as well as accurately predict different types of skin cancer. Most of the studies involving CNNs reported an average accuracy of over 90%. New techniques in the deep learning space make use of extreme learning machines. These models outperform state-of-the-art techniques, with reported accuracies of over 93%. While they return accurate results, they are susceptible to poorly augmented datasets, which can sharply decrease the accuracy of the model.

Table 5 summarizes the works discussed on deep learning models used for skin cancer diagnosis. Figure 8 shows the deep learning models in skin cancer diagnosis, as elucidated in this study.

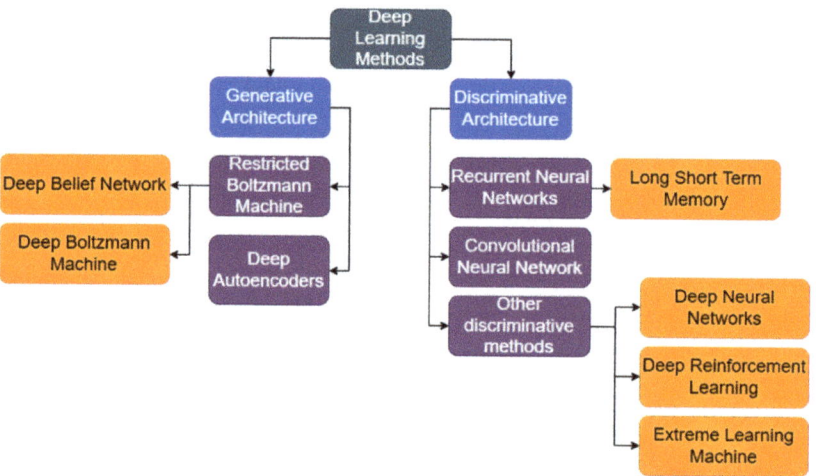

Figure 8. Current deep learning models for skin cancer diagnosis: tree illustration.

Table 5. Summary of works on deep learning models in skin cancer diagnosis.

Reference	Skin Cancer Category	Deep Learning Model	Description of Approach Used	Dataset	Key Contribution	Limitations	Performance Evaluation Metrics and Results
[72]	Melanoma skin cancer	Recurrent neural networks	Classification phases uses modified deep learning algorithm by coalescing optimization concepts from RNNs	PH2	Superior to existing algorithms in terms of optimal segmentation and classification for melanoma skin cancer	Heavy dependence on parameters for segmentation and classification	Algorithmic analysis including specificity: 0.94915, sensitivity: 0.83051, precision: 0.89091, F1-score: 0.85965, etc.
[76]	Skin cancer detection	Autoencoders	Dataset is reconstructed using autoencoder model, reconstruction and spiking networks contribute to enhanced performance	ISIC	Feature sets obtained from convolution model are suitable for merging	Model extracts many unnecessary and irrelevant features	Specificity: 0.9332, sensitivity: 0.9372, precision: 0.9450, F1-score: 0.9411, accuracy: 0.9354
[81]	Skin cancer diagnosis	Long short-term memory model	Tumor marker data values were used to train and test an LSTM model	Two independent medical centers	LSTM model demonstrates superiority while dealing with irregular data and can be used when time intervals between tests vary	Inability to analyze irregular tumor marker data for cancer screening	Time-to-cancer diagnosis in different risk groups, risk stratification
[87]	Binary classification, multi-class skin cancer diagnosis	Deep neural network	CNN architectures trained on large datasets and evaluated against algorithm-assisted clinicians' results	Edinburgh and SNU datasets	Model serves as an ancillary tool to enhance diagnostic accuracy of clinicians	Outcome of algorithm is significantly affected by composition of input images; performance is sub-optimal if input image quality is low	Improvement in sensitivity and specificity by 12.1% and 1.1%, respectively
[88]	Malignant tumor detection	Deep belief network	Analyze patient data from deep learning perspective, merged with patient attributes and case reports to construct an expert system helping to predict the probability of early cancer	Jiangsu Provincial Hospital of Traditional Chinese Medicine	Relatively effective dimensional reduction and noise cancellation technique, reduces missed clinician diagnoses during endoscopy and treatment	Medium runtime in comparison to other deep learning methods	Accuracy: 0.8148, precision: 0.8571, recall: 0.6, F1 score: 0.7059
[91]	Melanoma, carcinoma, keratosis	Deep convolutional neural network	Classifies skin cancer using ECOC SVM and deep CNN, images are cropped to reduce noise	Pretrained on ImageNet, Internet Images for fine-tuning	Multi-class skin cancer classification using fine-tuned pretrained ImageNet model	Model does not extend to ABCD (asymmetry, border, color, diameter) rule	Accuracy: 0.942, specificity: 0.9074, sensitivity: 0.9783
[96]	Tumor causing somatic mutations	Deep Boltzmann machine	Multi-modal deep Boltzmann machine approach for prediction of somatic mutation genes that undergo malignant transformation, model learns relation between germline and mutation profiles using data	—	Genome-based diagnostic test to monitor for the presence of cancer-driving mutations	Sample size of is limited, Whole Exome Sequencing (WES) data displayed at gene level	Average accuracy: 0.7176, p-value
[99]	Melanoma skin cancer	Extreme learning machine	After pre-processing, Otsu method is employed to segment region of interest, subsequently, feature extraction is applied to mine important characteristics, deep belief network is used to categorize and classify	ISIC for training, SIIM-ISIC melanoma for validation	Optimized Pipeline feature designed for efficient detection of melanoma from images, DBN uses Thermal Exchange Optimization Algorithm as new meta-heuristic method	Computationally very intensive and time consuming	Accuracy: 0.9265, specificity: 0.8970, sensitivity: 0.9118, PPV: 0.8676, NPV: 0.9412

4. Open Challenges in Skin Cancer Diagnosis

4.1. Communication Barrier between AI and Dermatologists

Giant strides in the field of Artificial Intelligence for skin cancer diagnosis mean it may have established its place in the scene for years to come, but it has still not been able to breach the communication barrier that exists between dermatologists and AI. In [103], it is suggested that dermatologists must embrace the potential shown by AI applications in various fields, such as clinical and research situations. The preconceived notion surrounding the use of AI in the cancer diagnosis domain that the introduction of technology may eventually downsize the workforce, has set the wrong precedent, and has brought about apprehensions about adopting AI for the same. It must be understood that, while AI has been ever improving and returns a higher accuracy with respect to diagnoses, clinicians are undoubtedly more skillful in identifying mimetics, as well as patterns that have not been made available to the models through the training datasets [103]. The authors of [103] reiterate that the role of dermatologists is not limited to detecting and identifying skin lesions, but also to extract valuable information and inferences from their observations. At present, the latter is not quite fine-tuned and is still in the rudimentary stages in machines. In a survey conducted on Chinese dermatologists [104], the majority of the participants believed that AI in the workplace assisted with daily activities involving diagnosis and treatment. In accordance with the claims made by the authors of [103], the survey results indicated that only 3% of the dermatologist participants believed that AI could and would replace their day-to-day work. Another survey in [105] indicated positive diagnosis results and a higher accuracy, as compared to traditional approaches, after dermatologists used the help of AI in making their decisions. The need to bridge the communication gap between AI and dermatologists is paramount, and efforts must be taken to involve the various functionalities offered by AIs in the workplace.

4.2. Dataset Availability and Features

Incorporating deep learning into cancer diagnosis in the real world comes with one major roadblock—the lack of availability of datasets. Machine learning and deep learning algorithms require huge amounts of datasets to be trained upon, without which the models will ultimately return subpar results. Some databases do not include benign lesions such as blisters and warts; these lesions are managed by dermatologists daily, making it a very common occurrence in day-to-day diagnoses. This poses the threat of missing skin cancer among benign lesions, as they are not included in the datasets. According to [7], most of the online publicly available datasets consist of only raw images. This essentially means that most of the headway must be generated by the researchers themselves. To tackle the prevalent issue of an imbalance in the datasets, researchers have started employing data augmentation techniques such as cropping, rotation, and filtering, which, in turn, increases the number of training images the models can use [8]. While the datasets provide a rich source of information for the researchers, the absence of clarity in the metadata for various characteristics, such as ethnicity and skin types, inhibits the utility of clinical images [33]. The future of datasets and the furthering of improvement in AI-based diagnostic methods have already been set in motion in the form of open science, such as providing clinical decision support for diagnoses and screening. To overcome the problems faced in obtaining datasets to a greater extent, the adoption of open science must gain traction.

4.3. Patient Perspectives on Artificial Intelligence

Artificial Intelligence is assured to change the way patients interact with healthcare-associated processes, but it has remained elusive in terms of patients' outlook and perspectives on AI in healthcare. The survey conducted in [106] aims to decipher the reception of Artificial Intelligence in healthcare by the patients. The central theme of most responses revolved around the diagnosis of the illness. This establishes a symbiotic relation between patients and the use of AI. While around 75% of the patients were keen to recommend AI in healthcare to family members, the apprehension of the remaining 25% is concerning. One way to tackle this is by ensuring that the response to conflict can be resolved by seeking a biopsy to complement the Artificial Intelligence decision-making. Apart from incorrect diagnoses, patients also are wary about their medical and clinical history being made available if used for datasets. Without properly labeled images, AI will be unable to train properly, leading to incorrect diagnosis results. Data analytics involving AI models for skin cancer diagnoses heavily use these labels to infer observations for future research [35]. By concealing the data, or submitting falsified information, this destroys the purpose of training an AI. This can be mitigated by ensuring that data collection organizations maintain non-disclosure policies.

4.4. Variation in Lesion Images

Skin cancer diagnosis using machine learning and deep learning involves multiple steps, out of which the primary step is skin lesion segmentation. As straightforward as it may seem, this task is commonly associated with setbacks that inhibit its smooth completion, namely the variations in lesion sizes, imprecise and indistinct boundaries, and different skin colors. The variation in different images, such as illumination difference, leads to uneven shadows and bright areas, making it tougher to segment the skin lesions [107]. Conventional algorithms such as CNNs and CNN-based approaches may perform superiorly in terms of labeling, but they still return a poor contrast between lesion and regular skin images. This is due to the deviations in the dataset, such as skin tone and aberrations, etc. The immense variation in datasets leads to the lack of inference drawn from the results, as suggested in [108]. A varying methodological quality shows higher amounts of specificity and sensitivity when compared to an expert's diagnosis, thus rendering the use of AI in healthcare less useful. The corresponding diagnostic score and criteria for qualifying as an expert have been covered in a review that studies optical coherence while diagnosing adult skin cancer [108]. To tackle the problem of the varying characteristics of skin lesions, AI models must look to maximize their diversification and intensification [109]. By employing such mechanisms, the models can overcome the stagnation faced due to the increasing variation. In addition, the diagnosis of skin cancer in people of color is put off until advanced stages, due to the variations in lesion images that engender from the difference in skin tones [122]. Furthermore, due to socio-economic factors such as care barriers, models are not trained on different skin tones [122]. They develop an inherent bias towards the dominant skin tone and lesion color that the model has been trained on, which ultimately compromises the quality of the skin cancer diagnosis.

4.5. Dermatological Image Acquisition

Image acquisition in dermatology generally deals with close-up images of lesions or dermatosis. In most cases, the anatomical context of such images is lost due to the exclusion of surrounding structures, while the primary focus of the image is the lesion. Furthermore, with the rapid adoption of digital skin imaging applications, the utilization of smartphone-acquired images in dermatology have also increased proportionally [123]. While many studies have proposed methods to detect melanomas from inconsistent dermoscopy images, most of them produce localized results that cannot be used universally due to the acquisitive conditions they are trained on, such as isolated datasets and specific illumination conditions, etc. [124]. In addition to these problems, the quality of the acquired images is significantly compromised due to the varying illumination conditions during the acquisition phase, such as specular reflection. In [125], a generative adversarial neural network is proposed to deal with the persisting present problem of color inconsistency. The wider adoption of such methods, and an increase in the novelty of ideas that overcome erratic dermoscopy images, are required for overcoming the challenges faced by image acquisition.

4.6. Ethical and Legal Perspectives

While the use of AI in the clinical practice and healthcare domains has lots of upsides, it raises many ethical challenges. The use of health AI, albeit for transforming the patient–clinician relationship, carries ambiguity around the use of informed consent. The clinicians are unaware about the circumstances under which they should or should not inform the patient about AI being a part of the relationship [110]. AI decisions carry lots of weight, and they come with the challenges of safety and transparency. While it is understood that no AI model can be correct all the time, incorrect decisions can prove to be fatal, as well as mold correct decisions as unsafe. This gives rise to the concern around model algorithms' fairness and bias. Models are trained on a particular set of data, making them biased to the characters they inferred from the dataset. It is virtually impossible for any dataset to exactly sample the world's population and thus raises a flag for a cause for concern. AI technology has been identified to have a tremendous capability to threaten patient preference [111]. Parallelly, the use of health-related AI inevitably intersects with the law in more than one way. The question of how liability should be attributed in the case of harmful treatment is still unanswered. Similarly, AI bias against historically disadvantaged groups can attract anti-discrimination and human rights laws [112]. It is yet unknown whether the existing privacy laws can protect patients undergoing AI-based healthcare. It is necessary to understand that, while the potential benefits of AI in healthcare are plenty, it cannot be adopted for commercial use unless the ethical and legal challenges are responded to, as they serve as the bedrock of the entire system.

Figure 9 visualizes the open problems in skin cancer diagnosis using machine-learning- and deep-learning-based techniques.

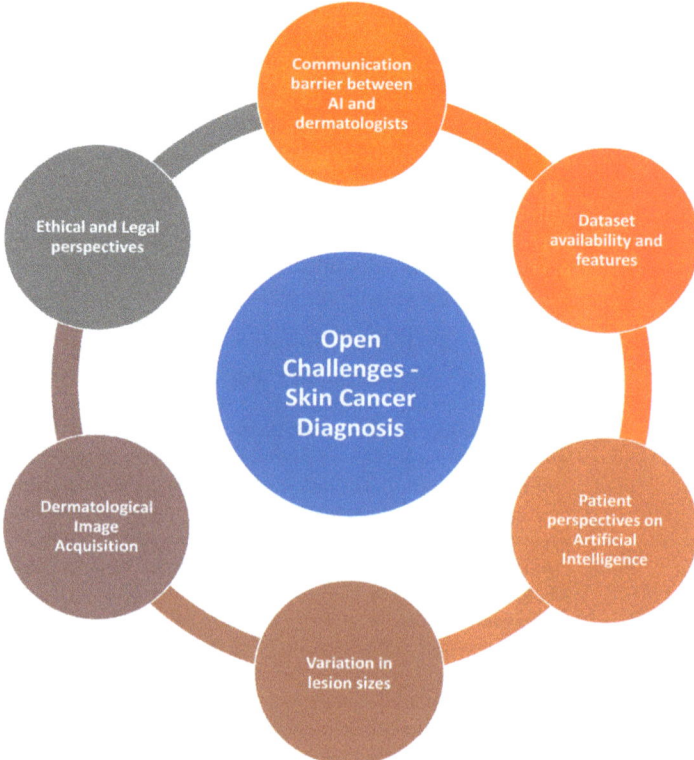

Figure 9. Open challenges in skin cancer diagnosis.

5. Future Research Directions

5.1. Combining AI with Next-Generation Sequencing for Refining Skin Cancer Diagnosis

Next-generation sequencing (NGS) technologies have progressed to facilitate the increase in data output and the efficiencies associated with it. NGS is categorized based on its respective read lengths [113]. NGS is used to determine the order of nucleotides in entire genomes or targeted regions in RNA and DNA. High-throughput DNA sequencing technology and methods have paved the way for commercializing new techniques [114]. The goal of DNA sequencing methods is to support speed while staying accurate, coupled with lower input rates of DNA and RNA input data. Squamous cell carcinoma (SCC) carries one of the highest tumor mutation burdens amongst all cancers. By employing the targeted next-generation sequencing of localized and metastatic high-risk SCCs, gene mutations can be compared with the intention of identifying key differences and improving targeted treatment alternatives [115]. Since the introduction of molecular tools, the discovery of new viruses, such as the papillomavirus, has been accelerated. NGS can be combined with improved protocols to help detect known and unknown human papillomaviruses [116].

5.2. AI-powered Automated Decision Support Systems for Skin Cancer Diagnosis

Decision support systems are computerized programs used to assist with decision-making and choosing the right course of action; Artificial-Intelligence-powered decision support systems can be used in the diagnosis of skin cancer. They provide options of flexibility in designing deep learning classification models by hinting at the common procedures and looping patterns [117]. Support systems can be initialized with pretrained deep neural network models combined with transfer learning to classify skin lesion localization and classification [118]. Present day decision support systems are fused with automated deep learning methods. These methods are fine-tuned and trained with the help of transfer learning using imbalanced data [119]. The model extracts the features using an average pooling layer, although the extracted features are not sufficient. By employing a modified genetic algorithm based on metaheuristics, relevant and significant features are extracted which can further be sent to a classifier that acts as a decision support system. As mentioned in [120], using AI-powered decision support systems can help clinicians diagnose and potentially replace invasive diagnostic techniques.

5.3. Smart Robotics for Skin Cancer Diagnosis

Robots can be used to improve the detection of skin cancer. Existing robots like Vectra WB360 combine 3D images with the corresponding sequential digital dermoscopic images, owing to the non-invasive tracking of melanoma and non-melanoma skin cancer. The photographic analysis of the WB360 allows for a global view of the skin surface and generates a body map to record the evolution of the lesions. This feature is very useful in detecting any suspicious developments promptly.

5.4. Wearable Computing for Skin Cancer Diagnosis

Wearable computing is a paradigm that involves the computation of accessories that can be worn by humans. Any small device capable of computing and processing data that can be worn on the body is categorized as a wearable computer. Wearable computers have been used in the field of cancer detection [121]. A few challenges that have not allowed for widespread clinical adoption yet are the high fragility, bendability, non-cooperative form factor of the sensors used, inappropriate connectivity, clinical inertia, and ultimately the awareness, as well as the cost, associated with wearable devices. Future research and corporations should aim to reduce the cost policy while tackling the challenges of using wearable computing as a vital alternative for cancer detection.

These event-driven tools are beneficial when concerning computational effectiveness, higher efficiency, power consumption, flexibility, and improved real-time performance. The possibility of incorporating these tools into wearable devices could be beneficial in terms of performance enhancement.

5.5. Teledermatology

Teledermatology is described as technology that supports healthcare from a distance [130]. Teledermatology aims to provide clinical services to patients, monitor their health, and provide resources through remote locations. This technology can be used for diagnosing, screening, and even managing skin cancer effectively. In total, three prospective solutions for implementing these are the store and forward method, real-time video conferencing, and a hybrid solution that includes both. At present, the store and forward method is widely in use with patients taking pictures and videos, which are then forwarded to the dermatologist. The ease of the convenience and the inexpensiveness make it a very popular choice. Real-time video conferencing uses the interaction between patient and physician through a video calling software to provide immediate advice. This simulates an in-person clinic experience, where the physician can verify medical data and history before prescribing anything. This method requires a stable internet connection and a high-quality video camera if it must be used for skin cancer. A low-quality camera may not fully capture the border and may eventually lead to erroneous diagnoses. The hybrid method mixes the advantages of both the methods: real-time video conferencing coupled with high-quality images sent to the dermatologist. Together, these serve as a beneficial way to consult and diagnose skin cancer. Teledermatology can be used with many machine learning and deep learning techniques to make the entire process much smoother. For instance, there are various CNN architectures which can be employed using transfer learning [131]. Doing so can help the dermatologist make decisions with a higher degree of confidence. Ensemble models can be incorporated into the pipeline for the store and forward method, enabling the system to be more accurate after the patient sends adequate-quality photos or videos.

Figure 10 illustrates the future directions for machine-learning- and deep-learning-enabled skin cancer diagnosis.

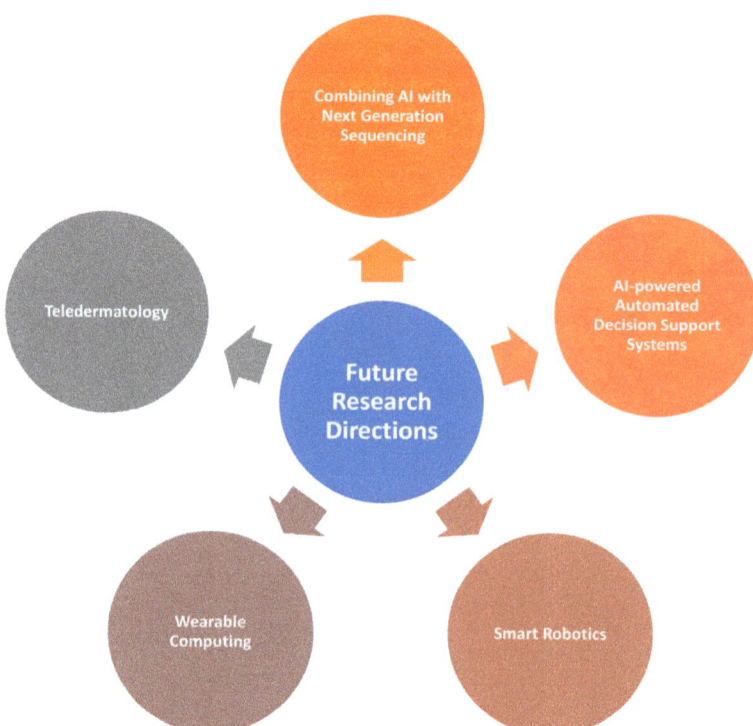

Figure 10. Future research directions of skin cancer diagnosis.

The internet of medical things (IoMT) and cloud computing will be the essential elements in upcoming mobile AI-powered healthcare-related decision support systems. In this framework, the event-driven tools can be beneficial when concerning computational effectiveness, real-time compression, data transmission efficiency, power consumption, and flexibility [135–137]. The possibility of incorporating these tools into contemporary mobile healthcare solutions can be investigated in the future.

6. Conclusions

A comprehensive survey is presented on machine learning and deep learning techniques, deployed for an automated skin cancer diagnosis. A comparison is made to the widely used skin cancer datasets and dominant studies. An insight discussion is had while exploring the lessons from prior works. Its aim is to set this survey as a benchmark for further studies in the field of skin cancer diagnosis by also including the limitations and benefits of the previous works. It is concluded that the Artificial Intelligence (AI)-based healthcare solutions come with many pre-requisites, dependencies and issues that must first be resolved before they can scale up. The AI research carries ethical and legal ambiguities, along with a lack of clinical data on all skin types, thereby inducing unintended bias in the model's prediction. Moreover, although AI is gaining traction in the dermatology discipline, it still has lots of room to grow and enhance further in terms of the sensitivity, specificity, and accuracy of detecting the skin lesions. Additionally, dermatologists must take the first step in accepting and embracing AI, not as a threat to their professions, but as an ancillary tool to complement their diagnoses. While considering the challenges for implanting end-to-end AI-based solutions in healthcare, there are lots of prospects, promises, and challenges. Wearable computing and robotics are evolving, and AI healthcare can be incorporated into these recent innovations to ease the apprehensive market. While the limited available data suggest a parity between those who are keen on adopting AI healthcare, and those aversive towards it, the room to improve automated skin cancer detection has been established.

Author Contributions: Conceptualization, N.M., K.S. and S.M.Q.; methodology, N.M., K.S. and S.M.Q.; implementation, N.M. and K.S.; validation, K.S., S.M.Q. and P.P.; investigation, N.M., K.S. and S.M.Q.; resources, K.S., S.M.Q. and P.P.; writing—original draft preparation, N.M. and K.S.; writing—review and editing, S.M.Q. and P.P.; visualization, N.M. and K.S.; supervision, K.S. and S.M.Q.; project administration, K.S., S.M.Q. and P.P.; funding acquisition, S.M.Q. and P.P. All authors have read and agreed to the published version of the manuscript.

Funding: This research received no external funding.

Acknowledgments: This work is technically supported by the Vellore Institute of Technology, Effat University, LINEACT CESI, Cracow University of Technology, and Polish Academy of Sciences. The authors are thankful to the Effat University, Cracow University of Technology and Polish Academy of Sciences for financially supporting this paper.

Conflicts of Interest: Regarding the publication of this paper, the authors affirm that there are no conflict of interest.

Appendix A

Table A1. List of abbreviations used in this manuscript along with their full form.

Acronym	Definition
AI	Artificial Intelligence
ANN	Artificial neural network
KNN	K-nearest neighbors
ABCD	Asymmetry, border, color, diameter
SVM	Support vector machine

Table A1. *Cont.*

Acronym	Definition
ROC	Receiver Operating Characteristic
AUC	Area under curve
RNN	Recurrent neural network
DHOA	Deer hunting optimization algorithm
LSTM	Long short-term memory
DBN	Deep belief network
CNN	Convolutional neural network
DBM	Deep Boltzmann machine
RL	Reinforcement learning
ELM	Extreme learning machine
NGS	Next generation sequencing
DNA	Deoxyribonucleic acid
RNA	Ribonucleic acid
SCC	Squamous cell carcinoma

References

1. Murugan, A.; Nair, S.A.H.; Preethi, A.A.P.; Kumar, K.P.S. Diagnosis of skin cancer using machine learning techniques. *Microprocess. Microsyst.* **2020**, *81*, 103727. [CrossRef]
2. Vijayalakshmi, M.M. Melanoma skin cancer detection using image processing and machine learning. *Int. J. Trend Sci. Res. Dev.* **2019**, *3*, 780–784.
3. Ozkan, I.A.; Koklu, M. Skin lesion classification using machine learning algorithms. *Int. J.-Telligent Syst. Appl. Eng.* **2017**, *5*, 285–289. [CrossRef]
4. Monika, M.K.; Vignesh, N.A.; Kumari, C.U.; Kumar, M.; Lydia, E.L. Skin cancer detection and classification using machine learning. *Mater. Today Proc.* **2020**, *33*, 4266–4270. [CrossRef]
5. Nahata, H.; Singh, S.P. Deep learning solutions for skin cancer detection and diagnosis. In *Machine Learning with Health Care Perspective*; Springer: Cham, Switzerland, 2020; pp. 159–182.
6. Das, K.; Cockerell, C.J.; Patil, A.; Pietkiewicz, P.; Giulini, M.; Grabbe, S.; Goldust, M. Machine Learning and Its Application in Skin Cancer. *Int. J. Environ. Res. Public Health* **2021**, *18*, 13409. [CrossRef]
7. Tufail, A.B.; Ma, Y.-K.; Kaabar, M.K.A.; Martínez, F.; Junejo, A.R.; Ullah, I.; Khan, R. Deep learning in cancer diagnosis and prognosis prediction: A minireview on challenges, recent trends, and future directions. *Comput. Math. Methods Med.* **2021**, *2021*, 9025470. [CrossRef]
8. Munir, K.; Elahi, H.; Ayub, A.; Frezza, F.; Rizzi, A. Cancer Diagnosis Using Deep Learning: A Bibliographic Review. *Cancers* **2019**, *11*, 1235. [CrossRef]
9. Goyal, M.; Knackstedt, T.; Yan, S.; Hassanpour, S. Artificial intelligence-based image classification methods for diagnosis of skin cancer: Challenges and opportunities. *Comput. Biol. Med.* **2020**, *127*, 104065. [CrossRef] [PubMed]
10. Li, H.; Pan, Y.; Zhao, J.; Zhang, L. Skin disease diagnosis with deep learning: A review. *Neurocomputing* **2021**, *464*, 364–393. [CrossRef]
11. Shastry, K.A.; Sanjay, H.A. Cancer diagnosis using artificial intelligence: A review. *Artif. Intell. Rev.* **2021**, *55*, 2641–2673. [CrossRef]
12. Painuli, D.; Bhardwaj, S.; Köse, U. Recent advancement in cancer diagnosis using machine learning and deep learning techniques: A comprehensive review. *Comput. Biol. Med.* **2022**, *146*, 105580. [CrossRef] [PubMed]
13. Naeem, A.; Farooq, M.S.; Khelifi, A.; Abid, A. Malignant Melanoma Classification Using Deep Learning: Datasets, Performance Measurements, Challenges and Opportunities. *IEEE Access* **2020**, *8*, 110575–110597. [CrossRef]
14. Haggenmüller, S.; Maron, R.C.; Hekler, A.; Utikal, J.S.; Barata, C.; Barnhill, R.L.; Beltraminelli, H.; Berking, C.; Betz-Stablein, B.; Blum, A.; et al. Skin cancer classification via convolutional neural networks: Systematic review of studies involving human experts. *Eur. J. Cancer* **2021**, *156*, 202–216. [CrossRef] [PubMed]
15. Adegun, A.; Viriri, S. Deep learning techniques for skin lesion analysis and melanoma cancer detection: A survey of state-of-the-art. *Artif. Intell. Rev.* **2020**, *54*, 811–841. [CrossRef]
16. Saba, T. Recent advancement in cancer detection using machine learning: Systematic survey of decades, comparisons and challenges. *J. Infect. Public Health* **2020**, *13*, 1274–1289. [CrossRef]
17. Usama, M.; Naeem, M.A.; Mirza, F. Multi-Class Skin Lesions Classification Using Deep Features. *Sensors* **2022**, *22*, 8311. [CrossRef]

18. Bratchenko, I.A.; Bratchenko, L.A.; Khristoforova, Y.A.; Moryatov, A.A.; Kozlov, S.V.; Zakharov, V.P. Classification of skin cancer using convolutional neural networks analysis of Raman spectra. *Comput. Methods Programs Biomed.* **2022**, *219*, 106755. [CrossRef]
19. Brinker, T.J.; Hekler, A.; Utikal, J.S.; Grabe, N.; Schadendorf, D.; Klode, J.; Berking, C.; Steeb, T.; Enk, A.H.; von Kalle, C. Skin Cancer Classification Using Convolutional Neural Networks: Systematic Review. *J. Med. Internet Res.* **2018**, *20*, e11936. [CrossRef]
20. Bakos, R.M.; Blumetti, T.P.; Roldán-Marín, R.; Salerni, G. Noninvasive Imaging Tools in the Diagnosis and Treatment of Skin Cancers. *Am. J. Clin. Dermatol.* **2018**, *19*, 3–14. [CrossRef]
21. Wakelin, S.H. Benign skin lesions. *Medicine* **2021**, *49*, 443–446. [CrossRef]
22. Fujisawa, Y.; Otomo, Y.; Ogata, Y.; Nakamura, Y.; Fujita, R.; Ishitsuka, Y.; Fujimoto, M. Deep-learning-based, computer-aided classifier developed with a small dataset of clinical images surpasses board-certified dermatologists in skin tumor diagnosis. *Br. J. Dermatol.* **2019**, *180*, 373–381. [CrossRef] [PubMed]
23. Papageorgiou, V.; Apalla, Z.; Sotiriou, E.; Papageorgiou, C.; Lazaridou, E.; Vakirlis, S.; Ioannides, D.; Lallas, A. The limitations of dermoscopy: False-positive and false-negative tumors. *J. Eur. Acad. Dermatol. Venereol.* **2018**, *32*, 879–888. [CrossRef] [PubMed]
24. Catalano, O.; Roldán, F.A.; Varelli, C.; Bard, R.; Corvino, A.; Wortsman, X. Skin cancer: Findings and role of high-resolution ultrasound. *J. Ultrasound* **2019**, *22*, 423–431. [CrossRef] [PubMed]
25. Jinnai, S.; Yamazaki, N.; Hirano, Y.; Sugawara, Y.; Ohe, Y.; Hamamoto, R. The development of a skin cancer classi-fication system for pigmented skin lesions using deep learning. *Biomolecules* **2020**, *10*, 1123. [CrossRef] [PubMed]
26. Ghazal, T.M.; Hussain, S.; Khan, M.F.; Said, R.A.T.; Ahmad, M. Detection of Benign and Malignant Tumors in Skin Empowered with Transfer Learning. *Comput. Intell. Neurosci.* **2022**, *2022*, 4826892. [CrossRef]
27. Giavina-Bianchi, M.; Cordioli, E.; Dos Santos, A.P. Accuracy of Deep Neural Network in Triaging Common Skin Diseases of Primary Care Attention. *Front Med.* **2021**, *8*, 670300. [CrossRef]
28. Korhonen, N.; Ylitalo, L.; Luukkaala, T.; Itkonen, J.; Häihälä, H.; Jernman, J.; Snellman, E.; Palve, J. Premalignant lesions, basal cell carcinoma and melanoma in patients with cutaneous squamous cell carcinoma. *Arch. Dermatol. Res.* **2020**, *313*, 879–884. [CrossRef]
29. Nauta, M.; Walsh, R.; Dubowski, A.; Seifert, C. Uncovering and Correcting Shortcut Learning in Machine Learning Models for Skin Cancer Diagnosis. *Diagnostics* **2021**, *12*, 40. [CrossRef]
30. Chan, S.; Reddy, V.; Myers, B.; Thibodeaux, Q.; Brownstone, N.; Liao, W. Machine Learning in Dermatology: Current Applications, Opportunities, and Limitations. *Dermatol. Ther.* **2020**, *10*, 365–386. [CrossRef]
31. Zhang, N.; Cai, Y.-X.; Wang, Y.-Y.; Tian, Y.-T.; Wang, X.-L.; Badami, B. Skin cancer diagnosis based on optimized convolutional neural network. *Artif. Intell. Med.* **2020**, *102*, 101756. [CrossRef]
32. Hekler, A.; Utikal, J.S.; Enk, A.H.; Hauschild, A.; Weichenthal, M.; Maron, R.C.; Berking, C.; Haferkamp, S.; Klode, J.; Schadendorf, D.; et al. Superior skin cancer classification by the combination of human and artificial intelligence. *Eur. J. Cancer* **2019**, *120*, 114–121. [CrossRef]
33. Wen, D.; Khan, S.M.; Xu, A.J.; Ibrahim, H.; Smith, L.; Caballero, J.; Zepeda, L.; Perez, C.D.B.; Denniston, A.K.; Liu, X.; et al. Characteristics of publicly available skin cancer image datasets: A systematic review. *Lancet Digit. Health* **2021**, *4*, e64–e74. [CrossRef] [PubMed]
34. Veta, M.; Heng, Y.J.; Stathonikos, N.; Bejnordi, B.E.; Beca, F.; Wollmann, T.; Rohr, K.; Shah, M.A.; Wang, D.; Rousson, M.; et al. Predicting breast tumor proliferation from whole-slide images: The TUPAC16 challenge. *Med. Image Anal.* **2019**, *54*, 111–121. [CrossRef] [PubMed]
35. Han, S.S.; Kim, M.S.; Lim, W.; Park, G.H.; Park, I.; Chang, S.E. Classification of the Clinical Images for Benign and Malignant Cutaneous Tumors Using a Deep Learning Algorithm. *J. Investig. Dermatol.* **2018**, *138*, 1529–1538. [CrossRef] [PubMed]
36. Sharma, A.N.; Shwe, S.; Mesinkovska, N.A. Current state of machine learning for non-melanoma skin cancer. *Arch. Dermatol. Res.* **2022**, *314*, 325–327. [CrossRef] [PubMed]
37. Murphree, D.H.; Puri, P.; Shamim, H.; Bezalel, S.A.; Drage, L.A.; Wang, M.; Comfere, N. Deep learning for dermatologists: Part I. Fundamental concepts. *J. Am. Acad. Dermatol.* **2020**, *87*, 1343–1351. [CrossRef] [PubMed]
38. Roffman, D.; Hart, G.; Girardi, M.; Ko, C.J.; Deng, J. Predicting non-melanoma skin cancer via a multi-parameterized artificial neural network. *Sci. Rep.* **2018**, *8*, 1–7. [CrossRef]
39. Sugiarti, S.; Yuhandri, Y.; Na'am, J.; Indra, D.; Santony, J. An artificial neural network approach for detecting skin cancer. *Telecommun. Comput. Electron. Control.* **2019**, *17*, 788–793. [CrossRef]
40. Lopez-Leyva, J.A.; Guerra-Rosas, E.; Alvarez-Borrego, J. Multi-Class Diagnosis of Skin Lesions Using the Fourier Spectral Information of Images on Additive Color Model by Artificial Neural Network. *IEEE Access* **2021**, *9*, 35207–35216. [CrossRef]
41. Xuyi, W.; Seow, H.; Sutradhar, R. Artificial neural networks for simultaneously predicting the risk of multiple co-occurring symptoms among patients with cancer. *Cancer Med.* **2020**, *10*, 989–998. [CrossRef]
42. Sutradhar, R.; Barbera, L. Comparing an Artificial Neural Network to Logistic Regression for Predicting ED Visit Risk Among Patients with Cancer: A Population-Based Cohort Study. *J. Pain Symptom Manag.* **2020**, *60*, 1–9. [CrossRef] [PubMed]
43. Alwan, O.F. Skin cancer images classification using naïve bayes. *Emergent J. Educ. Discov. Lifelong Learn.* **2022**, *3*, 19–29.
44. Balaji, V.R.; Suganthi, S.T.; Rajadevi, R.; Kumar, V.K.; Balaji, B.S.; Pandiyan, S. Skin disease detection and seg-mentation using dynamic graph cut algorithm and classification through Naive Bayes classifier. *Measurement* **2020**, *163*, 107922. [CrossRef]
45. Mobiny, A.; Singh, A.; Van Nguyen, H. Risk-Aware Machine Learning Classifier for Skin Lesion Diagnosis. *J. Clin. Med.* **2019**, *8*, 1241. [CrossRef]

46. Browning, A.P.; Haridas, P.; Simpson, M.J. A Bayesian Sequential Learning Framework to Parameterise Continuum Models of Melanoma Invasion into Human Skin. *Bull. Math. Biol.* **2018**, *81*, 676–698. [CrossRef]
47. Tanaka, T.; Voigt, M.D. Decision tree analysis to stratify risk of de novo non-melanoma skin cancer following liver transplantation. *J. Cancer Res. Clin. Oncol.* **2018**, *144*, 607–615. [CrossRef]
48. Sun, J.; Huang, Y. Computer aided intelligent medical system and nursing of breast surgery infection. *Microprocess. Microsyst.* **2020**, *81*, 103769. [CrossRef]
49. Quinn, P.L.; Oliver, J.B.; Mahmoud, O.M.; Chokshi, R.J. Cost-Effectiveness of Sentinel Lymph Node Biopsy for Head and Neck Cutaneous Squamous Cell Carcinoma. *J. Surg. Res.* **2019**, *241*, 15–23. [CrossRef]
50. Saba, T.; Khan, M.A.; Rehman, A.; Marie-Sainte, S.L. Region Extraction and Classification of Skin Cancer: A Het-erogeneous framework of Deep CNN Features Fusion and Reduction. *J. Med. Syst.* **2019**, *43*, 289. [CrossRef]
51. Ghiasi, M.M.; Zendehboudi, S. Application of decision tree-based ensemble learning in the classification of breast cancer. *Comput. Biol. Med.* **2021**, *128*, 104089. [CrossRef]
52. Alkhushayni, S.; Al-Zaleq, D.; Andradi, L.; Flynn, P. The Application of Differing Machine Learning Algorithms and Their Related Performance in Detecting Skin Cancers and Melanomas. *J. Ski. Cancer* **2022**, *2022*, 2839162. [CrossRef]
53. Ak, M.F. A Comparative Analysis of Breast Cancer Detection and Diagnosis Using Data Visualization and Machine Learning Applications. *Healthcare* **2020**, *8*, 111. [CrossRef]
54. Sivaraj, S.; Malmathanraj, R.; Palanisamy, P. Detecting anomalous growth of skin lesion using threshold-based segmentation algorithm and Fuzzy K-Nearest Neighbor classifier. *J. Cancer Res. Ther.* **2020**, *16*, 40–52. [CrossRef] [PubMed]
55. Oukil, S.; Kasmi, R.; Mokrani, K.; García-Zapirain, B. Automatic segmentation and melanoma detection based on color and texture features in dermoscopic images. *Ski. Res. Technol.* **2021**, *28*, 203–211. [CrossRef] [PubMed]
56. Nawaz, M.; Mehmood, Z.; Nazir, T.; Naqvi, R.A.; Rehman, A.; Iqbal, M.; Saba, T. Skin cancer detection from der-moscopic images using deep learning and fuzzy k-means clustering. *Microsc. Res. Tech.* **2022**, *85*, 339–351. [CrossRef] [PubMed]
57. Anas, M.; Gupta, K.; Ahmad, S. Skin cancer classification using K-means clustering. *Int. J. Tech. Res. Appl.* **2017**, *5*, 62–65.
58. Hossain, M.S.; Muhammad, G.; Alhamid, M.F.; Song, B.; Al-Mutib, K. Audio-Visual Emotion Recognition Using Big Data Towards 5G. *Mob. Networks Appl.* **2016**, *21*, 753–763. [CrossRef]
59. Khan, M.Q.; Hussain, A.; Rehman, S.U.; Khan, U.; Maqsood, M.; Mehmood, K.; Khan, M.A. *Classification of Melanoma and Nevus in Digital Images for Diagnosis of Skin Cancer*; IEEE: Washington, DC, USA, 2019; Volume 7, pp. 90132–90144.
60. Janney, B.; Roslin, E. Analysis of Skin Cancer using K-Means Clustering and Hybrid Classification Model. *Indian J. Public Health Res. Dev.* **2019**, *10*, 1371–1378. [CrossRef]
61. Murugan, A.; Nair, S.H.; Kumar, K.P.S. Detection of Skin Cancer Using SVM, Random Forest and kNN Classifiers. *J. Med. Syst.* **2019**, *43*, 269. [CrossRef]
62. Luu, N.T.; Le, T.-H.; Phan, Q.-H.; Pham, T.-T. Characterization of Mueller matrix elements for classifying human skin cancer utilizing random forest algorithm. *J. Biomed. Opt.* **2021**, *26*, 075001. [CrossRef] [PubMed]
63. Nandhini, S.; Sofiyan, M.A.; Kumar, S.; Afridi, A. Skin cancer classification using random forest. *Int. J. Manag. Humanit.* **2019**, *4*, 39–42. [CrossRef]
64. Dhivyaa, C.R.; Sangeetha, K.; Balamurugan, M.; Amaran, S.; Vetriselvi, T.; Johnpaul, P. Skin lesion classification using decision trees and random forest algorithms. *J. Ambient. Intell. Humaniz. Comput.* **2020**, 1–13. [CrossRef]
65. Melbin, K.; Raj, Y. Integration of modified ABCD features and support vector machine for skin lesion types classi-fication. *Multimed. Tools Appl.* **2021**, *80*, 8909–8929. [CrossRef]
66. Alsaeed, A.A.D. On the development of a skin cancer computer aided diagnosis system using support vector machine. *Biosci. Biotechnol. Res. Commun.* **2019**, *12*, 297–308.
67. Neela, A.G. Implementation of support vector machine for identification of skin cancer. *Int. J. Eng. Manuf.* **2019**, *9*, 42–52.
68. Arora, G.; Dubey, A.K.; Jaffery, Z.A.; Rocha, A. Bag of feature and support vector machine based early diagnosis of skin cancer. *Neural Comput. Appl.* **2020**, *34*, 8385–8392. [CrossRef]
69. Poovizhi, S.; Tr, G.B. An Efficient Skin Cancer Diagnostic System Using Bendlet Transform and Support Vector Machine. *An. Acad. Bras. Ciências* **2020**, *92*. [CrossRef]
70. Schaefer, G.; Krawczyk, B.; Celebi, M.E.; Iyatomi, H. An ensemble classification approach for melanoma diagnosis. *Memetic Comput.* **2014**, *6*, 233–240. [CrossRef]
71. Rahman, Z.; Hossain, M.S.; Islam, M.R.; Hasan, M.M.; Hridhee, R.A. An approach for multiclass skin lesion clas-sification based on ensemble learning. *Inform. Med. Unlocked* **2021**, *25*, 100659. [CrossRef]
72. Divya, D.; Ganeshbabu, T.R. Fitness adaptive deer hunting-based region growing and recurrent neural network for melanoma skin cancer detection. *Int. J. Imaging Syst. Technol.* **2020**, *30*, 731–752. [CrossRef]
73. Ahmad, B.; Usama, M.; Ahmad, T.; Khatoon, S.; Alam, C.M. An ensemble model of convolution and recurrent neural network for skin disease classification. *Int. J. Imaging Syst. Technol.* **2021**, *32*, 218–229. [CrossRef]
74. Patil, R.S.; Biradar, N. Automated mammogram breast cancer detection using the optimized combination of con-volutional and recurrent neural network. *Evol. Intell.* **2021**, *14*, 1459–1474. [CrossRef]
75. Alom, M.Z.; Aspiras, T.; Taha, T.M.; Asari, V.K. Skin cancer segmentation and classification with NABLA-N and inception recurrent residual convolutional networks. *arXiv* **2019**, arXiv:1904.11126.

76. Toğaçar, M.; Cömert, Z.; Ergen, B. Intelligent skin cancer detection applying autoencoder, MobileNetV2 and spiking neural networks. *Chaos Solitons Fractals* **2021**, *144*, 110714. [CrossRef]
77. Diame, Z.E.; ElBery, M.; Salem MA, M.; Roushdy, M.I. Experimental Comparative Study on Autoencoder Per-formance for Aided Melanoma Skin Disease Recognition. *Int. J. Intell. Comput. Inf. Sci.* **2022**, *22*, 88–97.
78. Majji, R.; Prakash, P.G.O.; Cristin, R.; Parthasarathy, G. Social bat optimisation dependent deep stacked auto-encoder for skin cancer detection. *IET Image Process.* **2020**, *14*, 4122–4131. [CrossRef]
79. Diame, Z.E.; Al-Berry, M.N.; Salem, M.A.-M.; Roushdy, M. Autoencoder Performance Analysis of Skin Lesion Detection. *J. Southwest Jiaotong Univ.* **2021**, *56*, 937–947. [CrossRef]
80. Srinivasu, P.N.; SivaSai, J.G.; Ijaz, M.F.; Bhoi, A.K.; Kim, W.; Kang, J.J. Classification of skin disease using deep learning neural networks with MobileNet V2 and LSTM. *Sensors* **2021**, *21*, 2852. [CrossRef]
81. Wu, X.; Wang, H.-Y.; Shi, P.; Sun, R.; Wang, X.; Luo, Z.; Zeng, F.; Lebowitz, M.S.; Lin, W.-Y.; Lu, J.-J.; et al. Long short-term memory model—A deep learning approach for medical data with irregularity in cancer predication with tumor markers. *Comput. Biol. Med.* **2022**, *144*, 105362. [CrossRef]
82. Elashiri, M.A.; Rajesh, A.; Pandey, S.N.; Shukla, S.K.; Urooj, S.; Lay-Ekuakille, A. Ensemble of weighted deep concatenated features for the skin disease classification model using modified long short term memory. *Biomed. Signal Process. Control.* **2022**, *76*, 103729. [CrossRef]
83. Liao, J.; Liu, L.; Duan, H.; Huang, Y.; Zhou, L.; Chen, L.; Wang, C. Using a Convolutional Neural Network and Convolutional Long Short-term Memory to Automatically Detect Aneurysms on 2D Digital Subtraction Angiography Images: Framework Development and Validation. *JMIR Public Health Surveill.* **2022**, *10*, e28880. [CrossRef] [PubMed]
84. Mazoure, B.; Mazoure, A.; Bédard, J.; Makarenkov, V. DUNEScan: A web server for uncertainty estimation in skin cancer detection with deep neural networks. *Sci. Rep.* **2022**, *12*, 1–10. [CrossRef] [PubMed]
85. Esteva, A.; Kuprel, B.; Novoa, R.A.; Ko, J.; Swetter, S.M.; Blau, H.M.; Thrun, S. Dermatologist-level classification of skin cancer with deep neural networks. *Nature* **2017**, *542*, 115–118. [CrossRef]
86. Khan, M.A.; Sharif, M.; Akram, T.; Kadry, S.; Hsu, C.-H. A two-stream deep neural network-based intelligent system for complex skin cancer types classification. *Int. J. Intell. Syst.* **2022**, *37*, 10621–10649. [CrossRef]
87. Han, S.S.; Park, I.; Chang, S.E.; Lim, W.; Kim, M.S.; Park, G.H.; Chae, J.B.; Huh, C.H.; Na, J.-I. Augmented Intelligence Dermatology: Deep Neural Networks Empower Medical Professionals in Diagnosing Skin Cancer and Predicting Treatment Options for 134 Skin Disorders. *J. Investig. Dermatol.* **2020**, *140*, 1753–1761. [CrossRef]
88. Wan, J.-J.; Chen, B.-L.; Kong, Y.-X.; Ma, X.-G.; Yu, Y.-T. An Early Intestinal Cancer Prediction Algorithm Based on Deep Belief Network. *Sci. Rep.* **2019**, *9*, 1–13. [CrossRef]
89. Al-Antari, M.A.; Al-Masni, M.; Park, S.-U.; Park, J.; Metwally, M.K.; Kadah, Y.M.; Han, S.-M.; Kim, T.-S. An Automatic Computer-Aided Diagnosis System for Breast Cancer in Digital Mammograms via Deep Belief Network. *J. Med. Biol. Eng.* **2017**, *38*, 443–456. [CrossRef]
90. Farhi, L.; Kazmi, S.M.; Imam, H.; Alqahtani, M.; Rehman, F.U. Dermoscopic Image Classification Using Deep Belief Learning Network Architecture. *Wirel. Commun. Mob. Comput.* **2022**, *2022*, 2415726. [CrossRef]
91. Dorj, U.-O.; Lee, K.-K.; Choi, J.-Y.; Lee, M. The skin cancer classification using deep convolutional neural network. *Multimedia Tools Appl.* **2018**, *77*, 9909–9924. [CrossRef]
92. Refianti, R.; Mutiara, A.B.; Priyandini, R.P. Classification of melanoma skin cancer using convolutional neural network. *Int. J. Adv. Comput. Sci. Appl.* **2019**, *10*, 409–417. [CrossRef]
93. Höhn, J.; Hekler, A.; Krieghoff-Henning, E.; Kather, J.N.; Utikal, J.S.; Meier, F.; Brinker, T.J. Integrating patient data into skin cancer classification using convolutional neural networks: Systematic review. *J. Med. Internet Res.* **2021**, *23*, e20708. [CrossRef]
94. Han, S.S.; Moon, I.J.; Lim, W.; Suh, I.S.; Lee, S.Y.; Na, J.-I.; Kim, S.H.; Chang, S.E. Keratinocytic Skin Cancer Detection on the Face Using Region-Based Convolutional Neural Network. *JAMA Dermatol.* **2020**, *156*, 29–37. [CrossRef] [PubMed]
95. Chaturvedi, S.S.; Tembhurne, J.V.; Diwan, T. A multi-class skin Cancer classification using deep convolutional neural networks. *Multimedia Tools Appl.* **2020**, *79*, 28477–28498. [CrossRef]
96. Li, Y.; Fauteux, F.; Zou, J.; Nantel, A.; Pan, Y. Personalized prediction of genes with tumor-causing somatic mutations based on multi-modal deep Boltzmann machine. *Neurocomputing* **2019**, *324*, 51–62. [CrossRef]
97. Peter Soosai Anandaraj, A.; Gomathy, V.; Amali Angel Punitha, A.; Abitha Kumari, D.; Sheeba Rani, S.; Sureshkumar, S. Internet of Medical Things (IoMT) Enabled Skin Lesion Detection and Classification Using Optimal Segmentation and Restricted Boltzmann Machines. In *Cognitive Internet of Medical Things for Smart Healthcare*; Springer: Cham, Switzerland, 2021; pp. 195–209.
98. Usmani, U.A.; Watada, J.; Jaafar, J.; Aziz, I.A.; Roy, A. A Reinforcement Learning Algorithm for Automated Detection of Skin Lesions. *Appl. Sci.* **2021**, *11*, 9367. [CrossRef]
99. Wang, S.; Hamian, M. Skin Cancer Detection Based on Extreme Learning Machine and a Developed Version of Thermal Exchange Optimization. *Comput. Intell. Neurosci.* **2021**, *2021*, 9528664. [CrossRef] [PubMed]
100. Sayed, G.I.; Soliman, M.M.; Hassanien, A.E. A novel melanoma prediction model for imbalanced data using optimized SqueezeNet by bald eagle search optimization. *Comput. Biol. Med.* **2021**, *136*, 104712. [CrossRef]
101. Afza, F.; Sharif, M.; Khan, M.A.; Tariq, U.; Yong, H.-S.; Cha, J. Multiclass Skin Lesion Classification Using Hybrid Deep Features Selection and Extreme Learning Machine. *Sensors* **2022**, *22*, 799. [CrossRef]

102. Khan, I.U.; Aslam, N.; Anwar, T.; Aljameel, S.S.; Ullah, M.; Khan, R.; Rehman, A.; Akhtar, N. Remote Diagnosis and Triaging Model for Skin Cancer Using EfficientNet and Extreme Gradient Boosting. *Complexity* **2021**, *2021*, 5591614. [CrossRef]
103. Alabdulkareem, A. Artificial intelligence and dermatologists: Friends or foes? *J. Dermatol. Dermatol. Surg.* **2019**, *23*, 57. [CrossRef]
104. Shen, C.; Li, C.; Xu, F.; Wang, Z.; Shen, X.; Gao, J.; Ko, R.; Jing, Y.; Tang, X.; Yu, R.; et al. Web-based study on Chinese dermatologists' attitudes towards artificial intelligence. *Ann. Transl. Med.* **2020**, *8*, 698. [CrossRef] [PubMed]
105. Maron, R.C.; Utikal, J.S.; Hekler, A.; Hauschild, A.; Sattler, E.; Sondermann, W.; Haferkamp, S.; Schilling, B.; Heppt, M.V.; Jansen, P.; et al. Artificial Intelligence and Its Effect on Dermatologists' Accuracy in Dermoscopic Melanoma Image Classification: Web-Based Survey Study. *J. Med. Internet Res.* **2020**, *22*, e18091. [CrossRef] [PubMed]
106. Nelson, C.A.; Pérez-Chada, L.M.; Creadore, A.; Li, S.J.; Lo, K.; Manjaly, P.; Mostaghimi, A. Patient perspectives on the use of artificial intelligence for skin cancer screening: A qualitative study. *JAMA Dermatol.* **2020**, *156*, 501–512. [CrossRef]
107. Sreelatha, T.; Subramanyam, M.V.; Prasad, M.N.G. A Survey work on Early Detection methods of Melanoma Skin Cancer. *Res. J. Pharm. Technol.* **2019**, *12*, 2589. [CrossRef]
108. di Ruffano, L.F.; Dinnes, J.; Deeks, J.J.; Chuchu, N.; Bayliss, S.E.; Davenport, C.; Takwoingi, Y.; Godfrey, K.; O'Sullivan, C.; Matin, R.N.; et al. Optical coherence tomography for diagnosing skin cancer in adults. *Cochrane Database Syst. Rev.* **2018**, *12*, CD013189. [CrossRef]
109. Tan, T.Y.; Zhang, L.; Lim, C.P. Intelligent skin cancer diagnosis using improved particle swarm optimization and deep learning models. *Appl. Soft Comput.* **2019**, *84*, 105725. [CrossRef]
110. Gerke, S.; Minssen, T.; Cohen, G. Ethical and legal challenges of artificial intelligence-driven healthcare. In *Artificial Intelligence in Healthcare*; Academic Press: Cambridge, MA, USA, 2020; pp. 295–336.
111. Rigby, M.J. Ethical Dimensions of Using Artificial Intelligence in Health Care. *AMA J. Ethic-* **2019**, *21*, E121–E124. [CrossRef]
112. Da Silva, M.; Horsley, T.; Singh, D.; Da Silva, E.; Ly, V.; Thomas, B.; Daniel, R.C.; Chagal-Feferkorn, K.A.; Iantomasi, S.; White, K.; et al. Legal concerns in health-related artificial intelligence: A scoping review protocol. *Syst. Rev.* **2022**, *11*, 1–8. [CrossRef]
113. Hu, T.; Chitnis, N.; Monos, D.; Dinh, A. Next-generation sequencing technologies: An overview. *Hum. Immunol.* **2021**, *82*, 801–811. [CrossRef]
114. Slatko, B.E.; Gardner, A.F.; Ausubel, F.M. Overview of Next-Generation Sequencing Technologies. *Curr. Protoc. Mol. Biol.* **2018**, *122*, e59. [CrossRef] [PubMed]
115. Lobl, M.B.; Clarey, D.; Higgins, S.; Sutton, A.; Hansen, L.; Wysong, A. Targeted next-generation sequencing of matched localized and metastatic primary high-risk SCCs identifies driver and co-occurring mutations and novel therapeutic targets. *J. Dermatol. Sci.* **2020**, *99*, 30–43. [CrossRef] [PubMed]
116. Brancaccio, R.N.; Robitaille, A.; Dutta, S.; Cuenin, C.; Santare, D.; Skenders, G.; Leja, M.; Fischer, N.; Giuliano, A.R.; Rollison, D.E.; et al. Generation of a novel next-generation sequencing-based method for the isolation of new human papillomavirus types. *Virology* **2018**, *520*, 1–10. [CrossRef] [PubMed]
117. Kadampur, M.A.; Al Riyaee, S. Skin cancer detection: Applying a deep learning based model driven architecture in the cloud for classifying dermal cell images. *Inform. Med. Unlocked* **2019**, *18*, 100282. [CrossRef]
118. Khan, M.A.; Akram, T.; Sharif, M.; Kadry, S.; Nam, Y. Computer Decision Support System for Skin Cancer Localization and Classification. *Comput. Mater. Contin.* **2021**, *68*, 1041–1064. [CrossRef]
119. Sharif, M.I.; Khan, M.A.; Alhussein, M.; Aurangzeb, K.; Raza, M. A decision support system for multimodal brain tumor classification using deep learning. *Complex Intell. Syst.* **2021**, *8*, 3007–3020. [CrossRef]
120. Abdar, M.; Acharya, U.R.; Sarrafzadegan, N.; Makarenkov, V. NE-nu-SVC: A New Nested Ensemble Clinical Decision Support System for Effective Diagnosis of Coronary Artery Disease. *IEEE Access* **2019**, *7*, 167605–167620. [CrossRef]
121. Ray, P.P.; Dash, D.; De, D. A Systematic Review of Wearable Systems for Cancer Detection: Current State and Challenges. *J. Med. Syst.* **2017**, *41*, 180. [CrossRef]
122. Gupta, A.K.; Bharadwaj, M.; Mehrotra, R. Skin Cancer Concerns in People of Color: Risk Factors and Prevention. *Asian Pac. J. Cancer Prev.* **2016**, *17*, 5257–5264. [CrossRef]
123. Sun, M.D.; Kentley, J.; Wilson, B.W.; Soyer, H.P.; Curiel-Lewandrowski, C.N.; Rotemberg, V.; ISIC Technique Working Group. Digital skin imaging applications, part I: Assessment of image acquisition technique features. *Ski. Res. Technol.* **2022**, *28*, 623–632. [CrossRef]
124. Barata, C.; Marques, J.S.; Celebi, M.E. Improving dermoscopy image analysis using color constancy. In *2014 IEEE International Conference on Image Processing (ICIP)*; IEEE: Washington, DC, USA, 2014; pp. 3527–3531.
125. Salvi, M.; Branciforti, F.; Veronese, F.; Zavattaro, E.; Tarantino, V.; Savoia, P.; Meiburger, K.M. DermoCC-GAN: A new approach for standardizing dermatological images using generative adversarial networks. *Comput. Methods Programs Biomed.* **2022**, *225*, 107040. [CrossRef] [PubMed]
126. Watson, M.; Holman, D.M.; Maguire-Eisen, M. Ultraviolet Radiation Exposure and Its Impact on Skin Cancer Risk. *Semin. Oncol. Nurs.* **2016**, *32*, 241–254. [CrossRef] [PubMed]
127. Wolner, Z.J.; Yélamos, O.; Liopyris, K.; Rogers, T.; Marchetti, M.A.; Marghoob, A.A. Enhancing Skin Cancer Diagnosis with Dermoscopy. *Dermatol. Clin.* **2017**, *35*, 417–437. [CrossRef] [PubMed]
128. A Comparison of Polarised and Nonpolarised Dermoscopy I DermNet. Available online: https://dermnetnz.org/topics/a-comparison-of-polarised-and-nonpolarised-dermoscopy (accessed on 30 January 2023).

129. Hone, N.L.; Grandhi, R.; Ingraffea, A.A. Basal Cell Carcinoma on the Sole: An Easily Missed Cancer. *Case Rep. Dermatol.* **2016**, *8*, 283–286. [CrossRef] [PubMed]
130. Pala, P.; Bergler-Czop, B.S.; Gwiżdż, J. Teledermatology: Idea, benefits and risks of modern age–a systematic review based on melanoma. *Adv. Dermatol. Allergol. Postępy Dermatol. I Alergol.* **2020**, *37*, 159–167. [CrossRef]
131. Veronese, F.; Branciforti, F.; Zavattaro, E.; Tarantino, V.; Romano, V.; Meiburger, K.; Salvi, M.; Seoni, S.; Savoia, P. The Role in Teledermoscopy of an Inexpensive and Easy-to-Use Smartphone Device for the Classification of Three Types of Skin Lesions Using Convolutional Neural Networks. *Diagnostics* **2021**, *11*, 451. [CrossRef]
132. Skin Cancer ISIC. Available online: https://www.kaggle.com/datasets/nodoubttome/skin-cancer9-classesisic (accessed on 30 November 2022).
133. Dermatology Data Set. Available online: https://archive.ics.uci.edu/ml/datasets/Dermatology?ref=datanews.io (accessed on 30 November 2022).
134. The HAM10000 Dataset, a Large Collection of Multi-Source Dermatoscopic Images of Common Pigmented Skin Lesions. Available online: https://dataverse.harvard.edu/dataset.xhtml?persistentId=doi:10.7910/DVN/DBW86T (accessed on 30 November 2022).
135. Hussain, S.F.; Qaisar, S.M. Epileptic seizure classification using level-crossing EEG sampling and en-semble of sub-problems classifier. *Expert Syst. Appl.* **2022**, *191*, 116356. [CrossRef]
136. Qaisar, S.M.; Alsharif, F.; Subasi, A.; Bensenouci, A. Appliance Identification Based on Smart Meter Data and Event-Driven Processing in the 5G Framework. *Procedia Comput. Sci.* **2021**, *182*, 103–108. [CrossRef]
137. Qaisar, S.M.; Khan, S.I.; Dallet, D.; Tadeusiewicz, R.; Pławiak, P. Signal-piloted processing metaheuristic optimization and wavelet decomposition based elucidation of arrhythmia for mobile healthcare. *Biocybern. Biomed. Eng.* **2022**, *42*, 681–694. [CrossRef]

Disclaimer/Publisher's Note: The statements, opinions and data contained in all publications are solely those of the individual author(s) and contributor(s) and not of MDPI and/or the editor(s). MDPI and/or the editor(s) disclaim responsibility for any injury to people or property resulting from any ideas, methods, instructions or products referred to in the content.

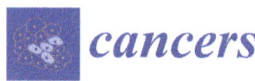

Review

The Role of Deep Learning in Advancing Breast Cancer Detection Using Different Imaging Modalities: A Systematic Review

Mohammad Madani [1,2], Mohammad Mahdi Behzadi [1,2] and Sheida Nabavi [2,*]

[1] Department of Mechanical Engineering, University of Connecticut, Storrs, CT 06269, USA
[2] Department of Computer Science and Engineering, University of Connecticut, Storrs, CT 06269, USA
* Correspondence: sheida.nabavi@uconn.edu

Simple Summary: Breast cancer is the most common cancer, which resulted in the death of 700,000 people around the world in 2020. Various imaging modalities have been utilized to detect and analyze breast cancer. However, the manual detection of cancer from large-size images produced by these imaging modalities is usually time-consuming and can be inaccurate. Early and accurate detection of breast cancer plays a critical role in improving the prognosis bringing the patient survival rate to 50%. Recently, some artificial-intelligence-based approaches such as deep learning algorithms have shown remarkable advancements in early breast cancer diagnosis. This review focuses first on the introduction of various breast cancer imaging modalities and their available public datasets, then on proposing the most recent studies considering deep-learning-based models for breast cancer analysis. This study systemically summarizes various imaging modalities, relevant public datasets, deep learning architectures used for different imaging modalities, model performances for different tasks such as classification and segmentation, and research directions.

Abstract: Breast cancer is among the most common and fatal diseases for women, and no permanent treatment has been discovered. Thus, early detection is a crucial step to control and cure breast cancer that can save the lives of millions of women. For example, in 2020, more than 65% of breast cancer patients were diagnosed in an early stage of cancer, from which all survived. Although early detection is the most effective approach for cancer treatment, breast cancer screening conducted by radiologists is very expensive and time-consuming. More importantly, conventional methods of analyzing breast cancer images suffer from high false-detection rates. Different breast cancer imaging modalities are used to extract and analyze the key features affecting the diagnosis and treatment of breast cancer. These imaging modalities can be divided into subgroups such as mammograms, ultrasound, magnetic resonance imaging, histopathological images, or any combination of them. Radiologists or pathologists analyze images produced by these methods manually, which leads to an increase in the risk of wrong decisions for cancer detection. Thus, the utilization of new automatic methods to analyze all kinds of breast screening images to assist radiologists to interpret images is required. Recently, artificial intelligence (AI) has been widely utilized to automatically improve the early detection and treatment of different types of cancer, specifically breast cancer, thereby enhancing the survival chance of patients. Advances in AI algorithms, such as deep learning, and the availability of datasets obtained from various imaging modalities have opened an opportunity to surpass the limitations of current breast cancer analysis methods. In this article, we first review breast cancer imaging modalities, and their strengths and limitations. Then, we explore and summarize the most recent studies that employed AI in breast cancer detection using various breast imaging modalities. In addition, we report available datasets on the breast-cancer imaging modalities which are important in developing AI-based algorithms and training deep learning models. In conclusion, this review paper tries to provide a comprehensive resource to help researchers working in breast cancer imaging analysis.

Keywords: artificial intelligence; breast cancer; deep learning; histopathology; imaging modality; mammography

Citation: Madani, M.; Behzadi, M.M.; Nabavi, S. The Role of Deep Learning in Advancing Breast Cancer Detection Using Different Imaging Modalities: A Systematic Review. *Cancers* 2022, 14, 5334. https://doi.org/10.3390/cancers14215334

Academic Editors: Marcin Woźniak and Muhammad Fazal Ijaz

Received: 1 October 2022
Accepted: 25 October 2022
Published: 29 October 2022

Publisher's Note: MDPI stays neutral with regard to jurisdictional claims in published maps and institutional affiliations.

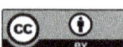

Copyright: © 2022 by the authors. Licensee MDPI, Basel, Switzerland. This article is an open access article distributed under the terms and conditions of the Creative Commons Attribution (CC BY) license (https://creativecommons.org/licenses/by/4.0/).

1. Introduction

Breast cancer is the second most fatal disease in women and is a leading cause of death for millions of women around the world [1]. According to the American Cancer Society, approximately 20% of women who have been diagnosed with breast cancer die [2,3]. Generally, breast tumors are divided into four groups: normal, benign, in situ carcinoma, and invasive carcinoma [1]. A benign tumor is an abnormal but noncancerous collection of cells in which minor changes in the structure of cells happen, and they cannot be considered cancerous cells [1]. However, in situ carcinoma and invasive carcinoma are classified as cancer [4]. In situ carcinoma remains in its organ and does not affect other organs. On the other hand, invasive carcinoma spreads to surrounding organs and causes the development of many cancerous cells in the organs [5,6]. Early detection of breast cancer is a determinative step for treatment and is critical to avoiding further advancement of cancer and its complications [7]. There are several well-known imaging modalities to detect and treat breast cancer at an early stage including mammograms (MM) [8], breast thermography (BTD) [9], magnetic resonance imaging (MRI) [10], positron emission tomography (PET) [11], computed tomography (CT) [11], ultrasound (US) [12], and histopathology (HP) [13]. Among these modalities, mammograms (MMs) and histopathology (HP), which involve image analysis of the removed tissue stained with hematoxylin and eosin to increase visibility, are widely used [14,15]. Mammography tries to filter a large-scale population for initial breast cancer symptoms, while histopathology tries to capture microscopic images with the highest possible resolution to find exact cancerous tissues at the molecular level [16,17]. In practice for breast cancer screening, radiologists or pathologists observe and examine breast images manually for diagnosis, prognosis, and treatment decisions [7]. Such screening usually leads to over- or under-treatment because of inaccurate detection, resulting in a prolonged diagnosis process [18]. It is worth noting that only 0.6% to 0.7% of cancer detections in women during the screening are validated and 15–35% of cancer screening fails due to errors related to the imaging process, quality of images, and human fatigue [19–21]. Several decades ago, computer-aided detection (CAD) systems were first employed to assist radiologists in their decision-making. CAD systems generally analyze imaging data and other cancer-related data alone or in combination with other clinical information [22]. Additionally, based on the statistical models, CADs can provide results about the probability of diseases such as breast cancer [23]. CAD systems have been widely used to help radiologists in patient care processes such as cancer staging [23]. However, conventional CAD systems, which are based on traditional image processing techniques, have been limited in their utility and capability.

To tackle these problems and enhance efficiency as well as decrease false cancer detection rates, precise automated methods are needed to complement the work of humans or replace them. AI is one of the most effective approaches capturing much attention in analyzing medical imaging, especially for the automated analysis and extraction of relevant information from imaging modalities such as MMs and HPs [24,25]. Many available AI-based tools for image recognition to detect breast cancer have exhibited better performance than traditional CAD systems and manually examining images by expert radiologists or pathologists due to the limitations of current manual approaches [26]. In other words, AI-based methods avoid expensive and time-consuming manual inspection and effectively extract key and determinative information from high-resolution image data [26,27]. For example, a spectrum of diseases is associated with specific features, such as mammographic features. Thus, AI can learn these types of features from the structure of image data and then detect the spectrum of the disease assisting the radiologist or histopathologist. It is worth noting that in contrast to human inspection, algorithms are mainly similar to the black box and cannot understand the context, mode of collection, or meaning of viewed images, resulting in the problem of "shortcut" learning [28,29]. Thus, building interpretable AI-based models is necessary. AI models can generally be categorized into two groups to interpret and extract information from image data: (1) Traditional machine learning algorithms which need to receive handcrafted features derived from raw image data as preprocessing steps. (2) Deep learning algorithms that process raw images and try to extract features by mathematical optimization and multiple-level abstractions [30]. Although both approaches have shown promising results in breast cancer detection, recently, the latter approach has attracted more interest mainly because of its capability to learn the most salient representations of the data without human intervention to produce superior performance [31,32]. This review assesses and compresses recent datasets and AI-based models, specifically created by deep learning algorithms, used on TBD, PET, MRI, US, HP, and MM in breast cancer screening and detection. We also highlight the future direction in breast cancer detection via deep learning. This study can be summarized as follows: (1) Review of different imaging modalities for breast cancer screening. (2) Comparison of different deep learning models proposed in the most recent studies and their achieved performances on breast cancer classification, segmentation, detection, and other analysis. (3) Lastly, the conclusion of the paper and suggestions for future research directions. The main contributions of this paper can be listed as follows:

1. We reviewed different imaging tasks such as classification, segmentation, and detection through deep learning algorithms, while most of the existing review papers focus on a specific task.
2. We covered all available imaging modalities for breast cancer analysis in contrast to most of the existing studies that focus on single or two imaging modalities.
3. For each imaging modality, we summarized all available datasets.
4. We considered the most recent studies (2019–2022) on breast cancer imaging diagnosis employing deep learning models.

2. Imaging Modalities and Available Datasets for Breast Cancer

In this study, we summarize well-known imaging modalities for breast cancer diagnosis and analysis. As many existing studies have shown, there are several imaging modalities, including mammography, histopathology, ultrasound, magnetic resonance imaging, positron emission tomography, digital breast tomosynthesis, and a combination of these modalities (multimodalities) [10,32,33]. There are various public or private datasets for these modalities. Approximately 70% of available public datasets are related to mammography and ultrasound modalities demonstrating the prevalence of these methods, especially mammography, for breast cancer screening [31,32]. On the other hand, the researcher also widely utilized other modalities such as histopathology and MRI to confirm cancer and deal with difficulties related to mammography and ultrasound imaging modalities such as large variations in the image's shape, morphological structure, and the density of breast tissues, etc. Here, we outline the aforementioned imaging modalities and available datasets for breast cancer detection.

2.1. Mammograms (MMs)

The advantages of mammograms, such as being cost-effective to detect tumors in the initial stage before development, mean that MMs are the most promising imaging screening technique in clinical practice. MMs are generally images of breasts produced by low-intensity X-rays (Figure 1) [33]. In this imaging modality, cancerous regions are brighter and more clear than other parts of breast tissue, helping to detect small variations in the composition of the tissues; therefore, it is used for the diagnosis and analysis of breast cancer [34,35] (Figure 1). Although MMs are the standard approach for breast cancer analysis, it is an inappropriate imaging modality for women with dense breasts [36], since the performance of MMs highly depends on specific tumor morphological characteristics [36,37]. To deal with this problem, using automated whole breast ultrasound (AWBU) or other methods are suggested with MMs to produce a more detailed image of breast tissues [38].

For various tasks in breast cancer analysis, such as breast lesion detection and classification, MMs are generally divided into two forms: screen film mammograms (SFM) and digital mammograms (DMM). DMM is widely categorized into three categories consisting of full-field digital mammograms (FFDM), digital breast tomosynthesis (DBT), and contrast-enhanced digital mammograms (CEDM) [39–44]. SFM was the standard imaging method in MMs because of its high sensitivity (100%) in the analysis and detection of lesions in breasts composed primarily of fatty tissue [45]. However, it has many drawbacks, including the following: (1) SFM imaging needs to be repeated with a higher radiation dose because some parts of the image in SFM have lesser contrast and cannot be further improved, and (2) various regions of the breast image are represented according to the characteristic response of the SFM [19,45]. Since 2010, DMM has replaced film as the primary screening modality. The main advantages of digital imaging over file systems are the higher contrast resolution and the ability to enlarge the image or change the contrast and brightness. These advantages help radiologists to detect subtle abnormalities, particularly in a background of dense breast tissue, more easily. Most studies comparing digital and film mammography performance have found little difference in cancer detection rates [46]. Digital mammography increases the chance of detecting invasive cancer in premenopausal and perimenopausal women and women with dense breasts. However, it increases false-positive findings as well [46]. Randomized mammographic trials/randomized controlled trials (RMT/RCT) represent the most important usage of MMs, through which large-scale screening for breast cancer analysis is performed. Despite the great capability of MMs for early-stage cancer detection, it is difficult to use MMs alone for detection. Because it requires additional screening tests along with mammographic trials/RMT such as breast self-examination (BSE) and clinical breast examination (CBE), which are more feasible methods to detect breast cancer at early stages to improve breast cancer survival [38,47,48]. Additionally, BSE and CBE avoid tremendous harm due to MMs screening, such as repeating the imaging process. More details about the advantages and disadvantages of MMs are provided in Table 1.

Table 1. Advantages and limitations of various imaging modalities.

Imaging Modalities	Advantages	Limitations
MM	- More than 70% of studies (computational and experimental) for breast cancer analysis. - Time- and cost-effective approach for image capturing and processing compared to other modalities - No need for highly professional radiologists for diagnosis and cancer detection compared to other methods	- Cannot capture micro-calcification because MMs are created via low-dose X-ray - Limited capability for diagnosis of cancer in dense breasts - Needs more testing for accurate diagnosis - Needs various pre-processing for classification because of considering many factors and structures such as the border of the breast, fibrous strands, hypertrophied lobules, etc. which may cause misunderstanding Problems in the visualization of cancer in high breast density
US	- A very efficient approach in reducing false negative rates for diagnosis because of its capability in capturing images from different views and angles. - A highly safe and most efficient approach for a routine checkup because the US is a non-invasive method - Ability to detect invasive cancer areas Highly recommended for the identification of breast lesion ROI because of its additional features such as color-coded SWE images	- Capturing low-quality images for examination of the larger amount of tissues - Difficult to understand SWE images - Single Nakagami parametric image cannot detect cancerous tissues Proper ROI estimation is very difficult because of the shadowing effect making the tumor contour unclear
MRI	- Safe method due to no exposure to harmful ionizing radiation - Captures images with more detail - Captures more suspicious areas for further analysis compared to other modalities Can be improved by adding contrast agents to represent images with more details	- Misses some tumors but can be used as a complement of MMs - Increases body temperature - May lead to some allergies Invasive method and dangerous

Table 1. Cont.

Imaging Modalities	Advantages	Limitations
HP	<ul><li>Produces color-coded images that help to detect cancer subtypes and early detection of cancer</li><li>Widely used in cancer diagnosis similar to MMs</li><li>Shows tissues in two forms including WSI and ROI extracted from WSI</li><li>Provides more reliable results for diagnosis than any other imaging modalities</li><li>ROI increases accuracy of cancer diagnosis and analysis</li><li>Can be stored for future analysis</li></ul>	<ul><li>Expensive and time-consuming method to analyze and need</li><li>Highly expert pathologist</li><li>It is tedious to extract ROI and analysis, so it may lead to a decrease in the accuracy of analysis because of fatigue</li><li>Analysis of HPs highly depends on many factors such as fixation, lab protocols, sample orientations, human expertise in tissue preparation, color variation</li><li>The hardest imaging modality for applying a DL approach for the classification of cancers, and it needs high computational resources for analysis</li></ul>
DBT	<ul><li>Increases cancer detection rate</li><li>Can find cancers that were entirely missed on MMs</li><li>Presents a unique opportunity for AI systems to help develop DBT-based practices from the ground up.</li><li>Captures a more detailed view of tissues by rotating the X-ray emitter to receive multiple images</li><li>Has great capability to distinguish small lesions which may obscure the projections obtained using MMs</li></ul>	<ul><li>Time consuming and expensive because of making 3D images</li><li>Lack of proper data curation and labeling</li><li>Decreasing accuracy of analysis when using 2D slices instead of 3D images</li><li>Looking only at 2D slices, it is still unclear whether AIModels operate better using abnormalities labeled</li><li>Using bounding boxes or tightly-drawn margins of lesions</li><li>DBT studies easily require more storage than MMs by order of magnitude or more.</li></ul>
PET	<ul><li>An efficient method in the analysis of small lesions</li><li>Great capability to detect metastasis at different sites and organs.</li><li>Checks up the entire patient for local recurrence, lymph node metastases, and distant metastases using a single injection of activity</li><li>Highly recommended for patients with dense breasts or implants</li></ul>	<ul><li>Poor detection rates for small or non-invasive breast cancers</li><li>Missed osteoblastic metastases showed lower metabolic activity</li></ul>

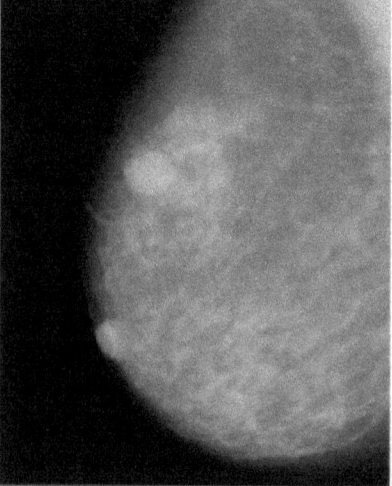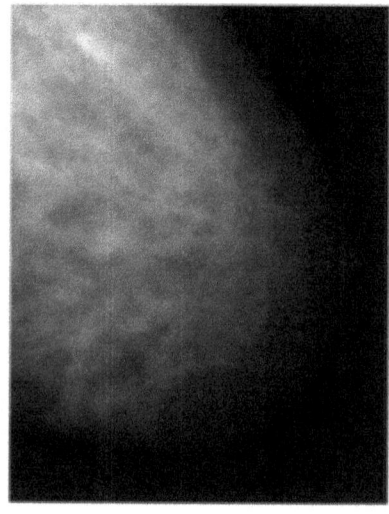

Figure 1. Example of breast cancer images using traditional film MMs. Reprinted/adapted with permission from [49]. 2021, Elsevier.

2.2. Digital Breast Tomosynthesis (DBT)

DBT is a novel imaging modality making 3D images of breasts by the utilization of X-rays captured from different angles [50]. This method is similar to what is performed in mammograms, except the tube with the X-ray moves in a circular arc around the breast [51–53] (Figure 2). Repeated exposures to the breast tissue at different angles produce DBT images in half-millimeter slices. In this method, computational methods are utilized to collect information received from X-ray images to produce z-stack breast images and 2D reconstruction images [53,54]. In contrast to the conventional FSM method, DBT can easily cover the imaging of tumors from small to large size, especially in the case of small lesions and dense breasts [55]. However, the main challenging issue regarding the DBT is the long reading time because of the number of mammograms, the z-stack of images, and the number of recall rates for architectural distortion type of breast cancer abnormality [56]. After FFDM, DBT is the commonly used method for imaging modalities. Many studies recently used this imaging modality for breast cancer detection due to its favorable sensitivity and accuracy in screening and producing better details of tissue in breast cancer [57–60]. Table 1 provides details of the pros and cons of DBT for breast cancer analysis.

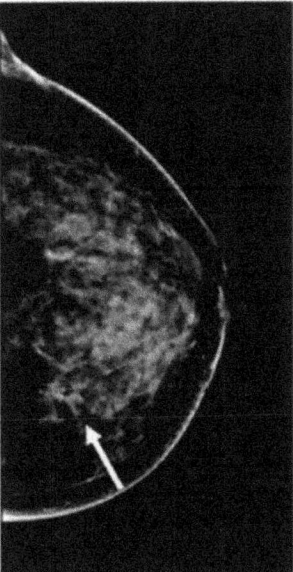 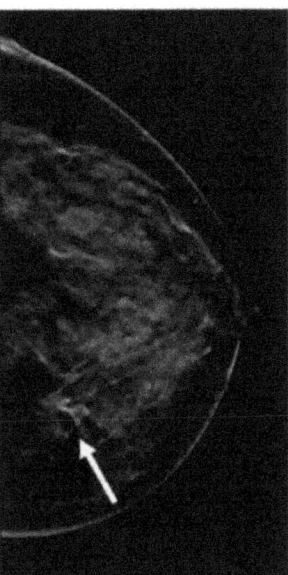

Figure 2. Images of cancerous breast tissue by DBT imaging modality [61]. Reprinted/adapted with permission from [61]. 2021, Elsevier.

2.3. Ultrasound (US)

All of the aforementioned modalities can endanger patients and radiologists because of possible overdosage of ionizing radiation, making these approaches slightly risky and unhealthy for certain sensitive patients [62]. Additionally, these methods show low specificity, meaning the low ability to correctly determine a tissue without disease as a negative case. Therefore, although the aforementioned imaging modalities are highly used for early breast cancer detection, the US as a safe imaging modality has been used [62–67] (Figure 3). Compared to MMs, the US is a more convenient method for women with dense breasts. It is also useful to characterize abnormal regions and negative tumors detected by MMs [68]. Some studies showed the high accuracy of the US in detecting and discriminating benign and malignant masses [69]. US images are used in three broad combinations, i.e., (i) simple two-dimensional grayscale US images, (ii) color US images with shear wave elastography

(SWE) added features, and (iii) Nakagami colored US images without any need for ionizing radiation [70,71]. It is worth noting that Nakagami-colored US images are responsible for the region of interest extraction by better detection of irregular masses in the breast. Moreover, US can be used as a complement to MMs owing to its availability, inexpensiveness compared to other modalities, and it being well tolerated by patients [70,72,73]. In a recent retrospective study, US breast imaging has shown high predictive value when combined with MMs images [74]. US images, along with MMs, improved the overall detection by about 20% and decreased unnecessary biopsy tasks by 40% in total [67]. Moreover, US is a reliable and valuable tool for metastatic lymph node screening in breast cancer patients. It is a cheap, noninvasive, easy-to-handle and cost-effective diagnostic method [75]. However, the US represents some limitations. For instance, the interpretation of US images is highly difficult and needs an expert radiologist to comprehensively understand these images. This is because of the complex nature of US images and the presence of speckle noise [76,77]. To deal with this issue, new technologies have been introduced in breast US imaging, such as automated breast ultrasound (ABUS). ABUS produces 3D images using wider probes. Shin et al. [78] improved how ABUS allows more appropriate image evaluation for large breast masses compared to conventional breast US. On the other hand, ABUS showed the lowest reliability in the prediction of residual tumor size and pCR (pathological complete response) [79]. Table 1 highlights more details about the weaknesses and strengths of the US imaging modality.

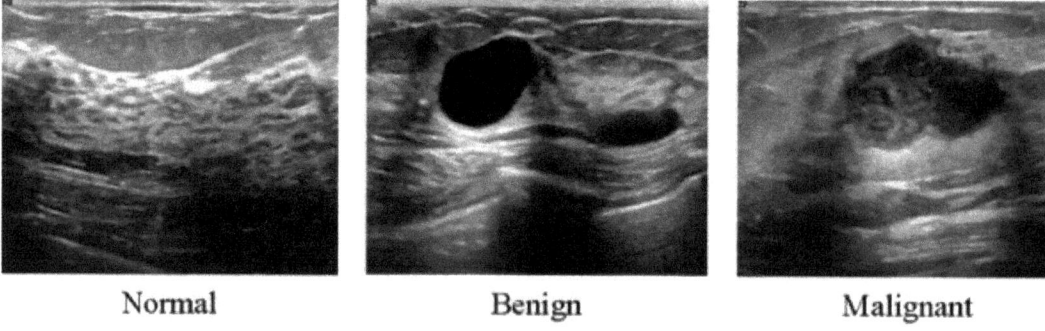

Figure 3. Ultrasound images from breast tissue for normal, benign, and malignant [80].

2.4. Magnetic Resonance Imaging (MRI)

MRI creates images of the whole breast and presents it as thin slices that cover the entire breast volume. It works based on radio frequency absorption of nuclei in the existence of potent magnetic fields. MRI uses a magnetic field along with radio waves to capture multiple breast images at different angles from a tissue [81–83] (Figure 4). By the combination of these images together, clear and detailed images of tissues are produced. Hence, MRI creates much clearer images for breast cancer analysis than other imaging modalities [84]. For instance, the MRI image shows many details clearly, leading to easy detection of lesions that are considered benign in other imaging modalities. Additionally, MRI is the most favorable method for breast cancer screening in women with dense breasts without any ionizing and other health risks, which we have seen in other modalities such as MMs [85,86]. Another interesting issue about MRI is its capability for producing high-quality images with a clearer view via the utilization of a contrast agent before taking MRI images [87,88]. Furthermore, MRI is more accurate than MM, DBT, and the US in evaluating residual tumors and predicting pCR [79,89], which helps clinicians to select appropriate patients for avoiding surgery after neoadjuvant chemotherapy (first-line treatment of breast cancer) when pCR is obtained [90,91]. Even though MRI exhibits promising advantages, such as high sensitivity, it shows low specificity, and it is time consuming and expensive, especially since its reading time is long [92,93]. It is worth noting that some new MRI-based methods, such as ultrafast breast MRI (UF-MRI), create much more efficient images with high screening specificity with short reading time [94,95]. Additionally, diffusion-weighted MR imaging (DWI-MRI) and dynamic contrast-enhanced MRI (DCE-MRI) provide higher volumetric resolution for better lesion visualization and lesion temporal pattern enhancement to use in breast cancer diagnosis and prognosis and correlation with genomics [53,81,96–98]. Details about various MRI-based methods and their pros and cons are available in Table 1.

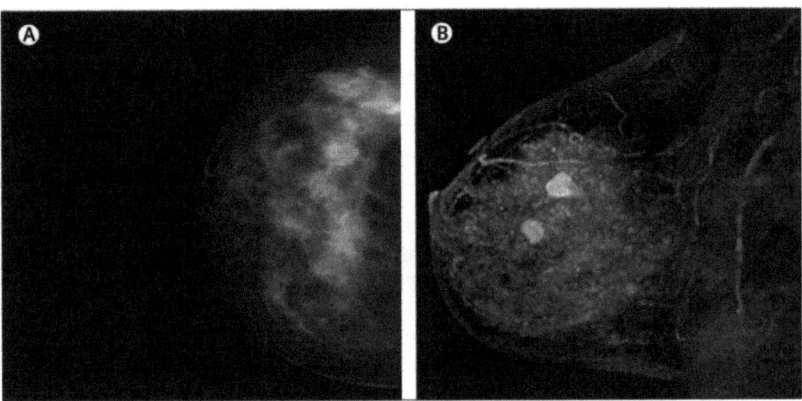

Figure 4. Dense cancerous breast tissue images conducted by MRI method from different angles. (**A**) Normal; (**B**) malignant [82]. Reprinted/adapted with permission from [82]. 2011, Elsevier.

2.5. Histopathology

Recently, various studies have confirmed that the gold standard for confirmation of breast cancer diagnosis, treatment, and management is given by the histopathological analysis of a section of the suspected area by a pathologist [99–101]. Histopathology consists of examining tissue lesion samples stained, for example, with hematoxylin and eosin (H&E) to produce colored histopathologic (HP) images for better visualization and detailed analysis of tissues [102–104] (Figure 5). Generally, HP images are obtained from a piece of suspicious human tissue to be tested and analyzed by a pathologist [105]. HP images are defined as gigapixel whole-slide images (WSI) from which some small patches are extracted to enhance the analysis of these WSI (Figure 5). In other words, pathologists try to extract small patches related to ROI from WSI to diagnose breast cancer subtypes, which is a great advantage of HPs, enabling them to classify multiple classes of breast cancer [106,107] for prognosis and treatment. Additionally, much more meaningful ROI can be derived from HPs, in contrast to other imaging modalities confirming outstanding authenticity for breast cancer classification, especially breast cancer subtype classification. Furthermore, one of the most important advantages of HPs is their capability to integrate multi-omics features to analyze and diagnose breast cancer with high confidence [108]. TCGA is the most favorable resource for breast histopathological images. The TCGA database is widely employed in multi-level omics integration investigations. In other words, within TCGA, HPs provide contextual features to extract morphological properties, while molecular information from omics data at different levels, including microRNA, CNV, and DNA methylation [108], are also available for each patient. Integrating morphology and multiomics information provides an opportunity to more accurately detect and classify breast cancer. Despite these advantages, HPs have some limitations. For example, analyzing multiple biopsy sections, such as converting an invasive biopsy to digital images, is a lengthy process requiring a high concentration level due to the cell structures' microscopic size [109]. More drawbacks and advantages of the HP imagining modality are summarized in Table 1.

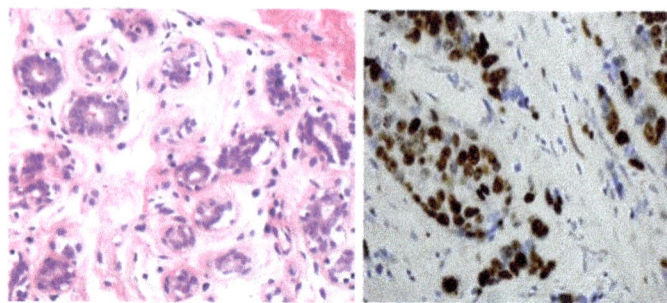

Figure 5. Images of the breast from H&E (haemotoxylin and eosin) stained image of a benign case provided by histopathology imaging modality [105]. Reprinted/adapted with permission from [105]. 2017, Elsevier.

2.6. Positron Emission Tomography (PET)

PET uses radiotracers for visualizing and measuring the changes in metabolic processes and other physiological activities, such as blood flow, regional chemical composition, and absorption. PET is a recent effective imaging method showing the promising capability to measure tissues' in vivo cellular, molecular, and biochemical properties (Figure 6). One of the key applications of PET is the analysis of breast cancer [110]. Studies highlighted that PET is a handy tool in staging advanced and inflammatory breast cancer and evaluating the response to treatment of the recurrent disease [34,35]. In contrast to the anatomic imaging method, PET highlights a more specific targeting of breast cancer with a larger margin between tumor and normal tissue, representing one step forward in cancer detection besides anatomic modalities [111–113]. Thus, the PET approach is used in hybrid modalities with CT for specific organ imaging to encourage the advantages of PET and improve spatial resolution, which is one of this modality's strengths. Additionally, PET uses the integration of radionuclides with some elements or pharmaceutical compounds to form radiotracers, improving the performance of PET [114]. Fluorodeoxyglucose (FDG), a glucose analog, is most commonly used for most breast cancer imaging studies as an effective radiotracer developed for PET imaging [115]. Recent studies clarified a specific correlation between the degree of FDG uptake and several phenotypic features containing a tumor histologic type and grade, cell receptor expression, and cellular proliferation [116,117]. These correlations lead to making the FDG-PET system for breast cancer analysis such as diagnosis, staging, re-staging, and treatment response evaluation [111,118,119]. Another PET system is a breast-dedicated high-resolution PET system designed in a hanging breast imaging modality. Some studies demonstrate that these PET-based modalities can detect almost all breast lesions and cancerous regions [120]. Table 1 summarizes some of PET-based imaging modalities' limitations and advantages. Also, in Table 2, we provided most commonly used public datasets for different imaging modalities in breast cancer detection.

Table 2. Public datasets for different imaging modalities for breast cancer analysis.

Imaging Modality	Public Dataset	Link of Dataset	Information about Dataset
MM	BCDR	https://www.medicmind.tech/cancer-imaging-data accessed date: 25 September 2022	426 benign and 310 malignant
	IRMA	https://www.medicmind.tech/cancer-imaging-data accessed date: 25 September 2022	1865 typical cases and 932 abnormal
	MIAS	https://www.medicmind.tech/cancer-imaging-data accessed date: 25 September 2022	133 abnormal and 189 of normal class
	DDSM	https://www.medicmind.tech/cancer-imaging-data accessed date: 25 September 2022	912 benign and 784 malignant
	INBreast	http://marathon.csee.usf.edu/Mammography/Database.html accessed date: 25 September 2022	410 malignant

Table 2. Cont.

Imaging Modality	Public Dataset	Link of Dataset	Information about Dataset
US	MBUD	https://www.kaggle.com/datasets/aryashah2k/breast-ultrasound-images-dataset accessed date: 25 September 2022	472 normal 278 abnormal
	OASBUD	http://bluebox.ippt.gov.pl/~hpiotrzk/ accessed date: 25 September 2022	48 benign 52 malignant
	BUSI	https://scholar.cu.edu.eg/?q=afahmy/pages/dataset accessed date: 25 September 2022	620 benign 210 malignant
	MT-small	https://www.kaggle.com/datasets/mohammedtgadallah/mt-small-dataset accessed date: 25 September 2022	200 benign 200 malignant
	UDIAT	https://datasets.bifrost.ai/info/1320 accessed date: 25 September 2022	110 benign 53 malignant
	STUHospital	https://github.com/xbhlk/STU-Hospital accessed date: 25 September 2022	42 malignant
MRI	DCE-MRI	https://mridiscover.com/dce-mri/ accessed date: 25 September 2022	559 malignant
	DWI	https://radiopaedia.org/articles/diffusion-weighted-imaging-2?lang=us accessed date: 25 September 2022	328 malignant
	RIDER	https://wiki.cancerimagingarchive.net/display/Public/RIDER+Collections accessed date: 25 September 2022	500 malignant
	DMR-IR	http://visual.ic.uff.br/dmi/ accessed date: 25 September 2022	267 normal 44 abnormal
	TCIA	https://www.cancerimagingarchive.net/ accessed date: 25 September 2022	91 malignant
HP	BreakHis	https://www.kaggle.com/datasets/ambarish/breakhis accessed date: 25 September 2022	2480 benign and 5429 malignant
	Camelyon	https://camelyon16.grand-challenge.org/Data/ accessed date: 25 September 2022	240 benign 160 malignant
	TUPAC	https://github.com/DeepPathology/TUPAC16_AlternativeLabels accessed date: 25 September 2022	50 benign 23 malignant
	BACH	https://zenodo.org/record/3632035#.Yxl8gnbMK3A accessed date: 25 September 2022	37 benign 38 malignant
	ICPR 2012	http://icpr2012.org/ accessed date: 25 September 2022	50 malignant
	IDC	https://imaging.datacommons.cancer.gov/ accessed date: 25 September 2022	162 malignant
	Wisconsin	https://archive.ics.uci.edu/ml/datasets/Breast+Cancer+Wisconsin+%28Diagnostic%29 accessed date: 25 September 2022	357 benign and 212 malignant
	DRYAD	https://datadryad.org/stash/dataset/doi:10.5061/dryad.05qfttf4t accessed date: 25 September 2022	173 malignant
	CRC	https://paperswithcode.com/dataset/crc accessed date: 25 September 2022	2031 normal 1974 malignant
	AMIDA	https://www.amida.com/index.html accessed date: 25 September 2022	23 malignant
	TCGA	https://portal.gdc.cancer.gov/ accessed date: 25 September 2022	1097 malignant
DBT	BCS-DBT	https://sites.duke.edu/mazurowski/resources/digital-breast-tomosynthesis-database/ accessed date: 25 September 2022	22,032 DBT volume from 5610 subjects (89 malignant, 112 benign, 5129 normal)

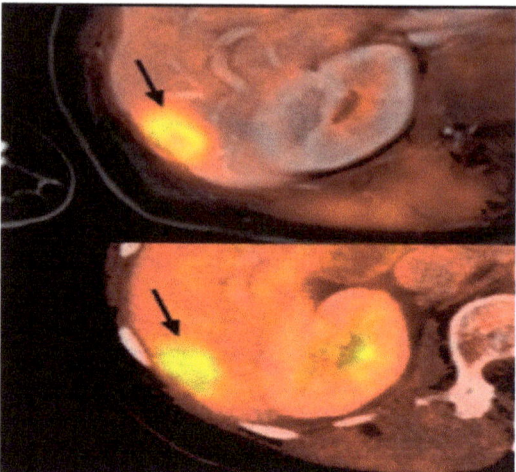

Figure 6. Example of PET images for breast cancer analysis [118]. Reprinted/adapted with permission from [118]. 2021, Elsevier.

3. Artificial Intelligence in Medical Image Analysis

Artificial intelligence (AI) has become very popular in the past few years because it adds human capabilities, e.g., learning, reasoning, and perception, to the software accurately and efficiently, and as a result, computers gain the ability to perform tasks that are usually carried out by humans. The recent advances in computing resources and availability of large datasets, as well as the development of new AI algorithms, have opened the path to the use of AI in many different areas, including but not limited to image synthesis [121], speech recognition [122,123] and engineering [124–126]. AI has been also employed in healthcare industries for applications such as protein engineering [127–130], cancer detection [131], and drug discovery [132,133]. More specifically, AI algorithms have shown an outstanding capability to discover complex patterns and extract discriminative features from medical images, providing higher-quality analysis and better quantitative results efficiently and automatically. AI has been a great help for physicians in imaging-related tasks, i.e., disease detection and diagnosis, to accomplish more accurate results [134]. Deep learning (DL) [30] is part of a broader family of AI which imitates the way humans learn. DL uses multiple layers to gain knowledge, and the complexity of the learned features increases hierarchically. DL algorithms have been applied in many applications, and in some of them, they could outperform humans. DL algorithms have also been used in various categories in the realm of cancer diagnosis using cancer images from different modalities, including detecting cancer cells, cancer type classification, lesion segmentation, etc. To learn more about DL, we refer interested readers to [135].

3.1. Benefits of Using DL for Medical Image Analysis

Comparing the healthcare area with others, it is safe to say that the decision-making process is much more crucial in healthcare systems than in other areas since it directly affects people's lives. For example, a wrong decision by a physician in diagnosing a disease can lead to the death of a patient. Complex and constrained clinical environments and workflows make the physician's decision-making very challenging, especially for image-related tasks since they require high visual perception and cognitive ability [136]. In these situations, AI can be a great tool to decrease the false-diagnosis rates by extracting specific and known features from the images or even helping the physician by giving an initial guess for the solution. Nowadays, more and more healthcare providers are encouraged to use AI algorithms due to the availability of computing resources, advancement in image analysis tools, and the great performance shown by AI methods.

3.2. Deep Learning Models for Breast Cancer Detection

This section briefly discusses the deep learning algorithms applied to images from each breast cancer modality.

3.2.1. Digital Mammography and Digital Breast Tomosynthesis (MM-DBT)

With the recent technology developments, MM images follow the same trend and take more advanced forms, e.g., digital breast tomosynthesis (DBT). Each MM form has been widely used for breast cancer detection and classification. One of the first attempts to use deep learning for MMs was carried out by [137]. The authors in [137] used a convolutional neural network (CNN)-based model to learn features from mammography images before feeding them to a support vector machine (SVM) classifier. Their algorithm could achieve 86% AUC in lesion classification, which had about 6% improvement compared to the best conventional approach before this paper. Following [137], more studies [138–140] have also used CNN-based algorithms for lesion classification. However, in these papers, the region of interest was extracted without the help of a deep learning algorithm, i.e., by employing traditional image processing methods [139] or by an expert [140]. More specifically, the authors in [138] first divided MM images into patches and extracted the features from the patches using a conventional image-processing algorithm, and then used the random forest classifier to choose good candidate patches for their CNN algorithm. Their approach could achieve an AUC of 92.9%, which is slightly better than the baseline method based on a conventional method with an AUC of 91%. With the advancement in DL algorithms and the availability of complex and powerful DL architectures, DL methods have been used to extract ROIs from full MM images. As a result, the input to the algorithm is no longer the small patches, and the full MM image could be used as input. For example, the proposed method in [131] uses YOLO [141], a well-known algorithm for detection and classification, to simultaneously extract and classify ROIs in the whole image. Their results show that their algorithm performs similarly to a CNN model trained on small patches with an AUC of 97%. Figure 7 shows the overall structure of the proposed model in [131].

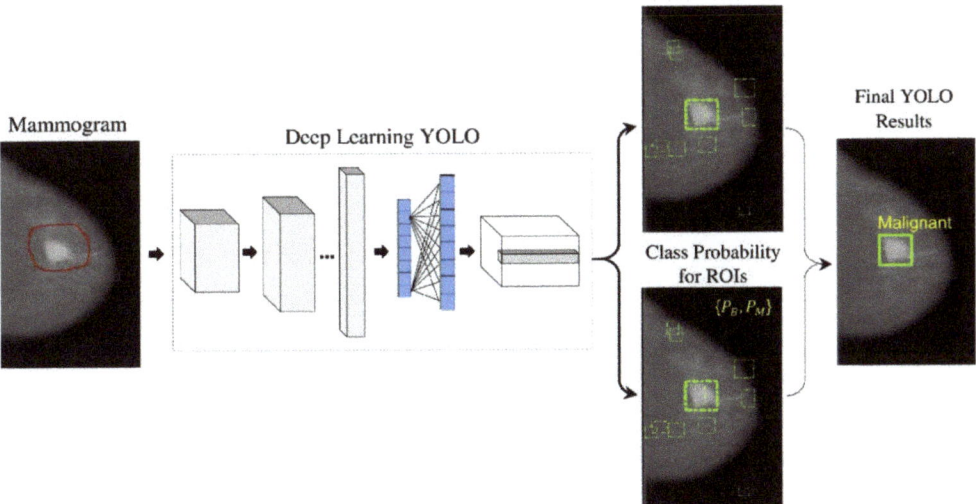

Figure 7. Schematic diagram of the proposed YOLO-based CAD system in [131]. Reprinted/adapted with permission from [131]. 2021, Elsevier.

To increase the accuracy of cancer detection, DBT has emerged as a predominant breast-imaging modality. It has been shown that DBT increases the cancer detection rate (CDR) while decreasing recall rates (RR) when compared to FFDM [142–144]. Following the same logic, some DL algorithms have been proposed to apply to DBT images for cancer detection [145–149]. For instance, the authors in [150] proposed a deep learning model based on ResNet architecture to classify the input images into normal, benign, high-risk, or malignant. They trained the model on an FFDM dataset, then fine-tuned the model using 2D reconstruction of DBT images obtained by applying the 2D maximum intensity projection (MIP) method. Their method achieved an AUC of 84.7% on the DBT dataset. A deep CNN has been developed in [145] that uses DBT volumes to classify the masses. Their proposed approach obtained an AUC of 84.7%, which is about 2% higher than the current CAD method with hand-crafted features.

Although deep learning models perform very well in medical image analysis, their major bottleneck is the thirst for training datasets. In the medical field, collecting and labeling data is very expensive. Some studies used transfer learning to overcome this problem. In the study by [151], the authors developed a two-stage transfer learning approach to classify DBT images as mass or normal. In the first stage, the authors fine-tuned a pretrained AlexNet [152] using FFDM images, and then the fine-tuned model was used to train a model using DBT images. The CNN model in the second stage was used as the feature extractor for DBT images, and the random forest classifier was used to classify the extracted features as mass or normal. They obtained an AUC of 90% on their test dataset. In another work in [153], the authors used a VGG19 [154] network trained on the ImageNet dataset as a feature extractor for FFDM and DBT images for malignant and benign classification. The extracted features were fed to an SVM classifier to estimate the probability of malignancy. Their method obtained an AUC of 98% and 97% on the DBT images in CC and MLO view, respectively. These methods show that by using a relatively small training dataset and employing transfer learning techniques, deep learning models can perform well. Most of the aforementioned studies compare their DL algorithms with traditional CAD methods. However, the best way to evaluate the performance of a DL method is to compare that with a radiologist directly. For example, the performance of DL systems on FFDM and DBT has been investigated in [155]. The study shows that a DL system can achieve comparable sensitivity as radiologists in FFDM images while decreasing the recall rate. Additionally, on DBT images, an AI system can have the same performance as radiologists, although the recall rate has increased.

Table 3 shows the list of recent DL-based models used for MM and DBT with their performances. The application of DL in breast cancer detection is not limited to mammography images. In the following section, we discuss the DL application in other breast cancer imaging modalities.

Table 3. The summary of the studies that used MM and DBT datasets.

Paper	Year	Task	Model	Type	Dataset	Evaluation
Agnes et al. [146]	2020	Classification	Multiscale All CNN	MM	MIAS	Acc = 96.47%
Shu et al. [156]	2020	Classification	CNN	MM	INbreast CBIS-DDSM	INbreast: Acc = 92.2% CBIS: Acc = 76.7%
Singh et al. [150]	2020	Classification	CNN	FFDM and DBT	Private	FFDM: AUC = 0.9 DBT: AUC = 0.85
Boumaraf et al. [157]	2020	Classification	DBN (Deep Belief Network)	MM	DDSM	Acc = 84.5%
Matthews et al. [158]	2021	Classification	Transfer learning based on ResNet	DBT	Private	AUC = 0.9
Zhang et al. [159]	2021	Classification	GNN (Graph Neural Network) + CNN	MM	MIAS	Acc = 96.1%
Li et al. [160]	2021	Classification	SVM (Support Vector Machine)	MM	INbreast	Acc = 84.6%
Saber et al. [161]	2021	Classification	CNN/Transfer learning	MM	MIAS	Acc = 98.87% F-score = 99.3%

Table 3. Cont.

Paper	Year	Task	Model	Type	Dataset	Evaluation
Malebary et al. [162]	2021	Classification	CNN	MM	DDSM MIAS	DDSM: Acc = 97% MIAS: Acc = 97%
Li et al. [163]	2021	Classification	CNN-RNN (Recurrent Neural Network)	MM	DDSM	ACC = 94.7%, Recall = 94.1% AUC = 0.968
Ueda et al. [164]	2022	Classification	CNN	MM	Private DDSM	AUC = 0.93
Mota et al. [165]	2022	Classification	CNN	DBT	VICTRE	AUC = 0.941
Bai et al. [166]	2022	Classification	GCN (Graph Convolutional Network)	DBT	BCS-DBT Private	Acc = 84% AUC = 0.87
Zhu et al. [167]	2018	Mass Segmentation	FCN (Fully Convolutional Network) + CRF (Conditional Random Field)	MM	INbreast DDSM-BCRP	INbreast: Dice = 90.97% DDSM-BCRP: Dice = 91.3%
Wang et al. [168]	2019	Mass Segmentation	MNPNet (Multi-Level Nested Pyramid Network)	MM	INbreast DDSM-BCRP	INbreast: Dice = 91.1% DDSM-BCRP: Dice = 91.69%
Saffari et al. [169]	2020	Dense tissue Segmentation/Classification	cGAN and CNN	MM	INbreast	S: Acc = 98% C: Acc = 97.85%
Ahmed et al. [170]	2020	Tumor Segmentation/Classification	DeepLab/mask RCNN	MM	MIAS CBIS-DDSM	DeepLab: C: Acc = 95% S: MAP = 72% Mask RCNN: C: Acc = 98% S: MAP = 80%
Buda et al. [171]	2020	Lesion detection	CNN	DBT	Private	Sensitivity = 65%
Cheng et al. [172]	2020	Mass Segmentation	Spatial Enhanced Rotation Aware Net	MM	DDSM	Dice = 84.3% IOU = 73.95%
Chen et al. [173]	2020	Mass Segmentation	Modified U-Net	MM	INbreast CBIS-DDSM	INbreast: Dice = 81.64% CBIS: Dice = 82.16%
Soleimani et al. [174]	2020	Breast-Pectoral Segmentation	CNN	MM	MIAS CBIS-DDSM INbreast	MIAS: Dice = 97.59% CBIS: Dice = 97.69% INbreast: Dice = 96.39%
Al-antari et al. [175]	2020	Breast lesions Segmentation/Classification	YOLO	MM	DDSM INbreast	S: DDSM: F1-score = 99.28% INbreast: F1-score = 98.02% C: DDSM: Acc = 97.5% INbreast: Acc = 95.32%
Li et al. [176]	2020	Mass Segmentation	Siamese-Faster-RCNN	MM	INbreast BCPKUPH(private) TXMD(private)	INbreast: TP = 0.88, BCPKUPH: TP = 0.85 TXMD: TP = 0.85
Peng et al. [177]	2020	Mass Segmentation	Faster RCNN	MM	CBIS-DDSM INbreast	CBIS: TP = 0.93 INbreast: TP = 0.95
Kavitha et al. [178]	2021	Mass Segmentation/Classification	CapsNet	MM	MIAS DDSM	MIAS: Acc = 98.5% DDSM: Acc = 97.55%
Shoshan et al. [179]	2021	Lesion detection	CNN	DBT	DBTex challenge	Avg. sensitivity = 0.91
Hossain et al. [180]	2022	Lesion detection	CNN	DBT	DBTex challenge	Avg. sensitivity = 0.815
Hossain et al. [181]	2022	Lesion detection	CNN	DBT	DBTex challenge	Avg. sensitivity = 0.84
Atrey et al. [182]	2022	Breast lesion Segmentation	CNN	MM	DDSM	Dice = 65%

3.2.2. Ultrasound (US)

As has been explained in Section 2, ultrasound performs much better in detecting cancers and reduces unnecessary biopsy operations [183]. Therefore, it is not surprising to see that the researchers use this type of image in their DL models for cancer detection [184–186]. For instance, a GoogleNet [187]-based CNN has been trained on the suspicious ROIs of US images in [184]. The proposed method in [184] achieved an AUC of 96%, which is 6% higher than the CAD-based method with hand-crafted features. The authors in [188–190] trained CNN models directly with whole US images without extracting the ROIs. For example, the authors in [190] combined VGG19 and ResNet152 and trained the ensemble network on US images. Their proposed method achieved an AUC of 95% on a balanced, independent test dataset. Figure 8 represents an example of CNN models for breast cancer subtype classification.

In comparison with datasets for mammography images, there are fewer datasets for US images, and they usually contain much fewer images. Therefore, most of the proposed DL models use some kind of data augmentation method, such as rotation, to increase the size of training data and improve the model performance. However, one should be careful about how to augment US images since some augmentation may decrease the model performance. For example, it has been shown in [186] that performing the image rotation or shift in the longitudinal direction can affect the model performance negatively. The generative adversarial networks (GANs) can also be used to generate synthetic US images with or without tumors [191]. These images can be added to the original training images to improve the model's accuracy.

The US images have also been used in lesion detection in which, when given an image, the CAD system decides whether the lesion is present. One of the challenges that the researcher faces in this type of problem with normal US images is that there is a need for a US doctor to manually select the images that have lesions for the models. This depends on the doctors' availability and is usually expensive and time-consuming. It also adds human errors to the system [192]. To solve this problem, a method has been developed in [193] to detect the lesions in real time during US scanning. Another type of US imaging is called the 3D automated breast US scan, which captures the entire breast [194,195]. The authors in [195] developed a CNN model based on VGGNet, ResNet [196], and DenseNet [197] networks. Their approach obtained an AUC of 97% on their private dataset and an AUC of 97.11% on the breast ultrasound image (BUSI) dataset [80].

Some methods combined the detection and classification of lesions in US images in one step [198]. An extensive study in [199] compares different DL architectures for US image detection and classification. Their results show that the DenseNet is a good candidate for classification analysis of US images, which provides accuracies of 85% and 87.5% for full image classification and pre-defined ROIs, respectively. The authors in [200] developed a weakly supervised DL algorithm based on VGG16, ResNet34, and GoogleNet trained using 1000 unannotated US images. They have reported an average AUC of 88%.

Some studies validate the performance of DL algorithms [201–203] using expert inference, showing that DL algorithms can greatly help radiologists. This is mostly in cases where the lesion was already detected by an expert, and the DL model is used to classify them. However, unlike the mammography studies, most of the studies are not validated by multiple physicians and do not show the generalizability of their method on multiple datasets which should be addressed in future validations. Table 4 shows the list of recent algorithms used for US images and their performances.

Table 4. The summary of the studies that used ultrasound dataset.

Paper	Year	Task	Model	Dataset	Evaluation
Byra et al. [204]	2019	Classification	Transfer learning based on VGG-19 and InceptionV3	OASBUD	VGG19: AUC = 0.822 InceptionV3: AUC = 0.857
Byra et al. [186]	2019	Classification	Transfer learning based on VGG 19	Private	AUC = 0.936
Hijab et al. [205]	2019	Classification	Transfer learning based on VGG16	Private	Acc = 97.4% AUC = 0.98
Zhang et al. [206]	2019	Classification	Deep Polynomial Network (DPN)	Private	Acc = 95.6% AUC = 0.961
Fujioka et al. [207]	2020	Classification	CNN	Private	AUC = 0.87

Table 4. *Cont.*

Paper	Year	Task	Model	Dataset	Evaluation
Wu et al. [208]	2020	Classification	Random Forest (RF)	Private	Acc = 86.97%
Wu et al. [209]	2020	Classification	Generalized Regression Neural Network (GRNN)	Private	Acc = 87.78% F1 score = 86.15%
Gong et al. [210]	2020	Classification	Multi-view Deep Neural Network Support Vector Machine (MDNNSVM)	Private	Acc = 86.36% AUC = 0.908
Moon et al. [195]	2020	Classification	VGGNet + ResNet + DenseNet (Ensemble loss)	SNUH BUSI	SNUH: Acc = 91.1% AUC = 0.9697 BUSI: Acc = 94.62% AUC = 0.9711
Zhang et al. [211]	2020	Classification	CNN	Private	AUC = 1
Yousef Kalaf et al. [212]	2021	Classification	Modified VGG16	Private	Acc = 93% F1 score = 94%
Misra et al. [213]	2022	Classification	Transfer learning based on AlexNet and ResNet	Private	Acc = 90%
Vakanski et al. [214]	2020	Tumor Segmentation	CNN	BUSI	Acc = 98% Dice score = 90.5%
Byra et al. [215]	2020	Mass Segmentation	CNN	Private	Acc = 97% Dice score = 82.6%
Singh et al. [216]	2020	Tumor Segmentation	CNN	Mendeley UDIAT	Mendeley: Dice = 0.9376 UDIAT: Dice = 86.82%
Han et al. [217]	2020	Lesion Segmentation	GAN	Private	Dice = 87.12%
Wang et al. [218]	2021	Lesion Segmentation	Residual Feedback Network	1-Ultrasound-cases.info and BUSI 2- UDIAT 3- Radiopaedia	1-Dice = 86.91% 2-Dice = 81.79% 3-Dice = 87%
Wang et al. [219]	2021	Segmentation	CNN	Ultrasoundcases.info BUSI STUHospital	Ultrasoundcases: Dice = 84.71% BUSI: Dice = 83.76% STUHospital: Dice = 86.52%
Li et al. [220]	2022	Tumor Segmentation + Classification	DeepLab3	Private	S: Dice = 77.3% C: Acc = 94.8%
Byra et al. [221]	2022	Mass Segmentation + Classification	Y-Net	Private	S: Dice = 64.0% C: AUC = 0.87

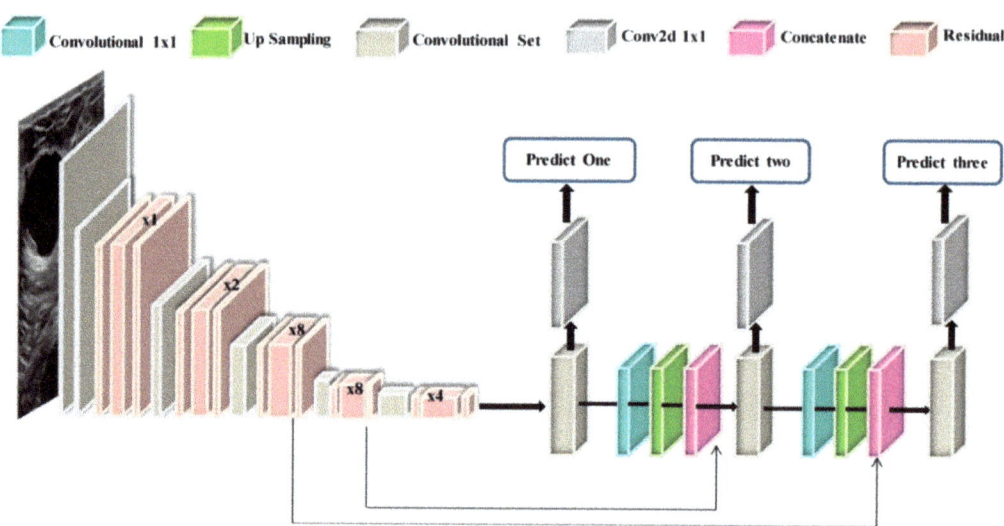

Figure 8. Example of a model architecture for breast cancer subtypes classification from US images via CNN models [222].

3.2.3. Magnetic Resonance Imaging (MRI)

As explained in Section 2, MRI has higher sensitivity for breast cancer detection in dense breasts [223] than MM and US images. However, the big difference between MRI and MM or US images is that the MRI is a 3D scan, but MM and US are 2D images. Moreover, MRI sequences are captured over time, increasing the MRI dimensionality to 4D (dynamic contrast-enhanced (DCE)-MRI). This makes MRI images more challenging for DL algorithms compared to MM and US images, as most of the current DL algorithms are built for 2D images. One way to address this challenge is to convert the 3D image to 2D by either dividing 3D MRIs into 2D slices [224,225] or using MIP to build a 2D representation [226]. Moreover, most DL algorithms have been developed for colored images, which are 3D images whose third dimension represents the color channels. However, the MRIs are grayscale images. Therefore, some developed MRI models put three consecutive slices of grayscale MRI together and build a 3D image [227,228]. Some other approaches modify the current 2D DL architecture to make them appropriate for MRI 3D scans [229].

All the above approaches have been used in lesion classification DL algorithms. For example, [230] uses 2D slices of the ROIs as input to their CNN model. They obtained an accuracy of 85% on their test dataset. The MIP technique is used in [231] which obtained an AUC of 89.5%. In the study carried out by Zhou et al. [229], the authors put the grayscale MRIs together and built 3D images for their DL methods. Their algorithm obtained an AUC of 92%. In another study presented in [193], the proposed algorithm uses the actual 3D MRI scans obtaining an AUC of 85.9% by the 3D version of DenseNet [197]. It is worth mentioning that the performance of 2D and 3D approaches cannot be compared since they used different datasets. However, some studies compared their proposed methods with radiologists' interpretations [228,229]. Figure 9 shows a schematic of a framework for cancer subtype classification with MRI.

Like in MM and US images, the DL methods have been widely used in lesion detection and segmentation problems in MRI images. A CNN algorithm based on RetinaNet [232] has been developed in [233] for detecting lesions from the 4D MR scans. Their method obtained a sensitivity of 95%. One study [234] used a mask-guided hierarchical learning (MHL) framework for breast tumor segmentation based on U-net architecture. Their method achieved the Dice similarity coefficient (DSC) of 0.72 for lesion segmentation. In another work [235], the authors proposed a U-net-based CNN model called 3TP U-net for the lesion segmentation task. Their algorithm obtained a Dice similarity coefficient of 61.24%. Alternatively, the authors in [236] developed a CNN-based segmentation model by refining the U-net architecture to segment the lesions in MRIs. Their proposed method achieved a Dice similarity coefficient of 86.5%. It has to be noted that in most lesion segmentation algorithms, there is a need for a mask that shows the pixels that belong to the breast as ground truth for training. These masks can help the models to focus on the right place and ignore the areas that do not have any information. Table 5 shows the list of recent algorithms used for MRI images and their performances.

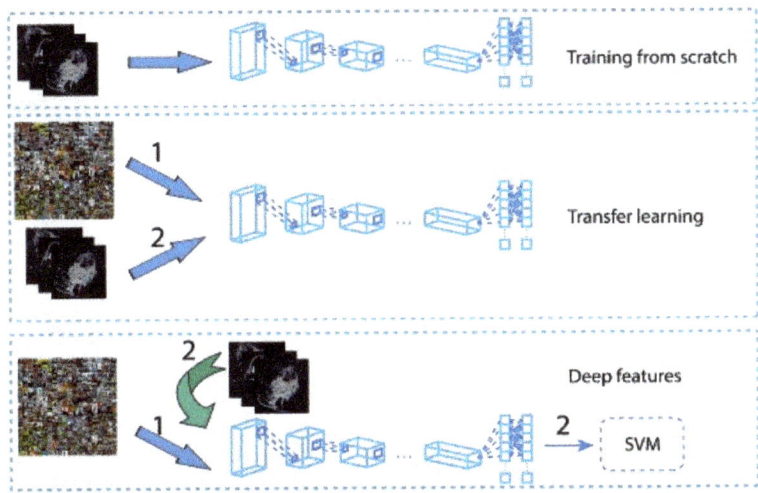

Figure 9. A model architecture for cancer subtypes prediction via ResNet 50 and CNN models from MRI images [237]. Reprinted/adapted with permission from [237]. 2019, Elsevier.

Table 5. Summary of the studies that used MRI datasets.

Paper	Year	Task	Model	Dataset	Evaluation
Ha et al. [238]	2019	Classification	CNN	Private	Acc = 70%
Ha et al. [239]	2019	Classification	CNN	Private	Acc = 88%
Fang et al. [240]	2019	Classification	CNN	Private	Acc = 70.5%
Zheng et al. [241]	2020	Classification	CNN	TCIA	Acc = 97.2%
Holste et al. [242]	2021	Classification	Fusion Deep learning	Private	AUC = 0.9
Winkler et al. [243]	2021	Classification	CNN	Private	ACC = 92.8%
Fujioka et al. [244]	2021	Classification	CNN	Private	AUC = 0.89
Liu et al. [245]	2022	Classification	Weakly ResNet-101	Private	AUC = 0.92 ACC = 94%
Bie et al. [246]	2022	Classification	CNN	Private	ACC = 92% Specificity = 94%
Jing et al. [247]	2022	Classification	U-NET and ResNet 34	Private	AUC = 0.81
Wu et al. [248]	2022	Classification	CNN	Private	Acc = 87.7% AUC = 91.2%
Verburg et al. [249]	2022	Classification	CNN	Private	AUC = 0.83
Dutta et al. [250]	2021	Tumor Segmentation	Multi-contrast D-R2UNet	Private	F1 score = 95%

Table 5. Cont.

Paper	Year	Task	Model	Dataset	Evaluation
Carvalho et al. [251]	2021	Tumor Segmentation	SegNet and UNet	QIN Breast DCE-MRI	Dice = 97.6% IOU = 95.3%
Wang et al. [252]	2021	Lesion Segmentation	CNN	Private	Dice = 76.4%
Nowakowska et al. [253]	2022	Segmentation of BPE area and non-enhancing tissue	CNN	Private	Dice = 76%
Khaled et al. [254]	2022	Lesion segmentation	3D U-Net	TCGA-BRCA	Dice = 68%
Yue et al. [255]	2022	Segmentation	Res_U-Net	Private	Dice = 89%
Rahimpour et al. [256]	2022	Tumor Segmentation	3D U-Net	Private	Dice = 78%
Zhu et al. [257]	2022	Lesion Segmentation/Classification	V-Net	Private	S: Dice = 86% C: Avg. AUC = 0.84

3.2.4. Histopathology

In contrast to other modalities, histopathology images are colored images that are provided either as the whole-slide images (WSI) or the extracted image patches from the WSI, i.e., ROIs that are extracted by pathologists. The histopathology images are a great means of diagnosing breast cancer types that are impossible to find with radiology images, i.e., MRIs. Moreover, these images have been used to detect cancer subtypes because of the details they have about the tissue. Therefore, they are widely used with DL algorithms for cancer detection. For example, Ref. [258] employed a CNN-based DL algorithm to classify the histopathology images into four classes: normal tissue, benign lesion, in situ carcinoma, and invasive carcinoma. They combined the classification results of all the image patches to obtain the final image-wise classification. They also used their model to classify the images into two classes, carcinoma, and non-carcinoma. An SVM has been trained on the features extracted by a CNN to classify the images. Their method obtained an accuracy of 77.8% on four-class classification and an accuracy of 83.3% on binary classification. In another work proposed in [259], two CNN models were developed, one for predicting malignancy and the other for predicting malignancy and image magnification levels simultaneously. They used images of size 700 × 460 with different magnification levels. Their average binary classification for benign/malignant is 83.25%. A novel framework was proposed in [260] that uses a hybrid attention-based mechanism to classify histopathology images. The attention mechanism helps to find the useful regions from raw images automatically.

The transfer learning approach has also been employed in analyzing histopathology images since the histopathology image datasets suffer from the lack of a large amount of data required for deep learning models. For example, the method developed in [261] uses pretrained Inception-V3 [187] and Inception-ResNet-V2 [262] and fine-tunes them for both binary and multiclass classification on histology images. Their approach obtained an accuracy of 97.9% in binary classification and an accuracy of 92.07% in the multi-classification task. In another work [263], the authors developed a framework for classifying malignant and benign cells that extracted the features from images using GoogleNet, VGGNet, and ResNet and then combined those features to use them in the classifier. Their framework obtained an average accuracy of 97%. The authors in [264] used a fine-tuned GoogleNet to extract features from the small patches of pathological images. The extracted features were fed to a bidirectional long short-term memory (LSTM) layer for classification. Their approach obtained an accuracy of 91.3%. Figure 10 shows the overview of the method proposed in [264]. GANs have also been combined with transfer learning to further increase classification accuracy. In work carried out in [265], StyleGAN [266] and Pix2Pix [267] were used to generate fake images. Then, VGG-16 and VGG-19 were fine-tuned to classify images. Their proposed method achieved an accuracy of 98.1% in binary classification.

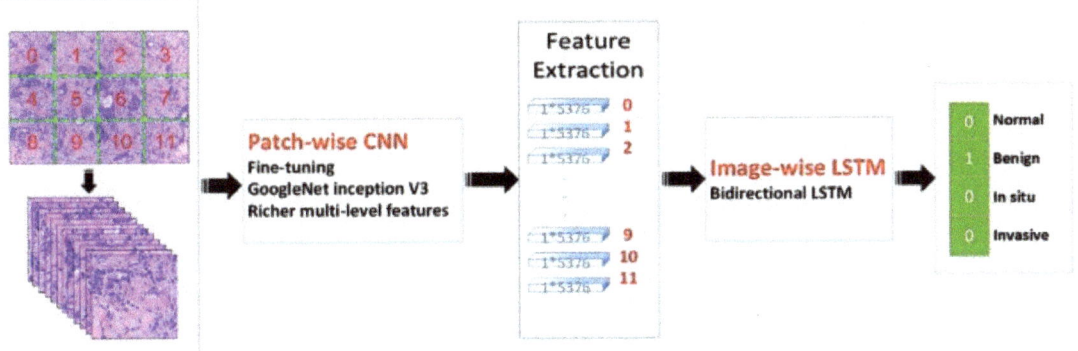

Figure 10. Prediction of breast cancer grades from extracted patches from histopathology images via patch-wise LSTM architecture [264]. Reprinted/adapted with permission from [264]. 2019, Elsevier.

Histopathology images have been widely used for nuclei detection and segmentation. For instance, in the work presented in [268], a novel framework called HASHI was developed that automatically detects invasive breast cancer in the whole slide images. Their framework obtained a Dice coefficient of 76% on their independent test dataset. In the other work performed in [269] for nuclei detection, a series of handcrafted features and features extracted from CNN were combined for better detection. The method used three different datasets and obtained an F-score of 90%. The authors in [270] presented a fully automated workflow for nuclei segmentation in histopathology images based on deep learning and the morphological properties extracted from the images. Their workflow achieved an accuracy and F1-score of 95.4% and 80.5%, respectively. In another work by [271], the authors first extracted the small patches from the high-resolution whole slides, then each small patch was segmented using a CNN along with an encoder-decoder; finally, to combine the local segmentation result, they used an improved merging strategy based on a fully connected conditional random field. Their algorithm obtained a segmentation accuracy of 95.6%. Table 6 shows the performance of recently developed DL methods in histology images.

3.2.5. Positron Emission Tomography (PET)/Computed Tomography (CT)

PET/CT is a nuclear medicine imaging technique that helps increase the effectiveness of detecting and classifying axillary lymph nodes and distant staging [272]. However, they have trouble detecting early-stage breast cancer. Therefore, it is not surprising that PET/CT is barely used with DL algorithms. However, PET/CT has some important applications that DL algorithms can be applied. For example, as discussed in [273], breast cancer is one of the reasons for most cases of bone metastasis. A CNN-based algorithm was developed in [274] to detect breast cancer metastasis on whole-body scintigraphy scans. Their algorithm obtained 92.5% accuracy in the binary classification of whole-body scans.

In the other application, PET/CT can be used to quantify the whole-body metabolic tumor volume (MTV) to reduce the labor and cost of obtaining MTV. For example, in the work presented in [275], a model trained on the MTV of lymphoma and lung cancer patients is used to detect the lesions in PET/CT scans of breast cancer patients. Their algorithm could detect 92% of the measurable lesions.

Table 6. The summary of the studies that used histopathology datasets.

Paper	Year	Task	Model	Dataset	Evaluation
Zainudin et al. [276]	2019	Breast Cancer Cell Detection/Classification	CNN	MITOS	Acc = 84.5% TP = 80.55% FP = 11.6%
Li et al. [277]	2019	Breast Cancer Cell Detection/Classification	Deep cascade CNN	MITOSIS AMIDA13 TUPAC16	MITOSIS: F-score = 56.2% AMIDA13: F-score = 67.3% TUPAC16: F-score = 66.9%
Das et al. [278]	2019	Breast Cancer Cell Detection/Classification	CNN	MITOS ATYPIA14	MITOS: F1-score = 84.05% ATYPIA14: F1-score = 59.76%
Gour et al. [279]	2020	Classification	CNN	BreakHis	Acc = 92.52% F1 score = 93.45%
Saxena et al. [280]	2020	Classification	CNN	BreakHis	Avg. Acc = 88%
Hirra et al. [281]	2021	Classification	DBN	DRYAD	Acc = 86%
Senan et al. [282]	2021	Classification	CNN	BreakHis	Acc = 95% AUC = 99.36%
Zewdie et al. [283]	2021	Classification	CNN	Private BreakHis Zendo	Binary Acc = 96.75% Grade classification Acc = 93.86%
Kushwaha et al. [284]	2021	Classification	CNN	BreakHis	Acc = 97%
Gheshlaghi et al. [285]	2021	Classification	Auxiliary Classifier GAN	BreakHis	Binary Acc = 90.15% Sub-type classification Acc = 86.33%
Reshma et al. [286]	2022	Classification	Genetic Algorithm with CNN	BreakHis	Acc = 89.13%
Joseph et al. [287]	2022	Classification	CNN	BreakHis	Avg. Multiclass Acc = 97%
Ahmad et al. [288]	2022	Classification	CNN	BreakHis	Avg. Binary Acc = 99% Avg. Multiclass Acc = 95%
Mathew et al. [289]	2022	Breast Cancer Cell Detection/Classification	CNN	ATYPIA MITOS	F1 score = 61.91%
Singh and Kumar [290]	2022	Classification	Inception ResNet	BHI BreakHis	BHI: Acc = 85.21% BreakHis: Avg. Acc = 84%
Mejbri et al. [291]	2019	Tissue-level Segmentation	DNNs	Private	U-Net: Dice = 86%, SegNet: Dice = 87%, FCN: Dice = 86%, DeepLab: Dice = 86%
Guo et al. [292]	2019	Cancer Regions Segmentation	Transfer learning based on Inception-V3 and ResNet-101	Camelyon16	IOU = 80.4% AUC = 96.2%
Priego-Torres et al. [271]	2020	Tumor Segmentation	CNN	Private	Acc = 95.62% IOU = 92.52%
Budginaitè et al. [293]	2021	Cell Nuclei Segmentation	Micro-Net	Private	Dice = 81%
Pedersen et al. [294]	2022	Tumor Segmentation	CNN	Norwegian cohort [295]	Dice = 93.3%
Khalil et al. [296]	2022	Lymph node Segmentation	CNN	Private	F1 score = 84.4% IOU = 74.9%

4. Discussion

Breast cancer plays a crucial role in the mortality of women in the world. Cancer detection in its early stage is an essential task to reduce mortality. Recently, many imaging modalities have been used to give more detailed insights into breast cancer. However, manual analysis of these imaging modalities with a huge number of images is a difficult and time-consuming task leading to inaccurate diagnoses and an increased false-detection rate. Thus, to tackle these problems, an automated approach is needed. The most effective and reliable approach for medical image analysis is CAD. CAD systems have been designed to help physicians to reduce their errors in analyzing medical images. A CAD system highlights the suspicious features in images (e.g., masses) and helps radiologists to reduce false-negative readings. Moreover, CAD systems usually detect more false features than true marks, and it is the radiologist's responsibility to evaluate the results. This characteristic of CAD systems increases the reading time and limits the number of cases that radiologists can evaluate. Recently, the advancement of AI, especially DL-based methods, could effectively speed up the image analysis process and help radiologists in early breast cancer diagnosis.

Considering the importance of DL-based CAD systems for breast cancer detection and diagnosis, in this paper, we have discussed the applications of different DL algorithms in breast cancer detection. We first reviewed the imaging modalities used for breast cancer screening and diagnosis. Besides a comprehensive discussion, we discussed the advantage and limitations of each imaging modality and summarize the public datasets available for each modality with the links to the datasets. We then reviewed the recent DL algorithms used for breast imaging analysis along with the detail of their datasets and results. The studies presented promising results from DL-based CAD systems. However, the DL-based CAD tools still face many challenges that prohibit them from clinical usage. Here, we discussed some of these challenges as well as the future direction for cancer detection studies.

One of the main obstacles to having a robust DL-based CAD tool is the cost of collecting medical images. The medical images used for DL algorithms should contain reliable annotated images from different patients. Data collection would be very costly for sufficient abnormal data compared to normal cases since the number of abnormal cases is much lower than the normal cases (e.g., several abnormal cases per thousand patients in the breast cancer screening population). The data collection also depends on the number of patients that takes a specific examination and the availability of equipment and protocols in different clinical settings. For example, MM datasets are usually very large datasets, including thousands of patients. However, the MRI or PET/CT datasets contain much fewer patients. Due to the existence of a large public dataset for MM, much more DL algorithms have been developed and validated for the MM modality than other datasets. One way to create a big dataset for different image modalities is multi-institutional collaboration. The dataset obtained from these collaborations covers a large group of patients with different characteristics, different imaging equipment, and clinical settings and protocols. These datasets make the DL algorithms more robust and reliable.

Currently available medical image datasets usually contain a small amount of data. On the other hand, employing DL and exploiting its capabilities on a small amount of training data is challenging. Because the DL algorithms should be trained on a large dataset to have a good performance. Some possible solutions can help to overcome the problems related to small datasets. For example, the datasets from different medical centers can be combined to create a bigger one. However, there are usually some patient privacy policies that should be addressed. Another solution to this problem is using federated learning [297] in which the algorithm is trained on datasets locally, but it should travel between the centers and be trained on the datasets in each center. The federated learning algorithms are not popular yet, and they are not widely implemented. In most cases, the training data cannot be publicly shared; therefore, there is no way to evaluate the DL methods and regenerate the results in the studies. Many studies used transfer learning to overcome the problem of small datasets. Some of the studies used a pre-trained model to extract features from the medical images and then, they used the extracted features to train a DL model for target tasks. However, other studies initialized their model with pre-trained model weights and then fine-tuned their models with the medical image datasets. Although transfer learning shows some improvement for the small datasets, the performance of the target model highly depends on the difference between the characteristics of source datasets and target datasets. In these cases, a negative transfer [298] may occur in which the source domain reduces the learning performance in the target domain. Some studies used data augmentation rather than transfer learning to increase the size of the dataset artificially and improve the model performance. However, one should note that augmenting data does not introduce the independent features to the model; therefore, it does not provide much new knowledge for the DL model compared to new independent images.

The shortage of datasets with comprehensive and fully labeled/annotated data is also another challenge that DL-based CAD systems face. Most of the DL methods are supervised algorithms, and they need fully labeled/annotated datasets. However, creating a large fully annotated dataset is a very challenging task since annotating medical images is time-consuming and may have human errors. To avoid the need for annotated datasets, some papers used unsupervised algorithms, but they obtained less accurate results compared to supervised algorithms.

Another important challenge is the generalizability of the DL algorithms. Most of the proposed approaches work on the datasets obtained with specific imaging characteristics and cannot be used for the datasets obtained from different populations, different clinical settings, or different imaging equipment and protocols. This is an obstacle to the wide use of AI methods in cancer detection in medical centers. Each health clinic should design and conduct a testing protocol for DL-based CAD systems using the data obtained from the local patient population before any clinical usage of these systems. During the testing period, the user should find the weaknesses and strengths of the system based on the output of the system for different input cases. The user should know that what is the characteristics of the failed and correct output and recognize when the system makes mistake and when it works fine. This testing procedure not only evaluates DL-based CAD models but also teaches the user the best way to use DL-based CAD systems.

Another limitation can be the interpretability of DL algorithms. Most DL algorithms are like a black box, and there are no suitable explanations for the decision, and feature selection happens during the training and learning processes. Radiologists usually do not prefer these uninterpretable DL algorithms because they need to understand the physical meaning of the decisions taken by the algorithms and which parts of images are highly discriminative. Recently, some DL-based algorithms such as DeepSHAP [299] were introduced to define an interpretable model to give more insight into the decision-making of DL algorithms in medical image analysis. Therefore, to increase physicians' confidence and reliability of the decision made by DL tools, the utilization of interpretable approaches and proper explanation of DL algorithms is required for breast cancer analysis, helping widely used DL technology in clinical care applications such as breast cancer analysis.

DL algorithms show outstanding performance in analyzing imaging data. However, as discussed, there are still many challenges that they face. Besides DL algorithms, some studies show that using omics data instead of imaging data may lead to higher classification accuracy [108,300]. The omics data contain fewer but more effective features than imaging data. Moreover, the DL methods may extract the features from the images that are not relevant to the final label and those features may decrease the model performance. On the other hand, processing omics data is more expensive than image processing. Moreover, there are much more algorithms available for image processing than omics processing. Additionally, there are much more imaging data available than omics data.

5. Conclusions

Cancer detection in its early stage can improve the survival rate and reduce mortality. The rapid developments in deep learning-based techniques in medical image analysis algorithms along with the availability of large datasets and computational resources made it possible to improve breast cancer detection, diagnosis, prognosis, and treatment. Moreover, due to the capability of deep learning algorithms particularly CNNs, they have been very popular among the research community. In this research, comprehensive detail of the most recently employed deep learning methods is provided for different image modalities in different applications (e.g., classification, and segmentation). Despite outstanding performance by deep learning methods, they still face many challenges that should be addressed before deep learning can eventually influence clinical practices. Besides the challenges, ethical issues related to the explainability and interpretability of these systems need to be considered before deep learning can be expanded to its full potential in the clinical breast cancer imaging practice. Therefore, it is the responsibility of the research community to make the deep learning algorithms fully explainable before considering these systems as decision-making candidates in clinical practice.

Author Contributions: Data curation, M.M. and M.M.B.; writing—original draft preparation, M.M. and M.M.B.; writing—review and editing, M.M., M.M.B. and S.N.; supervision, S.N. All authors have read and agreed to the published version of the manuscript.

Funding: This research received no external funding.

Conflicts of Interest: There are no conflict of interest.

References

1. Zhou, X.; Li, C.; Rahaman, M.M.; Yao, Y.; Ai, S.; Sun, C.; Wang, Q.; Zhang, Y.; Li, M.; Li, X.; et al. A comprehensive review for breast histopathology image analysis using classical and deep neural networks. *IEEE Access* **2020**, *8*, 90931–90956. [CrossRef]
2. Global Burden of 87 Risk Factors in 204 Countries and Territories, 1990–2019: A Systematic Analysis for the Global Burden of Disease Study 2019—ScienceDirect. Available online: https://www.sciencedirect.com/science/article/pii/S0140673620307522 (accessed on 21 July 2022).
3. Anastasiadi, Z.; Lianos, G.D.; Ignatiadou, E.; Harissis, H.V.; Mitsis, M. Breast cancer in young women: An overview. *Updat. Surg.* **2017**, *69*, 313–317. [CrossRef] [PubMed]
4. Chiao, J.-Y.; Chen, K.-Y.; Liao, K.Y.-K.; Hsieh, P.-H.; Zhang, G.; Huang, T.-C. Detection and classification the breast tumors using mask R-CNN on sonograms. *Medicine* **2019**, *98*, e15200. [CrossRef] [PubMed]
5. Cruz-Roa, A. Accurate and reproducible invasive breast cancer detection in whole-slide images: A Deep Learning approach for quantifying tumour extent. *Sci. Rep.* **2017**, *7*, 46450. [CrossRef]
6. Richie, R.C.; Swanson, J.O. Breast cancer: A review of the literature. *J. Insur. Med.* **2003**, *35*, 85–101.
7. Youlden, D.R.; Cramb, S.M.; Dunn, N.A.M.; Muller, J.M.; Pyke, C.M.; Baade, P.D. The descriptive epidemiology of female breast cancer: An international comparison of screening, incidence, survival and mortality. *Cancer Epidemiol.* **2012**, *36*, 237–248. [CrossRef]
8. Moghbel, M.; Ooi, C.Y.; Ismail, N.; Hau, Y.W.; Memari, N. A review of breast boundary and pectoral muscle segmentation methods in computer-aided detection/diagnosis of breast mammography. *Artif. Intell. Rev.* **2019**, *53*, 1873–1918. [CrossRef]
9. Moghbel, M.; Mashohor, S. A review of computer assisted detection/diagnosis (CAD) in breast thermography for breast cancer detection. *Artif. Intell. Rev.* **2013**, *39*, 305–313. [CrossRef]
10. Murtaza, G.; Shuib, L.; Wahab, A.W.A.; Mujtaba, G.; Nweke, H.F.; Al-Garadi, M.A.; Zulfiqar, F.; Raza, G.; Azmi, N.A. Deep learning-based breast cancer classification through medical imaging modalities: State of the art and research challenges. *Artif. Intell. Rev.* **2019**, *53*, 1655–1720. [CrossRef]
11. Domingues, I.; Pereira, G.; Martins, P.; Duarte, H.; Santos, J.; Abreu, P.H. Using deep learning techniques in medical imaging: A systematic review of applications on CT and PET. *Artif. Intell. Rev.* **2019**, *53*, 4093–4160. [CrossRef]
12. Kozegar, E.; Soryani, M.; Behnam, H.; Salamati, M.; Tan, T. Computer aided detection in automated 3-D breast ultrasound images: A survey. *Artif. Intell. Rev.* **2019**, *53*, 1919–1941. [CrossRef]
13. Saha, M.; Chakraborty, C.; Racoceanu, D. Efficient deep learning model for mitosis detection using breast histopathology images. *Comput. Med. Imaging Graph.* **2018**, *64*, 29–40. [CrossRef]
14. Suh, Y.J.; Jung, J.; Cho, B.-J. Automated Breast Cancer Detection in Digital Mammograms of Various Densities via Deep Learning. *J. Pers. Med.* **2020**, *10*, 211. [CrossRef] [PubMed]
15. Cheng, H.D.; Shi, X.J.; Min, R.; Hu, L.M.; Cai, X.P.; Du, H.N. Approaches for automated detection and classification of masses in mammograms. *Pattern Recognit.* **2006**, *39*, 646–668. [CrossRef]
16. Van Ourti, T.; O'Donnell, O.; Koç, H.; Fracheboud, J.; de Koning, H.J. Effect of screening mammography on breast cancer mortality: Quasi-experimental evidence from rollout of the Dutch population-based program with 17-year follow-up of a cohort. *Int. J. Cancer* **2019**, *146*, 2201–2208. [CrossRef] [PubMed]
17. Sutanto, D.H.; Ghani, M.K.A. A Benchmark of Classification Framework for Non-Communicable Disease Prediction: A Review. *ARPN J. Eng. Appl. Sci.* **2015**, *10*, 15.
18. Van Luijt, P.A.; Heijnsdijk, E.A.M.; Fracheboud, J.; Overbeek, L.I.H.; Broeders, M.J.M.; Wesseling, J.; Heeten, G.J.D.; de Koning, H.J. The distribution of ductal carcinoma in situ (DCIS) grade in 4232 women and its impact on overdiagnosis in breast cancer screening. *Breast Cancer Res.* **2016**, *18*, 47. [CrossRef]

19. Baines, C.J.; Miller, A.B.; Wall, C.; McFarlane, D.V.; Simor, I.S.; Jong, R.; Shapiro, B.J.; Audet, L.; Petitclerc, M.; Ouimet-Oliva, D. Sensitivity and specificity of first screen mammography in the Canadian National Breast Screening Study: A preliminary report from five centers. *Radiology* **1986**, *160*, 295–298. [CrossRef]
20. Houssami, N.; Macaskill, P.; Bernardi, D.; Caumo, F.; Pellegrini, M.; Brunelli, S.; Tuttobene, P.; Bricolo, P.; Fantò, C.; Valentini, M. Breast screening using 2D-mammography or integrating digital breast tomosynthesis (3D-mammography) for single-reading or double-reading–evidence to guide future screening strategies. *Eur. J. Cancer* **2014**, *50*, 1799–1807. [CrossRef]
21. Houssami, N.; Hunter, K. The epidemiology, radiology and biological characteristics of interval breast cancers in population mammography screening. *NPJ Breast Cancer* **2017**, *3*, 12. [CrossRef]
22. Massafra, R.; Comes, M.C.; Bove, S.; Didonna, V.; Diotaiuti, S.; Giotta, F.; Latorre, A.; La Forgia, D.; Nardone, A.; Pomarico, D.; et al. A machine learning ensemble approach for 5-and 10-year breast cancer invasive disease event classification. *PLoS ONE* **2022**, *17*, e0274691. [CrossRef] [PubMed]
23. Chan, H.P.; Samala, R.K.; Hadjiiski, L.M. CAD and AI for breast cancer—Recent development and challenges. *Br. J. Radiol.* **2019**, *93*, 20190580. [CrossRef] [PubMed]
24. Jannesari, M.; Habibzadeh, M.; Aboulkheyr, H.; Khosravi, P.; Elemento, O.; Totonchi, M.; Hajirasouliha, I. Breast Cancer Histopathological Image Classification: A Deep Learning Approach. In Proceedings of the 2018 IEEE International Conference on Bioinformatics and Biomedicine (BIBM), Madrid, Spain, 3–6 December 2018; pp. 2405–2412. [CrossRef]
25. Rodriguez-Ruiz, A.; Lång, K.; Gubern-Merida, A.; Broeders, M.; Gennaro, G.; Clauser, P.; Helbich, T.H.; Chevalier, M.; Tan, T.; Mertelmeier, T.; et al. Stand-alone artificial intelligence for breast cancer detection in mammography: Comparison with 101 radiologists. *JNCI J. Natl. Cancer Inst.* **2019**, *111*, 916–922. [CrossRef] [PubMed]
26. McKinney, S.M.; Sieniek, M.; Godbole, V.; Godwin, J.; Antropova, N.; Ashrafian, H.; Back, T.; Chesus, M.; Corrado, G.S.; Darzi, A.; et al. International evaluation of an AI system for breast cancer screening. *Nature* **2020**, *577*, 89–94. [CrossRef] [PubMed]
27. Obermeyer, Z.; Emanuel, E.J. Predicting the Future—Big Data, Machine Learning, and Clinical Medicine. *N. Engl. J. Med.* **2016**, *375*, 1216–1219. [CrossRef]
28. Geirhos, R.; Jacobsen, J.H.; Michaelis, C.; Zemel, R.; Brendel, W.; Bethge, M.; Wichmann, F.A. Shortcut learning in deep neural networks. *Nat. Mach. Intell.* **2020**, *2*, 665–673. [CrossRef]
29. Freeman, K.; Geppert, J.; Stinton, C.; Todkill, D.; Johnson, S.; Clarke, A.; Taylor-Phillips, S. Use of artificial intelligence for image analysis in breast cancer screening programmes: Systematic review of test accuracy. *BMJ* **2021**, *374*. [CrossRef]
30. LeCun, Y.; Bengio, Y.; Hinton, G. Deep learning. *Nature* **2015**, *521*, 436–444. [CrossRef]
31. Burt, J.R.; Torosdagli, N.; Khosravan, N.; RaviPrakash, H.; Mortazi, A.; Tissavirasingham, F.; Hussein, S.; Bagci, U. Deep learning beyond cats and dogs: Recent advances in diagnosing breast cancer with deep neural networks. *Br. J. Radiol.* **2018**, *91*, 20170545. [CrossRef]
32. Sharma, S.; Mehra, R. Conventional Machine Learning and Deep Learning Approach for Multi-Classification of Breast Cancer Histopathology Images—A Comparative Insight. *J. Digit. Imaging* **2020**, *33*, 632–654. [CrossRef]
33. Hadadi, I.; Rae, W.; Clarke, J.; McEntee, M.; Ekpo, E. Diagnostic performance of adjunctive imaging modalities compared to mammography alone in women with non-dense and dense breasts: A systematic review and meta-analysis. *Clin. Breast Cancer* **2021**, *21*, 278–291. [CrossRef] [PubMed]
34. Yassin, N.I.R.; Omran, S.; el Houby, E.M.F.; Allam, H. Machine learning techniques for breast cancer computer aided diagnosis using different image modalities: A systematic review. *Comput. Methods Programs Biomed.* **2018**, *156*, 25–45. [CrossRef] [PubMed]
35. Saslow, D.; Boetes, C.; Burke, W.; Harms, S.; Leach, M.O.; Lehman, C.D.; Morris, E.; Pisano, E.; Schnall, M.; Sener, S.; et al. American Cancer Society guidelines for breast screening with MRI as an adjunct to mammography. *CA A Cancer J. Clin.* **2007**, *57*, 75–89.
36. Park, J.; Chae, E.Y.; Cha, J.H.; Shin, H.J.; Choi, W.J.; Choi, Y.W.; Kim, H.H. Comparison of mammography, digital breast tomosynthesis, automated breast ultrasound, magnetic resonance imaging in evaluation of residual tumor after neoadjuvant chemotherapy. *Eur. J. Radiol.* **2018**, *108*, 261–268. [CrossRef] [PubMed]
37. Huang, S.; Houssami, N.; Brennan, M.; Nickel, B. The impact of mandatory mammographic breast density notification on supplemental screening practice in the United States: A systematic review. *Breast Cancer Res. Treat.* **2021**, *187*, 11–30. [CrossRef] [PubMed]
38. Cho, N.; Han, W.; Han, B.K.; Bae, M.S.; Ko, E.S.; Nam, S.J.; Chae, E.Y.; Lee, J.W.; Kim, S.H.; Kang, B.J.; et al. Breast cancer screening with mammography plus ultrasonography or magnetic resonance imaging in women 50 years or younger at diagnosis and treated with breast conservation therapy. *JAMA Oncol.* **2017**, *3*, 1495–1502. [CrossRef]
39. Arevalo, J.; Gonzalez, F.A.; Ramos-Pollan, R.; Oliveira, J.L.; Lopez, M.A.G. Convolutional neural networks for mammography mass lesion classification. In Proceedings of the 2015 37th Annual International Conference of the IEEE Engineering in Medicine and Biology Society (EMBC), Milan, Italy, 25–29 August 2015; pp. 797–800. [CrossRef]
40. Duraisamy, S.; Emperumal, S. Computer-aided mammogram diagnosis system using deep learning convolutional fully complex-valued relaxation neural network classifier. *IET Comput. Vis.* **2017**, *11*, 656–662. [CrossRef]
41. Khan, M.H.-M. Automated breast cancer diagnosis using artificial neural network (ANN). In Proceedings of the 2017 3rd Iranian Conference on Intelligent Systems and Signal Processing (ICSPIS), Shahrood, Iran, 20–21 December 2017; pp. 54–58. [CrossRef]

42. Hadad, O.; Bakalo, R.; Ben-Ari, R.; Hashoul, S.; Amit, G. Classification of breast lesions using cross-modal deep learning. In Proceedings of the 2017 IEEE 14th International Symposium on Biomedical Imaging (ISBI 2017), Melbourne, VIC, Australia, 18–21 April 2017; pp. 109–112. [CrossRef]
43. Kim, D.H.; Kim, S.T.; Ro, Y.M. Latent feature representation with 3-D multi-view deep convolutional neural network for bilateral analysis in digital breast tomosynthesis. In Proceedings of the 2016 IEEE International Conference on Acoustics, Speech and Signal Processing (ICASSP), Shanghai, China, 20–25 March 2016; pp. 927–931. [CrossRef]
44. Comstock, C.E.; Gatsonis, C.; Newstead, G.M.; Snyder, B.S.; Gareen, I.F.; Bergin, J.T.; Rahbar, H.; Sung, J.S.; Jacobs, C.; Harvey, J.A.; et al. Comparison of Abbreviated Breast MRI vs Digital Breast Tomosynthesis for Breast Cancer Detection Among Women with Dense Breasts Undergoing Screening. *JAMA* **2020**, *323*, 746–756. [CrossRef]
45. Debelee, T.G.; Schwenker, F.; Ibenthal, A.; Yohannes, D. Survey of deep learning in breast cancer image analysis. *Evol. Syst.* **2019**, *11*, 143–163. [CrossRef]
46. Screening for Breast Cancer—ClinicalKey. Available online: https://www.clinicalkey.com/#!/content/book/3-s2.0-B9780323640596001237 (accessed on 27 July 2022).
47. Chen, T.H.H.; Yen, A.M.F.; Fann, J.C.Y.; Gordon, P.; Chen, S.L.S.; Chiu, S.Y.H.; Hsu, C.Y.; Chang, K.J.; Lee, W.C.; Yeoh, K.G.; et al. Clarifying the debate on population-based screening for breast cancer with mammography: A systematic review of randomized controlled trials on mammography with Bayesian meta-analysis and causal model. *Medicine* **2017**, *96*, e5684. [CrossRef]
48. Vieira, R.A.d.; Biller, G.; Uemura, G.; Ruiz, C.A.; Curado, M.P. Breast cancer screening in developing countries. *Clinics* **2017**, *72*, 244–253. [CrossRef]
49. Abdelrahman, L.; al Ghamdi, M.; Collado-Mesa, F.; Abdel-Mottaleb, M. Convolutional neural networks for breast cancer detection in mammography: A survey. *Comput. Biol. Med.* **2021**, *131*, 104248. [CrossRef] [PubMed]
50. Hooley, R.J.; Durand, M.A.; Philpotts, L.E. Advances in Digital Breast Tomosynthesis. *Am. J. Roentgenol.* **2017**, *208*, 256–266. [CrossRef] [PubMed]
51. Gur, D.; Abrams, G.S.; Chough, D.M.; Ganott, M.A.; Hakim, C.M.; Perrin, R.L.; Rathfon, G.Y.; Sumkin, J.H.; Zuley, M.L.; Bandos, A.I. Digital breast tomosynthesis: Observer performance study. *Am. J. Roentgenol.* **2009**, *193*, 586–591.
52. Østerås, B.H.; Martinsen, A.C.T.; Gullien, R.; Skaane, P. Digital Mammography versus Breast Tomosynthesis: Impact of Breast Density on Diagnostic Performance in Population-based Screening. *Radiology* **2019**, *293*, 60–68. [CrossRef]
53. Zhang, J.; Ghate, S.V.; Grimm, L.J.; Saha, A.; Cain, E.H.; Zhu, Z.; Mazurowski, M.A. February. Convolutional encoder-decoder for breast mass segmentation in digital breast tomosynthesis. In *Medical Imaging 2018: Computer-Aided Diagnosis*; SPIE: Bellingham, WA, USA, 2018; Volume 10575, pp. 639–644.
54. Poplack, S.P.; Tosteson, T.D.; Kogel, C.A.; Nagy, H.M. Digital breast tomosynthesis: Initial experience in 98 women with abnormal digital screening mammography. *AJR Am. J. Roentgenol.* **2007**, *189*, 616–623. [CrossRef]
55. Mun, H.S.; Kim, H.H.; Shin, H.J.; Cha, J.H.; Ruppel, P.L.; Oh, H.Y.; Chae, E.Y. Assessment of extent of breast cancer: Comparison between digital breast tomosynthesis and full-field digital mammography. *Clin. Radiol.* **2013**, *68*, 1254–1259. [CrossRef]
56. Lourenco, A.P.; Barry-Brooks, M.; Baird, G.L.; Tuttle, A.; Mainiero, M.B. Changes in recall type and patient treatment following implementation of screening digital breast tomosynthesis. *Radiology* **2015**, *274*, 337–342. [CrossRef]
57. Heywang-Köbrunner, S.H.; Jänsch, A.; Hacker, A.; Weinand, S.; Vogelmann, T. Digital breast tomosynthesis (DBT) plus synthesised two-dimensional mammography (s2D) in breast cancer screening is associated with higher cancer detection and lower recalls compared to digital mammography (DM) alone: Results of a systematic review and meta-analysis. *Eur. Radiol.* **2021**, *32*, 2301–2312.
58. Alabousi, M.; Wadera, A.; Kashif Al-Ghita, M.; Kashef Al-Ghetaa, R.; Salameh, J.P.; Pozdnyakov, A.; Zha, N.; Samoilov, L.; Dehmoobad Sharifabadi, A.; Sadeghirad, B. Performance of digital breast tomosynthesis, synthetic mammography, and digital mammography in breast cancer screening: A systematic review and meta-analysis. *JNCI J. Natl. Cancer Inst.* **2020**, *113*, 680–690. [CrossRef]
59. Durand, M.A.; Friedewald, S.M.; Plecha, D.M.; Copit, D.S.; Barke, L.D.; Rose, S.L.; Hayes, M.K.; Greer, L.N.; Dabbous, F.M.; Conant, E.F. False-negative rates of breast cancer screening with and without digital breast tomosynthesis. *Radiology* **2021**, *298*, 296–305. [CrossRef] [PubMed]
60. Alsheik, N.; Blount, L.; Qiong, Q.; Talley, M.; Pohlman, S.; Troeger, K.; Abbey, G.; Mango, V.L.; Pollack, E.; Chong, A.; et al. Outcomes by race in breast cancer screening with digital breast tomosynthesis versus digital mammography. *J. Am. Coll. Radiol.* **2021**, *18*, 906–918. [CrossRef] [PubMed]
61. Boisselier, A.; Mandoul, C.; Monsonis, B.; Delebecq, J.; Millet, I.; Pages, E.; Taourel, P. Reader performances in breast lesion characterization via DBT: One or two views and which view? *Eur. J. Radiol.* **2021**, *142*, 109880. [CrossRef] [PubMed]
62. Fiorica, J.V. Breast Cancer Screening, Mammography, and Other Modalities. *Clin. Obstet. Gynecol.* **2016**, *59*, 688–709. [CrossRef] [PubMed]
63. Jesneck, J.L.; Lo, J.Y.; Baker, J.A. Breast Mass Lesions: Computer-aided Diagnosis Models with Mammographic and Sonographic Descriptors. *Radiology* **2007**, *244*, 390–398. [CrossRef]
64. Cheng, H.D.; Shan, J.; Ju, W.; Guo, Y.; Zhang, L. Automated breast cancer detection and classification using ultrasound images: A survey. *Pattern Recognit.* **2010**, *43*, 299–317. [CrossRef]
65. Maxim, L.D.; Niebo, R.; Utell, M.J. Screening tests: A review with examples. *Inhal. Toxicol.* **2014**, *26*, 811–828. [CrossRef]

66. Han, J.; Li, F.; Peng, C.; Huang, Y.; Lin, Q.; Liu, Y.; Cao, L.; Zhou, J. Reducing unnecessary biopsy of breast lesions: Preliminary results with combination of strain and shear-wave elastography. *Ultrasound Med. Biol.* **2019**, *45*, 2317–2327. [CrossRef]
67. Zhi, H.; Ou, B.; Luo, B.-M.; Feng, X.; Wen, Y.-L.; Yang, H.-Y. Comparison of Ultrasound Elastography, Mammography, and Sonography in the Diagnosis of Solid Breast Lesions. *J. Ultrasound Med.* **2007**, *26*, 807–815. [CrossRef]
68. Corsetti, V.; Houssami, N.; Ghirardi, M.; Ferrari, A.; Speziani, M.; Bellarosa, S.; Remida, G.; Gasparotti, C.; Galligioni, E.; Ciatto, S. Evidence of the effect of adjunct ultrasound screening in women with mammography-negative dense breasts: Interval breast cancers at 1 year follow-up. *Eur. J. Cancer* **2011**, *47*, 1021–1026. [CrossRef]
69. Shin, S.Y.; Lee, S.; Yun, I.D.; Kim, S.M.; Lee, K.M. Joint Weakly and Semi-Supervised Deep Learning for Localization and Classification of Masses in Breast Ultrasound Images. *IEEE Trans. Med. Imaging* **2018**, *38*, 762–774. [CrossRef] [PubMed]
70. Becker, A.S.; Mueller, M.; Stoffel, E.; Marcon, M.; Ghafoor, S.; Boss, A. Classification of breast cancer in ultrasound imaging using a generic deep learning analysis software: A pilot study. *Br. J. Radiol.* **2017**, *91*, 20170576. [CrossRef] [PubMed]
71. Youk, J.H.; Gweon, H.M.; Son, E.J. Shear-wave elastography in breast ultrasonography: The state of the art. *Ultrasonography* **2017**, *36*, 300–309. [CrossRef] [PubMed]
72. MARIBS study group. Screening with magnetic resonance imaging and mammography of a UK population at high familial risk of breast cancer: A prospective multicentre cohort study (MARIBS). *Lancet* **2005**, *365*, 1769–1778. [CrossRef]
73. Kelly, K.; Dean, J.; Comulada, W.; Lee, S.-J. Breast cancer detection using automated whole breast ultrasound and mammography in radiographically dense breasts. *Eur. Radiol.* **2009**, *20*, 734–742. [CrossRef]
74. Makanjuola, D.I.; Alkushi, A.; al Anazi, K. Defining radiologic complete response using a correlation of presurgical ultrasound and mammographic localization findings with pathological complete response following neoadjuvant chemotherapy in breast cancer. *Eur. J. Radiol.* **2020**, *130*, 109146. [CrossRef]
75. Bove, S.; Comes, M.C.; Lorusso, V.; Cristofaro, C.; Didonna, V.; Gatta, G.; Giotta, F.; La Forgia, D.; Latorre, A.; Pastena, M.I.; et al. A ultrasound-based radiomic approach to predict the nodal status in clinically negative breast cancer patients. *Sci. Rep.* **2022**, *12*, 7914. [CrossRef]
76. Stavros, A.T.; Thickman, D.; Rapp, C.L.; Dennis, M.A.; Parker, S.H.; Sisney, G.A. Solid breast nodules: Use of sonography to distinguish between benign and malignant lesions. *Radiology* **1995**, *196*, 123–134. [CrossRef]
77. Yap, M.H. Automated breast ultrasound lesions detection using convolutional neural networks. *IEEE J. Biomed. Health Inform.* **2017**, *22*, 1218–1226. [CrossRef]
78. Shin, H.J.; Kim, H.H.; Cha, J.H. Current status of automated breast ultrasonography. *Ultrasonography* **2015**, *34*, 165–172. [CrossRef]
79. Kolb, T.M.; Lichy, J.; Newhouse, J.H. Comparison of the performance of screening mammography, physical examination, and breast US and evaluation of factors that influence them: An analysis of 27,825 patient evaluations. *Radiology* **2002**, *225*, 165–175. [CrossRef] [PubMed]
80. Al-Dhabyani, W.; Gomaa, M.; Khaled, H.; Fahmy, A. Dataset of breast ultrasound images. *Data Brief* **2019**, *28*, 104863. [CrossRef] [PubMed]
81. Antropova, N.O.; Abe, H.; Giger, M.L. Use of clinical MRI maximum intensity projections for improved breast lesion classification with deep convolutional neural networks. *JMI* **2018**, *5*, 014503. [CrossRef] [PubMed]
82. Morrow, M.; Waters, J.; Morris, E. MRI for breast cancer screening, diagnosis, and treatment. *Lancet* **2011**, *378*, 1804–1811. [CrossRef]
83. Kuhl, C.K.; Schrading, S.; Strobel, K.; Schild, H.H.; Hilgers, R.-D.; Bieling, H.B. Abbreviated Breast Magnetic Resonance Imaging (MRI): First Postcontrast Subtracted Images and Maximum-Intensity Projection—A Novel Approach to Breast Cancer Screening With MRI. *JCO* **2014**, *32*, 2304–2310. [CrossRef]
84. Morris, E.A. Breast cancer imaging with MRI. *Radiol. Clin. N. Am.* **2002**, *40*, 443–466. [CrossRef]
85. Teh, W.; Wilson, A.R.M. The role of ultrasound in breast cancer screening. A consensus statement by the European Group for breast cancer screening. *Eur. J. Cancer* **1998**, *34*, 449–450. [CrossRef]
86. Sardanelli, F.; Giuseppetti, G.M.; Panizza, P.; Bazzocchi, M.; Fausto, A.; Simonetti, G.; Lattanzio, V.; Del Maschio, A. Sensitivity of MRI Versus Mammography for Detecting Foci of Multifocal, Multicentric Breast Cancer in Fatty and Dense Breasts Using the Whole-Breast Pathologic Examination as a Gold Standard. *Am. J. Roentgenol.* **2004**, *183*, 1149–1157. [CrossRef]
87. Rasti, R.; Teshnehlab, M.; Phung, S.L. Breast cancer diagnosis in DCE-MRI using mixture ensemble of convolutional neural networks. *Pattern Recognit.* **2017**, *72*, 381–390. [CrossRef]
88. Mann, R.M.; Kuhl, C.K.; Kinkel, K.; Boetes, C. Breast MRI: Guidelines from the European Society of Breast Imaging. *Eur. Radiol.* **2008**, *18*, 1307–1318. [CrossRef]
89. Pasquero, G.; Surace, A.; Ponti, A.; Bortolini, M.; Tota, D.; Mano, M.P.; Arisio, R.; Benedetto, C.; Baù, M.G. Role of Magnetic Resonance Imaging in the Evaluation of Breast Cancer Response to Neoadjuvant Chemotherapy. *Vivo* **2020**, *34*, 909–915. [CrossRef]
90. Kim, Y.; Sim, S.H.; Park, B.; Chae, I.H.; Han, J.H.; Jung, S.-Y.; Lee, S.; Kwon, Y.; Park, I.H.; Ko, K.; et al. Criteria for identifying residual tumours after neoadjuvant chemotherapy of breast cancers: A magnetic resonance imaging study. *Sci. Rep.* **2021**, *11*, 634. [CrossRef] [PubMed]
91. Massafra, R.; Comes, M.C.; Bove, S.; Didonna, V.; Gatta, G.; Giotta, F.; Fanizzi, A.; La Forgia, D.; Latorre, A.; Pastena, M.I.; et al. Robustness Evaluation of a Deep Learning Model on Sagittal and Axial Breast DCE-MRIs to Predict Pathological Complete Response to Neoadjuvant Chemotherapy. *J. Pers. Med.* **2022**, *12*, 953. [CrossRef] [PubMed]

92. Houssami, N.; Cho, N. Screening women with a personal history of breast cancer: Overview of the evidence on breast imaging surveillance. *Ultrasonography* **2018**, *37*, 277–287. [CrossRef] [PubMed]
93. Greenwood, H.I. Abbreviated protocol breast MRI: The past, present, and future. *Clin. Imaging* **2019**, *53*, 169–173. [CrossRef]
94. Van Zelst, J.C.M.; Vreemann, S.; Witt, H.-J.; Gubern-Merida, A.; Dorrius, M.D.; Duvivier, K.; Lardenoije-Broker, S.; Lobbes, M.B.; Loo, C.; Veldhuis, W.; et al. Multireader Study on the Diagnostic Accuracy of Ultrafast Breast Magnetic Resonance Imaging for Breast Cancer Screening. *Investig. Radiol.* **2018**, *53*, 579–586. [CrossRef]
95. Heller, S.L.; Moy, L. MRI breast screening revisited. *J. Magn. Reson. Imaging* **2019**, *49*, 1212–1221. [CrossRef]
96. Rauch, G.M.; Adrada, B.E.; Kuerer, H.M.; Van La Parra, R.F.D.; Leung, J.W.T.; Yang, W.T. Multimodality Imaging for Evaluating Response to Neoadjuvant Chemotherapy in Breast Cancer. *Am. J. Roentgenol.* **2016**, *208*, 290–299. [CrossRef]
97. Mahrooghy, M.; Ashraf, A.B.; Daye, D.; McDonald, E.S.; Rosen, M.; Mies, C.; Feldman, M.; Kontos, D. Pharmacokinetic Tumor Heterogeneity as a Prognostic Biomarker for Classifying Breast Cancer Recurrence Risk. *IEEE Trans. Biomed. Eng.* **2015**, *62*, 1585–1594. [CrossRef]
98. Mazurowski, M.A.; Grimm, L.J.; Zhang, J.; Marcom, P.K.; Yoon, S.C.; Kim, C.; Ghate, S.V.; Johnson, K.S. Recurrence-free survival in breast cancer is associated with MRI tumor enhancement dynamics quantified using computer algorithms. *Eur. J. Radiol.* **2015**, *84*, 2117–2122. [CrossRef]
99. Jiang, Y.; Chen, L.; Zhang, H.; Xiao, X. Breast cancer histopathological image classification using convolutional neural networks with small SE-ResNet module. *PLoS ONE* **2019**, *14*, e0214587. [CrossRef] [PubMed]
100. Yan, R.; Ren, F.; Wang, Z.; Wang, L.; Ren, Y.; Liu, Y.; Rao, X.; Zheng, C.; Zhang, F. A hybrid convolutional and recurrent deep neural network for breast cancer pathological image classification. In *2018 IEEE International Conference on Bioinformatics and Biomedicine (BIBM)*; IEEE: Piscataway, NJ, USA, 2018; pp. 957–962.
101. Bejnordi, B.E.; Zuidhof, G.C.A.; Balkenhol, M.; Hermsen, M.; Bult, P.; Van Ginneken, B.; Karssemeijer, N.; Litjens, G.; Van Der Laak, J. Context-aware stacked convolutional neural networks for classification of breast carcinomas in whole-slide histopathology images. *J. Med. Imaging* **2017**, *4*, 044504. [CrossRef] [PubMed]
102. Jimenez-del-Toro, O.; Otálora, S.; Andersson, M.; Eurén, K.; Hedlund, M.; Rousson, M.; Müller, H.; Atzori, M. Analysis of Histopathology Images: From Traditional Machine Learning to Deep Learning. In *Biomedical Texture Analysis*; Academic Press: Cambridge, MA, USA, 2017; pp. 281–314.
103. Roy, K.; Banik, D.; Bhattacharjee, D.; Nasipuri, M. Patch-based system for Classification of Breast Histology images using deep learning. *Comput. Med. Imaging Graph.* **2018**, *71*, 90–103. [CrossRef] [PubMed]
104. Tellez, D.; Balkenhol, M.; Karssemeijer, N.; Litjens, G.; van der Laak, J.; Ciompi, F. March. H and E stain augmentation improves generalization of convolutional networks for histopathological mitosis detection. In *Medical Imaging 2018: Digital Pathology*; SPIE: Bellingham, WA, USA, 2018; Volume 10581, pp. 264–270.
105. Aswathy, M.A.; Jagannath, M. Detection of breast cancer on digital histopathology images: Present status and future possibilities. *Inform. Med. Unlocked* **2017**, *8*, 74–79. [CrossRef]
106. Araújo, T.; Aresta, G.; Castro, E.M.; Rouco, J.; Aguiar, P.; Eloy, C.; Polónia, A.; Campilho, A. Classification of breast cancer histology images using Convolutional Neural Networks. *PLoS ONE* **2017**, *12*, e0177544. [CrossRef]
107. Bardou, D.; Zhang, K.; Ahmad, S.M. Classification of Breast Cancer Based on Histology Images Using Convolutional Neural Networks. *IEEE Access* **2018**, *6*, 24680–24693. [CrossRef]
108. Wu, C.; Zhou, F.; Ren, J.; Li, X.; Jiang, Y.; Ma, S. A Selective Review of Multi-Level Omics Data Integration Using Variable Selection. *High-Throughput* **2019**, *8*, 4. [CrossRef]
109. Zeiser, F.A.; da Costa, C.A.; Roehe, A.V.; Righi, R.D.R.; Marques, N.M.C. Breast cancer intelligent analysis of histopathological data: A systematic review. *Appl. Soft Comput.* **2021**, *113*, 107886. [CrossRef]
110. Flanagan, F.L.; Dehdashti, F.; Siegel, B.A. PET in breast cancer. *Semin. Nucl. Med.* **1998**, *28*, 290–302. [CrossRef]
111. Groheux, D.; Hindie, E. Breast cancer: Initial workup and staging with FDG PET/CT. *Clin. Transl. Imaging* **2021**, *9*, 221–231. [CrossRef]
112. Fowler, A.M.; Strigel, R.M. Clinical advances in PET–MRI for breast cancer. *Lancet Oncol.* **2022**, *23*, e32–e43. [CrossRef]
113. Vercher-Conejero, J.L.; Pelegrí-Martinez, L.; Lopez-Aznar, D.; Cózar-Santiago, M.D.P. Positron Emission Tomography in Breast Cancer. *Diagnostics* **2015**, *5*, 61–83. [CrossRef] [PubMed]
114. Gillies, R. In vivo molecular imaging. *J. Cell. Biochem.* **2002**, *87*, 231–238. [CrossRef] [PubMed]
115. Mankoff, D.A.; Eary, J.F.; Link, J.M.; Muzi, M.; Rajendran, J.G.; Spence, A.M.; Krohn, K.A. Tumor-specific positron emission tomography imaging in patients: [18F] fluorodeoxyglucose and beyond. *Clin. Cancer Res.* **2007**, *13*, 3460–3469. [CrossRef]
116. Avril, N.; Menzel, M.; Dose, J.; Schelling, M.; Weber, W.; Janicke, F.; Nathrath, W.; Schwaiger, M. Glucose metabolism of breast cancer assessed by 18F-FDG PET: Histologic and immunohistochemical tissue analysis. *J. Nucl. Med.* **2001**, *42*, 9–16.
117. Pijl, J.P.; Nienhuis, P.H.; Kwee, T.C.; Glaudemans, A.W.J.M.; Slart, R.H.; Gormsen, L.C. Limitations and Pitfalls of FDG-PET/CT in Infection and Inflammation. *Semin. Nucl. Med.* **2021**, *51*, 633–645. [CrossRef]
118. Han, S.; Choi, J.Y. Impact of 18F-FDG PET, PET/CT, and PET/MRI on Staging and Management as an Initial Staging Modality in Breast Cancer. *Clin. Nucl. Med.* **2021**, *46*, 271–282. [CrossRef]
119. Le Boulc'h, M.; Gilhodes, J.; Steinmeyer, Z.; Molière, S.; Mathelin, C. Pretherapeutic Imaging for Axillary Staging in Breast Cancer: A Systematic Review and Meta-Analysis of Ultrasound, MRI and FDG PET. *J. Clin. Med.* **2021**, *10*, 1543. [CrossRef]

120. Koolen, B.B.; Aukema, T.S.; González Martínez, A.J.; Vogel, W.V.; Caballero Ontanaya, L.; Vrancken Peeters, M.J.; Vroonland, C.J.; Rutgers, E.J.; Benlloch Baviera, J.M.; Valdés Olmos, R.A. First clinical experience with a dedicated PET for hanging breast molecular imaging. *Q. J. Nucl. Med. Mol. Imaging* **2013**, *57*, 92–100. [CrossRef]
121. Rombach, R.; Blattmann, A.; Lorenz, D.; Esser, P.; Ommer, B. High-Resolution Image Synthesis with Latent Diffusion Models. 2022, pp. 10684–10695. Available online: https://openaccess.thecvf.com/content/CVPR2022/html/Rombach_High-Resolution_Image_Synthesis_With_Latent_Diffusion_Models_CVPR_2022_paper.html (accessed on 24 July 2022).
122. Baevski, A.; Hsu, W.-N.; Conneau, A.; Auli, M. Unsupervised Speech Recognition. In *Advances in Neural Information Processing Systems*; MTI Press: Cambridge, MA, USA, 2021; Volume 34, pp. 27826–27839.
123. Shahamiri, S.R. Speech Vision: An End-to-End Deep Learning-Based Dysarthric Automatic Speech Recognition System. *IEEE Trans. Neural Syst. Rehabil. Eng.* **2021**, *29*, 852–861. [CrossRef]
124. Behzadi, M.M.; Ilies, H.T. GANTL: Towards Practical and Real-Time Topology Optimization with Conditional GANs and Transfer Learning. *J. Mech. Des.* **2021**, *144*, 1–32. [CrossRef]
125. Behzadi, M.M.; Ilieş, H.T. Real-Time Topology Optimization in 3D via Deep Transfer Learning. *Comput. Des.* **2021**, *135*, 103014. [CrossRef]
126. Madani, M.; Tarakanova, A. Molecular Design of Soluble Zein Protein Sequences. *Biophys. J.* **2020**, *118*, 45a. [CrossRef]
127. Madani, M.; Lin, K.; Tarakanova, A. DSResSol: A sequence-based solubility predictor created with Dilated Squeeze Excitation Residual Networks. *Int. J. Mol. Sci.* **2021**, *22*, 13555. [CrossRef]
128. Madani, M.; Behzadi, M.M.; Song, D.; Ilies, H.; Tarakanova, A. CGAN-Cmap: Protein contact map prediction using deep generative adversarial neural networks. *bioRxiv* **2022**. [CrossRef]
129. Kunkel, G.; Madani, M.; White, S.J.; Verardi, P.H.; Tarakanova, A. Modeling coronavirus spike protein dynamics: Implications for immunogenicity and immune escape. *Biophys. J.* **2021**, *120*, 5592–5618. [CrossRef]
130. Madani, M.; Tarakanova, A. Characterization of Mechanics and Tunability of Resilin Protein by Molecular Dynamics Simulation. *Biophys. J.* **2020**, *118*, 45a–46a. [CrossRef]
131. Dildar, M.; Akram, S.; Irfan, M.; Khan, H.U.; Ramzan, M.; Mahmood, A.R.; Alsaiari, S.A.; Saeed, A.H.M.; Alraddadi, M.O.; Mahnashi, M.H. Skin Cancer Detection: A Review Using Deep Learning Techniques. *Int. J. Environ. Res. Public Health* **2021**, *18*, 5479. [CrossRef]
132. Kim, J.; Park, S.; Min, D.; Kim, W. Comprehensive Survey of Recent Drug Discovery Using Deep Learning. *Int. J. Mol. Sci.* **2021**, *22*, 9983. [CrossRef]
133. Zhang, L.; Tan, J.; Han, D.; Zhu, H. From machine learning to deep learning: Progress in machine intelligence for rational drug discovery. *Drug Discov. Today* **2017**, *22*, 1680–1685. [CrossRef]
134. Kumar, Y.; Koul, A.; Singla, R.; Ijaz, M.F. Artificial intelligence in disease diagnosis: A systematic literature review, synthesizing framework and future research agenda. *J. Ambient Intell. Humaniz. Comput.* **2022**, 1–28. [CrossRef] [PubMed]
135. Goodfellow, I.; Bengio, Y.; Courville, A. *Deep Learning*; MIT Press: Cambridge, MA, USA, 2016.
136. Fitzgerald, R. Error in Radiology. *Clin. Radiol.* **2001**, *56*, 938–946. [CrossRef] [PubMed]
137. Kooi, T.; Gubern-Merida, A.; Mordang, J.J.; Mann, R.; Pijnappel, R.; Schuur, K.; Heeten, A.D.; Karssemeijer, N. A comparison between a deep convolutional neural network and radiologists for classifying regions of interest in mammography. In Proceedings of the International Workshop on Breast Imaging, Malmö, Sweden, 19–22 June 2016; Springer: Cham, Switzerland, 2016; pp. 51–56.
138. Kooi, T.; Litjens, G.; van Ginneken, B.; Gubern-Mérida, A.; Sánchez, C.I.; Mann, R.; den Heeten, A.; Karssemeijer, N. Large scale deep learning for computer aided detection of mammographic lesions. *Med. Image Anal.* **2017**, *35*, 303–312. [CrossRef] [PubMed]
139. Samala, R.K.; Chan, H.-P.; Hadjiiski, L.M.; Cha, K.; Helvie, M.A. Deep-learning convolution neural network for computer-aided detection of microcalcifications in digital breast tomosynthesis. In *Medical Imaging 2016: Computer-Aided Diagnosis*; SPIE: Bellingham, WA, USA, 2016; Volume 9785, pp. 234–240. [CrossRef]
140. Huynh, B.Q.; Li, H.; Giger, M.L. Digital mammographic tumor classification using transfer learning from deep convolutional neural networks. *J. Med. Imaging* **2016**, *3*, 034501. [CrossRef]
141. Redmon, J.; Divvala, S.; Girshick, R.; Farhadi, A. You Only Look Once: Unified, Real-Time Object Detection. In Proceedings of the 2016 IEEE Conference on Computer Vision and Pattern Recognition (CVPR), Las Vegas, NV, USA, 27–30 June 2016; pp. 779–788. [CrossRef]
142. Skaane, P.; Sebuødegård, S.; Bandos, A.I.; Gur, D.; Østerås, B.H.; Gullien, R.; Hofvind, S. Performance of breast cancer screening using digital breast tomosynthesis: Results from the prospective population-based Oslo Tomosynthesis Screening Trial. *Breast Cancer Res. Treat.* **2018**, *169*, 489–496. [CrossRef]
143. Skaane, P.; Bandos, A.I.; Niklason, L.T.; Sebuødegård, S.; Østerås, B.H.; Gullien, R.; Gur, D.; Hofvind, S. Digital Mammography versus Digital Mammography Plus Tomosynthesis in Breast Cancer Screening: The Oslo Tomosynthesis Screening Trial. *Radiology* **2019**, *291*, 23–30. [CrossRef]
144. Haas, B.M.; Kalra, V.; Geisel, J.; Raghu, M.; Durand, M.; Philpotts, L.E. Comparison of Tomosynthesis Plus Digital Mammography and Digital Mammography Alone for Breast Cancer Screening. *Radiology* **2013**, *269*, 694–700. [CrossRef]
145. Pinto, M.C.; Rodriguez-Ruiz, A.; Pedersen, K.; Hofvind, S.; Wicklein, J.; Kappler, S.; Mann, R.M.; Sechopoulos, I. Impact of artificial intelligence decision support using deep learning on breast cancer screening interpretation with single-view wide-angle digital breast tomosynthesis. *Radiology* **2021**, *300*, 529–536. [CrossRef]

146. Kooi, T.; Karssemeijer, N. Classifying symmetrical differences and temporal change for the detection of malignant masses in mammography using deep neural networks. *J. Med. Imaging* **2017**, *4*, 044501. [CrossRef]
147. Wu, N.; Phang, J.; Park, J.; Shen, Y.; Huang, Z.; Zorin, M.; Jastrzebski, S.; Fevry, T.; Katsnelson, J.; Kim, E.; et al. Deep Neural Networks Improve Radiologists' Performance in Breast Cancer Screening. *IEEE Trans. Med. Imaging* **2019**, *39*, 1184–1194. [CrossRef]
148. Loizidou, K.; Skouroumouni, G.; Pitris, C.; Nikolaou, C. Digital subtraction of temporally sequential mammograms for improved detection and classification of microcalcifications. *Eur. Radiol. Exp.* **2021**, *5*, 40. [CrossRef] [PubMed]
149. Yang, Z.; Cao, Z.; Zhang, Y.; Tang, Y.; Lin, X.; Ouyang, R.; Wu, M.; Han, M.; Xiao, J.; Huang, L.; et al. MommiNet-v2: Mammographic multi-view mass identification networks. *Med. Image Anal.* **2021**, *73*, 102204. [CrossRef] [PubMed]
150. Singh, S.; Matthews, T.P.; Shah, M.; Mombourquette, B.; Tsue, T.; Long, A.; Almohsen, R.; Pedemonte, S.; Su, J. Adaptation of a deep learning malignancy model from full-field digital mammography to digital breast tomosynthesis. In *Medical Imaging 2020: Computer-Aided Diagnosis*; SPIE: Bellingham, WA, USA, 2020; Volume 11314, pp. 25–32.
151. Samala, R.K.; Chan, H.-P.; Hadjiiski, L.M.; A Helvie, M.; Richter, C.; Cha, K. Evolutionary pruning of transfer learned deep convolutional neural network for breast cancer diagnosis in digital breast tomosynthesis. *Phys. Med. Biol.* **2018**, *63*, 095005. [CrossRef] [PubMed]
152. Krizhevsky, A.; Sutskever, I.; Hinton, G.E. ImageNet classification with deep convolutional neural networks. *Commun. ACM* **2017**, *60*, 84–90. [CrossRef]
153. Mendel, K.; Li, H.; Sheth, D.; Giger, M. Transfer Learning from Convolutional Neural Networks for Computer-Aided Diagnosis: A Comparison of Digital Breast Tomosynthesis and Full-Field Digital Mammography. *Acad. Radiol.* **2019**, *26*, 735–743. [CrossRef]
154. Simonyan, K.; Zisserman, A. Very Deep Convolutional Networks for Large-Scale Image Recognition. In Proceedings of the 3rd International Conference on Learning Representations (ICLR 2015), San Diego, CA, USA, 7–9 May 2015; Computational and Biological Learning Society: New York, NY, USA, 2015; pp. 1–14.
155. Romero-Martín, S.; Elías-Cabot, E.; Raya-Povedano, J.L.; Gubern-Mérida, A.; Rodríguez-Ruiz, A.; Álvarez-Benito, M. Stand-Alone Use of Artificial Intelligence for Digital Mammography and Digital Breast Tomosynthesis Screening: A Retrospective Evaluation. *Radiology* **2022**, *302*, 535–542. [CrossRef]
156. Shu, X.; Zhang, L.; Wang, Z.; Lv, Q.; Yi, Z. Deep Neural Networks with Region-Based Pooling Structures for Mammographic Image Classification. *IEEE Trans. Med. Imaging* **2020**, *39*, 2246–2255. [CrossRef]
157. Boumaraf, S.; Liu, X.; Ferkous, C.; Ma, X. A New Computer-Aided Diagnosis System with Modified Genetic Feature Selection for BI-RADS Classification of Breast Masses in Mammograms. *BioMed Res. Int.* **2020**, *2020*, e7695207. [CrossRef]
158. Matthews, T.P.; Singh, S.; Mombourquette, B.; Su, J.; Shah, M.P.; Pedemonte, S.; Long, A.; Maffit, D.; Gurney, J.; Hoil, R.M.; et al. A Multisite Study of a Breast Density Deep Learning Model for Full-Field Digital Mammography and Synthetic Mammography. *Radiol. Artif. Intell.* **2021**, *3*, e200015. [CrossRef]
159. Zhang, Y.-D.; Satapathy, S.C.; Guttery, D.S.; Górriz, J.M.; Wang, S.-H. Improved Breast Cancer Classification Through Combining Graph Convolutional Network and Convolutional Neural Network. *Inf. Process. Manag.* **2020**, *58*, 102439. [CrossRef]
160. Li, H.; Mukundan, R.; Boyd, S. Novel Texture Feature Descriptors Based on Multi-Fractal Analysis and LBP for Classifying Breast Density in Mammograms. *J. Imaging* **2021**, *7*, 205. [CrossRef] [PubMed]
161. Saber, A.; Sakr, M.; Abo-Seida, O.M.; Keshk, A.; Chen, H. A Novel Deep-Learning Model for Automatic Detection and Classification of Breast Cancer Using the Transfer-Learning Technique. *IEEE Access* **2021**, *9*, 71194–71209. [CrossRef]
162. Malebary, S.J.; Hashmi, A. Automated Breast Mass Classification System Using Deep Learning and Ensemble Learning in Digital Mammogram. *IEEE Access* **2021**, *9*, 55312–55328. [CrossRef]
163. Li, H.; Niu, J.; Li, D.; Zhang, C. Classification of breast mass in two-view mammograms via deep learning. *IET Image Process.* **2020**, *15*, 454–467. [CrossRef]
164. Ueda, D.; Yamamoto, A.; Onoda, N.; Takashima, T.; Noda, S.; Kashiwagi, S.; Morisaki, T.; Fukumoto, S.; Shiba, M.; Morimura, M.; et al. Development and validation of a deep learning model for detection of breast cancers in mammography from multi-institutional datasets. *PLoS ONE* **2022**, *17*, e0265751. [CrossRef]
165. Mota, A.M.; Clarkson, M.J.; Almeida, P.; Matela, N. Automatic Classification of Simulated Breast Tomosynthesis Whole Images for the Presence of Microcalcification Clusters Using Deep CNNs. *J. Imaging* **2022**, *8*, 231. [CrossRef]
166. Bai, J.; Jin, A.; Jin, A.; Wang, T.; Yang, C.; Nabavi, S. Applying graph convolution neural network in digital breast tomosynthesis for cancer classification. In Proceedings of the 13th ACM International Conference on Bioinformatics, Computational Biology and Health Informatics, Northbrook, IL, USA, 7–10 August 2022; pp. 1–10. [CrossRef]
167. Zhu, W.; Xiang, X.; Tran, T.D.; Hager, G.D.; Xie, X. Adversarial deep structured nets for mass segmentation from mammograms. In Proceedings of the 2018 IEEE 15th International Symposium on Biomedical Imaging (ISBI 2018), Washington, DC, USA, 4–7 April 2018; pp. 847–850. [CrossRef]
168. Wang, R.; Ma, Y.; Sun, W.; Guo, Y.; Wang, W.; Qi, Y.; Gong, X. Multi-level nested pyramid network for mass segmentation in mammograms. *Neurocomputing* **2019**, *363*, 313–320. [CrossRef]
169. Saffari, N.; Rashwan, H.A.; Abdel-Nasser, M.; Kumar Singh, V.; Arenas, M.; Mangina, E.; Herrera, B.; Puig, D. Fully automated breast density segmentation and classification using deep learning. *Diagnostics* **2020**, *10*, 988. [CrossRef]
170. Ahmed, L.; Iqbal, M.M.; Aldabbas, H.; Khalid, S.; Saleem, Y.; Saeed, S. Images data practices for Semantic Segmentation of Breast Cancer using Deep Neural Network. *J. Ambient Intell. Humaniz. Comput.* **2020**, 1–17. [CrossRef]

171. Buda, M.; Saha, A.; Walsh, R.; Ghate, S.; Li, N.; Święcicki, A.; Lo, J.Y.; Mazurowski, M.A. Detection of masses and architectural distortions in digital breast tomosynthesis: A publicly available dataset of 5,060 patients and a deep learning model. *arXiv* **2020**, arXiv:2011.07995.
172. Cheng, Y.; Gao, Y.; Xie, L.; Xie, X.; Lin, W. Spatial Enhanced Rotation Aware Network for Breast Mass Segmentation in Digital Mammogram. *IEEE Access* **2020**, 1. [CrossRef]
173. Chen, J.; Chen, L.; Wang, S.; Chen, P. A Novel Multi-Scale Adversarial Networks for Precise Segmentation of X-ray Breast Mass. *IEEE Access* **2020**, *8*, 103772–103781. [CrossRef]
174. Soleimani, H.; Michailovich, O.V. On Segmentation of Pectoral Muscle in Digital Mammograms by Means of Deep Learning. *IEEE Access* **2020**, *8*, 204173–204182. [CrossRef]
175. Al-Antari, M.A.; Han, S.-M.; Kim, T.-S. Evaluation of deep learning detection and classification towards computer-aided diagnosis of breast lesions in digital X-ray mammograms. *Comput. Methods Programs Biomed.* **2020**, *196*, 105584. [CrossRef] [PubMed]
176. Li, Y.; Zhang, L.; Chen, H.; Cheng, L. Mass detection in mammograms by bilateral analysis using convolution neural network. *Comput. Methods Programs Biomed.* **2020**, *195*, 105518. [CrossRef]
177. Peng, J.; Bao, C.; Hu, C.; Wang, X.; Jian, W.; Liu, W. Automated mammographic mass detection using deformable convolution and multiscale features. *Med. Biol. Eng. Comput.* **2020**, *58*, 1405–1417. [CrossRef]
178. Kavitha, T.; Mathai, P.P.; Karthikeyan, C.; Ashok, M.; Kohar, R.; Avanija, J.; Neelakandan, S. Deep Learning Based Capsule Neural Network Model for Breast Cancer Diagnosis Using Mammogram Images. *Interdiscip. Sci. Comput. Life Sci.* **2021**, *14*, 113–129. [CrossRef]
179. Shoshan, Y.; Zlotnick, A.; Ratner, V.; Khapun, D.; Barkan, E.; Gilboa-Solomon, F. Beyond Non-maximum Suppression—Detecting Lesions in Digital Breast Tomosynthesis Volumes. In *Medical Image Computing and Computer Assisted Intervention—MICCAI 2021*; Springer: Cham, Switzerland, 2021; pp. 772–781. [CrossRef]
180. Hossain, B.; Nishikawa, R.M.; Lee, J. Developing breast lesion detection algorithms for Digital Breast Tomosynthesis: Leveraging false positive findings. *Med. Phys.* **2022**. [CrossRef]
181. Hossain, B.; Nishikawa, R.M.; Lee, J. Improving lesion detection algorithm in digital breast tomosynthesis leveraging ensemble cross-validation models with multi-depth levels. In *Medical Imaging 2022: Computer-Aided Diagnosis*; SPIE: Bellingham, WA, USA, 2022; Volume 12033, pp. 91–97. [CrossRef]
182. Atrey, K.; Singh, B.K.; Roy, A.; Bodhey, N.K. Real-time automated segmentation of breast lesions using CNN-based deep learning paradigm: Investigation on mammogram and ultrasound. *Int. J. Imaging Syst. Technol.* **2021**, *32*, 1084–1100. [CrossRef]
183. Shen, S.; Zhou, Y.; Xu, Y.; Zhang, B.; Duan, X.; Huang, R.; Li, B.; Shi, Y.; Shao, Z.; Liao, H.; et al. A multi-centre randomised trial comparing ultrasound vs mammography for screening breast cancer in high-risk Chinese women. *Br. J. Cancer* **2015**, *112*, 998–1004. [CrossRef]
184. Han, S.; Kang, H.-K.; Jeong, J.-Y.; Park, M.-H.; Kim, W.; Bang, W.-C.; Seong, Y.-K. A deep learning framework for supporting the classification of breast lesions in ultrasound images. *Phys. Med. Biol.* **2017**, *62*, 7714. [CrossRef]
185. Shi, J.; Zhou, S.; Liu, X.; Zhang, Q.; Lu, M.; Wang, T. Stacked deep polynomial network based representation learning for tumor classification with small ultrasound image dataset. *Neurocomputing* **2016**, *194*, 87–94. [CrossRef]
186. Byra, M.; Galperin, M.; Ojeda-Fournier, H.; Olson, L.; O'Boyle, M.; Comstock, C.; Andre, M. Breast mass classification in sonography with transfer learning using a deep convolutional neural network and color conversion. *Med. Phys.* **2018**, *46*, 746–755. [CrossRef] [PubMed]
187. Szegedy, C.; Liu, W.; Jia, Y.; Sermanet, P.; Reed, S.; Anguelov, D.; Erhan, D.; Vanhoucke, V.; Rabinovich, A. Going deeper with convolutions. In Proceedings of the IEEE Conference on Computer Vision and Pattern Recognition, Boston, MA, USA, 7–12 June 2015; pp. 1–9.
188. Shi, X.; Cheng, H.D.; Hu, L.; Ju, W.; Tian, J. Detection and classification of masses in breast ultrasound images. *Digit. Signal Process.* **2010**, *20*, 824–836. [CrossRef]
189. Fujioka, T.; Kubota, K.; Mori, M.; Kikuchi, Y.; Katsuta, L.; Kasahara, M.; Oda, G.; Ishiba, T.; Nakagawa, T.; Tateishi, U. Distinction between benign and malignant breast masses at breast ultrasound using deep learning method with convolutional neural network. *Jpn. J. Radiol.* **2019**, *37*, 466–472. [CrossRef] [PubMed]
190. Tanaka, H.; Chiu, S.-W.; Watanabe, T.; Kaoku, S.; Yamaguchi, T. Computer-aided diagnosis system for breast ultrasound images using deep learning. *Phys. Med. Biol.* **2019**, *64*, 235013. [CrossRef]
191. Fujioka, T.; Kubota, K.; Mori, M.; Katsuta, L.; Kikuchi, Y.; Kimura, K.; Kimura, M.; Adachi, M.; Oda, G.; Nakagawa, T.; et al. Virtual Interpolation Images of Tumor Development and Growth on Breast Ultrasound Image Synthesis with Deep Convolutional Generative Adversarial Networks. *J. Ultrasound Med.* **2020**, *40*, 61–69. [CrossRef]
192. Liu, B.; Cheng, H.D.; Huang, J.; Tian, J.; Tang, X.; Liu, J. Fully automatic and segmentation-robust classification of breast tumors based on local texture analysis of ultrasound images. *Pattern Recognit.* **2010**, *43*, 280–298. [CrossRef]
193. Zhang, X.; Lin, X.; Zhang, Z.; Dong, L.; Sun, X.; Sun, D.; Yuan, K. Artificial Intelligence Medical Ultrasound Equipment: Application of Breast Lesions Detection. *Ultrason. Imaging* **2020**, *42*, 191–202. [CrossRef]
194. Chiang, T.-C.; Huang, Y.-S.; Chen, R.-T.; Huang, C.-S.; Chang, R.-F. Tumor Detection in Automated Breast Ultrasound Using 3-D CNN and Prioritized Candidate Aggregation. *IEEE Trans. Med. Imaging* **2018**, *38*, 240–249. [CrossRef]

195. Moon, W.K.; Lee, Y.; Ke, H.-H.; Lee, S.H.; Huang, C.-S.; Chang, R.-F. Computer-aided diagnosis of breast ultrasound images using ensemble learning from convolutional neural networks. *Comput. Methods Programs Biomed.* **2020**, *190*, 105361. [CrossRef] [PubMed]
196. He, K.; Zhang, X.; Ren, S.; Sun, J. Deep Residual Learning for Image Recognition. *arXiv* **2015**, arXiv:1512.03385. Available online: http://arxiv.org/abs/1512.03385 (accessed on 17 March 2021).
197. Huang, G.; Liu, Z.; van der Maaten, L.; Weinberger, K.Q. Densely Connected Convolutional Networks. In Proceedings of the 2017 IEEE Conference on Computer Vision and Pattern Recognition (CVPR), Honolulu, HI, USA, 21–26 July 2017; pp. 2261–2269. [CrossRef]
198. Huang, Y.; Han, L.; Dou, H.; Luo, H.; Yuan, Z.; Liu, Q.; Zhang, J.; Yin, G. Two-stage CNNs for computerized BI-RADS categorization in breast ultrasound images. *Biomed. Eng. Online* **2019**, *18*, 8. [CrossRef]
199. Cao, Z.; Duan, L.; Yang, G.; Yue, T.; Chen, Q. An experimental study on breast lesion detection and classification from ultrasound images using deep learning architectures. *BMC Med. Imaging* **2019**, *19*, 51. [CrossRef]
200. Kim, J.; Kim, H.J.; Kim, C.; Lee, J.H.; Kim, K.W.; Park, Y.M.; Kim, H.W.; Ki, S.Y.; Kim, Y.M.; Kim, W.H. Weakly-supervised deep learning for ultrasound diagnosis of breast cancer. *Sci. Rep.* **2021**, *11*, 24382. [CrossRef] [PubMed]
201. Choi, J.S.; Han, B.-K.; Ko, E.S.; Bae, J.M.; Ko, E.Y.; Song, S.H.; Kwon, M.-R.; Shin, J.H.; Hahn, S.Y. Effect of a Deep Learning Framework-Based Computer-Aided Diagnosis System on the Diagnostic Performance of Radiologists in Differentiating between Malignant and Benign Masses on Breast Ultrasonography. *Korean J. Radiol.* **2019**, *20*, 749–758. [CrossRef]
202. Park, H.J.; Kim, S.M.; La Yun, B.; Jang, M.; Kim, B.; Jang, J.Y.; Lee, J.Y.; Lee, S.H. A computer-aided diagnosis system using artificial intelligence for the diagnosis and characterization of breast masses on ultrasound: Added value for the inexperienced breast radiologist. *Medicine* **2019**, *98*, 546–552. [CrossRef] [PubMed]
203. Xiao, M.; Zhao, C.; Zhu, Q.; Zhang, J.; Liu, H.; Li, J.; Jiang, Y. An investigation of the classification accuracy of a deep learning framework-based computer-aided diagnosis system in different pathological types of breast lesions. *J. Thorac. Dis.* **2019**, *11*, 5023. [CrossRef]
204. Byra, M.; Sznajder, T.; Korzinek, D.; Piotrzkowska-Wróblewska, H.; Dobruch-Sobczak, K.; Nowicki, A.; Marasek, K. Impact of ultrasound image reconstruction method on breast lesion classification with deep learning. In *Iberian Conference on Pattern Recognition and Image Analysis*; Springer: Berlin/Heidelberg, Germany, 2019; pp. 41–52.
205. Hijab, A.; Rushdi, M.A.; Gomaa, M.M.; Eldeib, A. Breast Cancer Classification in Ultrasound Images using Transfer Learning. In Proceedings of the 2019 the Fifth International Conference on Advances in Biomedical Engineering (ICABME), Tripoli, Lebanon, 17–19 October 2019; pp. 1–4. [CrossRef]
206. Zhang, Q.; Song, S.; Xiao, Y.; Chen, S.; Shi, J.; Zheng, H. Dual-mode artificially-intelligent diagnosis of breast tumours in shear-wave elastography and B-mode ultrasound using deep polynomial networks. *Med. Eng. Phys.* **2019**, *64*, 1–6. [CrossRef]
207. Fujioka, T.; Katsuta, L.; Kubota, K.; Mori, M.; Kikuchi, Y.; Kato, A.; Oda, G.; Nakagawa, T.; Kitazume, Y.; Tateishi, U. Classification of breast masses on ultrasound shear wave elastography using convolutional neural networks. *Ultrason. Imaging* **2020**, *42*, 213–220. [CrossRef]
208. Wu, J.-X.; Chen, P.-Y.; Lin, C.-H.; Chen, S.; Shung, K.K. Breast Benign and Malignant Tumors Rapidly Screening by ARFI-VTI Elastography and Random Decision Forests Based Classifier. *IEEE Access* **2020**, *8*, 54019–54034. [CrossRef]
209. Wu, J.-X.; Liu, H.-C.; Chen, P.-Y.; Lin, C.-H.; Chou, Y.-H.; Shung, K.K. Enhancement of ARFI-VTI Elastography Images in Order to Preliminary Rapid Screening of Benign and Malignant Breast Tumors Using Multilayer Fractional-Order Machine Vision Classifier. *IEEE Access* **2020**, *8*, 164222–164237. [CrossRef]
210. Gong, B.; Shen, L.; Chang, C.; Zhou, S.; Zhou, W.; Li, S.; Shi, J. Bi-modal ultrasound breast cancer diagnosis via multi-view deep neural network svm. In *2020 IEEE 17th International Symposium on Biomedical Imaging (ISBI)*; IEEE: Piscataway, NJ, USA, 2020; pp. 1106–1110.
211. Zhang, X.; Liang, M.; Yang, Z.; Zheng, C.; Wu, J.; Ou, B.; Li, H.; Wu, X.; Luo, B.; Shen, J. Deep Learning-Based Radiomics of B-Mode Ultrasonography and Shear-Wave Elastography: Improved Performance in Breast Mass Classification. *Front. Oncol.* **2020**, *10*, 1621. [CrossRef] [PubMed]
212. Yousef Kalaf, E.; Jodeiri, A.; Kamaledin Setarehdan, S.; Lin, N.W.; Rahman, K.B.; Aishah Taib, N.; Dhillon, S.K. Classification of breast cancer lesions in ultrasound images by using attention layer and loss ensembles in deep convolutional neural networks. *arXiv* **2021**, arXiv:2102.11519.
213. Misra, S.; Jeon, S.; Managuli, R.; Lee, S.; Kim, G.; Yoon, C.; Lee, S.; Barr, R.G.; Kim, C. Bi-Modal Transfer Learning for Classifying Breast Cancers via Combined B-Mode and Ultrasound Strain Imaging. *IEEE Trans. Ultrason. Ferroelectr. Freq. Control* **2021**, *69*, 222–232. [CrossRef]
214. Vakanski, A.; Xian, M.; Freer, P.E. Attention-Enriched Deep Learning Model for Breast Tumor Segmentation in Ultrasound Images. *Ultrasound Med. Biol.* **2020**, *46*, 2819–2833. [CrossRef]
215. Byra, M.; Jarosik, P.; Szubert, A.; Galperin, M.; Ojeda-Fournier, H.; Olson, L.; O'Boyle, M.; Comstock, C.; Andre, M. Breast mass segmentation in ultrasound with selective kernel U-Net convolutional neural network. *Biomed. Signal Process. Control* **2020**, *61*, 102027. [CrossRef]
216. Singh, V.K.; Abdel-Nasser, M.; Akram, F.; Rashwan, H.A.; Sarker, M.K.; Pandey, N.; Romani, S.; Puig, D. Breast tumor segmentation in ultrasound images using contextual-information-aware deep adversarial learning framework. *Expert Syst. Appl.* **2020**, *162*, 113870. [CrossRef]

217. Han, L.; Huang, Y.; Dou, H.; Wang, S.; Ahamad, S.; Luo, H.; Liu, Q.; Fan, J.; Zhang, J. Semi-supervised segmentation of lesion from breast ultrasound images with attentional generative adversarial network. *Comput. Methods Programs Biomed.* **2019**, *189*, 105275. [CrossRef]
218. Wang, K.; Liang, S.; Zhang, Y. Residual Feedback Network for Breast Lesion Segmentation in Ultrasound Image. In *Medical Image Computing and Computer Assisted Intervention—MICCAI 2021*; Springer: Cham, Switzerland, 2021; pp. 471–481. [CrossRef]
219. Wang, K.; Liang, S.; Zhong, S.; Feng, Q.; Ning, Z.; Zhang, Y. Breast ultrasound image segmentation: A coarse-to-fine fusion convolutional neural network. *Med. Phys.* **2021**, *48*, 4262–4278. [CrossRef]
220. Li, Y.; Liu, Y.; Huang, L.; Wang, Z.; Luo, J. Deep weakly-supervised breast tumor segmentation in ultrasound images with explicit anatomical constraints. *Med. Image Anal.* **2022**, *76*, 102315. [CrossRef] [PubMed]
221. Byra, M.; Jarosik, P.; Dobruch-Sobczak, K.; Klimonda, Z.; Piotrzkowska-Wroblewska, H.; Litniewski, J.; Nowicki, A. Joint segmentation and classification of breast masses based on ultrasound radio-frequency data and convolutional neural networks. *Ultrasonics* **2022**, *121*, 106682. [CrossRef] [PubMed]
222. Jabeen, K.; Khan, M.A.; Alhaisoni, M.; Tariq, U.; Zhang, Y.-D.; Hamza, A.; Mickus, A.; Damaševičius, R. Breast Cancer Classification from Ultrasound Images Using Probability-Based Optimal Deep Learning Feature Fusion. *Sensors* **2022**, *22*, 807. [CrossRef] [PubMed]
223. Berg, W.A.; Zhang, Z.; Lehrer, D.; Jong, R.A.; Pisano, E.D.; Barr, R.G.; Böhm-Vélez, M.; Mahoney, M.C.; Evans, W.P.; Larsen, L.H.; et al. Detection of breast cancer with addition of annual screening ultrasound or a single screening MRI to mammography in women with elevated breast cancer risk. *JAMA* **2012**, *307*, 1394–1404.
224. Maicas, G.; Carneiro, G.; Bradley, A.P.; Nascimento, J.C.; Reid, I. Deep reinforcement learning for active breast lesion detection from DCE-MRI. In Proceedings of the International Conference on Medical Image Computing and Computer-Assisted Intervention, Quebec City, QC, Canada, 11–13 September 2017; Springer: Cham, Switzerland, 2017; pp. 665–673.
225. Zhou, J.; Zhang, Y.; Chang, K.; Lee, K.E.; Wang, O.; Li, J.; Lin, Y.; Pan, Z.; Chang, P.; Chow, D.; et al. Diagnosis of Benign and Malignant Breast Lesions on DCE-MRI by Using Radiomics and Deep Learning with Consideration of Peritumor Tissue. *J. Magn. Reson. Imaging* **2019**, *51*, 798–809. [CrossRef]
226. Daimiel Naranjo, I.; Gibbs, P.; Reiner, J.S.; Lo Gullo, R.; Thakur, S.B.; Jochelson, M.S.; Thakur, N.; Baltzer, P.A.; Helbich, T.H.; Pinker, K. Breast lesion classification with multiparametric breast MRI using radiomics and machine learning: A comparison with radiologists' performance. *Cancers* **2022**, *14*, 1743. [CrossRef]
227. Antropova, N.; Huynh, B.Q.; Giger, M.L. A deep feature fusion methodology for breast cancer diagnosis demonstrated on three imaging modality datasets. *Med. Phys.* **2017**, *44*, 5162–5171. [CrossRef]
228. Truhn, D.; Schrading, S.; Haarburger, C.; Schneider, H.; Merhof, D.; Kuhl, C. Radiomic versus Convolutional Neural Networks Analysis for Classification of Contrast-enhancing Lesions at Multiparametric Breast MRI. *Radiology* **2019**, *290*, 290–297. [CrossRef]
229. Zhou, J.; Luo, L.; Dou, Q.; Chen, H.; Chen, C.; Li, G.; Jiang, Z.; Heng, P.A. Weakly supervised 3D deep learning for breast cancer classification and localization of the lesions in MR images. *J. Magn. Reson. Imaging* **2019**, *50*, 1144–1151. [CrossRef]
230. Feng, H.; Cao, J.; Wang, H.; Xie, Y.; Yang, D.; Feng, J.; Chen, B. A knowledge-driven feature learning and integration method for breast cancer diagnosis on multi-sequence MRI. *Magn. Reson. Imaging* **2020**, *69*, 40–48. [CrossRef]
231. Fujioka, T.; Yashima, Y.; Oyama, J.; Mori, M.; Kubota, K.; Katsuta, L.; Kimura, K.; Yamaga, E.; Oda, G.; Nakagawa, T.; et al. Deep-learning approach with convolutional neural network for classification of maximum intensity projections of dynamic contrast-enhanced breast magnetic resonance imaging. *Magn. Reson. Imaging* **2020**, *75*, 1–8. [CrossRef]
232. Lin, T.Y.; Goyal, P.; Girshick, R.; He, K.; Dollar, P. Focal Loss for Dense Object Detection. In Proceedings of the IEEE International Conference on Computer Vision, Venice, Italy, 22–29 October 2017; p. 9.
233. Ayatollahi, F.; Shokouhi, S.B.; Mann, R.M.; Teuwen, J. Automatic breast lesion detection in ultrafast DCE-MRI using deep learning. *Med. Phys.* **2021**, *48*, 5897–5907. [CrossRef] [PubMed]
234. Zhang, J.; Saha, A.; Zhu, Z.; Mazurowski, M.A. Hierarchical Convolutional Neural Networks for Segmentation of Breast Tumors in MRI With Application to Radiogenomics. *IEEE Trans. Med. Imaging* **2019**, *38*, 435–447. [CrossRef] [PubMed]
235. Piantadosi, G.; Marrone, S.; Galli, A.; Sansone, M.; Sansone, C. DCE-MRI Breast Lesions Segmentation with a 3TP U-Net Deep Convolutional Neural Network. In Proceedings of the 2019 IEEE 32nd International Symposium on Computer-Based Medical Systems (CBMS), Cordoba, Spain, 5–7 June 2019; pp. 628–633. [CrossRef]
236. Lu, W.; Wang, Z.; He, Y.; Yu, H.; Xiong, N.; Wei, J. Breast Cancer Detection Based on Merging Four Modes MRI Using Convolutional Neural Networks. In Proceedings of the ICASSP 2019—2019 IEEE International Conference on Acoustics, Speech and Signal Processing (ICASSP), Brighton, UK, 12–17 May 2019; pp. 1035–1039. [CrossRef]
237. Zhu, Z.; Albadawy, E.; Saha, A.; Zhang, J.; Harowicz, M.R.; Mazurowski, M.A. Deep learning for identifying radiogenomic associations in breast cancer. *Comput. Biol. Med.* **2019**, *109*, 85–90. [CrossRef] [PubMed]
238. Ha, R.; Mutasa, S.; Karcich, J.; Gupta, N.; Van Sant, E.P.; Nemer, J.; Sun, M.; Chang, P.; Liu, M.Z.; Jambawalikar, S. Predicting Breast Cancer Molecular Subtype with MRI Dataset Utilizing Convolutional Neural Network Algorithm. *J. Digit. Imaging* **2019**, *32*, 276–282. [CrossRef] [PubMed]
239. Ha, R.; Chin, C.; Karcich, J.; Liu, M.Z.; Chang, P.; Mutasa, S.; Van Sant, E.P.; Wynn, R.T.; Connolly, E.; Jambawalikar, S. Prior to Initiation of Chemotherapy, Can We Predict Breast Tumor Response? Deep Learning Convolutional Neural Networks Approach Using a Breast MRI Tumor Dataset. *J. Digit. Imaging* **2018**, *32*, 693–701. [CrossRef]

240. Fang, Y.; Zhao, J.; Hu, L.; Ying, X.; Pan, Y.; Wang, X. Image classification toward breast cancer using deeply-learned quality features. *J. Vis. Commun. Image Represent.* **2019**, *64*, 102609. [CrossRef]
241. Zheng, J.; Lin, D.; Gao, Z.; Wang, S.; He, M.; Fan, J. Deep Learning Assisted Efficient AdaBoost Algorithm for Breast Cancer Detection and Early Diagnosis. *IEEE Access* **2020**, *8*, 96946–96954. [CrossRef]
242. Holste, G.; Partridge, S.C.; Rahbar, H.; Biswas, D.; Lee, C.I.; Alessio, A.M. End-to-end learning of fused image and non-image features for improved breast cancer classification from mri. In Proceedings of the IEEE/CVF International Conference on Computer Vision, Montreal, BC, Canada, 11–17 October 2021; pp. 3294–3303.
243. Eskreis-Winkler, S.; Onishi, N.; Pinker, K.; Reiner, J.S.; Kaplan, J.; Morris, E.A.; Sutton, E.J. Using Deep Learning to Improve Nonsystematic Viewing of Breast Cancer on MRI. *J. Breast Imaging* **2021**, *3*, 201–207. [CrossRef]
244. Işın, A.; Direkoğlu, C.; Şah, M. Review of MRI-based brain tumor image segmentation using deep learning methods. *Procedia Comput. Sci.* **2016**, *102*, 317–324. [CrossRef]
245. Liu, M.Z.; Swintelski, C.; Sun, S.; Siddique, M.; Desperito, E.; Jambawalikar, S.; Ha, R. Weakly Supervised Deep Learning Approach to Breast MRI Assessment. *Acad. Radiol.* **2021**, *29*, S166–S172. [CrossRef] [PubMed]
246. Bie, C.; Li, Y.; Zhou, Y.; Bhujwalla, Z.M.; Song, X.; Liu, G.; van Zijl, P.C.; Yadav, N.N. Deep learning-based classification of preclinical breast cancer tumor models using chemical exchange saturation transfer magnetic resonance imaging. *NMR Biomed.* **2022**, *35*, e4626. [CrossRef]
247. Jing, X.; Wielema, M.; Cornelissen, L.J.; van Gent, M.; Iwema, W.M.; Zheng, S.; Sijens, P.E.; Oudkerk, M.; Dorrius, M.D.; van Ooijen, P. Using deep learning to safely exclude lesions with only ultrafast breast MRI to shorten acquisition and reading time. *Eur. Radiol.* **2022**. [CrossRef] [PubMed]
248. Wu, Y.; Wu, J.; Dou, Y.; Rubert, N.; Wang, Y.; Deng, J. A deep learning fusion model with evidence-based confidence level analysis for differentiation of malignant and benign breast tumors using dynamic contrast enhanced MRI. *Biomed. Signal Process. Control* **2021**, *72*, 103319. [CrossRef]
249. Verburg, E.; van Gils, C.H.; van der Velden, B.H.M.; Bakker, M.F.; Pijnappel, R.M.; Veldhuis, W.B.; Gilhuijs, K.G.A. Deep Learning for Automated Triaging of 4581 Breast MRI Examinations from the DENSE Trial. *Radiology* **2022**, *302*, 29–36. [CrossRef] [PubMed]
250. Dutta, K.; Roy, S.; Whitehead, T.; Luo, J.; Jha, A.; Li, S.; Quirk, J.; Shoghi, K. Deep Learning Segmentation of Triple-Negative Breast Cancer (TNBC) Patient Derived Tumor Xenograft (PDX) and Sensitivity of Radiomic Pipeline to Tumor Probability Boundary. *Cancers* **2021**, *13*, 3795. [CrossRef]
251. Carvalho, E.D.; Silva, R.R.V.; Mathew, M.J.; Araujo, F.H.D.; de Carvalho Filho, A.O. Tumor Segmentation in Breast DCE-MRI Slice Using Deep Learning Methods. In Proceedings of the 2021 IEEE Symposium on Computers and Communications (ISCC), Athens, Greece, 5–8 September 2021; pp. 1–6. [CrossRef]
252. Wang, H.; Cao, J.; Feng, J.; Xie, Y.; Yang, D.; Chen, B. Mixed 2D and 3D convolutional network with multi-scale context for lesion segmentation in breast DCE-MRI. *Biomed. Signal Process. Control* **2021**, *68*, 102607. [CrossRef]
253. Nowakowska, S.; Borkowski, K.; Ruppert, C.; Hejduk, P.; Ciritsis, A.; Landsmann, A.; Macron, M.; Berger, N.; Boss, A.; Rossi, C. Deep Learning for Automatic Segmentation of Background Parenchymal Enhancement in Breast MRI. In Proceedings of the Medical Imaging with Deep Learning (MIDL), Zürich, Switzerland, 6–8 July 2022.
254. Khaled, R.; Vidal, J.; Vilanova, J.C.; Martí, R. A U-Net Ensemble for breast lesion segmentation in DCE MRI. *Comput. Biol. Med.* **2021**, *140*, 105093. [CrossRef]
255. Yue, W.; Zhang, H.; Zhou, J.; Li, G.; Tang, Z.; Sun, Z.; Cai, J.; Tian, N.; Gao, S.; Dong, J.; et al. Deep learning-based automatic segmentation for size and volumetric measurement of breast cancer on magnetic resonance imaging. *Front. Oncol.* **2022**, *12*, 984626. [CrossRef]
256. Rahimpour, M.; Martin, M.-J.S.; Frouin, F.; Akl, P.; Orlhac, F.; Koole, M.; Malhaire, C. Visual ensemble selection of deep convolutional neural networks for 3D segmentation of breast tumors on dynamic contrast enhanced MRI. *Eur. Radiol.* **2022**. [CrossRef]
257. Zhu, J.; Geng, J.; Shan, W.; Zhang, B.; Shen, H.; Dong, X.; Liu, M.; Li, X.; Cheng, L. Development and validation of a deep learning model for breast lesion segmentation and characterization in multiparametric MRI. *Front. Oncol.* **2022**, *12*, 946580. [CrossRef] [PubMed]
258. Wang, D.; Khosla, A.; Gargeya, R.; Irshad, H.; Beck, A.H. Deep learning for identifying metastatic breast cancer. *arXiv* **2016**, arXiv:1606.05718.
259. Bayramoglu, N.; Kannala, J.; Heikkilä, J. Deep learning for magnification independent breast cancer histopathology image classification. In Proceedings of the 2016 23rd International Conference on Pattern Recognition (ICPR), Cancún, Mexico, 4–8 December 2016. [CrossRef]
260. Xu, B.; Liu, J.; Hou, X.; Liu, B.; Garibaldi, J.; Ellis, I.O.; Green, A.; Shen, L.; Qiu, G. Look, investigate, and classify: A deep hybrid attention method for breast cancer classification. In *2019 IEEE 16th International Symposium on Biomedical Imaging (ISBI 2019)*; IEEE: Piscataway, NJ, USA, 2019; pp. 914–918.
261. Xie, J.; Liu, R.; Luttrell, J.I.; Zhang, C. Deep Learning Based Analysis of Histopathological Images of Breast Cancer. *Front. Genet.* **2019**, *10*, 80. Available online: https://www.frontiersin.org/articles/10.3389/fgene.2019.00080 (accessed on 7 August 2022). [CrossRef] [PubMed]
262. Szegedy, C.; Ioffe, S.; Vanhoucke, V.; Alemi, A. Inception-v4, Inception-ResNet and the Impact of Residual Connections on Learning. *arXiv* **2016**, arXiv:1602.07261. [CrossRef]

263. Khan, S.; Islam, N.; Jan, Z.; Din, I.U.; Rodrigues, J.J.P.C. A novel deep learning based framework for the detection and classification of breast cancer using transfer learning. *Pattern Recognit. Lett.* **2019**, *125*, 1–6. [CrossRef]
264. Yan, R.; Ren, F.; Wang, Z.; Wang, L.; Zhang, T.; Liu, Y.; Rao, X.; Zheng, C.; Zhang, F. Breast cancer histopathological image classification using a hybrid deep neural network. *Methods* **2019**, *173*, 52–60. [CrossRef]
265. Thuy, M.B.H.; Hoang, V.T. Fusing of deep learning, transfer learning and gan for breast cancer histopathological image classification. In Proceedings of the International Conference on Computer Science, Applied Mathematics and Applications, Hanoi, Vietnam, 19–20 December 2019; Springer: Berlin/Heidelberg, Germany, 2019; pp. 255–266.
266. Karras, T.; Laine, S.; Aila, T. A Style-Based Generator Architecture for Generative Adversarial Networks. *arXiv* **2019**. [CrossRef]
267. Isola, P.; Zhu, J.-Y.; Zhou, T.; Efros, A.A. Image-to-Image Translation with Conditional Adversarial Networks. In Proceedings of the 2017 IEEE Conference on Computer Vision and Pattern Recognition (CVPR), Honolulu, HI, USA, 21–26 July 2017; pp. 5967–5976. [CrossRef]
268. Cruz-Roa, A.; Gilmore, H.; Basavanhally, A.; Feldman, M.; Ganesan, S.; Shih, N.; Tomaszewski, J.; Madabhushi, A.; González, F. High-throughput adaptive sampling for whole-slide histopathology image analysis (HASHI) via convolutional neural networks: Application to invasive breast cancer detection. *PLoS ONE* **2018**, *13*, e0196828. [CrossRef]
269. Albarqouni, S.; Christoph, B.; Felix, A.; Vasileios, B.; Stefanie, D.; Nassir, N. Aggnet: Deep learning from crowds for mitosis detection in breast cancer histology images. *IEEE Trans. Med. Imaging* **2016**, *35*, 1313–1321. [CrossRef]
270. Naylor, P.; Laé, M.; Reyal, F.; Walter, T. Nuclei segmentation in histopathology images using deep neural networks. In Proceedings of the 2017 IEEE 14th International Symposium on Biomedical Imaging (ISBI 2017), Melbourne, VIC, Australia, 18–21 April 2017; pp. 933–936. [CrossRef]
271. Priego-Torres, B.M.; Sanchez-Morillo, D.; Fernandez-Granero, M.A.; Garcia-Rojo, M. Automatic segmentation of whole-slide H&E stained breast histopathology images using a deep convolutional neural network architecture. *Expert Syst. Appl.* **2020**, *151*, 113387. [CrossRef]
272. Ming, Y.; Wu, N.; Qian, T.; Li, X.; Wan, D.Q.; Li, C.; Li, Y.; Wu, Z.; Wang, X.; Liu, J.; et al. Progress and Future Trends in PET/CT and PET/MRI Molecular Imaging Approaches for Breast Cancer. *Front. Oncol.* **2020**, *10*, 1301. [CrossRef] [PubMed]
273. Macedo, F.; Ladeira, K.; Pinho, F.; Saraiva, N.; Bonito, N.; Pinto, L.; Gonçalves, F. Bone metastases: An overview. *Oncol. Rev.* **2017**, *11*, 321. [PubMed]
274. Papandrianos, N.; Papageorgiou, E.; Anagnostis, A.; Feleki, A. A Deep-Learning Approach for Diagnosis of Metastatic Breast Cancer in Bones from Whole-Body Scans. *Appl. Sci.* **2020**, *10*, 997. [CrossRef]
275. Weber, M.; Kersting, D.; Umutlu, L.; Schäfers, M.; Rischpler, C.; Fendler, W.P.; Buvat, I.; Herrmann, K.; Seifert, R. Just another "Clever Hans"? Neural networks and FDG PET-CT to predict the outcome of patients with breast cancer. *Eur. J. Pediatr.* **2021**, *48*, 3141–3150. [CrossRef] [PubMed]
276. Zainudin, Z.; Shamsuddin, S.M.; Hasan, S. Deep Layer CNN Architecture for Breast Cancer Histopathology Image Detection. In Proceedings of the International Conference on Advanced Machine Learning Technologies and Applications (AMLTA2019), Cairo, Egypt, 28–30 March 2019; Springer: Berlin/Heidelberg, Germany, 2020; pp. 43–51. [CrossRef]
277. Li, C.; Wang, X.; Liu, W.; Latecki, L.J.; Wang, B.; Huang, J. Weakly supervised mitosis detection in breast histopathology images using concentric loss. *Med. Image Anal.* **2019**, *53*, 165–178. [CrossRef] [PubMed]
278. Das, D.K.; Dutta, P.K. Efficient automated detection of mitotic cells from breast histological images using deep convolution neutral network with wavelet decomposed patches. *Comput. Biol. Med.* **2018**, *104*, 29–42. [CrossRef]
279. Gour, M.; Jain, S.; Kumar, T.S. Residual learning based CNN for breast cancer histopathological image classification. *Int. J. Imaging Syst. Technol.* **2020**, *30*, 621–635. [CrossRef]
280. Saxena, S.; Shukla, S.; Gyanchandani, M. Pre-trained convolutional neural networks as feature extractors for diagnosis of breast cancer using histopathology. *Int. J. Imaging Syst. Technol.* **2020**, *30*, 577–591. [CrossRef]
281. Hirra, I.; Ahmad, M.; Hussain, A.; Ashraf, M.U.; Saeed, I.A.; Qadri, S.F.; Alghamdi, A.M.; Alfakeeh, A.S. Breast Cancer Classification from Histopathological Images Using Patch-Based Deep Learning Modeling. *IEEE Access* **2021**, *9*, 24273–24287. [CrossRef]
282. Senan, E.M.; Alsaade, F.W.; Al-mashhadani, M.I.A.; Aldhyani, T.H.H.; Al-Adhaileh, M.H. Classification of Histopathological Images for Early Detection of Breast Cancer Using Deep Learning. *J. Appl. Sci. Eng.* **2021**, *24*, 323–329. [CrossRef]
283. Zewdie, E.T.; Tessema, A.W.; Simegn, G.L. Classification of breast cancer types, sub-types and grade from histopathological images using deep learning technique. *Heal. Technol.* **2021**, *11*, 1277–1290. [CrossRef]
284. Kushwaha, S.; Adil, M.; Abuzar, M.; Nazeer, A.; Singh, S.K. Deep learning-based model for breast cancer histopathology image classification. In Proceedings of the 2021 2nd International Conference on Intelligent Engineering and Management (ICIEM), London, UK, 28–30 April 2021; pp. 539–543. [CrossRef]
285. Gheshlaghi, S.H.; Kan, C.N.E.; Ye, D.H. Breast Cancer Histopathological Image Classification with Adversarial Image Synthesis. In Proceedings of the 2021 43rd Annual International Conference of the IEEE Engineering in Medicine & Biology Society (EMBC), Virtual Conference, 1–5 November 2021; pp. 3387–3390. [CrossRef]
286. Reshma, V.K.; Arya, N.; Ahmad, S.S.; Wattar, I.; Mekala, S.; Joshi, S.; Krah, D. Detection of Breast Cancer Using Histopathological Image Classification Dataset with Deep Learning Techniques. *BioMed Res. Int.* **2022**, *2022*, 8363850. [CrossRef] [PubMed]
287. Joseph, A.A.; Abdullahi, M.; Junaidu, S.B.; Ibrahim, H.H.; Chiroma, H. Improved multi-classification of breast cancer histopathological images using handcrafted features and deep neural network (dense layer). *Intell. Syst. Appl.* **2022**, *14*, 200066. [CrossRef]

288. Ahmad, N.; Asghar, S.; Gillani, S.A. Transfer learning-assisted multi-resolution breast cancer histopathological images classification. *Vis. Comput.* **2021**, *38*, 2751–2770. [CrossRef]
289. Mathew, T.; Ajith, B.; Kini, J.R.; Rajan, J. Deep learning-based automated mitosis detection in histopathology images for breast cancer grading. *Int. J. Imaging Syst. Technol.* **2022**, *32*, 1192–1208. [CrossRef]
290. Singh, S.; Kumar, R. Breast cancer detection from histopathology images with deep inception and residual blocks. *Multimed. Tools Appl.* **2021**, *81*, 5849–5865. [CrossRef]
291. Mejbri, S.; Franchet, C.; Reshma, I.A.; Mothe, J.; Brousset, P.; Faure, E. Deep Analysis of CNN Settings for New Cancer whole-slide Histological Images Segmentation: The Case of Small Training Sets. In Proceedings of the 6th International conference on BioImaging (BIOIMAGING 2019), Prague, Czech Republic, 22–24 February 2019; pp. 120–128. [CrossRef]
292. Guo, Z.; Liu, H.; Ni, H.; Wang, X.; Su, M.; Guo, W.; Wang, K.; Jiang, T.; Qian, Y. A Fast and Refined Cancer Regions Segmentation Framework in Whole-slide Breast Pathological Images. *Sci. Rep.* **2019**, *9*, 882. [CrossRef]
293. Budginaitė, E.; Morkūnas, M.; Laurinavičius, A.; Treigys, P. Deep Learning Model for Cell Nuclei Segmentation and Lymphocyte Identification in Whole Slide Histology Images. *Informatica* **2021**, *32*, 23–40. [CrossRef]
294. Pedersen, A.; Smistad, E.; Rise, T.V.; Dale, V.G.; Pettersen, H.S.; Nordmo, T.-A.S.; Bouget, D.; Reinertsen, I.; Valla, M. H2G-Net: A multi-resolution refinement approach for segmentation of breast cancer region in gigapixel histopathological images. *Front. Med.* **2022**, *9*, 971873. [CrossRef]
295. Engstrøm, M.J.; Opdahl, S.; Hagen, A.I.; Romundstad, P.R.; Akslen, L.A.; Haugen, O.A.; Vatten, L.J.; Bofin, A.M. Molecular subtypes, histopathological grade and survival in a historic cohort of breast cancer patients. *Breast Cancer Res. Treat.* **2013**, *140*, 463–473. [CrossRef]
296. Khalil, M.-A.; Lee, Y.-C.; Lien, H.-C.; Jeng, Y.-M.; Wang, C.-W. Fast Segmentation of Metastatic Foci in H&E Whole-Slide Images for Breast Cancer Diagnosis. *Diagnostics* **2022**, *12*, 990. [CrossRef] [PubMed]
297. Yang, Q.; Liu, Y.; Cheng, Y.; Kang, Y.; Chen, T.; Yu, H. Federated Learning. *Synth. Lect. Artif. Intell. Mach. Learn.* **2019**, *13*, 1–207. [CrossRef]
298. Zhang, W.; Deng, L.; Zhang, L. A Survey on Negative Transfer. *IEEE Trans. Neural Netw. Learn. Syst.* **2021**, *13*, 1–25.
299. Ribeiro, M.T.; Singh, S.; Guestrin, C. "Why Should I Trust You?": Explaining the Predictions of Any Classifier. *arXiv* **2016**, arXiv:1602.04938. Available online: http://arxiv.org/abs/1602.04938 (accessed on 20 September 2022).
300. Wu, C.; Ma, S. A selective review of robust variable selection with applications in bioinformatics. *Brief. Bioinform.* **2015**, *16*, 873–883. [CrossRef]

MDPI
St. Alban-Anlage 66
4052 Basel
Switzerland
www.mdpi.com

Cancers Editorial Office
E-mail: cancers@mdpi.com
www.mdpi.com/journal/cancers

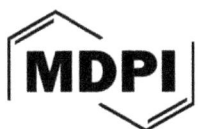

Disclaimer/Publisher's Note: The statements, opinions and data contained in all publications are solely those of the individual author(s) and contributor(s) and not of MDPI and/or the editor(s). MDPI and/or the editor(s) disclaim responsibility for any injury to people or property resulting from any ideas, methods, instructions or products referred to in the content.

www.ingramcontent.com/pod-product-compliance
Lightning Source LLC
LaVergne TN
LVHW070122100526
838202LV00016B/2213